PEDIATRIC NUTRITION

Incorporating National and International Recommendations

(IAP, NNF, GOI's DOWCD, BPNI, FOGSI, ICMR, AAP, IPA, NFI, IBFAN, WABA, ACASH, UNICEF, WHO, etc.)

Second Edition

Excerpts from Book Reviews:

"......a very comprehensive and up-to-date book on child nutrition, especially relevant to the readers of the Indian subcontinent......Special feature of the book is incorporation of the national and international recommendations......will serve the pediatricians, both from academic and practising background, for a long time to come."

–Indian Pediatrics
New Delhi, India

"......an outstanding well-illustrated spotlight on the best in the pediatric nutrition globally with supportive references at the end of each and every chapter....strongly recommended for the target audience."

–Tropical and Subtropical Pediatrics
Kuala Lumpur, Malaysia

PEDIATRIC NUTRITION

Incorporating National and International Recommendations

(IAP, NNF, GOI's DOWCD, BPNI, FOGSI, ICMR, AAP, IPA, NFI, IBFAN, WABA, ACASH, UNICEF, WHO, etc.)

Second Edition

Edited by

Suraj Gupte

MD, FIAP

Professor and Head

Postgraduate Department of Pediatrics
Narayana Medical College and Hospitals
Nellore-524002, South India

E-mail: drsurajgupte@gmail.com, recentadvances@yahoo.co.uk
surajgupte@rediffmail.com

Honorary Director

Pediatric Education Network

Editor-in-Chief

Recent Advances in Pediatrics (International Series)
The Short Textbook of Pediatrics
Pediatric Emergencies
Neonatal Emergencies
Pediatric Gastroenterology,
Hepatology and Nutrition
Influenza: Complete Spectrum ...etc

Author

Instructive Case Studies in Pediatrics
Differential Diagnosis in Pediatrics
Pediatric Drug Directory
Influenza, Perspectives in Influenza
Speaking of Child Care etc.

E-mail: recentadvances@yahoo.co.uk
drsurajgupte@gmail.com, surajgupte@rediffmail.com

Co-editor

Asian Journal of Maternity and Child Health
(Manila, Philippines)

Section Editor

Pediatrics Today (New Delhi, India)

Editorial Adviser

Asian Journal of Pediatric Practice (New Delhi, India)

Editorial Advisory Board Member/Reviewer

Indian Journal of Pediatrics (New Delhi, India)
Synopsis: A Current Survey of World Literature in Pediatrics (Detroit, USA), Indian Journal of Pediatric Gastroenterology, Hepatology and Nutrition (Jaipur, India), Maternal and Child Nutrition (Preston, UK), Journal of Infectious Diseases (Turkey)

Examiner

National Board of Examinations (NBE) for DNB, New Delhi, All India Institute of Medical Sciences (AIIMS), New Delhi, Postgraduate Institute of Medical Education and Research (PGIMER), Chandigarh, Sher-i-Kashmir Institute of Medical Sciences (SKIMS) and several universities

Pediatric Faculty Selection Expert

All India Institute of Medical Sciences, New Delhi
Punjab Public Service Commission,
Jammu and Kashmir Public Service Commission,
Union Public Service Commission

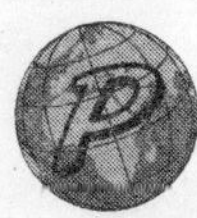

PEEPEE

PUBLISHERS AND DISTRIBUTORS (P) LTD.

Pediatric Nutrition

Published by
Pawaninder P. Vij

Peepee Publishers and Distributors (P) Ltd.
Head Office: 160, Shakti Vihar, Pitam Pura, Delhi-110 034 (India)

Correspondence Address:
7/31, First Floor, Ansari Road, Daryaganj
New Delhi-110 002 (India)

Ph: 65195868, 9811156083, 23246245

e-mail: peepee160@yahoo.co.in

e-mail: peepee160@rediffmail.com

e-mail: peepee160@gmail.com

www.peepeepub.com

First Edition: **2006**

Second Edition: 2012

ISBN: 978-81-8445-108-5

To

All healthcare providers contributing towards the excellence in child nutrition in particular and maternal nutrition in general, especially in the Indian subcontinent

Foreword

Malnutrition in childhood continues to dominate the health scenario in India and other developing countries especially in the South-East Asia. Over the last few decades, its prevalence has come down but rather slowly and to an unsatisfactory level only. Now, we see less frequently frank cases of advanced protein-energy malnutrition (PEM) like kwashiorkor, marasmus or marasmic-kwashiorkor and are successful in saving many infants and children who otherwise would have succumbed to severe acute malnutrition (SAM). Similar is the situation with regard to LBW babies, who may survive but with many unfavorable problems.

Most of these survivors however suffer from "nutritional stunting" with multiple handicaps including cognitive subnormality.

Talking about the academic literature in pediatric nutrition, undoubtedly we have innumerable monographs, booklets and educational material concerning child nutrition and malnutrition. However, these are usually limited to particular area(s) in child nutrition or have become obsolete with passage of time. Undoubtedly, there is a crying need for a community-oriented comprehensive and yet concise book that provides detailed essential information, inputs and practical guidelines for academicians, medical students and teachers, nutritionists and healthcare providers with a spotlight on improvement in overall nutrition, health and quality of life rather than sheer survival.

Dr. Suraj Gupte, a renowned pediatric educationist, researcher and author of national and international standing known for his worthy contribution to child nutrition did Herculean academic venture in publishing the much needed "Textbook of Pediatric Nutrition" in 2006. Inspired by works of the eminent authorities like Profs. D.B. Jelliffe, C.A. Gopalan and Dr. Shanti Ghosh plus by his own crave for perfection, the treatise met with high academic standards.

Now, its well executed second edition, rechristened **Pediatric Nutrition** provides a versatile platform for as many as 55 experts from India, United Kingdom, United States, Jamaica, etc. The comprehensive and state-of-the-art updates in 47 well-written chapters on nearly all aspects of child nutrition and nutrition deficiency states, are indeed very thought-provoking and timely.

A remarkable feature of the new edition is incorporation of excellent new chapter on 2006-07 WHO growth charts plus growth tables that are now required to be consulted and followed globally for assessment of nutritional status both at clinical level and for research studies, have been included, in addition.

The changing concepts in the management of SAM are explicitly dealt with emphasis on medical nutritional therapy. An independent chapter provides a superb description of ready-to-use therapeutic food (RUTF) that has revolutionized the nutritional therapy of SAM in Africa and is now making inroads in India and other countries of the South-East Asian Region (SEAR).

A commendable plus point of the book is a special accent on the relevance of descriptions to the Indian subcontinent rather than hifi theoretical discussions.

In short, the new edition of the book may aptly be described as a true reader-friendly compendium of changing and new concepts in child nutrition, undernutrition and overnutrition (that again is a sort of malnutrition) globally, providing recommendations from national and international organizations that are proactive in the field.

I sincerely feel that the second edition of **Dr. Suraj Gupte's Pediatric Nutrition** is set to offer enormous benefit to the professionals interested in maternal and child nutrition. This reader friendly textbook is strongly recommended to the pediatric residents, pediatric teachers, practitioners and healthcare providers in the field of maternal and child health, nutritionists, researchers, policy makers, etc.

Dr. Uday Bodhankar
Secretary General
Commonwealth Association for Health and Disability, United Kingdom
International Council Member, ASPR, Japan
Management Council Member MUHS
Ramdaspeth, Nagpur-440012 Maharashtra, India
Ph:(H) 0091 - 712 - 2459090 / 2422505
Fax: 0091 - 712 - 2428145
E-mail: ubodhankar@hotmail.com bodhankr ngp@bsnl.in

Preface to the Second Edition

We are pleased to offer the second revised and updated edition of the **"Pediatric Nutrition"**. This has become possible consequent upon the warm reception accorded to the first edition that was released at the 44th National Conference of the Indian Academy of Pediatrics (PEDICON 2006) held at the Hotel Ashok, New Delhi, India, consistent demand, changing recommendations in the field and the enthusiasm of the publishers.

On the suggestion from various quarters that the book is not addressed just to those involved in academics but is broad-based with appeal to all sections involved in nutrition of the child, including, clinicians and nutritionists, the prefix "Textbook" has been dropped. Secondly, in order that the book caters to the needs of the average readers, its size has been reduced without significantly affecting the core contents.

Over and above various revisions, new additions include **"Severe Acute Malnutrition (SAM)"**, **"Medical Therapeutic Foods"**, **"New (2006 and 2007) WHO Growth Standards and Charts"**, etc. These shall keep the readers abreast of the latest developments.

Hopefully, the revised, updated and improved new edition shall receive yet warmer reception from the readers in and outside India. Of course, feedback aimed at further improvement in the contents shall be most welcome to enable us work for a yet better next edition.

Suraj Gupte
MD, FIAP

Preface to the First Edition

Over three decades back, the noted *American Journal of Clinical Nutrition,* had posed this question to the experts in the field of child health and nutrition: Why does the Third World continue to have so much of child malnutrition?

The best response came from the doyen of international nutrition, Prof Derick B Jellife, pointing out "…. factors ranging from unequal distribution of food at international, national, community and family levels through poverty, ignorance, superstitions, erroneous beliefs, lack of knowledge of those involved in delivery of healthcare to wrong priorities and lopsided mindset of the policy-makers".

Interestingly, even today, this observation of Prof Jellife seemingly holds good. Nevertheless, over the years, the scenario with regard to prevalence of child malnutrition has undergone a perceptible change. As for example, it has in totality shown a significant reduction in Africa and Latin America. In the Indian subcontinent, gross reduction in prevalence of severe forms and some reduction in that of mild-moderate forms have occurred, though at a slow pace. Except iron deficiency anemia (IDA), incidence of micronutrient and vitamin deficiencies has been cut down to a large extent. The resultant fall in morbidity, mortality and improved child survival has been documented by such agencies as National Nutrition Monitoring Bureau and National Family Health Surveys I and II. Unfortunately, a large proportion of the survivors suffer from mild-moderate malnutrition that eventually ends up in "stunting" (nutritional dwarfing or short stature). These substandard survivors are likely to suffer from poor cognitive development and learning skills besides other handicaps, thereby expanding the pool of poor quality citizens in the long run.

The most important cause for this substandard survival, as duly emphasized time and again by the eminent nutritionist, Professor C. Gopalan, and the leading pediatric educationist and expert, Dr. Shanti Ghosh, revolves round bad infant and child-feeding and child-rearing practices. There has got to be an aggressive attack on this front if we are to have children who should not only survive but also grow into physically strong and mentally alert adults contributing to the welfare of the society and the nation.

Healthcare providers (of all grades) in general and pediatricians in particular, well sensitized and trained in infant and child nutrition, can contribute in a big way to attain this goal. Equally important is the actual involvement of the community in the endeavors. Enhanced emphasis on child nutrition not only in the teaching curriculum, both at undergraduate and postgraduate level in medical colleges/institutes but also in schools and colleges and in community activities too is needed.

With this background, need for an up-to-date, comprehensive and well-written textbook in child nutrition relevant to the settings in the Indian subcontinent has been widely felt.

This state-of-the-art and comprehensive pioneering textbook of pediatric nutrition from Indian subcontinent sets out to fill this felt gap. Its objective is not only to provide updated knowledge in the field but also to sensitize the healthcare providers, administrators and policy-makers to the nutritional needs of the community and, thereby, assist in attaining good nutritional status of our child population.

The reader-friendly book is the outcome of coordinated expertise, dedicated efforts, hard work and thoughtfulness of as many as 85 distinguished contributors constituting a multidisciplinary author team drawn from India and other countries. All the 69 chapters are written in a simple, straightforward and easy-to-understand style. Each chapter is to-the-point, keeping in mind the settings in the Indian subcontinent.

The treatise indeed is a dependable source to find by and large complete and authoritative guidance on various aspects of child nutrition. The contents, presentation and structure blend to provide a thoroughly readable, enjoyable, problem-oriented and evidence-based textbook of child nutrition.

I wish to express my thanks to the distinguished contributors, drawn from India and several other countries, for the rich quality of its contents and for reposing confidence in my editorship.

My wife, Shamma, daughter, Novy, a final year MBBS student, Government Medical College, Jammu, and son, Manu, an 8th semester BE student, MBS College of Engineering and Technology, Jammu, helped me in their own ways in working through the project successfully.

Finally, thanks are due to Mr. Pawaninder P. Vij, Director, Peepee Publishers and Distributors (P) Ltd. for commissioning this project, for handling its publication efficiently and for the skillful publishing qualities of the book.

Suraj Gupte

Acknowledgements

Grateful acknowledgements are due to:

- My wife, Shamma, who graciously assisted me so much in taking this important project to its logical conclusion despite her own preoccupations.
- My daughter, Dr. Novy, and son, Er Manu, for undertaking the tough responsibility of Executive Editors of the project.
- Dr. P. Narayana, Chairman, Dr. B. A. Ramakrishna, Principal, Dr. S. Vijay Kumar, Coordinator, and Dr. M. Veera Prasad, Medical Superintendent, Narayana Medical College and Hospitals for providing moral support and motivation for completing the project.
- The distinguished contributors, drawn from various countries globally for responding to our queries while the scripts were under process.
- The peer-reviewers who enhanced the excellence of the book though their objective comments, suggestions and recommendations.
- The reviewers/Journals, both from India and abroad, for appreciating the project and warmly recommending the book to the readers.
- Dr. Uday Bodhankar, a friend and philosopher, for his graciousness in penning "Foreword" and warmly recommending the treatise.
- The Publishers, Peepee Publishers and Distributors, New Delhi, for the skillful production qualities of the book.

Suraj Gupte
MD, FIAP

Contributors

Stephen Abil
Assistant Professor
Department of Infant and Child Nutrition
Institute of Child and Adolescent Health
London, United Kingdom
Ch 13: Feeding of the Low Birthweight Infants

Pankaj Abrol
Senior Professor and Head
Department of Pediatrics II
Pt. BD Sharma Postgraduate Institute of Medical Sciences
Rohtak, Haryana, India
Ch 20: Vitamin B Complex Deficiencies

B Adhisivam
Assistant Professor
Department of Pediatrics
Jawaharlal Postgraduate Institute of Medical
Sciences and Research (JIPMER)
Pondicherry, Union Territory, India
Ch 16: Malnutrition and Infection
Ch 26: Zinc in Child Nutrition

Samta Agrawal (Malik)
Practising Pediatrician
Malik Nursing Home, Chhindwara
Maharashtra, India
Ch 11: Complementary Feeding

Sugandha Arya
Pediatrician
Department of Pediatrics
Vardhman Mahavir Medical College and Safdarjung Hospital
New Delhi, India
Ch 8: Breastfeeding: The Supreme Gift

Akash A Bang
Pediatric Intensivist
Associate Professor in Pediatrics
Mahatma Gandhi Institute of Medical Sciences (MGIMS)
Sevagram, Maharashtra, India
Ch 1: Nutritional Requirements

Louise A Baur
Consultant
Department of Pediatrics
The Chinese University of Hong Kong and
Prince of Wales Hospital
Hong Kong, China
Ch 36: The Child with Obesity

Sandeep B Bavdekar
Professor
Department of Pediatrics
Seth GS Medical College and KEM Hospital
Parel, Mumbai, India
Ch 38: Immunonutrition

Lalit Bharedia
Consultant Pediatric Gastroenterologist
Department of Pediatrics and Neonatology
Fortis Escorts Hospital
Jaipur, Rajasthan, India
Ch 42: Nutrition in Liver Disease

B Vishnu Bhat
Professor
Department of Pediatrics
Jawaharlal Postgraduate Institute of Medical Sciences
and Research (JIPMER)
Pondicherry, Union Territory, India
Ch 15: Immunology of Malnutrition
Ch 16: Malnutrition and Infection
Ch 26: Zinc in Child Nutrition
Ch 47: Parenteral Nutrition

Uday Bodhankar
Consultant Pediatrician and Neonatologist
Ramdaspeth, Nagpur, Maharashtra, India
Ch 34: The Child with Failure to Thrive

Millie Boettcher
Division of Pediatric Gastroenterology and Nutrition
Alfred 1. DuPont Hospital for Children
Wilmington, United States
Ch 44: Nutrition in Inflammatory Bowel Disease

Harish Chellani
Associate Professor
Department of Pediatrics
Vardhman Mahavir Medical College and
Safdarjung Hospital
New Delhi, India
Ch 8: Breastfeeding: The Supreme Gift

Javed Chowdhary
Professor and Head
Department of Pediatrics
Government Medical College
Srinagar, Jammu and Kashmir, India
Ch 12: Low Birthweight Infants: Overview

EW Christopher
Assistant Professor
Division of Pediatric Endocrinology
Children's Hospital of Winconsin
Winconsin, USA
Ch 35: The Child with Short Stature

JP Dadhich
Senior Consultant
Division of Neonatology
Department of Pediatrics
SL Jain Hospital, Delhi, India
Ch 14: Fortification of Breast Milk

KE Elizabeth
Consultant in Nutrition and Genetics
Professor of Pediatrics
Government Medical College and SAT Hospital
Thiruvananthapuram, Kerala, India
Ch 23: Micronutrient Deficiency Disorders (MDDs)
Ch 37: Nutrition in Health and Illness
Ch 41: Nutritional Support in Cystic Fibrosis

Sabeena Farhath
Division of Pediatric Gastroenterology and Nutrition
Alfred 1. DuPont Hospital for
Children and Nutrition
Wilmington, United States
Ch 44: Nutrition in Inflammatory Bowel Disease

Kara Feigenbaum
Registered Nutritionist
Division of Pediatric Gastroenterology and Nutrition
Alfred 1. DuPont Hospital for Children and Nutrition
Wilmington, United States
Ch 43: Nutritional Management of Diabetes in Children

Swati Gadewar
Pediatrician
Division of Pediatric Gastroenterology and Nutrition
Department of Pediatrics
University of Maryland School of Medicine
Baltimore, Maryland, United States
Ch 45: Nutritional Management in HIV
Ch 46: Enteral Nutrition

Ajay Gaur
Associate Professor and Head
Department of Pediatrics, GR Medical College
Gwalior, Madhya Pradesh, India
Ch 39: Nutrition of the High-Risk Neonate

Swati Ghosh
Consultant
Center for Human Nutrition, Jamaica, West Indies
Ch 29: Protein-Energy Malnutrition: Overview

Meenakshi Girish
Consultant Pediatrician
Lata Mangeshkar Hospital
Nagpur, Maharashtra, India
Ch 34: The Child with Failure to Thrive

EM Gomez
Associate Clinical Professor
Department of Infant and Child Nutrition
Institute of Child and Adolescent Health
London, United Kingdom
Ch 12: Low Birthweight Infants: Overview
Ch 29: Protein-Energy Malnutrition: Overview
Ch 30: Various Classifications of Protein-Energy Malnutrition
Ch 35: The Child with Short Stature

Mary Gomez
Senior Research Fellow
Institute of Child and Adolescent Health
London, England
Ch 32: Severe Acute Malnutrition (SAM): State-of-the-art Management

CA Gopalan
Additional Chief Nutritionist
Department of Infant and Child Nutrition
Institute of Child and Adolescent Health
London, United Kingdom
Ch 18: Prevention and Control of Malnutrition

Lokesh Guglani
Senior Resident
Department of Pediatrics
All India Institute of Medical Sciences (AIIMS)
New Delhi, India
Ch 17: Nutrition, Malnutrition and Brain Development

Sheffali Gulati
Additional Professor
Division of Pediatric Neurology
Department of Pediatrics
All India Institute of Medical Sciences (AIIMS)
New Delhi, India
Ch 17: Nutrition, Malnutrition and Brain Development

Ravinder K Gupta
Associate Professor
Department of Pediatrics
Acharya Shri Chandar College of Medical Sciences (ASCOMS)
Sidhra, Jammu, Jammu and Kashmir, India
Ch 9: Breastfeeding and Maternal Medication
Ch 31: Mild-moderate Protein-energy Malnutrition: Nutritional Rehabilitation

Ritu Gupta
Assistant Professor
Department of Physiology
Government Medical College
Jammu, Jammu and Kashmir, India
Ch 9: Breastfeeding and Maternal Medication
Ch 31: Mild-moderate Protein-energy Malnutrition: Nutritional Rehabilitation

SK Gupta
Professor and Neurologist
Department of Medicine, Government Medical College
Jammu, Jammu and Kashmir, India
Ch 27: Infantile Tremor Syndrome (ITS)

Sanjeev Gupta
Senior Resident
Department of Pediatrics, Dayanand Medical College
Ludhiana, Punjab, India
Ch 21: Scurvy
Ch 22: Rickets

Novy Gupte
Resident, Postgraduate Department of Pharmacology, Therapeutics and Toxicology
Government Medical College and Associated Hospitals, Jammu
Jammu and Kashmir, India
Ch 33: Medical Nutrition Therapy in Severe Acute Malnutrition (SAM)
Ch 35: The Child with Short Stature

Suraj Gupte
Professor and Head
Postgraduate Department of Pediatrics
Narayana Medical College and Hospitals
Nellore, Andhra Pradesh, India
Ch 2: Assessment of Nutritional Status
Ch 6: New (2006-07) WHO Child Growth Standards and Charts
Ch 12: Low Birthweight Infants: Overview
Ch 13: Feeding of Low Birthweight Infants
Ch 18: Prevention and Control of Malnutrition
Ch 27: Infantile Tremor Syndrome (ITS)
Ch 28: Acrodermatitis Enteropathica
Ch 29: Protein-Energy Malnutrition: Overview
Ch 30: Various Classifications of Protein-Energy Malnutrition
Ch 32: Severe Acute Malnutrition (SAM): State-of-the-art Management
Ch 33: Medical Nutrition Therapy in Severe Acute Malnutrition (SAM)
Ch 35: The Child with Short Stature

Karoly Horvath
Director
Division of Pediatric Gastroenterology and Nutrition
Alfred I. DuPont Hospital for Children
Wilmington, Delaware, United States
Ch 40: Nutrition in Celiac Disease
Ch 44: Nutrition in Inflammatory Bowel Disease
Ch 45: Nutritional Management in HIV
Ch 46: Enteral Nutrition

Pratibha Kale
Associate Professor
Department of Pediatrics
Medical College
Amravati, Maharashtra, India
Ch 11: Complementary Feeding

Shivani Kansal
Senior Resident
Department of Pediatrics
Dayanand Medical College
Ludhiana, Punjab, India
Ch 21: Scurvy
Ch 22: Rickets
Ch 24: Iron Deficiency Anemia

Umesh Kapil
Professor and Head
Department of Human Nutrition
All India Institute of Medical Sciences (AIIMS)
New Delhi, India
Ch 19: Vitamin A Deficiency (VAD) Disorders
Ch 25: Iodine Deficiency and Its Health Consequences

BP Karunakara
Professor and Head
Department of Pediatrics
MS Ramaiah Medical College and Teaching Hospital
Bangalore, Karnataka, India
Ch 5: Nutrition and Growth

Deonath Mahto
Associate Professor of Pediatrics
Kalawati Saran Children's Hospital
Lady Hardinge Medical College
New Delhi, India
Ch 15: Immunology of Malnutrition
Ch 47: Parenteral Nutrition

PP Maiya
Professor and Head (Ex)
Department of Pediatrics
MS Ramaiah Medical College and Teaching Hospital
Bangalore, Karnataka, India
Ch 5: Nutrition and Growth

Anjali Malkani
Clinical Assistant Professor of Pediatrics
Division of Pediatric Gastroenterology and Nutrition
Department of Pediatrics
University of Maryland School of Medicine
Baltimore, Maryland, United States
Ch 46: Enteral Nutrition

Meenakshi Mehta
Professor and Head (Ex)
Department of Pediatrics
LTM Medical College and LTMG Hospital
Mumbai, India
Ch 3: Nutrition Education

EAS Nelson
Professor
Department of Pediatrics
The Chinese University of Hong Kong and
Prince of Wales Hospital
Hong Kong, China
Ch 36: The Child with Obesity

Mohinder Pal
Assistant Professor (Ex)
Government Medical College
Jammu, Jammu and Kashmir, India
Ch 13: Feeding of the Low Birthweight Infants
Ch 27: Infantile Tremor Syndrome (ITS)

Priyali Shah (Pathak)
Research Scientist
Department of Human Nutrition
All India Institute of Medical Sciences
New Delhi, India
Ch 19: Vitamin A Deficiency (VAD) Disorders

AK Patwari
Professor (Ex)
Department of Pediatrics
Kalawati Saran Children's Hospital
Lady Hardinge Medical College
New Delhi, India
Ch 10: Lactation Failure and Relactation

NC Prajapati
Professor
Department of Pediatrics
SN Medical College
Agra, UP, India
Ch 4: Maternal Nutrition and the Fetus and the Infant
Ch 7: Nutrition and Cognitive Development

Priyanka Rohtagi
Chief Clinical Nutritionist
Apollo Hospitals
Bangalore, Karnataka, India
Ch 42: Nutrition in Liver Disease

KR Sangra
B-Grade Pediatric Specialist
Directorate of Health Services
Jammu, Jammu and Kashmir, India
Ch 27: Infantile Tremor Syndrome (ITS)

Harmesh Singh Bains
Professor and Head
Department of Pediatrics
Dayanand Medical College
Ludhiana, Punjab, India
Ch 21: Scurvy
Ch 22: Rickets

Preeti Singh
Research Scientist
Department of Human Nutrition
All India Institute of Medical Sciences (AIIMS)
New Delhi, India
Ch 25: Iodine Deficiency and Its Health Consequences

Praveen C Sobti
Professor
Department of Pediatrics
Dayanand Medical College
Ludhiana, India
Ch 24: Iron Deficiency Anemia

Jyoti Suvarna
Pediatrician
Department of Pediatrics
Seth GS Medical College and
KEM Hospital, Parel
Mumbai, Maharashtra, India
Ch 38: Immunonutrition

Satish K Tiwari
Professor
Department of Pediatrics
Medical College
Amravati, Maharashtra, India
Ch 1: Nutritional Requirements
Ch 11: Complementary Feeding

Contents

Section 9: Other Nutrition-Related States

Section 10: Nutrition/Diet in Health and Disease

Section 11: Specialized Administration Techniques in Nutrition

Appendices

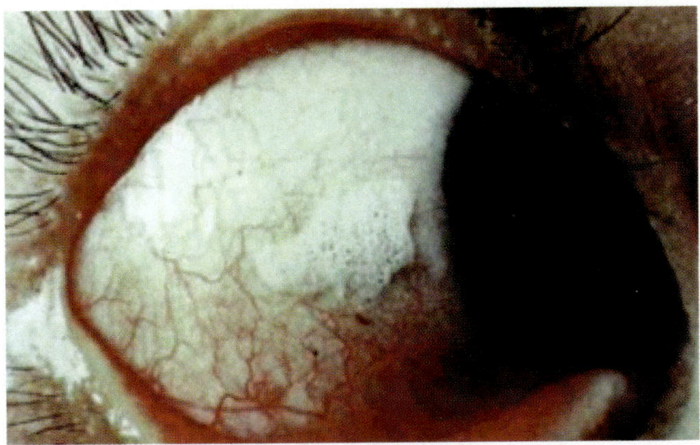

Fig. 19.1: VAD. Note the Bitot's spot (X1B) on temporal side of right cornea (See page 147)

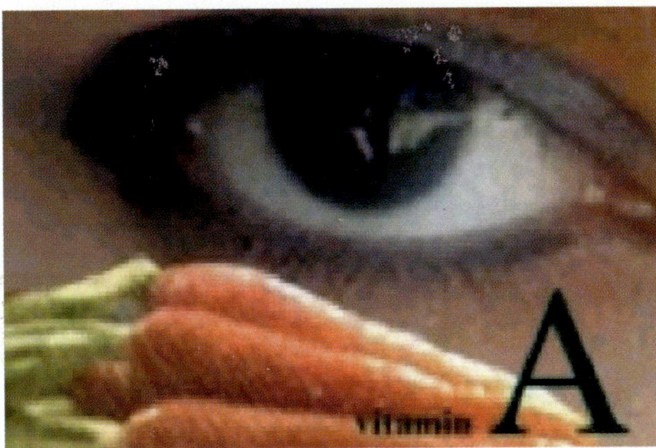

Fig. 19.2: Carrots are good source of vitamin A and therefore, vision-friendly (See page 149)

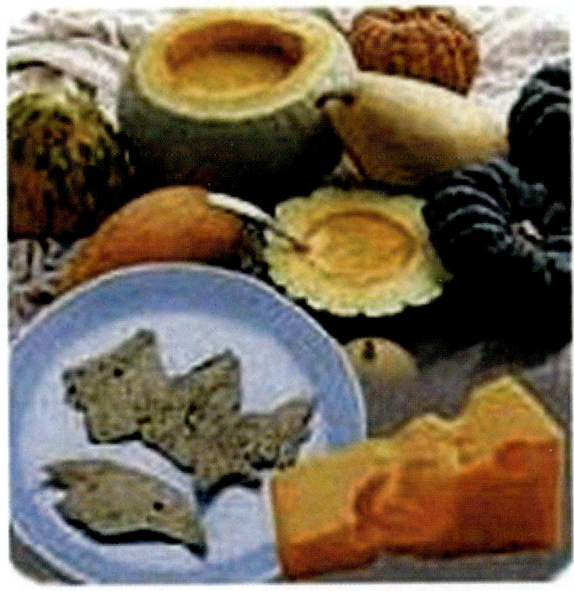

Fig. 19.3: Fruits and vegetables are a good source of vitamin A (See page 149)

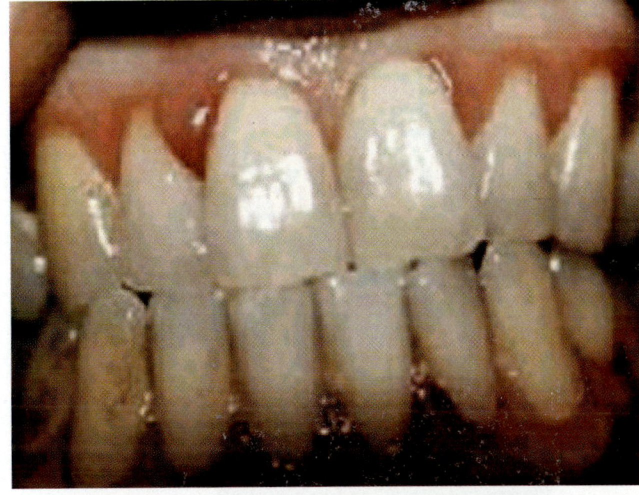

Fig. 21.1: Spongy gums in scurvy (See page 160)

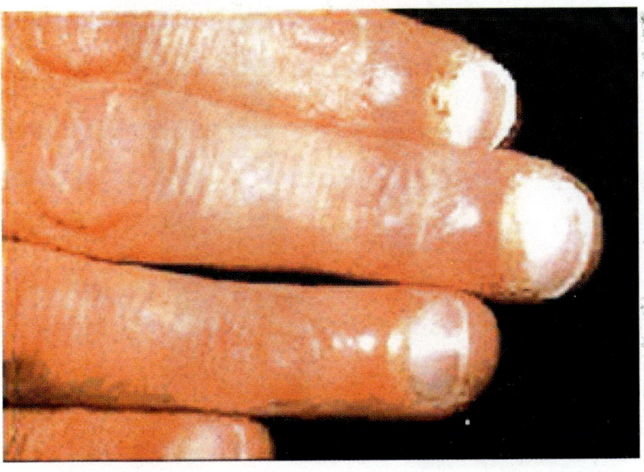

Fig. 21.2: Periungual hemorrhage in scurvy (See page 161)

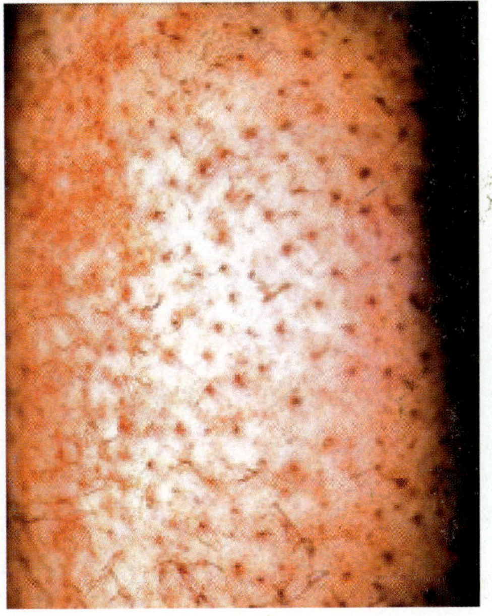

Fig. 21.3: Corkscrew skin in scurvy (See page 161)

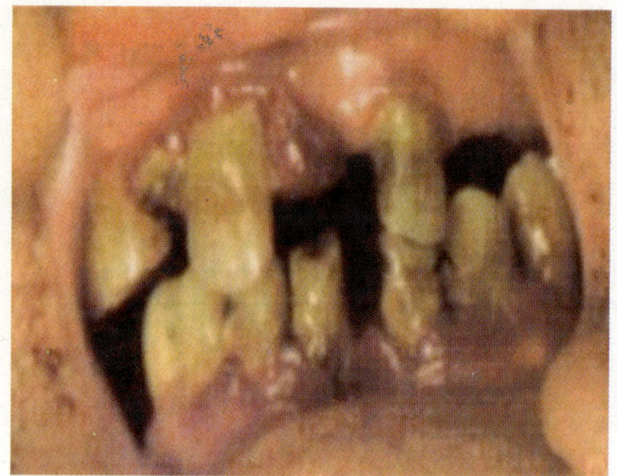

Fig. 21.4: Severe scurvy (See page 161)

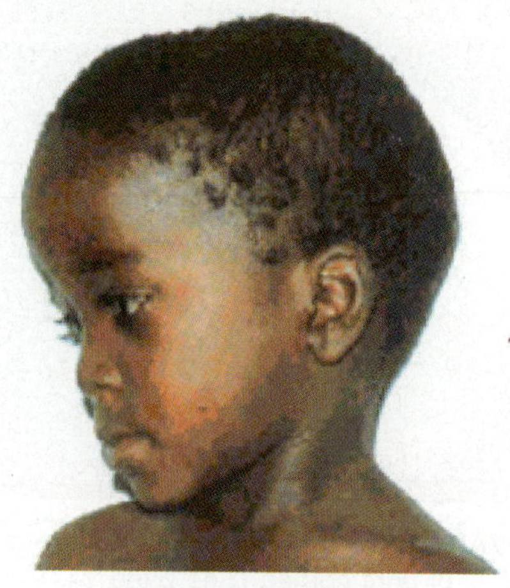

Fig. 22.1: Bossing of skull (See page 164)

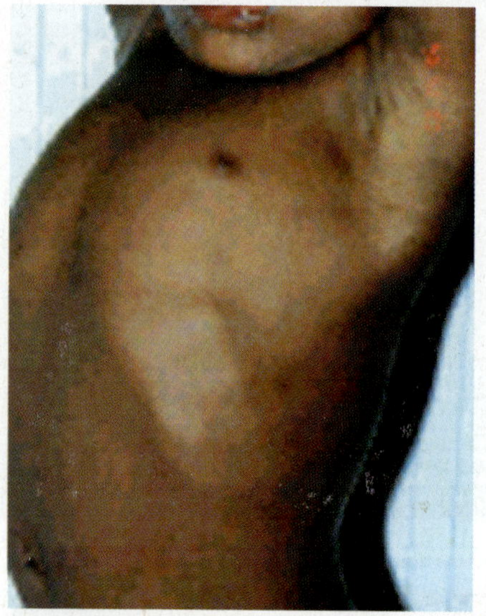

Fig. 22.2: Rachitic rosary (See page 165)

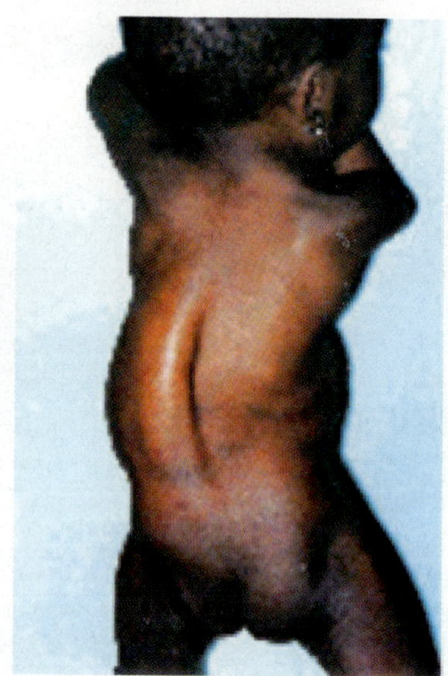

Fig. 22.3: Scoliosis in rickets (See page 165)

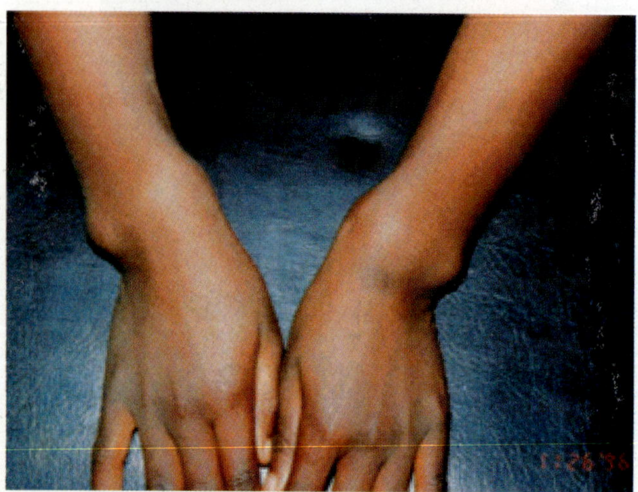

Fig. 22.4: Widening of wrist joints (See page 165)

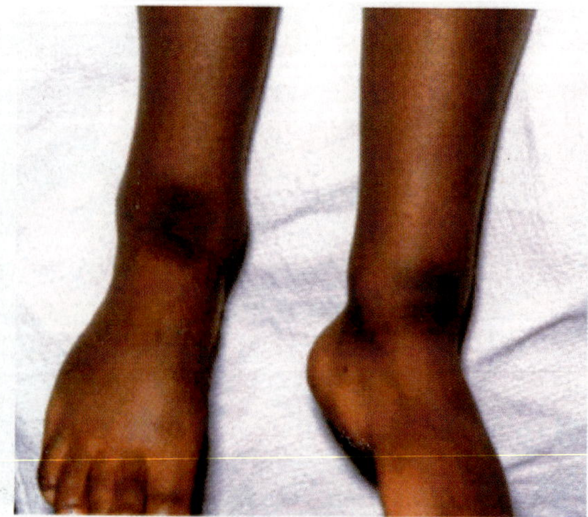

Fig. 22.5: Widening of ankle joints (See page 165)

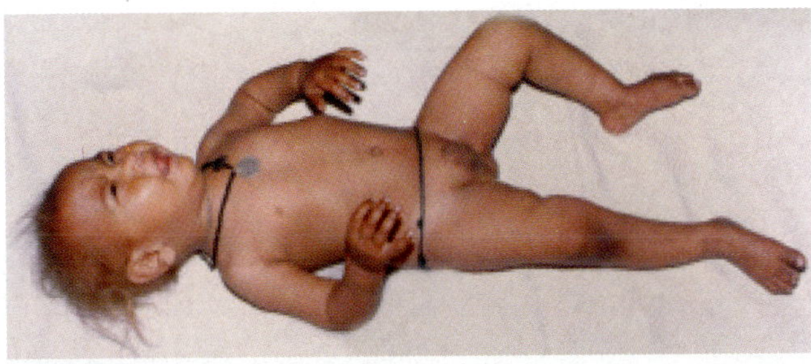

Fig. 29.1: Kwashiorkor: Note the characteristic features, including psychomotor change, oedema and hair changes (See page 219)

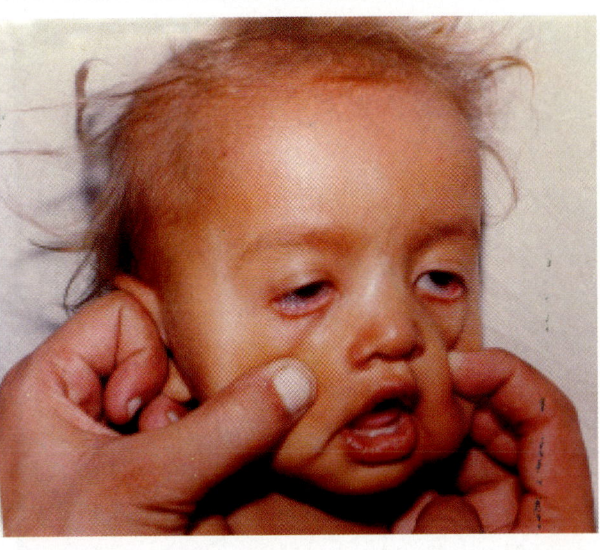

Fig. 29.2: Kwashiorkor: Note the hair changes and pallor. He had pedal edema with minimal ascitis (See page 219)

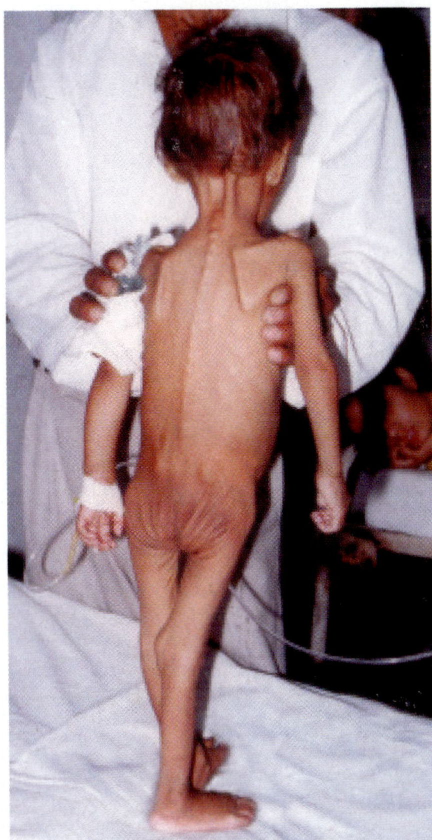

Fig. 29.3

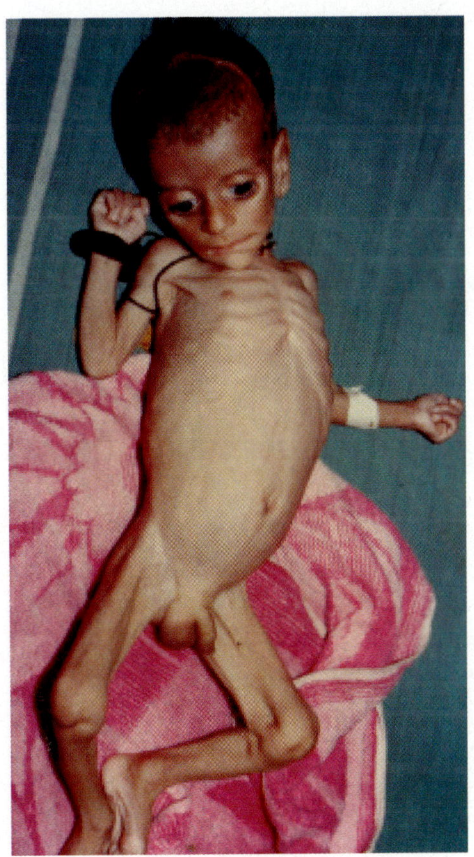

Fig. 29.4

Figs 29.3 and 29.4: Nutritional marasmus: Note the remarkable wasting (both muscle and subcutaneous fat) in two children who were hospitalized with severe PEM (See page 221)

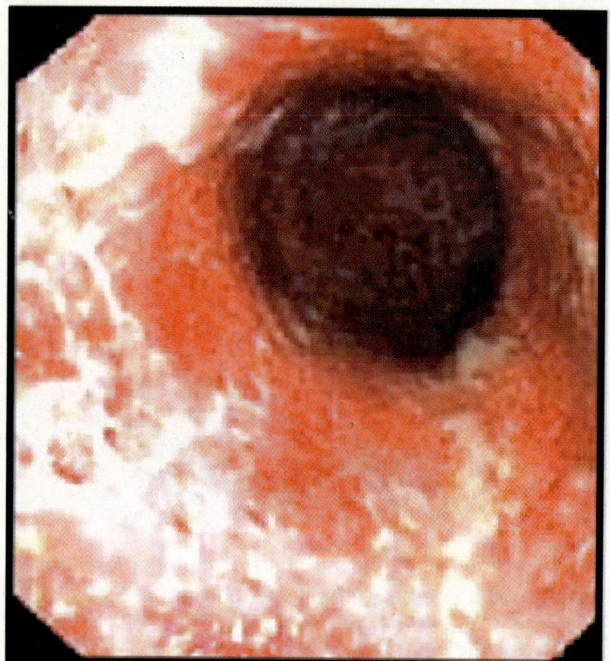

A. Ulcerative colitis

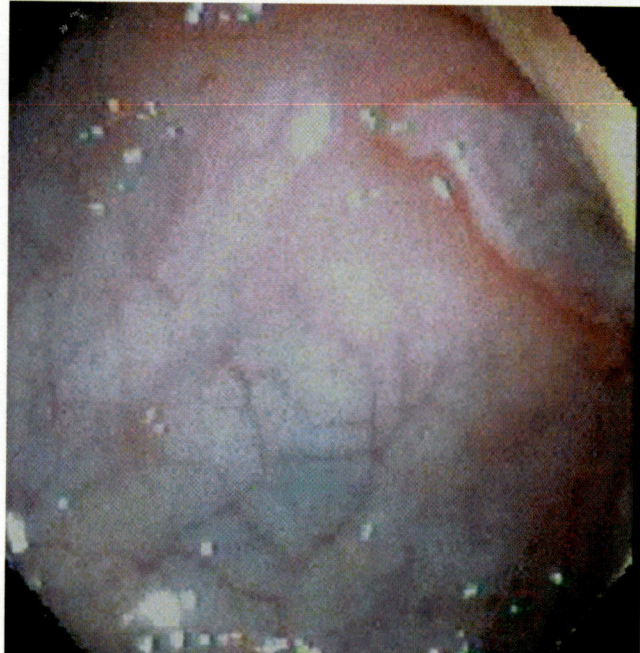

B. Crohn's disease

Fig. 44.1: Endoscopic pictures of children with IBD (A) Ulcerative colitis showing diffuse involvement of the colon; (B) Crohn's disease with typical ulceration and skip area (See page 342)

Akash A Bang • Satish K Tiwari

1 Nutritional Requirements

INTRODUCTION

Adequate growth and development of the child needs an appropriate and continuous supply of proper nutrients, especially in the first 3 years of life when growth is most rapid and the child is by and large totally dependent on his caretakers.

Food is the major medium through which every living being receives all these nutrients. In addition to supplying energy, which is required for the growth, physical activity and various metabolic needs of the body, food also supplies various substrates for metabolism and energy production. It also provides various vitamins and minerals many of which are required for synthesis of different hormones and enzymes in human body.

ENERGY

Energy value of foods is measured in kilocalorie (denoted as Cal) which is the amount of heat required to raise the temperature of 1kg of water by one degree from 14.5°C–15.5°C. The production of energy varies according to the oxidation of different foods. Oxidation of the following food components provide respective energy values:

- 1 g of carbohydrate 4 Cal
- 1 g of protein 4 Cal
- 1 g of fat 9 Cal
  - 1 g short-chain fatty acid 5.3 Cal
  - 1 g medium-chain fatty acid 8.3 Cal
  - 1 g long chain-fatty acid 9 Cal

Functions

The energy thus produced is used for various purposes. The average energy expenditure is as follows:

- 50% for basal metabolism.
- 25% for physical activity.
- 12% for growth.
- 8% as fecal loss mainly as unabsorbed fat.
- 4% for the Specific Dynamic Action (SDA), that is the increase in the metabolism over the BMR caused by the ingestion and assimilation of foods.

Recommended Daily Allowance (RDA)

The total caloric requirement can be calculated from the expected weight of a child by the Holliday and Segar formula as approximately 100 Cal/kg body weight for the first 10 kg of weight, 50 Cal/kg for each kg between 11-20 kg body weight and 20 Cal/kg for each kg of weight above 20 kg. Thus the caloric requirement of a child whose expected weight is about 24 kg would be (100*10) + (50*10) + (20*4) i.e. around 1580 Cal.

If weight of the child is not known, his caloric requirement can also be roughly calculated from age as follows:

During first year 110-120 Cal/kg/day
At 1 year 1000 Cal/kg/day

After 1 year, add around 100 Cal for each year till 12 years.

Thus at 2 years 1100 Cal/kg/day
3 years 1200 Cal/kg/day
4 years 1300 Cal/kg/day
5 years 1400 Cal/kg/day
6 years 1500 Cal/kg/day
7-9 years 1600-1800 Cal/kg/day
10-12 years 1900-2100 Cal/kg/day
Adolescent girl–2100 Cal/kg/day
Adolescent boy–2400 Cal/kg/day

In a routine diet, carbohydrates, fats and proteins are the major energy yielding nutrients and hence called as *macronutrients.* In contrast, vitamins and minerals do not provide significant energy. But, all the same, these are needed for various cellular functions. These are called as *micronutrients.*

A balanced diet is a diet, which provides all the macronutrients and micronutrients and also the non-nutrient components like fiber in adequate proportions—both quantitatively and qualitatively. In a balanced diet, roughly 50% calories are provided by carbohydrates, 35% by fats and around 15% by proteins. An imbalanced diet may cause the deficiency of the nutrients, which are quantitatively or qualitatively lesser than required or may cause toxicity of some other nutrients, which are in excess.

I. MACRONUTRIENTS

Proteins

Proteins are the second most abundant component of the human body after water. All the proteins are basically made up of 20 amino acids and differ only in their arrangement and total content of amino acids. The **essential amino acids** (EAA) include methionine, threonine, tryptophan, valine, leucine, isoleucine, phenylalanine and lysine. Histidine and arginine are called semi-essential aminoacids, as their synthesis rate is inadequate during infancy. Taurine and cystine are essential for babies borne with low birth weight.

Function

1. They act as the building blocks of various body tissues due to the amino acids present in them, which are needed for synthesis of all body proteins.
2. Thus they help in growth and development.
3. They are needed to compensate for wear and tear of the tissues.
4. Also act as energy source.
5. Needed for production and proper functioning of various enzymes, hormones, plasma proteins, hemoglobin, vitamins, and digestive juices.
6. Also act as powerful buffers to maintain acid base balance in the body.
7. Excess proteins which are neither used for energy production nor for synthesis of structural or functional proteins can be converted to fat and stored in liver so that it can be used in times of need in future.

Recommended Daily Allowance[1]

Following (Table 1.1) are the approximate ICMR recommendations for protein intake (grams proteins per kg of body weight per day) which are in terms of mixed vegetable proteins contained in Indian diet:

Table 1.1: Recommended daily allowance of proteins

Age	*Protein RDA*	*Age*	*Protein RDA*
0–3 months	2.3	4 – 6 years	1.6
3–6 months	1.9	6 – 9 years	1.55
6–9 months	1.7	9 – 12 years	1.5
9–12 months	1.5	12 – 15 years	1.4 Males
1–2 years	1.8		1.33 Females
2–3 years	1.7	15 – 18 years	1.3 Males
3–4 years	1.65		1.2 Females

Quality of Dietary Proteins

A complete protein is a protein, which contains all the essential amino acids in adequate quantities for the human growth and development. Dietary proteins can be animal or vegetable in origin. Animal proteins like those in meat, eggs, milk, fish etc. classified as complete proteins as they have higher contents of EAA. Vegetable proteins are relatively incomplete. Hence certain amounts of animal proteins are necessary in addition to vegetable proteins.

Cereals supply about 7-12 g proteins per 100 g weight and are poor in lysine. Maize lacks tryptophan. Pulses supply about 20-24 g proteins per 100 g weight (exception being soya which provides around 40 g proteins per 100 g weight) but are poor in methionine and threonine. Such lacking amino acids, called as limiting amino acids, can be overcome in a good mixed and balanced diet.

Biological Value (BV) of a protein refers to the fraction of the absorbed nitrogen that is retained in the body and thus is calculated as:

BV = Retained Nitrogen / Absorbed Nitrogen * 100

Egg protein is considered a reference protein with a BV of 100, as it is well digestible and complete in essential amino acids. BV of most cereals is around 65, whereas most pulses have a BV of about 75.

Net protein utilization (NPU) is the fraction of ingested nitrogen that is retained in the body and thus also takes into consideration digestion and absorption unlike BV.

NPU = Retained Nitrogen/Ingested nitrogen * 100

Carbohydrates

Carbohydrates can be simple which include monosaccharides (glucose, fructose, galactose etc) and disaccharides (sucrose, lactose, maltose) or they can also be complex which include various polysaccharides like starch, fiber, glycogen, dextrin, gum etc. Cereals are the richest source of carbohydrates. Other dietary sources include sugars, honey, jaggery, milk, tubers, roots, legumes etc.

Functions

1. Act as main source of energy due to their sheer bulk (50-60%) in a normal diet.
2. Excess is converted to glycogen and stored in liver and muscles and is thus a source of reserve energy.
3. Contribute to the taste, bulk and texture of foods.
4. Help in preservation of foods.
5. Are essential for digestion and assimilation of other food items as they act as carrier molecules for transport of ions like sodium.
6. Help in preventing the use of proteins for energy production and thus sparing them for vital growth and tissue repair functions, which is extremely important during rapid growth spurts like infancy and adolescence.

7. By sparing fats from being used for energy production, they also have anti-ketogenic properties.

Recommended Daily Allowance

Carbohydrates should contribute to about 50-60% of the total energy intake. This requires about 10-15 g carbohydrates per kg of body weight. They should preferably be obtained from sources like grains, legumes, vegetables and fruits, which are also rich in dietary fiber, vitamins and minerals and low in fat and total energy intake. Such diets, which are low in fat, monosaccharides and disaccharides, prevent tooth decay, obesity and cardiovascular diseases.

Fats

Functions

1. Act as concentrated source of energy in food and thus increase the total calorie intake without significant increase in the bulk.
2. Increase heat production and provide insulation against cold.
3. Act as important medium for absorption of fat-soluble vitamins.
4. Triglycerides act as storage form of energy.
5. They are important components of the cell membranes.
6. Omega-3 fatty acids like Eicosapentanoic acid (EPA) and Docosahexaenoic acid (DHA) lower blood cholesterol and triglycerides.
7. Essential fatty acids especially EPA and DHA act as precursors for various eicosanoids (prostaglandins, thromboxane and leucotriens) which have an important role as inflammatory mediators, regulation of blood pressure and immune response.
8. Cholesterol acts as precursor molecule for synthesis of a variety of compounds like bile salts, vitamin D and various steroid hormones etc.

Sources of saturated fatty acids (e.g. palmitic acid, stearic acid) are primarily animal fats with exception of coconut oil. They can also be produced in the body from carbohydrates and proteins.

Sources of unsaturated fatty acids are mainly vegetables, nuts or seeds. Monounsaturated fatty acids or MUFA (e.g. oleic acid) can also be produced in the body. However, the polyunsaturated fatty acids or PUFA cannot be produced in the body and hence needs to be supplemented from dietary sources. Hence these are called as essential fatty acids (EFA). PUFA consists of two types viz. omega-6 fatty acids (linoleic acid, arachidonic acid) and omega-3 fatty acids (linolenic acid, EPA, DHA). Normal balanced and mixed diet with some amount of vegetable oils is sufficient in omega-6 fatty acids but lack enough amounts of omega-3 fatty acids. Fish and other seafoods are rich in these omega-3 fatty acids, especially EPA and DHA. Breast milk is also rich in essential fatty acids.

Sources of cholesterol include animal fats like eggs, meat, ghee and cheese. It can also be produced in the body from carbohydrates and proteins.

Recommended Daily Allowance[2]

In a balanced diet, total fat intake should provide not more than about 30-35% of total calorie intake. Saturated fats should not exceed 10% of the total fat intake. And total cholesterol must be restricted to a maximum of 300 mg per day. Order of priority is to avoid excess total fats followed by saturated fats followed by cholesterol. A minimum of 3% of energy must be derived from linoleic acid and a minimum of 0.3% energy from linolenic acid.

II. MICRONUTRIENTS

The nutrients, which largely do not contribute to the energy intake but still are needed in very small amounts for healthy living are called as micronutrients, and include vitamins, minerals and trace elements.

Vitamins are organic compounds required as cofactors in various enzyme systems and thereby for normal growth and life. They are divided into two main groups:

1. Fat soluble vitamins—Vitamins A, D, E and K.
2. Water soluble vitamins—Vitamin B complex and vitamin C.

Minerals are small inorganic elements, which are indestructible unlike the macronutrients or vitamins and include the cations calcium, magnesium, sodium and potassium and the anions phosphorus, sulphur and chloride. These are sometimes also called as *macro-minerals* as they are required in amounts more than 100 mg per day.

Trace elements, sometimes also called as *micro-minerals*, include elements, which don't exceed 100-250 ug per g of matrix. These include iron, iodine, cobalt, zinc, copper, selenium, molybdenum, chromium etc. The sources, deficiency symptoms and signs, RDA, treatment associated with various minerals and vitamins are presented in Tables 1.2 and 1.3.

III. SPECIAL SITUATIONS

I. Nutritional Needs in Adolescence

Adolescents are especially prone to various kinds of nutritional problems due to the physical, mental and behavioral changes that they experience. The fast food, junk food, physical inactivity, smoking, alcohol intake, endocrine imbalances etc. may predispose them to obesity. On the other hand, there can be malnutrition and micronutrient deficiencies due to various factors like a fast life with career and study pressures leading to hurried and inadequate food intake, gender discrimination, aversion to certain foods due to strong likes and dislikes, psychiatric

Table 1.2: RDA, sources, deficiency features, treatment etc. of vitamins[3-5,7]

Name	RDA	Deficiency	Treatment	Sources	Dependency syndromes and Hypervitaminosis /toxicity	Remarks
1. Vitamin A	1000-3000 IU	Night blindness, xerophthalmia, skin lesions, infections of GIT, RT and Urinary tracts, growth retardation, calculi	>1yr- 2lac IU oral <1yr- 1lac IU oral IM dose half. Given on 0,1,14-28 d	Green + yellow vegetables and fruits, milk, egg, cheese, fish	Darrier disease ***Hypervitaminosis:*** pseudotumor cerebri **Acute:** 3lac U; **Chronic:**1lac U/d for 6 months	**Prevention:** 5 meg doses (as in t/t) 6 months apart from 9 mth-3 yr
2. Vitamin D	400 IU	Rickets, osteomalacia	6 lac IU IM	Egg-yolk, fish, skin exposed to sunlight	Vit D dependent rickets	
3. Vitamin E	5-15 IU	Hemolytic anemia in preterms, myopathies? retinopathy of prematurity, oxidative stress		Green leaves, nuts, plants, seeds, egg-yolk, vegetable oils	–	**Prevention:** 15-25 IU/d in preterms and fat malabsorption
4. Vitamin K	–	Hemorrhagic disease of newborn, hypoprothrombinemia, decreased hepatic production of factors II, VII, IX, X	2-5 mg in HDN; OD for 3 days in liver diseases, Monthly doses in liver diseases, malabsorptions, PEM	K_1-(Natural) cabbage, liver, spinach, tomato. K_2-intestinal flora K_3-synthetic	–	**Prevention:** 1mg IM in all neonates, 0.5 mg if wt<1.5 kg
5. Vitamin C	40 mg	Scurvy, bleeding, delayed wound healing, Iron deficiency anemia	500-1000 mg/d	Citrus fruits, amla, guava, pulses, sprouting cereals, potatos	Chediak Higashi Syndrome	**Prevention:** Lactating mothers -200-500 mg/d
6. Vitamin B_1 (Thiamine / Aneurine)	0.5-1.5 mg (1mg/ 1000 Cal)	Beriberi, CCF, peripheral neuritis, encephalopathy	25 mg IV, then IM, then 20 mg OD-BD	Yeast, outer layer of cereals, pulses, nuts	Leigh's disease, Maple syrup urine disease, Wernicke Korsakoff Syndrome	
7. Vitamin B_2 (Riboflavin)	0.5-1.5 mg	Cheilosis, angular stomatitis, atrophic glossitis, corneal neo-vascularization, nasolabial and scrotal dyssebacea and dermatitis	5-10 mg/d for a week	Egg, milk, milk products, liver, wheat, green leafy vegetables	Pyruvate kinase deficiency, Glutaric acidemia	
8. Niacin (Nicotinic acid)	5-15 mg	Pellagra, diarrhea, dementia, dermatitis (necklace, glove, boot)	50-300 mg/d	Cereals, nuts, meat	Hartnup disease	
9. Vitamin B_6 (Pyridoxine)	0.5-1.5 mg	Peripheral neuritis, convulsions, anemia, Seborrheic dermatitis, Cheilosis, glossitis, growth retardation, anorexia, abdominal discomfort	Seizures: 100 mg IM, then 2-10 mg/d according to severity of dependency	Meat, liver, vegetables, cereals	B_6 responsive anemia, B_6 responsive seizures, Homocystinuria, Oxaluria, Grey atrophy of choroid, Xanthinurenic aciduria, Cystathioninuria	
10. Folic acid	50-200 ug	Megaloblastic anemia	5mg/d orally or IM for 2-3 wks	Liver, pulses, vegetables	Formiminotransferase deficiency, Folate reductase deficiency, Homocystinuria	
11. Vit B_{12} (Cyno-cobalamine)	0.5-2 ug	Megaloblastic anemia, Sub acute combined degeneration of cord, hyper pigmentation of extremities, Infantile tremor syndrome	1mg/d IM for 2 wks	Animal food, fish, milk	Methylmalonic acidemia	

Table 1.3: RDA, sources, deficiency features, treatment etc. of macrominerals and trace elements[3,4]

Name	*RDA*	*Deficiency manifestations*	*Treatment*	*Sources*
1. **Calcium**	500-1000 mg	Hypo-calcemic tetany, seizures	100-200 mg/kg/d PO or 10% Inj Ca gluconate IV 0.5-1ml/kg	Milk, milk products, millets, greens, fish, crabs, oysters
2. **Magnesium**	200-300 mg	Hypo-magnesemia, seizures	0.1-0.2 ml/kg 50% $MgSo_4$ IM 12 hourly for 2-3 d	Cereals, nuts, legumes, greens
3. **Sodium**	1000-3000 mg	Hyponatremia, hypotension, dehydration, shock, lethargy, seizures	3% NaCl. In acute cases, raise serum Na by 5mEq/L immediately. In chronic cases, slow correction over 48 hrs	Common salt, green vegetables, cereals
4. **Potassium**	2-3 mEq/kg/d	Hypokalemia, hypotonia, paralytic ileus, flaccid paralysis	3-4 mEq/kg/d	Fruits, chocolates, tomato, milk, potato, banana, coconut water
5. **Phosphorus**	800-1000 mg	Isolated deficiency rare, Type II (hypophosphatemic rickets)	Oral phosphate 0.5-4 g/d in 4-6 divided doses with vit D	Cereals, milk, oil seeds, nuts, legumes, milk products
6. **Iron**	10-20 mg	Anemia, cognitive impairment, ADHD, koilonychias, dysphagia	3-6 mg/kg/d Iron orally. May consider blood transfusion SOS, but must treat the cause	Liver, meat, fish, egg yolk, legumes, jaggery, potatoes, dried fruits, green vegetables
7. **Iodine**	50-150 ug	Goiter, hypothyroidism, cretinism, learning disability, mental retardation	—	Sea foods, drinking water, iodized salt
8. **Zinc**[6]	5-15 mg	Growth retardation, anorexia, gonadal failure, alopecia, acral dermatitis, diarrhea, anosmia, reduced taste sensation, eye lesions, delayed wound healing, increased infections due to impaired cell mediated immunity, acrodermatitis enteropathica	1-2 mg/kg/d	Liver, meat, fish, legumes, cereals, nuts, cheese
9. **Copper**	1-2 mg	Hypochromic anemia, neutropenia, hypopigmentation of hairs, bony defects, vascular abnormalities, osteoporosis	—	Liver, meat, fish, legumes, nuts, oyster
10. **Selenium**	100 ug	Keshan cardiomyopathy, Kashinbeck osteoarthritis, myalgia, growth retardation, liver necrosis, risk of cancers		Green vegetables, meat, fish, liver, garlic
11. **Molybdenum**	200-500 ug	CNS abnormalities, Risk of GIT cancers, tachycardia, coma, central scotoma, irritability	—	Green vegetables, legumes, meat, fish, liver
12. **Chromium**	10 ug	Hyperglycemia, encephalopathy, peripheral neuropathy	180 ug stat	Yeast, liver, cereals, nuts, cocoa
13. **Cobalt**	Not known	Hypothyroidism, goiter, anemia	—	Meat, fish, liver
14. **Fluoride**	1-5 mg	Dental caries		Drinking water, sea foods, tea, cheese
15. **Manganese**	1-5 mg	Growth retardation, reddening of hairs, increased prothrombin time, hypocholesterolemia		Cereals, legumes, green vegetables, tea

problems like anorexia nervosa, increased demands due to the growth spurt, menarche and menorrhagia.

A balanced and mixed healthy diet is the most important and effective way to deal with most of the problems and hence must be promoted. The ideal pre-pregnancy weight and height recommended by UNICEF are 45 kg and 145 cm respectively and should be targeted in late childhood. Iron supplementation especially to girls in form of one tablet a week prevents anemia. Zinc supplementation improves weight and height gain in malnourished children and improves gonadal function. Other nutrients, which must be adequately supplemented in doses described earlier include vitamins A, E, C, calcium, iodine, fluoride, copper, selenium etc.

II. Nutritional Needs in Various Diseases[3,8]

1. **Congestive Cardiac Failure (CCF)**
   Acyanotic congenital heart diseases like PDA, VSD are the most common to cause growth retardation. Cyanotic diseases, though rarer, cause even a larger degree of growth retardation than the acyanotic ones. Due to this growth retardation and the associated infections and a hyper-catabolic state, 10-30% extra calories should be given over and above the RDA. Proteins in the diet should contribute upto 10-15% of total calories and should be of high biological value. In presence of CCF, fluid intake should be restricted to around 2/3 of the daily maintenance and salt intake to around 0.5 to 1 gm daily. Salty foods other than routine pulse and vegetables should be avoided.
2. **Hepatic Encephalopathy[9]**
   In the acute phase, proteins should be avoided orally. 10-20% extra calories are needed above the RDA. As much of this as possible should be given as 10% dextrose. This can be enriched with 25% dextrose. Vit. K should be supplemented. Branched chain amino acids viz. valine, leucine, isoleucine help in liver regeneration and should be supplemented as they are metabolized in muscles and kidney unlike other non-branched chain amino acids which require hepatic functioning for their metabolism.

   In the recovery phase, protein should be gradually added starting from around 10 gm/day and slowly increasing upto 1-1.5 gm/kg/day. These should mainly be provided using the proteins of vegetable origin. Fat content should be kept low as high fat decreases gastric emptying and may cause nausea. Medium chain triglycerides (MCT) are better tolerated and hence should be considered especially if there is decreased bile flow. Phospholipids extracts of soya is also helpful as it helps in liver regeneration and builds appetite.
3. **Chronic Liver Disease**
   Calorie intake should be increased to 10-20% extra calories to account for the malabsorption and deranged hepatic metabolism. No protein restriction is advocated and hence proteins should be given according to the RDA unless there is hepatic coma. In presence of cholestasis leading to fat malabsorption, fats should be restricted and should be given liberally as MCT. Fat malabsorption also leads to deficiency of fat—soluble vitamins, which must be supplemented in high doses. Vitamin A 10000-15000/d, Vitamin D 1000 U/kg/d (about 5000-8000/d), Vitamin E 15-25 U/kg/d (about 50-400U/d) should be given. Vitamin K injections should be given about 5 mg twice a month. Apart from these, all the water- soluble vitamins should be given in the doses of about twice their RDA.
4. **Acute Renal Failure[10]**
   Total fluid should be restricted to insensible losses (about 400 ml/M^2 Body Surface Area) + last day's output. 10-15% extra calories over the RDA need to be given for the stress caused by the infection/illness. Upto 45% of the caloric requirement can be derived from fats. Proteins should be restricted to 0.5 – 1.25 gm/kg/day. Mainly essential amino acids should be provided. No added salt should be given. Other supportive or medical measures include giving aluminium hydroxide and calcium salts to prevent hyperphosphataemia, prevention of hyperkalemia, treating anemia, hypertension, infections and coagulopathy.
5. **Chronic Renal Failure[11]**
   About 20% extra calories above the RDA are recommended. Excess protein intake precipitates acidosis, hyperkalemia and hyperphosphataemia and so proteins are restricted according to the severity of CRF. Animal proteins should be avoided, as milk is rich in phosphate whereas meat is rich in potassium. Salt should be taken in near normal amounts (No added salts, but excess should be avoided as it may cause hypertension). Potassium intake should be restricted and hyper- or hypo-kalemia should be promptly treated. Fruit juices can be given if serum potassium is low or normal.
6. **Diabetes Mellitus[12]**
   A balanced diet with adequate ratio of carbohydrates, fats and proteins is necessary. Optimal proportion will be approximately 50-60% caloric intake through carbohydrates, 20-30% through fats and 10-15% through proteins. To avoid severe blood sugar fluctuations, the gap between two meals should not be too much and at any one time too much should not be eaten. (Avoid fasting and feasting!). The composition should keep on changing to avoid monotony. This is achieved by spreading the total calorie intake (RDA) between 3 major meals and 3 minor snacks. An ideal diet schedule would include a breakfast, a lunch and a dinner providing about 20%, 20% and 30% of the expected total calorie intake respectively and a mid-morning, a mid-afternoon and an evening snack, each providing about 10% of the total expected calorie intake. If snacks are not possible these frequently, they can be clubbed with the nearest major meal and the calories in that meal should be increased.

   Carbohydrates should be given in form of starches as their glucose supply is slow and sustained. Rapidly absorbed mono or disaccharides like glucose, sugar, honey, sweets etc should be avoided. The diet should be rich in fiber (20-35g fiber/day) as it delays carbohydrate absorption. The fiber helps also by increasing insulin receptors, decreasing insulin requirement, decreasing cholesterol by binding to bile salts and promoting their excretion. Whole cereals, fruits, green vegetables, salads, pulses etc are examples of fiber rich foods. The diet should be low in **fat** to avoid hyper-lipidemia and its complications. In presence of good glycemic control half to one fruit can be allowed daily in place of a snack or if some extra exercise is done.

To avoid monotony, an exchange system is used where each exchange unit supplies about 10 g of carbohydrate. These units can be exchanged amongst themselves to increase the variety of food, e.g. half bread slice can be replaced with a medium size apple or orange OR a small potato OR half banana OR a glass of milk. Non-nutritive sweeteners like saccharin or aspartame can be used to enhance the palatability. However, their long-term side-effects like carcinogenicity still remain controversial.

7. **Phenylketonuria**[13]
Deficiency of phenylalanine hydroxylase leads to accumulation of excess phenylalanine in tissues. Earlier concept of "phenylalanine free diet" is now abandoned because phenylalanine is an essential amino acid and is required normally for adequate brain growth. Hence its total elimination from the diet may further aggravate the neural problems. The diet of choice is low phenylalanine diet. The goal should be to maintain serum phenylalanine levels between 3-15 mg%. The diet can be relaxed slightly after 6-8 yrs of age when neural maturation is almost complete. An ideal diet would avoid high protein items like fish, meat, eggs, cheese; limit medium protein items like pulses, cereals etc and liberally include low phenylalanine items like tubers, vegetables and fruits.

8. **Homocystinuria**
Methionine should be restricted in the diet to 20-25 mg/kg. For this, food items rich in proteins (e.g. dairy, poultry products, animal proteins etc) should be avoided. Legumes, which lack methionine, can be safely given. Adequate calorie intake in form of carbohydrates and fats must be ensured along with vitamins and minerals. Large doses of B_{12} (1-2 mg/d), B_6 (0.2-1g/d) and folic acid (1-5 mg/d) are beneficial.

9. **Galactosemia**
The importance of diet in galactosemia lies in the fact that it is probably the only preventable form of cataract besides diabetic cataract, which can be totally prevented by dietary modification. There is excess accumulation of galactose in the tissues and hence, dietary galactose must be omitted. As lactose is a disaccharide that consists of glucose and galactose, all types of milks and milk products should be avoided. Though "Non dairy creams" prepared from Soya protein isolates may be used as a substitute, whole soya flour preparations are best avoided as galactose may be present in some complex starches present in whole soya products apart from peas or vegetables. In the meat, liver should be avoided. Strict dietary restriction is necessary in the early years, but can be relaxed later on.

10. **Myoclonic Seizures**
A *ketogenic diet* benefits various myoclonic seizure syndromes of childhood. It produces its effect by increasing the inhibitory neurotransmitter GABA. In this type of diet, 80% calories are supplied by the fat and rest as carbohydrates. Proteins are restricted. Out of the total fat intake as large as 60% can be as MCT. This is accompanied with adequate supplementation of vitamins and minerals. Such diets can be extremely unpalatable and hence may not be tolerated by older children.

11. **Persistent Diarrhea**[8]
Dietary therapy is the cornerstone of treatment of persistent diarrhea. Breastfeeding must be continued. The initial diet A is a reduced lactose diet. It is prepared by mixing milk, sugar and puffed rice powder/cooked rice/sooji, and adding boiled water and oil to mix well. Alternatives include rice with curds. The rationale is that total elimination of milk is neither desired nor necessary at this stage. Hence the daily intake of milk is restricted to 50-60 ml/kg. And for this, instead of diluting milk with water, it is mixed with cereals and oil. The diet A can be started in 6-7 feeds per day at a calorie intake of minimum 100-120 Cal/kg/d. This should be slowly increased to 150 Cal/kg/d if weight gain is needed.

Some 30-35% children do not improve on diet A and require diet B, which is a lactose free, reduced starch diet. This is prepared by adding puffed rice powder/cooked rice, glucose, oil to well whipped egg white followed by addition of boiled water slowly with rapid mixing to avoid clumps. The rationale is that the children who don't respond to diet A may have impaired digestion of starch and other non-lactose disaccharides. For this, lactose is completely eliminated, starch is reduced, and carbohydrates are provided partially by the reduced starch and also partially by the added glucose. Proteins (which are primarily provided by milk in diet A) are provided by the egg white. Complete substitution of starch by glucose is avoided as it increases osmolarity tremendously and may lead to osmotic diarrhea.

A total of about 15-20% children may not be benefited by even diet B and require diet C, which is a starch free, monosaccharides based diet. It is prepared by mixing chicken puree or egg white with glucose, oil and boiled water slowly to make a smooth paste. The rationale is that these children don't tolerate even the reduced quantity of starch in the diet B and hence starch is completely replaced with glucose and oil is added for building up the energy intake.

Each diet should at least be tried for 7 days. If there is no weight gain by day 7 OR if signs of dehydration return anytime after starting the diet OR if there is a marked increase in stool frequency anytime after the initial 48 hours after starting a particular diet, this is labelled as treatment failure and the diet is changed to the next in order, provided there are no initial or hospital acquired infections.

Other dietary supplementation should include vitamin A, zinc. All other vitamins and minerals should be given in the dose of twice the RDA for 2-4 weeks to all children. If there is associated severe PEM, Magnesium sulfate (0.2 ml/kg of 50% solution IM BD for 3 days) and potassium (5-6 mEq/kg/d) should especially be supplemented.

12. **Severe Malnutrition[14-16]**

Initially the total volume of each feed should be less with a total of 12 feeds given 2 hourly. Later each feed can be increased in volume and spaced more i.e. 6-8 feeds daily given 3-4 hourly. Initially milk based diets are the most suitable, if tolerated. Sugar and oils can be used to provide extra calories. If milk based diets are not tolerated, reduced lactose diets as in the dietary therapy of persistent diarrhea may be followed. Initially the calorie and protein intake should be kept at the maintenance dose i.e. about 80-100 Cal/kg/d and 0.7 g protein/kg/d (of the present weight) to avoid CCF due to excess dietary sodium and rapid expansion of ECF volume due to intake and also due to reactivated sodium pump secondary to increased energy supply. In a week, this should be increased to 150 Cal/kg/d and 2-3 g protein/kg/d.

After about a week of initiation of feeding, further energy dense feeding is required for the optimum growth of severely malnourished child. In this phase, energy and protein intake is increased upto 150-200 cal/kg/d and 4-5g/kg/d respectively.

13. **Obesity[17]**

Total calorie intake should be reduced. Mid-time snacks in between the major meals should be decreased. Oily, junk foods, soft drinks with empty calories should be curtailed. Consumption of high calorie foods like ice creams, toffees, sweets should be decreased. High fiber diet, which is low in calorie intake, should be encouraged especially before the main meals. This includes sprouted grains or pulses, vegetable salads etc.

14. **Nephrotic Syndrome**

Normal protein diet is advised till there is proteinuria to replace the protein losses and at the same time avoid the hyper filtration renal injury and rise in blood urea nitrogen seen in high protein diets. High protein diets like pulses, egg white etc should be started immediately after the proteinuria is stopped. Dietary cholesterol should be kept low and hence whole eggs, meats, fish etc are not advised. Salt is restricted to the usual amounts used in routine cooking with no added salts allowed.

Free Oxygen Radicals and Antioxidants[18]

Free oxygen radicals are the highly unstable and reactive molecules containing one or more unpaired electrons, which are formed due to addition or removal of an electron to or from a stable bio-molecule, mostly during cellular oxidation processes. They have important role in killing of phagocytosed microbes, detoxification processes etc. However, increased production of free oxygen radical's results in damage and degeneration of various tissues. Such mechanism of injury has been implicated many diseases like kwashiorkor, rheumatoid, arthritis, cystic fibrosis, inflammatory bowel diseases, cancers, storage disorders, autoimmune hepatitis, retinopathy of prematurity, necrotizing enterocolitis, bronchopulmonary dysplasia etc.

Antioxidants are the substances, which balance and counteract the free oxygen radicals and thus form the natural defense system of body. They act by lysing and inactivating free radicals, detaching free radicals from the susceptible molecules and finally, rapid repair of the damage done by the free radicals. The endogenous antioxidants can be intracellular (catalase, glutathione peroxidase, superoxide dysmutase), extracellular (bilirubin, transferring, albumin, uric acid, haptoglobin, ceruloplasmin) or membrane components (vitamin E, b-carotenoids, coenzyme Q).

Many exogenous substances can work as antioxidants and thus help in fighting the oxidative stress and counterbalance the harmful effects of free oxygen radicals. This includes natural dietary components like b-carotenoids, vitamin E, vitamin C, selenium etc. and also some drugs like allopurinol, desferrioxamine etc.

In spite of all this, exogenous supplementation of antioxidants has not been proved to have a definite role in disease prevention. Hence, the best way to ensure an adequate supply of natural antioxidants is a mixed and well-balanced diet with ample amounts of vegetables and fruits and adequate intake of all-important vitamins and minerals.

The nutritional needs of the child must be closely monitored. There is no need for strict calculations but simple weight record may give clue to the optimal intake of food. Balanced diet as per the choice, affordability and availability will help in proper growth and development of the child.

REFERENCES

1. Indian Council of Medical Research. *Nutrient Requirements and Recommended Dietary Allowances for Indians: A Report of the Expert Group of the Indian Council of Medical Research.* Hyderabad: National Institute of Nutrition/ICMR 1990.
2. National Cholesterol Education Program (NCEP). Reports of the Expert Panel on Blood Cholesterol in Children and Adolescents. *Pediatrics* 1992; 89(suppl):525-535.
3. Elizabeth KE. *Nutrition and Child Development,* 2nd edn. Hyderabad: Paras 2002:86-114.
4. Viswanathan J, Desai AB. *Achar's Textbook of Pediatrics,* 3rd edn. Chennai: Orient Longman, 1989.
5. Heird WC. Vitamin deficiencies and excesses. In: Behrman RE, Kliegman RM, Jenson HB, Stanton BF (eds): *Nelson Textbook of Pediatrics*, 18th edn. Philadelphia; Saunders 2008:177-190.
6. Black MM. The evidence linking zinc deficiency with children's cognitive and motor functioning. *J Nutr* 2003;133:1473S-1476S.
7. Arthur JR, Beckett GJ. New metabolic roles for selenium. *Proc Nut Soc* 1994;53:616-624.
8. Gupte S, Vani S. Pediatric nutritional requirements. In: Gupte S (ed) *The Short Textbook of Pediatrics,* 11th edn. New Delhi: Jaypee 2009:109-114.
9. Kelly D. Managing liver failure. *Postgrad Med J* 2002;78:660-667.
10. Filler G. Acute renal failure in children: Etiology and management. *Pediatr Drugs* 2001;3:783-792.
11. Moudgil A, Bagga A. Evaluation and treatment of chronic failure. *Indian J Pediatr* 1999;66:241-253.
12. Gowers C. Changing recommendations in diabetes mellitus. *Am Chron Diabetol* 2001;7:101-109.
13. Cederbaum S. Phenylketonuria: An update. *Curr Opin Pediatr* 2002;14:702-706.
14. Bhan MK, Bhandari N, Bahl R. Management of the severely malnourished child: Perspective from developing countries. *BMJ* 2003;326:146-151.
15. Shah D, Gupta P. Management of severe malnutrition: Facilitating learning. *Lancet* 2003;361:2088.
16. WHO. *Management of Severe Malnutrition: A Manual for Physicians and Other Senior Health Workers.* Geneva: World Health Organization 1999.
17. WHO. Obesity: Preventing and Managing the Global Epidemic. Geneva: World Health Organization, WHO Technical Report Series, No. 894, 2002.
18. Shah D, Garg K, Choudhary P. Oxidants and antioxidants in pediatric nutrition and disease. *Nutrisearch* 2001;8:1-8.

Suraj Gupte

2 Assessment of Nutritional Status

INTRODUCTION

Though frank cases of kwashiorkor and marasmus cause little difficulty in their identification, assessment of nutritional status may be rather difficult, especially in borderline nutritional disturbances such as mild or even moderate malnutrition.[1-3]

Assessment of nutritional status is at two levels:[3-5]

1. *Individual Level:* It is affected by several factors, especially by adequacy of intake of food (in quantity as well as quality) by the individual and his overall health status.
2. *Community Level:* It is the sum-total of the nutritional status of the individuals comprising the community. The community level assessment aims at collecting precise information on prevalence and geographical distribution of the nutritional problems of the community and identification of individuals or population groups at risk or in greatest need of assistance. This assists in formulating nutrition/health care program(s) that would improve the nutrition of the said population. Further, the assessment also assists in evaluation of effectiveness of such programs. In the absence of such an information, it becomes difficult to define the problems afflicting the community and develop policies to overcome these problem(s).

   It is pertinent to remember that, in assessment of nutritional status at the community level, it is not necessary to examine all the individuals comprising the community. Instead, representative samples are enough to draw conclusions.

Quite a few methods are involved in assessment of the nutritional status, including:

1. Dietary history and intake.
2. Clinical examination for presence of deficiency signs.
3. Anthropometry.
4. Biochemical evaluation and other investigations.
5. Functional assessment.
6. Associated disorders.
7. Vital heath statistics.
8. Ecological assessment.

As appropriately stressed by several authorities, these methods should be considered complementary to each other rather than independent as such.

DIETARY HISTORY AND INTAKE

The assessment must begin with the dietary history. Details about intake of cereals, vegetables, pulses, fruits, eggs, meat, etc. and thereby average daily consumption of proteins and calories should be obtained. A rough idea about the adequacy of vitamins and minerals in the diet should also be formed.

A diet survey provides information on direct assessment of food consumption. It may be conducted by:

- Weightment of raw foods.
- Weightment of cooked foods.
- Oral questionnaire technique.

CLINICAL SIGNS

Evaluation for clinical signs, simplest and most practical way, should be considered an essential feature of nutritional assessment. Deficiency signs such as hair changes, anemia, xerosis, Bitot's spots, cheilosis, angular stomatitis, rachitic rosary, bleeding spongy gums, dental caries, etc. should be actively looked for.

Table 2.1 gives WHO classification of clinical signs in assessment of nutritional status which may be modified according to pediatric needs.

The observations on the deficiency signs should, however, be interpreted very cautiously. As for instance, phrynoderma (toad skin), though traditionally thought to be due to vitamin A deficiency, may also be a feature of scurvy and deficiency of linoleic acid.

Table 2.1: WHO classification of clinical signs in assessment of nutritional status

Signs Unrelated to Nutrition

- Alopecia
- Pyorrhea
- Pterygium

Signs Needing Further Investigations

- Malar pigmentation
- Corneal vascularization
- Geographic tongue

Signs of Definitive Value

- Angular stomatitis
- Bitot's spots
- Calf tenderness
- Absence of knee or ankle jerks (beriberi)
- Thyroid gland enlargement (endemic goiter)

Note: This categorization is general rather than child-oriented and may be modified for use in assessment of pediatric nutritional status.

ANTHROPOMETRY[3, 6-9]

Anthropometry is a very valuable index for evaluation of nutritional status. In fact, for practical purposes, it is the most useful method. Even a non-medico, given reasonable training, can collect these data. Recorder over a period of time, anthropometric data serve as a mirror of pattern of growth of children and its deviations from the normal.

Weight is by far the simplest, the most widely used and the most reliable index, provided that it is recorded correctly and is related to the correct age of the individual. Also, what is more important is the serial record of child's weight periodically on a *growth chart.*

Since, it is often difficult to find true age of the child in the underprivileged and ignorant sections of society, the following truly or relatively *age-independent indices of nutritional status* are recommended.

Weight for height, which is only partially age-independent, is calculated as follows:

$$\text{Percentage weight for height} = \frac{\text{Actual weight}}{\text{Expected weight for actual height}} \times 100$$

Height for age is useful for malnutrition spread over a prolonged period (chronic malnutrition). Since change in height occurs only gradually compared to weight, early detection of malnutrition or diagnosis of acute malnutrition is not workable by this parameter. It is calculated as:

$$\text{Percentage height for age} = \frac{\text{Actual height}}{\text{Expected height for Actual age}} \times 100$$

Midarm circumference (MAC) is measured midway between the point of the shoulder (acromian) and olecranon process. For all practical purposes, the maximum circumference of the upper arm measured when the left arm is hanging by the side of the body would do. Between 1-6 years of age, it is said to remain constant between 16.25 to 16.75 cm. According to new guidelines, any child in this age group with a circumference below 11.5 cm of the reference standard (new i.e. 2006, WHO growth standards) is to be considered suffering from severe malnutrition. MAC between 11.5-12.5 cm denotes moderatre malnutrition. Mild malnutrition is denoted by a MAC of 12.5-13.5 cm.

Midarm muscle circumference is calculated by the following formula:

$$\text{MAMC} = \text{MAC} - \pi \times \text{triceps skin fold thickness.}$$

Triceps skin fold thickness is measured by a standard caliper (Lange, Herpenden or Best). On an average it exceeds 10 mm in 1 to 6 years age group.

A measurement between 6 to 10 mm points to mild malnutrition and under 6 mm to moderate to gross malnutrition.

Head/chest circumference ratio is a useful index of malnutrition. For measuring chest circumference, the tape is placed at the level of the nipple in a plane at right angle to the spine. The measurement in midrespiration is recorded.

At birth, head circumference is larger than chest circumference by about 2.5 cm. By 6 to 12 months, both are equal. After first year, chest circumference tends to take over the head circumference. By 2 years, it is larger by 2.5 cm. By the age of 5 years, it is more or less 5 cm greater in size than the head circumference.

Body Mass Index (BMI) correlates well with the subcutaneous fat and the total body fat and, yet allows a variation in the lean body mass. It is given by the following formula:

$$\text{BMI} = \frac{\text{Weight (kg)}}{\text{Height (met)}^2} \times \text{kg/met}^2$$

BMI remains constant upto the age of 5 years. A BMI > 95th percentile or > 30 kg/met^2 establishes existence of obesity. A BMI < 15 kg/met^2 points to malnutrition.

Quetlet index based on relationship between weight and height is expressed as:

$$\frac{\text{Weight (kg)}}{\text{Height (cm)}^2} \times 100$$

Normal value varies between 0.14 to 0.16. In gross malnutrition, it is less than 0.14. It is quite reliable.

Ponderal index is given by the formula:

$$\text{PI} = \frac{\text{Weight (g)}}{\text{Length (cm)}^3} \times 100$$

Normal value is > 2.5. In infants of LBW of SGA (SFD) type (IUGR), it is <2.

Dugdale index too is based on relationship between weight and height. It is expressed as:

$$\frac{\text{Weight (kg)}}{\text{Height}^2\text{ (cm)}} \times 1.6$$

Normal value varies between 0.88 to 0.97. An index of less than 0.79 suggests malnutrition.

Rao's weight/height ratio is expressed as:

$$\frac{\text{Weight (kg)}}{\text{Height}^2\text{ (cm)}} \times 100$$

Normal value is above 0.15.

Mid-upper-arm/height ratio of less than 0.29 indicates gross malnutrition, the normal being 0.32 to 0.33.

Quac-stick method is a simple, easy, inexpensive and yet reliable method of detecting early malnutrition of acute onset. Quac-stick is an abbreviation of Quacker arm circumference measuring stick. The instrument consists of a stick graduated with figures for midarm circumference in relation to height. For this test, maximum left arm circumference—the arm hanging by the side of the body—is recorded. Then, the child is made to stand in front of the Quac-stick. From the graduations in the stick, his nutritional status in terms of 50, 60, 70 or 80% of the standard can be easily read.

Shakir tape method is another simple and age-independent tool for assessing malnutrition. This special tape has colored zones: red, yellow and green, corresponding to less than 12.5 cm (wasted), 12.5 to 13.5 cm (borderline) and over 13.5 cm (normal) midarm circumference.

Bangle method, another method not needing age and useful in preschool children, consists in slipping a bangle with a diameter of 4 cm up the forearm. An attempt is made to move it over to the upper arm. In case it can slip over the elbow, malnutrition is present. The method, though simple and easy, is not quite reliable.

BIOCHEMICAL AND OTHER INVESTIGATIONS[3,5]

Laboratory investigations include hemoglobin, serum proteins, blood levels of nutrients like vitamins, iron, etc. and amino acid level in blood and urine.

Serum amino acid patterns: Distortion of amino acid pattern is measured by comparing concentrations of two groups of amino acids using per chromatography as shown:

$$\text{Ratio} = \frac{\text{Glycine + Serine + Glutamin + Taurine}}{\text{Valine + Leucine + Isoleucine + Methionine}}$$

Mean ratio in normal children is 1.5. In subclinical malnutrition, it is between 2.0 to 4.0. In kwashiorkor, it is 3.5.

Urinary urea/creatine ratio: This ratio can be expressed by any of the two formulas:

$$\text{I. U/C} = \frac{\text{mg urea nitrogen ml}}{\text{mg creatinine nitrogen ml}^{-1}}$$

$$\text{2. U/C} = \frac{\text{mg urea nitrogen ml}^{-1}}{\text{mg creatinine ml}}$$

The reduced ratio is a measure of average protein intake rather than the exact nutritional status.

Urinary hydroxyproline index: The formula for calculating hydroxyproline index is as follows:

$$\text{HOP Index} = \frac{\text{memol hydroxyproline ml}^{-1}}{\text{memol creatinine ml– body weight}}$$

Normal value varies between 2.0 and 5.0. An index of less than 2.0 reflects growth retardation.

Urinary hydroxyproline creatinine ratio: It is supposed to be better than the HOP index. Its main flaw is that it varies considerably with age. Standard values for different ages are available.

Urinary creatinine-height index: It is the ratio between the creatinine excreted by the subject in 24 hours and the daily creatinine output of the average normal child of the same height:

$$\text{CHI} = \frac{\text{24-hour urine creatinine}}{\text{24-hour urine creatinine for a normal child of the same height}}$$

In kwashiorkor and marasmic kwashiorkor, value varies between 0.25 and 0.75. In nutritional marasmus, it ranges between 0.33 to 0.85. Normal children and those having fully recovered from malnutrition show an index of around unity.

3-Methyl histidine excretion 24-hour urinary excretion of 3-methyl histidine/kg body weight in malnourished children is reduced to around 33% of that of normal children. With beginning of nutritional rehabilitation, values speedily return to normal.

Salivary protein, salivary ferritin and free alpha-amino **nitrogen in leukocyte** are reduced in malnutrition.

All said and done, the real value of biochemical tests is to detect subclinical malnutrition that could not be revealed by anthropometry. How far these tests are of concrete value in practice remains to be convincingly substantiated.

Radiology may reveal some retardation of bone age, osteoporosis or classical signs of scurvy or rickets. Some workers have described transverse lines of arrested growth at the growing ends of long bones months prior to onset of frank PEM.

FUNCTIONAL ASSESSMENT

Of late, use of functional indices (Table 2.2) has been proposed as a valuable tool for assessment of nutritional status.

Table 2.2: Some indices employed for functional assessment of nutritional status

Indices	*Nutrients*
Structural Integrity	
• Erythrocyte fragility	Vitamin E, Selinium
• Capillary fragility	Vitamin C
• Tensile strength	Copper
Host Defence	
• Leukocyte chemotaxis	P/E Zinc
• Leukocyte phagocytic capacity	P/E Iron
• Leukocyte bactericidal capacity	P/E Selenium
• T cell blastogenesis	P/E zinc
• Delayed cutaneous hypersensitivity	P/E Zinc
Hemostasis	
• Prothrombin time	Vitamin K
Nerve Function	
• Nerve conduction	P/E, vitamin B_1 and B_{12}
• Dark adaptation	Vitamin A, Zinc
• EEG	P/E

ASSOCIATED DISORDERS

While assessing the nutritional status, one must look for signs pertaining to malabsorption, intestinal parasitic infestations, tuberculosis, measles, diarrheal disease, etc.

VITAL HEALTH STATISTICS

For evaluation of the nutritional status of a community, the above measures should be supported by vital statistics:

- *Mortality data* such as infant mortality, neonatal mortality, perinatal mortality, stillbirth rate, second year mortality, 1 to 4 years mortality (specifically related to malnutrition) and life expectancy as also the ecological background. It has been suggested that LBW rate should be considered a key index of nutritional status of a country.
- *Morbidity data* such as from hospital or community health and morbidity surveys related to PEM, nutritional anemia, vitamin A and other vitamin and micronutrient deficiencies, endemic goiter, etc.

There is substantial evidence that vital health statistics are influenced by nutritional status. Hence they may help as indices of malnutrition. Nevertheless, they need not be considered as very satisfactory parameter.

ECOLOGIC FACTORS

Since PEM is the consequence of a multiplicity of ecologic factors, it is important to collect information on such factors in the community, especially:

- Food consumption by the community through the so-called "food balance sheet" which consists in finding levels of food consumption in terms of per capita supply availability.
- Socio-economic factors, e.g., knowledge, practices, beliefs about feeding, education, income.
- Health and education services, e.g., feeding programs, immunization facilities.
- Conditioning influences, e.g., infections (viral, bacterial, parasitic) that are known to precipitate or aggravate malnutrition.[6-9]

REFERENCES

1. Ghosh S. Current nutrition scenario. In: Gupte S (ed): *Recent Advances in Pediatrics (Special Vol. 1: Nutrition, Growth and Development.* New Delhi: Jaypee 1997:1-17.
2. Gomez EM. Child nutrition: Changing scenario. *Nutrition* 2005;7:234-239.
3. Gupte S. Gomez EM. Protein-energy-malnutrition. In: Gupte S (ed): The *Short Textbook of Pediatrics,* 11th edn. New Delhi: Jaypee 2004: 129-154.
4. Park K. Nutrition and health. In: *Park's Textbook of Preventive and Social Medicine,* 18th edn. Jabalpur: Banarsidas Bhanot 2005: 438-487.
5. Alleyne GAO, Hay RW, Picou JP, Stanfield JP, Whitehead RG. *Protein-Energy Malnutrition.* London: Edward Arnold 1989.
6. Jeliffe *DB. The Assessment of the Nutritional Status of the Community.* Geneva: WHO 1966.
7. Jeliffe DB, Jeliffe EB. Community Nutritional Assessment. Oxford: Oxford University Press 1990.
8. Waterlow JC. *Protein-Energy Malnutrition.* London: Edward-Arnold 1992.
9. World Health Organization (WHO) Working Group. Use and interpretation of anthropometric indicators of nutritional status. *Bull WHO* 1986;64: 929-941.

Meenakshi Mehta

3 Nutrition Education

INTRODUCTION

Good nutrition forms the basic foundation of health, particular for good growth and development, survival and maintenance of health throughout life. The crucial child health and development is directly proportional to the maternal health and nutrition during pregnancy, and the nutrition received from the mother, after the birth, from breast milk. With increase in the growth rate of population, rural to urban migration and rapid industrialization, hundreds of millions of children, especially from the underprivileged strata of society, continue to silently develop malnutrition.[1]

Malnutrition is like an iceberg, we see only tip on the surface above water (serious cases) whereas those hidden under the water (milder cases), though not seen, are potentially dangerous and vulnerable to infection, high morbidity and mortality.

WHY NUTRITION EDUCATION?

Malnutrition does not start only after the birth. It may well be a continuation of intrauterine malnutrition which leads to chronic growth retardation. Some 24-40 percent of babies born in India have low birthweight (LBW). With such a bad start before life and poor beginning at birth, child has continuing malnutrition which is most damaging, particularly in the first five years of life.[2]

An equally important repercussion of modern development is unplanned urbanization. Most of the migrants of the cities are the unemployed or underemployed rural poor seeking livelihood in cities. They have come to cities not because they already have found secure jobs but only to look for them.

According to one estimate, over two decades back, around 200 million people lived in urban areas under conditions of absolute poverty characterized by lack of access to housing, potable water, sewerage and adequate nutrition.[13] About 56 percent of these were estimated to live in Asia, 24 percent in Latin America and 20 percent in Africa. Nutrition surveys in Colombia and Moracco had revealed that the nutritional status of the poorest urban socio-economic groups was worst than that of the corresponding poor rural groups in those countries. Because of uncertainty of job or poorly paid jobs, the "mothers" also try to hunt for jobs to supplement the family income. This results in the children being left alone at home, quite often the eldest child, frequently a girl child, "mothering" the younger sibs. This is compounded by effects of overcrowding, environmental pollution and less time which mothers find to look after their children.[4] In the absence of care and love usually offered by grandparents, aunts, or other family members in joint families at home in the villages (to which the mother has no access in this new urban setup), the change in feeding practices and the child rearing crops up. Almost always for the worse (vide infra)!

Mothers tend to use commercial milk foods and precooked ready-to-use cereals in infant feeding and cheap ready-to-eat but nutritionally poor snacks for younger children. Since these milk or milk foods are expensive, mothers dilute them in more than recommended proportion so that the formula lasts for the longer time, occasionally for the entire month till she is able to purchase the new stock. The baby is fed this diluted milk or cereal in an unhygienic way by bottle by the elder sib and is, hence, exposed to increased risk of recurrent diarrhea due to gastrointestinal infections. Malnutrition rapidly sets in due to inadequate nutrition and recurrent diarrhea. Unchecked, this progresses to severe malnutrition, growth retardation and decreased immunity in advanced cases, and occasionally, death.

The paradox of nutritional problems is that they are preventable but still exist in such a large magnitude. This affects the socioeconomic development of the community and the country and leads to social inequality and poverty.

Undoubtedly, poverty is the main limiting factor in buying enough food. Nevertheless, the widely prevalent malnutrition is not entirely due to poverty. There is a widespread ignorance about the essentials of child care and child rearing including nutritional requirements and the common foods that supply the necessary nutrients. Most mothers and health workers know very little of how much food a child needs for adequate growth and development. Hence, the advice given is inaccurate and often conflicting.

Quite often, the foods suggested are commercial, expensive and beyond the reach of the major sections of the community. The elaborate recipes are time-consuming, besides requiring additional resources. In addition, there is heavy influence of advertisements through TV, radio, popular magazines, newspapers, etc., on commercial instant weaning foods, and other foods which are expensive and are not suitable for all age groups.

Understandably, there is a real need for parental education for sound and correct child-rearing practices and, in particular, advice on *how, when* and *why* and with to feed the child from what is easily available in the household, provided enough of it is given. Thus, improving families 'knowledge, attitudes, skills, and practices will become the key to improved child nutrition. Perhaps, in no other branch of medicine, parental education plays such a crucial role as it is on the nutrition education of the parents.

DEFINITION AND CONCEPT

Unlike other subjects, there cannot be any definition on this subject. However, there should be a concept on parental nutrition education. It should encompass enough information and knowledge about the amount and the quality of food for the growing child for different age groups, provide practical background, knowledge to all those concerned with health and nutrition of children; it should also cover role of preventive care and improvement in the comprehensive child care and how best it can be achieved. Needless to add that some advice of household culinary techniques and nutritional care of pregnant and lactating mother indirectly will have invaluable implications on total child health including nutrition. In addition, it should also include advice on related aspects like immunization, growth, common illnesses, etc. which could have direct or indirect influence on the nutrition of the child as well as changes in diet during various childhood illnesses and diseases.

WHAT IS A HEALTHY CHILD

Health is not mere absence of signs and symptoms of illness or disease. We may recall that as WHO has defined health as "Health is a state of complete physical, mental and social wellbeing and not merely an absence of disease or infirmity". Thus, a healthy "child" is one who is active, happy, cheerful and playful. He has good appetite, eats well, and grows well. He has developed physically, mentally, emotionally and socially appropriate for his age. He can understand, comprehend and function properly as expected for his age and if in the age group of schooling he can study well. He does not fall sick frequently or needs medical attention. In other words a healthy child is happy and contented. His arms bend, legs are firm and strong, neither too thin nor too fat or swollen with water (edematous). The skin is smooth, without spots, or cracks. The eyes are bright, lips and tongue are pink. Head is neither too big nor too small with fairly good hair which are black and shiny and do not fall easily. The bones are strong, he does not become ill frequently and is able to play or study properly without getting fatigued.[5,6]

As protective substances to help the body resist disease and to function properly.

THE DAILY GUIDE TO GOOD EATING

We have learned which foods are building foods, which are protective and which are energy foods. Now you need to know how much of each kind of food should be advised to the mother to be given to the child too optimum nutrition. A balanced diet is that which contains different foods in the right proportions and amounts so that all the nutrients are provided in required quantities. To ensure a balanced diet one must include in the diet:

- A mixture of cereals (rice, wheat, jowar, bajra, etc.).
- Pulses (greengram, dal, turdal, etc.).
- At least one green leafy vegetables and other vegetables and fruits.
- One fruit daily.
- Fats and oils.
- A glass of milk daily if possible.
- Meat or fish or egg (if non-vegetarian).

To meet the protein requirements vegetarians must consume more legumes as compared to the meat/fish consumed by the non-vegetarians. The amount of different foods will vary depending on the age of the growing child which will be discussed later.[6]

FOOD AND HEALTH

The foods that we eat play an important role in maintaining good health. We have many foods to choose from the health of an individual depends upon the type and quality of foods he chooses to eat. However, for maintaining good health it is essential that the food eaten should be in balanced proportions, containing the required nutrients. To ensure a balanced diet, one should include in the diet all the types of foods:

- A mixture of cereals (rice, wheat, jowar, bajra, etc.).
- Pulses (green gram dal, bengal gram, etc.).
- At least one green leafy vegetable and other vegetables.
- A fruit daily.
- Fats and oils.
- A glass of milk everyday.
- An egg a day (if possible and acceptable).
- Meat or fish (if non-vegetarian).

However, when the food consumed is not adequate or not proper in quality or in right proportions, it affects the health. The effect of improper nutrition on the various organs are as follows:[6]

Skin: Normal healthy skin is smooth and glossy. The skin of a poorly nourished person is likely to be dull, scaly and tough. When the diet does not include enough of green leafy vegetables, egg, milk or pulses, the skin of the individual may become pale and rough.

Teeth: The foods rich in calcium like milk, cheese and green leafy vegetables such as amaranth, palak, etc. help in preventing tooth decay.

Eyes: Healthy eyes are bright, clear with good vision. If the diet does not contain sufficient quantities of vitamin A rich foods (e.g. green leafy vegetables) the eyes are affected. The individual is unable to see in dim light. In children this deficiency can lead to total blindness, as vitamin A is required for good, healthy eyes.

Hair: Normal, healthy hair is easy to manage, smooth and shiny. If the food eaten does not contain enough protein or vitamins, the hair may fall easily or become dull, dry and difficult to manage. In severe cases there may also be a change in color from black to light brown (hypochromotrichia). In fact, such a hair change is a sign of advanced protein-energy malnutrition in children (kwashiorkor).

Body size: Good food is required for the growth of various parts of the body including the size. In the absence of adequate and proper quality of food (especially calorie and protein) children fail to grow properly. This is commonly seen in children between 1-4 years. After 4-6 months of age when breast milk alone is not sufficient, additional foods—top milk, semi-solid foods should be added. Infants in whom weaning is started late or those who do not get supplementary foods in proper amount and quality and do not develop well. They become stunted in height, weak and do not even develop properly. In severe causes such children may become mentally retarded.

Bones: When children do not receive adequate food containing calcium and vitamin C and D, there is a great danger to the growth of their bones. Besides if the children do not receive adequate sunlight by which the provitamin D in the skin gets converted to active vitamin D, the children develop bony deformities known as rickets, clinically manifested by knocked knees, bow legs, deformed chest, big head, deformity of pelvis and, in extreme cases, poor muscle tone of legs.

Brain: Brain is the most important organ of our body. It controls all the functions of the other organs. Since the growth of brain is maximum in the first six years of life, it is very essential that receives adequate nutrition. Individuals with deficiency of proteins, carbohydrates—particularly glucose and essential amino acids and fatty acids are at the risk of poor neurological development and if prolonged may develop irreversible mental retardation.

COOKING AND PROCESSING OF FOOD[3,7]

Most foods except fruits and a few vegetables are cooked before they are eaten. The methods used for food processing which include cooking, are often distinguishing features of a country's traditional culture. There are many reasons for processing of food. These include:

- To improve the taste, flavour, appearance, palatability and digestibility and reduce the bulk and water content.
- To destroy disease causing bacteria and to prevent deterioration during storage and transportation particularly of the more perishable foods like meat, fish, vegetables and fruits.
- To remove toxins.
- To preserve foods for times of storage.
- To give variety to the family diet.

Cooking meat makes it softer and capable of being chewed. Pulses and legumes become more digestible when cooked. The biological value of proteins in some foods also improves with cooking.

Boiling results in a comparatively greater loss of nutrients, particularly when the ater is thrown away, as in the case of rice or some vegetables, as the water soluble vitamins are lost. Steaming vegetables prevents loss of nutrients due to leaching. If root vegetables such as potatoes are boiled along with their skin, the losses are relatively small. Ordinary cooking of cereals, pulses and meats does not result in a significant loss of protein, fat and carbohydrates. Some protein is lost when vegetables are boiled in water particularly when the salt is used while cooking and the water thrown away. Boiling milk makes it safer by destroying the bacteria. It also softens the proteins and makes them easier to digest, particularly for a young infant. Vitamin C, however, is destroyed by boiling. Esposure to light also destroys riboflavin and vitamin C. Addition of soda while cooking, it facilitates cooking and preserves the colour but destroys most of the thiamine. On the other hand a highly acidic substance like tamarind preserves the vitamins. The longer the food is cooked, the greater is the loss of nutrients, particularly thiamine and vitamin C. But if the water used for cooking is not discarded the loss is negligible. If more water is used, the same may be used for other preparations as it contains minerals like sodium and potassium. Cooking with the lid on preserves vitamin C. Steaming food preserves the nutrients as in the case of pressure cooking. In addition, it preserves the food value and saves a lot of time and fuel.

Cutting and trimming: Vegetables should be washed and then peeled, and not cut too small in order to minimise nutrient losses. The finer the vegetable is cut, the greater the loss. Removing leaves does away with a good source of carotene. As far as possible the leaves of radish and outer leaves of cabbage and cauliflower should be utilised.

Sprouting of legumes is common in many parts of India. It improves the nutritive value and digestibility and some toxins are also destroyed. Vitamin C and riboflavin are synthesized but cooking destroys much of vitamin C.

Malting breaks down the starch in the grains and converts it into sugar. About 100 gm of any whole cereals grain is first immersed overnight in two or three times its volume of water. The excess water is drained and the most swollen seeds are germinated in a moist and dark environment for 1 to 2 days till the sprouts are removed by hand abrasion and the grain is powdered and stored in a tight container. This contains high amount of amylase rich powder (ARF) 1/2 to 1 tsf (2-5 gm) of this to any porridge liquify as it and reduces its viscosity. Thus, this is a very good way of feeding small children without increasing the bulk. The malting process increases the riboflavin, niacin and iron content. Ragi malt is commonly used in South India as weaning food.

Fermentation increases digestibility and adds a distinctive flavour to the food. A common fermented food is curd, which is eaten all over India. It is very useful in certain disorders like lactose intolerance when milk is not tolerated because of its lactose content. The lactose of curd is broken down during the process of fermentation. The dal and rice mixtures used to make idli or dhokla are popular in South India and Gujarat. Fermentation involves the growth of micro-organisms which improves the nutritional value of the product.

Drying: By drying, the shelf-life of food is increased. Fish is commonly dried in coastal regions. Seasonal vegetables are also dried, but the common methods involved may lead to loss of nutrients. This can be diminished by putting the vegetables first in boiling water and then dried.

Milling: Milling involves making grains into powder form. This is commonly processed to make flour out of cereals. Finer the flour (maida) more is the loss of nutrients, although such a fine flour is more whiter and easily absorbable. That is why less refined atta is used for bread which has a better nutritional value.

Parboiling involves first soaking the rice in water, then steaming and drying. This process drives the nutrients into the interior of the grain and subsequent milling does not destroy as much vitamin B and minerals. Parboiled rice is more resistant to insects and fungus. The disadvantage is that it has a peculiar smell which may be due to inappropriate processing. Parboiling rice is common in South India. Similarly, parboiled wheat (Bulgar wheat) is used in nutritional supplementary programs. Kesari dal is also parboiled to destroy toxins which are responsible for causing lathyrism.

Storage: Before storage the grain should be dried properly and should be free from fungus-aflatoxin. If pesticides are added for preservation the grain should be thoroughly washed and dried before eating.

FEEDING (OF GIRLS AND WOMEN) AT DIFFERENT PHASES

Women face high risks of malnutrition and disease at all the three critical stages viz. infancy and childhood, adolescence and reproductive phase. Child mortality rate figures show high rates for female children than their male counterparts. This is perhaps indicative of social prejudices leading to neglect of female babies.

Adolescence

When girls attain adolescence they go through a second spurt of growth and their bodies grow much more rapidly to prepare them for child bearing. But, unfortunately, the intake of nutrients during this period is significantly low, the calories and protein gaps ranging from 300-400 calories and 2-22 g of protein respectively. The daily intake of vitamin A and iron by all age group is much lower than the recommended levels. Iron requirements in the adolescent girls and women of child bearing age should be considered. Keeping in mind the iron loss through the menstrual bleeding and the vicious cycle of pregnancy and lactation, poor nutritional status in a girl child continues in adolescence and leads to suboptimal anemic in adult women. She gets married and conceives in the anemic and malnourished status *per se*. No wonder that such a mother gives birth to a low birthweight baby! The sordid state of affairs is compounded by national poverty, gender bias, cultural practices and less priority to girls, women in terms of food and nutrition education and total well-being.

A developing country like India must start investing in her young growing girls, so that the future mother to be are healthy and are able to give birth to healthy neonates. The components of diet needing particular attention in this period are calories, proteins, iron, vitamin A and calcium. All efforts must be made to provide these recommended nutrients to the adolescent girls.

Pregnancy

We do not realise that by the time an infant is born, it is already nine months old. The infant in fact grows more rapidly in mother's womb than after birth and it follows therefore that for infants to be healthy the mothers should also be healthy. Thus, mother's nutrition has a direct relationship with birthweight, foetal stores of iron and fat soluble vitamin A and D and thiamine. Many surveys have shown that most mothers are underweight (less than 40 kg) and have a calorie deficit of 500 to 600 calories per day. Many mothers of poor communities continue to do hard physical work throughout pregnancy and it is estimated that they would need, on average, about 300 extracalories a day during the last trimester of pregnancy. Anemia is widely prevalent and over 50 percent women in their third trimester have Hb levels less than 11 g/dl, the minimal level recommended by World Health Organization (WHO). These women tire easily, are more susceptible to infections, are more likely to miscarriages and also prone to deliver low birthweight babies.[3] Needless to say pregnant women must take more food with iron and folate. There are two types of iron source: Heme sources—such as meat and poultry-easily absorbed by the body than the non-heme sources such as cereals, tubers, vegetables, and pulses. Hence greater amounts of non-heme sources enhances the iron absorption from non-heme source. Phytates present in wheat and other cereals, inhibit iron absorption, while ascrobic acid (vitamin C) enhances it. Egg yolk, tea and coffee also inhibit iron absorption. It is important to eat foods rich in vitamin C along with main meals, e.g. raw vegetables, sprouted legumes, mint chutney, fruits like guava, orange, lemon and amla (Indian goose berry). Tea and coffee should be avoided with and soon after a meal. As per the anemia prophylactic program of the Government of India launched in 1970, tablets of 60 mg of elemental iron and 500 mg of folic acid are given to pregnant women for 100 days. However, the utilization is very low and all efforts must be made to motivate pregnant women at all contact places, antenatal clinics, ICDS clinics immunization and supplementary food program centers. Similarly, care should be taken to give vitamin B complex and A by advising to eat green leafy vegetables milk and pulses.

Weight gain during pregnancy in India is much less than that found in the developed countries. Most women from lower socioeconomic strata gain around 3 to 5 kg as against 10 kg in the case of the more affluent women. Of this 10 kg about half is contributed by the weight of the fetus, placenta and amniotic fluid, and the other half by the deposition of fat which provides a store that can be used during lactation. The latter is not present in Indian women from low socioeconomic groups, as a result of which their body tissues are depleted during lactation. Poor maternal nutrition leads to low birthweight (LBW) babies. In most parts of India the birthweight is between 2700-2900 g which is more by 200-300 g in higher socioeconomic society, but less than 2500 g in women of underpreviledged societies accounting for about 1/3rd of all live births. These low birthweight babies are handicapped in several ways.

The recommended dietary intake during pregnancy in calories (kcal) 2500, proteins (g) 6.5, iron (mg) 38, calcium (mg) 1000, vitamin A (mg), retinol 600, B-carotene (mg) 2400.

Lactation

The dietary intake of lactating mothers belonging to low income groups is far below that recommended. Direct evidence of the amount of milk these women can produce is difficult to obtain, but is well-known. These women are not able to secrete adequate milk as seen from inadequate weight gain of their infants after the age of 9-5 months. Many well-nourished mothers can produce about 400 ml milk a day for a period of 6 months to a year and 100 to 150 ml in the second year. Maternal malnutrition affects the quality of milk produced, and the concentration of fat, vitamins A, B and C are lower than in well-fed women. The concentrations of iron and calcium, however, appear to be normal. The lactating women not only needs foods for her own requirements but also to compensate for the loss of energy in producing breast milk for her baby. A healthy mother cannot only provide abundant milk, but can also look after her baby because she herself is fit. The recommended dietary allowances during pregnancy and lactation given in Table 3.1.[3]

Table 3.1: Recommended dietary allowances during pregnancy and lactation

	Pregnancy	*Lactation*
Calories (kcal)	2500	2750
Proteins (g)	6.5	7.5
Iron (mg)	38	30
Calcium (mg)	1000	1000
Vitamin A/retinol (mg)	600 (μg)	950
B-carotene (μg)	2400	

NUTRITIONAL NEEDS OF CHILDREN

Adequate food is the most important requisite for growth, more so in the first five years of life when rapid growth occurs. Insufficient food will not only result in under-nutrition but will also hinder growth and may predispose to infections. The recommended nutritional requirements for different age groups is depicted in Table 3.2.

With net protein utilization 65 relatives to egg. In the previous units in this course you have learnt in detail about breastfeeding, feeding of young child, weaning, etc. Here, we should only stress on the aspects of young child feeding and nutrition which the parents should know and follow.

BREASTFEEDING

We are aware that currently great stress is being laid on breastfeeding. Unlike developed countries where breast-

Table 3.2: Recommended daily requirements of energy and protein

Age group	*Energy kcal per kg*	*Protein g/kg*
0 to 3 months	116	2.3*
3 to 6 months	99	1.85*
6 to 9 months	95	1.65**
9 to 12 months	101	1.50**
	Total daily requirements	
1 to 3 years	1240	21
4 to 6 years	1690	29
7 to 9 years	1950	40
10 to 12 years (boys)	2194	51.9
(girls)	1965	55
13 to 15 years (boys)	2450	67
(girls)	2060	62
16 to 18 years (boys)	2640	75
(girls)	2060	60

* In terms of milk protein alone.
** In terms of mixed vegetables protein.

feeding is optional, in Third World countries, breastfeeding is very much practised easily by majority of women. Although bottle feeding has penetrated even in rural areas, breastfeeding is practised by many mothers both in urban and rural societies. The qualities of breast milk, scientific, social and economic advantages are well-known. It needs to be stressed that mothers must exclusively breastfeed their babies at least for 4-6 months after which supplementary feeding can be introduced. To breastfeed successfully, a woman (especially primiparous) must feed confident. That means she must believe that she can do it. She needs encouragement, guidance and advice from family members, friends and relatives.

Important Messages for Parents on Breastfeeding[3]

1. Composition of breast milk is ideally suited to the requirements of the baby. A breastfed baby does not need to drink any extra water, even in hot weather.
2. Breast milk has several substances which protect the baby against diarrhea and other infections.
3. The baby's sucking makes the breast produce milk. The more he sucks the more milk is secreted.
4. A colostrum protects the baby from infections, breastfeeding should be started soon after birth.
5. It is important to put the baby to the breast in correct position.
6. A baby should be fed whenever he seems hungry both at day and night.
7. Exclusive breastfeeding should be promoted from birth to four to six months of age. No water, ghutti, fresh animal milk, infant formula or other liquids should be given before the age of four months.
8. A growing baby is getting enough breast milk.
9. Advise the mother about her own diet as this is beneficial for both her and the baby.
10. Engorgement is uncommon among mothers who feed exclusively from the breast and who feed frequently both day and night.
11. Prevent the formation of breast abscess by timely action against engorgement and mastitis.
12. Put the baby to the breast in correct position to prevent score and cracked nipples, washing the nipples with soap should be avoided.
13. Mother's milk is the best food for low birthweight babies.
14. Breast milk can be continued even if baby is sick, i.e. diarrhea, fever, etc.

COMPLEMENTARY FEEDING

After six months, many mothers do not have enough breast milk to suffice as the sole source of food to the baby. Thus, some other food will have to be started in addition. Since the baby is small and used to liquids, artificial food item. The type of milk is either cow, bufallo or goat milk, depending on how easily it is available. The dilution will depend upon which milk is used. In general the milk should be boiled, cream removed and then diluted 3:1 (3 part milk + 1 part of boiled water) for the first two months of age. Sugar may be added (1 tsf supplying 15 kcal), to about 100 ml of milk + water. Milk should be fed with cup and spoon (palada, bondla) traditional feeding vessel. Care must be taken to teach mother about the sterilization of the feeding utensils.

Important Messages for Parents on Artificial Feeding

1. A bottle is very difficult to clean and is a source of infection. Do not use a bottle, use a cup and spoon instead.
2. Artificially fed babies have a high risk of infection, which in turn leads to malnutrition and even death. Exclusive breastfeeding should be encouraged for the first four to six months. Any addition to breast milk (even water) greatly increases the risk of infection and increases the likelihood of the mother failing to produce enough milk. For the same reason commercial infant foods are unsafe.

Addition of Solids and Semi-solids

When the breast milk alone is not enough after first 4-6 months, addition of semi-solids or artificial milk is advisable. This can be achieved by giving seasonal fruits, vegetables mixed with milk or diluted with water and offered to the child. Delay in introduction of solids or semi-solids may lead to malnutrition and if prolonged growth and developmental retardation. Foods offered should be common home-made foods, easily made from locally available cereals, pulses, seasonal fruits, vegetables, in a soft semi-solid form, easily accepted by the infant. Oil or ghee and sugar or jaggery can be added to supply extra calories and palatability. To start with initially one serving can be given which later can be increased to two or three times a day. The entire process of offering and accepting this food should be an enjoyable activity for the baby. Mothers should be discouraged to buy commercial preparations as they are expensive. The articles of diet used can be dal and rice-khichdi, suji, nachni, rice-flakes, millet, fortified with oil. Seasonal fruits like banana, mosambi, oranges, papaya and DGLV-dark green leafy vegetables as a source of B-carotene should be added. The amount and frequency of feed to be gradually increased as the child grows.[14]

As most foods are bulky malted cereals ARF-amylase rich food can be added to decrease the viscosity and make the feed calorie dense. Care should be taken to prepare it hygienically and preserve carefully to avoid spoiling it.

FEEDING THE PRESCHOOL CHILD

Between the first and third years, the child must take about two to three glasses of milk. Pulses at least twice a day or fresh foods should be included daily. Eggs about four per week may be given if acceptable, as eggs contain proteins and vitamins essential for the growing child. Boiled vegetables and green leafy vegetables and seasonal fruits should be given twice in the day. To provide energy tubers and cereals must be given two to three times in the day. To improve acceptability, a variety of foodstuff should be offered. General hygienic precautions must be taken to prevent infective illnesses from the consumption of contamination of foods.

IMPORTANT MESSAGES FOR PARENTS ON ADDITION OF SEMI-SOLIDS AND SOLIDS

1. No one food is a 'must' for a child (except breast milk).
2. Semi-solids should be introduced when the baby is six months old. Continue to give him breast milk as well.
3. Small babies need to be fed five to six times a day. Add 1 to 2 teaspoons of oil to the food to increase energy density.
4. A child of 1 to 2 years needs half the amount of food that his mother eats.

COMMON DEFICIENCY, DISORDERS AND THEIR PREVENTION

Vitamin A Deficiency (VAD)

It is the most common cause of blindness among young children, particularly under the age of six years and is more common with protein energy malnutrition. It is estimated that five to seven percent of children suffer from eye signs of VAD and approximately 20,000 children become blind every year. Vitamin A helps in keeping the eyes and skin healthy and it has protective effect in prevention of recurrent gastrointestinal and respiratory infections. Milk, butter, yellow of egg, liver, fish, liver oil—particularly shark liver oil are rich sources of vitamin A and green leafy or yellow orange vegetables and fruits are rich in B-carotene, the precursor of vitamin A. Deficiency of above articles in diet of a young child leads to VAD. VAD may also occur in infants whose mothers are deficient in vitamin A, because the foetal stores are not built up. The colostrum is a rich source of vitamin A. Similarly, a breastfed baby commonly does not develop VAD as he gets all the required vitamin A from the breast milk. Hence, babies who do not get adequate breast milk or those who are weaned from the breastfeeds before four months and who do not receive the required vitamin A develop VAD. Night blindness can also occur as one of the early signs of VAD. When VAD takes a serious turn, apart from night blindness to undergo some changes. In a normal eye, the white ball which is bright and moist becomes dull and dry (xerosis) and in more advanced stage triangular spots appear in the eye (Bitot's spots). Even though vision may not be affected at this stage, blindness may set in if vitamin A is not given.

Prevention of Vitamin A Deficiency[3]

1. Every mother must know how to protect her child from this danger. A pregnant and lactating mother must regularly eat like green leafy vegetables, pumpkin, carrot, pappaya, mango, orange. Whenever possible milk and milk products must be taken. If possible the mother should learn to cultivate such green leafy vegetables for easy availability. Similarly, when weaning is introduced a mother must feed her child with above dietary articles. Feeding of colostrum and breast milk as long as possible must be encouraged.
2. Administering massive doses of vitamin A. Despite all the efforts and advice quite often children under six years do not get adequate dietary vitamin A, under such situations it is safe and wiser to prevent VAD in children with the administration of massive dose of vitamin A. Vitamin A is stored in the body for prolonged periods and hence periodic administration of massive doses ensures adequate vitamin A in the body. Under vitamin A massive dose programs the following doses are recommended:

   1 to 5 years—200,000 IU every six months.

   Infants 6 to 11 months—one dose of 100,000 IU every six months.

   Infants less than 6 months—50,000 IU once.

Since measles can worsen vitamin A deficiency, children having measles also should receive this.

Anemia[3]

Anemia is mainly due to iron deficiency, but folic acid (a B vitamin) and vitamin B_{12} deficiency may also play a part. A large number of our population are suffering from different degrees of anemia. Poverty and consequent inability to afford nutritious food are the main causes of anemia in our country. Some people are ignorant in the choice of right foods and anemia might result from this. Apart from nutritional deficiency, malaria and hookworm infestation also can lead to anemia. Recurrent pregnancy and lactation without adequate nutrition can aggravate anemia. Growing children especially under the age of six years and adolescent children are more vulnerable to develop anemia because their rapid growth and requirement of proper nutrition. Anemic children are lethargic, lack energy and get tired soon. They have short attention span and poor performance at school and have profound significance on learning ability. The child looks pale and conjunctiva, lips, tongue are pale, nails may become flat and in advance cases spoon-shaped. Anemia can be diagnosed by the assessment of hemoglobin normal levels are 14-15 g percent. Values below 11 g percent are diagnostic of anemia.

Prevention of Anemia

Advice should be given to consume dietary articles rich in iron-leafy vegetables, like drumstick leaves, gogu, amaranthus, palak, etc, beetroot, dates, jaggery etc. and liver. Since proteins help in formation of blood-milk, pulses, liver and eggs should also be eaten. Vitamins B and C help in iron absorption. Vitamin C is available from citrous fruits and vitamin B from grains, pulses, liver, and milk.[8]

Along with the diet treatment of hookworm infestation must be given. Suitable preparations of iron. Ferrous sulphate is as good as any other iron expensive salt. One tablet of 200 mg containing 40 mg of elemental iron is enough for a child upto five years. Because of world spread prevalence of anemia it is better to give iron as prophylactic 10 mg in first year and 20 mg in subsequent years.[3]

Iodine Deficiency

One out of every five people in India lives in iodine deficiency areas and is at risk of being affected by iodine deficiency disorders (IDD). Iodine is essential for the normal growth, development and functioning of the brain and body. A lack of iodine can give rise to goitre and make a person dull and easily tired and more important can lead to permanent mental retardation and stunting in a growing and developing child. A pregnant woman with iodine deficiency can produce a child who will grow up to mentally retarded. The average daily requirement for an adult is 150 mg a day. Iodine is present in the soil and water and our requirements come from crops growth in iodine rich soils. When the soil lacks iodine, the crops too are deficient in iodine and deficiency develops. The most visible and easily recognizable sign of iodine deficiency is goitre—an enlarged swelling of thyroid gland in front of the neck. IDD forms a spectrum of abnormalities which includes goiter, mental retardation and deafness. Iodine deficient women are likely to develop abortions or still births. Their children may be born deformed, mentally deficient or even cretin. In mild deficiency, the child may show poor performance at school. Although severe iodine deficiency belt is prevalent in sub-Himalayan region, it is present all over India, with new pockets being discovered in all the states. The regular consumption of iodized salt (15 mg iodine per g) provides protection against IDD. All health workers must motivate the community about the benefits of iodized salt.[3]

NUTRITION AND HEALTH EDUCATION

In a developing country like India, there are many constraints to better living and adequate nutrition. Incomes are low, housing is inadequate, there is over crowding, poor environmental sanitation and water supply, illiteracy is widespread. Communicable and infectious illnesses are rampant. Most of these problems are beyond the scope of the health worker and yet the community can be helped in many ways.

Principles[9]

Nutrition education, relevant to the needs, reaching to the homes and capable of being applied in family food patterns, is the ultimate road to good nutrition. It is, therefore, a means rather than an end. It should be practical and applied, adapted to economic and agricultural possibilities and in harmony with the socio-cultural setting. Nutrition education should include effective demonstration and sometimes supplementary feeding of vulnerable groups and practise by the mothers in food preparation. It can be an invaluable part of the community development, both in urban and rural areas. The emphasis should be on building better health through better food habits (and better food production) as well as preventing malnutrition and diseases. The nutrition education can be imparted at many places and by various techniques the most important aspects being reaching and involving the community for whom it is targeted. The community can be reached by the following:

The Home

The home is the ideal place, because by actually seeing the home set-up, environmental, water supply, sanitation, neighbourhood, cooking and washing facilities, one can get first hand information of all the aspects of the family life. It also generates confidence in the women folk and establishes a good rapport between the health worker (HW) and the family. The advice given on health and nutrition would thus be as it is related to that particular family, rather than general in approach. Mother could be guided on cooking, cleaning hygiene and later follow-up visits can enhance the co-operation of the family in a positive way. Further the visit could be adjusted as the convenient time of the mother so that she is able to discuss and learn to ease, while attending to her household chores. The HW must have a friendly approach and should be careful in not criticising the cultural beliefs and traditions. A few harmful practices like delayed weaning, starvation during diarrhea or isolation and non-feeding with measles, neglect weaning during diarrhea, attribute to feeding, use of unboiled water for drinking during monsoon, etc. can be discouraged with tact and skill. The head of family, grandparents should also be interviewed and complimented for their co-operation. This will help in allowing the mother to follow all the nutrition and health education advise imparted to her by the health worker.[3]

The Community

Community participation and involvement is the key to successful health and nutrition program. The community religious leaders, priests, politicians, respected members of community, school principals, women groups leaders, social workers and activists can also be brought on a common platform to decide the priorities of the community and for planning and implementing the programs. The priorities initially may not be directly related to nutrition like availability of water supply or enough toilets or building for school but which have long-term implications on the health and well-being of the community can be tackled first. This will win the confidence of the community and the subsequents, direct programs related to nutrition will be dealt by them in a much better way.

Nutrition Education for Urban and Rural Set-ups

The urban and rural set-ups and living are very different and the HW must appreciate the vast differences, while approaching these communities. What is suitable for urban practice is not suitable for rural and vice versa. While giving cooking demonstration, the type of fuel used, or the vegetables or cereals purchased or grown by the families in rural setting, type of milk available or water supply must be taken into account so that the mothers are able to practise the same without difficulty. In urban areas the migration of families from villages, or mothers also going for work and child looked after by siblings or neighbors or caretakers should be considered while advising the mother on nutrition advice.

Role of Health Worker (HW) in Nutrition Education

The HW is the keyperson in imparting nutrition education. Her age, her way of speaking and tone, language, her behavior, her way of dressing, her own background-educational and marital status has a great influence on the person to whom the HW is imparting education. For example an unmarried teenage HW advising the mother on breastfeeding or family planning, and similarly a male advising a pregnant woman or lactating mother will not be accepted culturally and will have a negative effect rather than a positive effect. Hence, care should be taken to consider these aspects while delegating the HW for particular role or area of nutrition education.

What to Emphasize in Relation to Nutrition Education?

Nutrition: The prime messages to be given to the mothers, during pregnancy and lactation and for the nutrition of the infants and children, i.e. breastfeeding, artificial feeding and addition of semi-solids and solids have already been highlighted earlier.

There are some additional aspects which have indirect relevance to better nutrition and health. These are:

Prevention of Infection

To lay stress on:

1. The importance of washing hands.
2. The importance of safe drinking water.
3. Use of the lavatory.
4. Environment cleanliness.
5. Common causes of diarrhea, parasitic infestations and ways to prevent these.
6. Prevention against other infections.
7. Immunization.

Treatment of Common Illnesses

To teach parents on:

1. How to prevent diarrheal dehydration through use of home available fluids or oral rehydration salt (ORS) solution? To prevent diarrhea, safe and hygienic eating habits and consumption of clean food and water (non-contaminated) is the approach.
2. How to deal with cases of fever by tepid sponging, cold packs on forehead and abdomen, good ventilation to allow hot air from the body to evaporate and giving the child orally any simple antipyretic tablets/syrup of paracetamol or aspirin or brufen, etc.?
3. How to identify children with cough and fever who have developed restlessness and rapid breathing?

Those who are breathless must be attended immediately. Preferably the child should be taken to the family physician or pediatrician who may admit/keep the child under close observation. He might give moist oxygen, an antibiotic, and if required, bronchodilators. If acute asthma is strongly suspected, he may give nebulization using specific drugs like salbutamol, etc.

Growth

The mothers can be explained the importance of growth—especially its relation to nutrition, the upward trend of growth on road to health and usefulness of growth monitoring on road to health charts on cards (See picture weighing—growth monitoring).

Care of the Mother

1. Need for extra diet during pregnancy and lactation has already been emphasized earlier.
2. Importance of prenatal care.
3. Reduction of hard physical work during the 3rd trimester.
4. Need for treatment of anemia.
5. Tetanus toxoid for prevention of tetanus in the mother as well as neonate in case of unsterile deliveries.
6. Delivery by a trained person.
7. Adequate spacing of children, advantages of family planning and small family.
8. Last but important need for female education.

Safe Drinking Water

The water should be taken from the municipal system, a deep well or a deep bore with a hand pump. It should be stored in covered pots and use with long handed ladles to avoid contamination with contaminated hands or environment. If the source of water is not safe, to teach mother about importance of use of boiled and cooled water for drinking and to educate the community for slow and filtration, chlorination, use of tincture iodine, potassium permanganate. Rain water can be stored and used as required.

Environmental Sanitation

This is very essential to reduce the incidence of diseases.

The parents must be taught to:

1. Proper collection and disposal of refuse and to use as compost.
2. Proper drainage, ideally linked to a kitchen or community garden.
3. Keeping the surroundings of well clean.
4. Preventing cattle near drinking water, not allowing bathing.
5. Discouraging defecation in open to avoid contamination of soil and water supply—which in turn may result in intestinal infections and parasitic infestation.

Kitchen Garden

As green vegetables may be expensive beyond the seasonal availability, mothers may be motivated to grow this and consume this to prevent VAD. Similarly fruits also can be grown.

Poultry

Egg is an excellent source of first class protein and vitamin A. Since the poorer families cannot afford it, it would be useful to train the mothers to cultivate hen so that eggs are easily available for the children.

Community Participation

The importance and relevance of community involvement and participation is the key to success of the entire nutrition education. This has already been emphasized in the beginning.[3]

Modes of Nutrition Education (NE)[9-15]

There are several methods of Nutrition Education. No one method which is a magic method. The most effective methods and techniques for educating mothers on nutrition are as follows:

1. Discussion with help of audiovisual equipment lectures, panel discussion on nutrition education.
2. Demonstration and practice classes.
3. Role playing.
4. Charts-games.

A wide variety of educational materials can be used as instructional aids, but they need to be carefully selected, adapted and relevant to the local conditions. They should simplify the subject and make it more concrete rather than more complicated and abstract. The materials used could be aesthetic, easily handled, cheap, light, pretested and preferably homemade. Most people retain only 10 percent of what they read, only 20 percent of what they hear; but 50 percent or more what they see and hear together, if integrated properly, and up to 90 percent they participate actively in practical work.[16-18]

Guidelines for Effective Nutrition Education

The success of nutrition education depends on the various factors of the educator. She must be friendly, yet firm, she should be enthusiastic but yet disciplined. The setting of nutrition education class-setting, timings, use of material for demonstration and advice. The HW should have the know-how of majority of Indian communities so that the mothers can be approached and understood well.

MONITORING AND EVALUATION

A nutrition program should be monitored and evaluated to judge its success. Evaluation often involves change in knowledge, attitudes, practices and eventually the nutritional status of children. If results are disappointed, the entire planning, etc. will have to be revised and those which are good will have to continued and encouraged. Thus nutrition education is an art; success will depend on how much interest the health worker takes.

It has been very aptly said by a Nobel laureate, "Underlying every condition is malnutrition, due to both, energy and protein deficiency… though poverty is the main contributing cause, it is greatly aggravated by lack of proper dietary knowledge."[18]

REFERENCES

1. Mehta MN, Kulkarni MV. Child nutrition: The Indian scene (ed). *Proceedings National Symposium-cum-Workshop on Child Nutrition*, Mumbai 1991.
2. Udani PM. Nutritional problems in children (Keynote address). *Processings National Symposium-cum-Workshop on Child Nutrition,* Mumbai 1991.
3. Ghosh S. *The Feeding and Care of Infants and Young Children* 6th edn. New Delhi: Voluntary Health Association of India 1992.
4. Gopalan C. The effect of developmental programs on the nutrition of population. In: *Nutrition, Health and National Development of India*. New Delhi: Media Workshop 1989;1-25.
5. Margaret AP. The healthy welfed person. In: *Feeding the Family*. Nairobi: East African Literature Bureau, 1970;1-5.
6. Srikantia SG. *A Manual of Nutrition*. Hyderabad: National Institute of Nutrition, Indian Council of Medical Research,1988.
7. Cameron M, Hefyander Y. *Manual on Feeding Infants and Young Children.* New Delhi: Oxford Medical Publishers, 1983.
8. Srilakshmi K, Shastri RBV, Murthy VR. *Food and Health* Hyderabad: National Institute of Nutrition, Indian Council of Medical Research 1973.
9. World Health Organization. *The Health Aspects of Food and Nutrition. A Manual for the Developing Countries in the Western Pacific Region*. Manila: WHO Western-Pacific Regional Office 1978.
10. Gupte S. *Infant Feeding,* New Delhi: Jaypee 1981.
11. Gupte S. Perspective in infant nutrition: In: Gupte S (ed): *Newer Horizons in Tropical Pediatrics*, 2nd edn. New Delhi: Jaypee 1986.
12. Gupte S. Update on protein-energy malnutrition. In: Gupte S (ed): *Newer Horizons in Tropical Pediatrics*, 2nd edn. New Delhi: Jaypee 1986.
13. Sweemer CD, Sen Gupta NK, Takuliea S. *Manual for Child Nutrition in Rural India*, New Delhi: Voluntary Health Association of India 1978.
14. Holmes AC. *Visual Aids in Nutrition Education*. Rome: Food and Agricultural Organization 1968.
15. Indian Council of Medical Research: *Nutrient Requirements and Recommended Dietary Allowances for Indians,* New Delhi: ICMR 1992.
16. Morley D, Woodland M *See How They Grow. A Tropical Community Health Manual,* London: Macmillan 1980.
17. Kig M. *Medical Care in Developing Countries*: Nairobi: Oxford University Press 1972.
18. Gupte S. Nutrition education, the pediatrician and the community: A 2-decades' experience. *International Congress of Community Awareness*, Singapore 1993.

NC Prajapati

4 Maternal Nutrition and the Fetus and the Infant

INTRODUCTION

Through centuries food has been recognized as important for human beings for health and disease. Great advances in the knowledge of nutrition and its practical application in the last 50-60 years have helped us identify specific nutritional diseases and methods to control them.

Nutritional problems are not just medical problems. They have a great impact in sectors of development like education, demography etc. Association of nutrition with infection, immunity, fertility, and maternal and child health is now well documented. Impact of maternal nutritional status on fetal and neonatal health and outcome has, therefore, attracted the attention of researchers involved in improving child survival status.[1, 2]

NUTRITIONAL REQUIREMENTS DURING PREGNANCY

Variety of terms have been used to define the amount of nutrients needed by the body such as optimum requirement / minimum requirement / recommended intake or allowances and safe level of intake. Of these, the term RDA (Recommended Dietary Allowance or Intake) has been widely accepted. It means the amount of nutrients sufficient for the maintenance of health in nearly all people and is based on the defined minimum requirements plus a safety margin.[1]

Energy

The energy requirement of women is increased by 300 Kcal throughout pregnancy and in lactation by 550 Kcal for the 1st 6 months and by 400 Kcal daily during the next 6 months over and above the normal requirements. This is to provide for the extra energy needs associated with the deposition of tissues or secretion of milk at rates consistent with good health.[1]

Protein requirements: The ICMR Expert Group suggests an intake of 1 g of protein per kilogram of bodyweight which are increased during pregnancy by about 14 g per day and during lactation by about 25 g per day (0-6 months) over and above the normal requirements.[3]

Fat

The daily requirement of fat is not known with certainty. ICMR Expert Group has recommended an intake of 20% of the total energy intake as fat of which at least 50% should consist of vegetable oil rich in essential fatty acids (Table 4.1).

Table 4.1: Summary of RDA for Indian women[3]

Particulars	*Sedentary work*	*Moderate work*	*Heavy work*	*Pregnancy*	*Lactation 0-6 months*	*Lactation 6-12 months*
Body weight	50 Kg	50 Kg	50 Kg	50 Kg	50 Kg	50 Kg
Calories	1875	2225	2925	+300	+550	+400
Protein (g/d)	50	50	50	+15	+25	+18
Fat	20	20	20	30	45	45
Ca^{++} (mg/d)	400	400	400	1000	1000	1000
Iron (mg/d)	30	30	30	38	30	30
Vit A (mg/d)	600	600	600	600	950	950
Thiamin (mg/d)	0.9	1.1	1.2	+0.2	+0.3	+0.2
Riboflavin (mg/d)	1.1	1.3	1.5	+0.2	+4	+0.2
Nicotinic acid (mg/d)	12	14	16	+2	+3	+3
Pyridoxine (mg/d)	2.0	2.0	2.0	2.5	2.5	2.5
Ascorbic acid (mg/d)	40	40	40	40	80	80
Folic acid (mg/d)	100	100	100	400	150	150
Vit B_{12} (mg/d)	1	1	1	1	1.5	1.5

Carbohydrates

The recommended intake is 50-70% of the total energy intake. Most Indian diets contain amounts more than this, providing as much as 90% of the total energy intake. This makes the diet imbalanced.

Overall, a pregnancy in total consumes about 60,000 kcal over and above normal metabolic requirements. A pregnant Indian lady requires 300 kcal, 15 g protein and 10 g fat daily in addition to her daily requirements. In terms of vitamins and other micronutrients she needs an additional 600 mg calcium, 8 mg iron, 300 mcg folic acid, 0.2 mg each of vitamin B_1 and B_2, 0.5 mg of pyridoxine and 2 mg of nicotinic acid over and above her daily requirements.[1,2] Magnesium and zinc are also required in increased amounts. The requirement is further increased during the days of lactation as the nutritional requirement of the growing infant is ever increasing, and the infant is totally dependent on mother, at least for initial 4-6 months of life. Table 4.2 summarizes the daily needs of a pregnant and lactating mother in comparison to a normal female.

Table 4.2: Maternal BMI and LBW [6]

BMI	*LBW*
<16.0	53.1
16.0-17.0	41.4
17.0-18.5	35.9
18.5-20.0	27.7
20.0-25.0	26.4
25.0-30.0	14.7
>30.0	20.0

EFFECT OF MATERNAL NUTRITION ON GROWTH OF FETUS

Birthweight is an important marker of adverse perinatal events (events occurred in the past) as well as future neonatal and infantile outcome future growth and development of (an infant). As for example, low birthweight is an important risk factor for neonatal sepsis as well as a major determinant of malnutrition during infancy.

Several studies have documented that extremes of maternal nutritional status are likely to adversely affect the fetus in the form of fetal maldevelopment, fetal death, untimely termination of pregnancy, IUGR, etc. Majority of neonatal problems occur in LBW babies. Also infants with neonatal problems or LBW are less likely to attain their full potential in terms of subsequent growth, development and intelligence. Interventions to improve neonatal outcome must start much before the childbirth. As maternal nutrition is a modifiable factor, timely intervention can help improve fetal wellbeing. Maternal nutrition before and during pregnancy has direct relation with fetal growth.[4-9]

Studies show that the nutritional status of a woman before conception and her weight gain during the period of pregnancy are both equally important determinants of fetal growth. Mothers who are overweight but have slow weight gain give birth to more deprived babies than do the mothers who were undernourished but have high weight gain. Type 1 IUGR (symmetric growth retardation) is primarily due to long-term malnutrition amongst mothers (poverty and chronic poor living conditions).[10-13]

A recent review[14] on relationship between maternal nutrition and the survival of the fetus and infant conclude that:

i. Maternal weight and weight gain are remarkably resistant to either dietary intake or supplementation.
ii. Nutritionally-induced increased birthweight does not universally increase the chances of survival of the offspring. (Pre-pregnancy weight, at least in affluent, industrialized societies while associated with increased birthweight, is also associated with higher perinatal mortality).
iii. While dietary supplements during pregnancy do have a modest effect on birthweight, in contrast to a large effect in famine or near-famine conditions, this is not mediated by maternal energy deposition; and
iv. Declining peripheral fat stores in late pregnancy are associated with accelerated fetal growth, and improved nutrition can lead to lower fat stores. Rather, the component of maternal weight gain associated with fetal growth is water, and presumably plasma volume.

The author believes that the studies documenting lower perinatal, primarily fetal mortality by maternal feeding both in famine and non-famine conditions are not likely to have been due only to acceleration of fetal growth.

Maternal malnutrition affects the birthweight and infant mortality through two main mechanisms:

1. Maternal malnutrition may lead to a smaller placental size and decrease nutrient supply to the fetus, resulting in developmental retardation during intrauterine life, or
2. Maternal malnutrition may result in suboptimal lactation performance, thus contributing to malnutrition and growth retardation of the child.[15]

Maternal nutrition is as important a determinant of birthweight as is the caloric supplementation during pregnancy. Infant mortality can be lowered and LBW babies prevented by ensuring adequate levels of maternal nutrition during pregnancy. However, efforts to improve maternal nutrition should start in childhood for optimum infant survival.[16]

MATERNAL VITAMIN AND TRACE ELEMENT DEFICIENCIES AND THE GROWTH OF FETUS

Apart from calorie and protein, vitamins and trace element deficiencies have also been documented to play an important role in determination of the fetal outcome. Therefore, micronutrient supplementation is not only important for all pregnant women, but absolutely essential where women are poorly nourished or anemic.[17, 18]

The evidence base for individual micronutrients benefit on neonatal morbidity, mortality, growth and development is patchy and often contradictory. Single micronutrient supplementations have not been shown to consistently affect size at birth or duration of gestation. The evidence linking maternal micronutrient deficiency to children's cognitive and motor functioning also lacks a clear consensus except for iodine in endemic areas.

Micronutrient imbalance can affect pregnancy outcome through alterations in maternal and conceptus metabolism, as a consequence of their essential role in enzymes and transcription factor and through their involvement in signal transduction pathways that regulate development.[5]

Vitamin A

Vitamin A deficiency (VAD) is associated with reduced fetal survival in animal models but this correlation has not been proved in humans.[19, 20] The results of large cluster randomized trial in Nepal has also showed no effect of vitamin A supplementation on neonatal morbidity. Daily intake of vitamin A recommended by ICMR (1990).[3,5,19,20]

Vitamin D and Vitamin E

Available data is not sufficient for evaluation of the effects of vitamin D and vitamin E on the growth of fetus and birthweight. The published trials were either of small sizes or gave conflicting results. One study on white mothers in France, showed no benefit of vitamin D supplementation on birthweight. Another study on Asian mothers in U.K., more likely to be vitamin D deficient, showed a higher mean birthweight in the vitamin D supplementation group but these differences were not statistically significant and length, head circumference or skin fold thickness did not increase. The intervention group had fewer cases of neonatal hypocalcemia.[21]

Vitamins B_1, B_2, B_3, B_6, B_{12}

Deficiency of thiamin, riboflavin and niacin during pregnancy might result in marked metabolic effects in the mother and impaired fetal growth since these are essential cofactors for certain enzymes involved in energy metabolism. Specific active transport systems maintain concentration gradient for thiamin and riboflavin in favor of the fetus across the placenta. The deficiency in pregnancy is common but the observational studies show widely differing findings. In a study in Kenya, better riboflavin status was associated with higher birthweight. Most observational studies for pyridoxine (B_6) have found no correlation with birthweight but in one study the Taiwanese mothers supplemented with 2 mg/d had higher birthweight infants.[22-27]

Vitamin B_{12} deficiency is more common in vegetarian people because it is mainly derived from animal sources. But the data is lacking as to the effect of vitamin B_{12} deficiency on the growth of fetus.

Vitamin C

Vitamin C supplementation has been shown to be associated positively with birthweight.[28, 29]

Folic Acid

The association between preconception folate deficiency and neural tube defects is well known. Folic acid is highly recommended for preventing neural tube defects but it is essential that folic acid is taken before or immediately after conception. Most experts recommend that all women of child-bearing age should consume 400 mcg of folic acid daily to prevent the occurrence of neural tube defects. Most of the trials in developed countries have shown no effect on birthweight but one study from India showed that infants born to mothers receiving folate supplements in addition to iron were heavier than those born to mothers receiving iron alone.[5, 30-32]

Iron

WHO Expert Group proposed that anemia of deficiency should be considered to exist when hemoglobin is below the following level: adult nonpregnant -12 g%, adult pregnant -11 g%. Hemoglobin of 10-11 g% has been defined as early anemia and level below 10 g% is marked anemia.[1] Iron deficiency anemia (IDA) during pregnancy is associated with an increased risk of intrauterine growth retardation (IUGR). The mechanism by which iron deficiency anemia causes growth retardation in fetus has not been clearly established. The possible explanation can be that the fetus becomes hypoxic due to maternal anemia and oxygen availability. Alternatively, iron deficiency may cause growth retardation more directly affecting the activity of the enzymes requiring Fe as a cofactor.[32-35]

Studies from developed countries showed that the highest birthweights were at the levels of hemoglobin below the cut-off for anemia, which might reflect plasma volume expansion as a favorable maternal adaptation to increase uteroplacental perfusion. However, data from developing countries shows that maternal iron deficiency is associated with low birthweight and poor outcome.[36,37]

Iodine

Deficiency of iodine has a clear link with thyroid dysfunction in pregnancy and results in cretinism. The effect of iodine deficiency on birthweight has not been studied and reported clearly. A trial of iodine supplementation have reported reduced rates of abortions and still births and significantly higher birthweights in supplemented mothers.[36-38]

Zinc

Role of zinc in fetal neural growth and development has been demonstrated in animal models. Zinc fingers (loops within the DNA binding domain of receptors for hormones, other vitamins and protein transcription factors) are active ion embryo genesis, cell differentiation and proliferation. In a review of data from over 40 observational studies including many from developing countries, approximately one half showed association between low zinc status and low birthweight. A large study of US women with low serum zinc concentration showed a significant increase in birthweight, head circumference and limb length in the supplemented group and the effect size was greater in thinner women.[2,39-41]

Calcium

There are very few studies that show an increase in mean birthweight after supplementation of calcium. The Cochrane meta-analysis showed a significant effect on low birthweight probably because of prolongation of gestation rather than enhanced fetal growth.[21]

Magnesium

Magnesium is another mineral for which studies have been conducted but focusing mainly on hypertension in mothers as an outcome. The Cochrane meta-analysis showed a beneficial effect on low birthweight and SGA babies. A positive correlation between magnesium intake in the first trimester of pregnancy with the birthweight but no effect of supplementation during 2nd and 3rd trimesters has also been documented.[21, 42]

Copper

Copper deficiency has been reported to result in structural and biochemical abnormalities in the fetus. Studies from developed countries have documented a significant correlation between low copper in drinking water and the occurrence of neural tube defects, making an impression that a primary deficiency of copper could result in birth defects like anencephaly in humans.[43-46]

The role of other trace elements like selenium, chromium, magnesium, and molybdenum in human pregnancy is not known.

In summary, there is no good evidence that single micronutrient supplementation leads to improvements in fetal growth and neonatal survival in undernourished population. Approach of multiple micronutrient supplements or improved overall micronutrient quality of mother's diet has not been logically tested. Since women in developing countries are likely to suffer from multiple micronutrient deficiencies, providing a full complement of micronutrients is expected to optimize functional and health benefits to the mother and infant.[5]

Regarding food supplementation, regardless of the controversy, most studies recommend an additional dietary allowance of 300 Kcal during the third trimester. The Indian National Maternal Supplementation Program is based on the same logic.[47-49]

BARKER'S HYPOTHESIS OF "FETAL ORIGIN OF ADULTHOOD DISEASES"[1,50]

Mother's health and nutritional status affect the child's health and nutritional status. This in turn has been influenced by her living conditions and nutritional history during her own childhood. During early life and development the embryo, fetus and infant are relatively plastic in terms of metabolic function. The effect of any adverse environmental exposure is likely to be more marked than at later stages and the influence is more likely to exert a fundamental effect on the development of metabolic capacity.

Nutrition is the major intrauterine environmental factor that alters expression of the fetal genome and may have life-long consequences. This phenomenon, termed "fetal programming" has led to the recent theory of "fetal origin of adulthood diseases" or the "early origin hypothesis of Barker".[51] The "fetal origins" hypothesis postulates that conditions, most likely nutritional, "program" the fetus for the development of chronic diseases in adulthood. Barker has shown that the size and shape of the infant at birth has considerable statistical power to predict the risk of chronic diseases in later life. Associations between the newborn's size at birth and various determinants or consequences of chronic diseases have been identified in many, but not all, of the available studies.[4,52]

Observational studies first showed an association between lower birthweight and higher rates of coronary diseases in the 1980s in England and Scandinavia. Later, it was confirmed in many experimental studies from different parts of the world, including the USA and India. Strong association has also been found for the risk factors for heart disease, diabetes and hypertension, the intermediary markers for heart disease, blood cholesterol and fibrinogen, bone disease, allergic disease and some aspects of brain function. Similarly a reverse relationship of birthweight and systolic blood pressure was shown in men and women, in developed as well as developing countries, and in all age groups, although it was less consistent in adolescents.

Insulin resistant and type–II diabetes have also been found to be independently related to small size at birth in several studies around the world. The association of small birth size with chronic disease tends to increase with catch-up growth and obesity, and usually persists after adjusting for confounding factors such as age, family history, and socio-economic history. Several twin studies lend support to the hypothesis. There is a tendency for lighter members of twin pairs to have a higher blood pressure, and more diabetes.

Pregnancy and lactation are energy-consuming events and this requirement is met with by increasing the intake but it has been observed that partitioning of energy to the fetus and mother depends upon the energy reserves of the mother before pregnancy.[53] This implies that the malnutrition amongst young and adolescent girls is more likely to cause growth retardation or other congenital or developmental problems in the fetus.

Scientists are now also looking further to find a possibility of the "programming" across the generations, or the involvement of embryo and oocyte. They are also endeavoring to describe the role of environment of grandmothers and mothers in predisposing offspring to health or illness in later life because an oocyte that becomes an adult human develops in the uterus of its grandmother.[54]

SPECTRUM OF NUTRITIONAL PROBLEMS DURING PREGNANCY

Nutrition is concerned primarily with the part played by nutrients in body growth, development, and maintenance. Good nutrition means "maintaining a nutritional status that enables us to grow well and enjoy good health". Malnutrition has been defined as "a pathological state resulting from a relative or absolute deficiency or excess of one or more essential nutrients". The spectrum of nutritional problems during pregnancy or at any other time can range from undernutrition (when insufficient food is eaten over an extended period of time), to overnutrition (resulting from the consumption of excessive quantity of food over an extended period of time), having in between the imbalance state (resulting from a disproportion amongst essential nutrients with or without the absolute deficiency of any nutrient), and the specific deficiency (resulting from a relative or absolute lack of an individual nutrient).

ASSESSMENT METHODS OF MATERNAL NUTRITION

Proper assessment of nutritional status demands a multi-angled approach. Various methods adopted are:

A. *Clinical examination for physical signs (both specific and non-specific) associated with malnutrition*: However, malnutrition cannot be quantified on the basis of clinical signs. Many deficiencies are unaccompanied by physical signs and lack of specificity and subjective nature of most of the physical signs.

B. *Anthropometry*: Height, weight, skin fold thickness, etc. are valuable indicators of nutritional status.

C. *Laboratory and biochemical assessment:* Tests like Hb, serum iron, serum retinol time consuming and expensive. Most biochemical tests reveal only the current nutritional status but they are useful to quantify malnutrition.[1]

BMI (based on maternal weight for height ratio) is very useful in predicting LBW. Other advantage of this is that it is not influenced by mother's age and parity. Its association with LBW is depicted in Table 4.2.[6]

Prepregnancy Weight and Fetal Outcome

Pre-pregnancy weight has been demonstrated to have a direct influence on birthweight and perinatal outcome. Maternal weight of less than 45 kg is a high risk factor.[7, 55]

Prepregnancy Height

Maternal height, an indirect evidence of heredity, socio-environmental and nutritional status has a determining influence on fetal and neonatal weight and mortality. In India ICMR multicentric reports have recorded height of less than 140 cms as a high risk factor.[7, 55]

Mid-arm Circumference

It has been used to identify women at risk. A higher incidence of LBW has been reported with a mid-arm circumference of <22.7 cm.

In India, during pregnancy, a weight gain of 9 kg is expected. It may, however, range from 6.7 to 18.0 kg. Inadequate maternal weight gain is associated with higher occurrence of LBW and perinatal mortality. Low weight gain after 20 wks of gestation may result in pre-term birth while slow or low weight gain throughout the pregnancy is associated with SGA infant.[7,8,56]

EFFECT OF MATERNAL NUTRITION ON BREAST MILK[57-61]

Exclusive breastfeeding for the 1st 4-6 months life is an integral part of safe motherhood program in India.

Breast milk is influenced by maternal intake of lipids, selenium, iodine and certain vitamins. The composition is also influenced by infant's birthweight and gestation, as each mother produces breast milk most suitable for infants requirements. The volume of breast milk and other

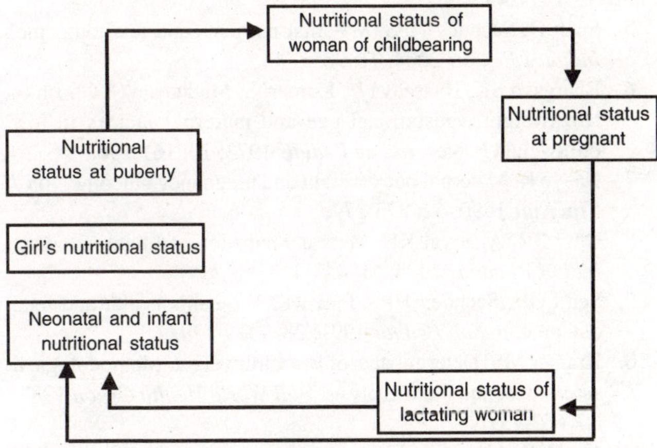

Fig. 4.1: Influence of each generation's nutritional status on the next generation[50]

Section 2

macronutrients are hardly influenced by maternal dietary intake. However, even chronically malnourished women are capable of producing adequate milk for their infants. So, "Not enough milk" is hardly ever a problem associated with maternal nutrition or malnutrition. Even a mother with somewhat malnutrition can produce enough milk to meet the needs of her baby. But yes, severe degrees of malnutrition amongst mothers can be associated with reduced amounts of milk production. In majority of cases the cause of "Not enough milk" is non-nutritional.

However, the quality of breast milk in terms of essential vitamins and micronutrients, which are essential for the proper growth of an infant, can be lacking even if a mother is producing sufficient quantity of milk. Lactating women are more likely to experience micronutrient deficiencies than a shortage of dietary energy or protein. Micronutrient deficiencies are also more likely to affect breast milk composition and the development and nutritional status of breast feeding infant. Dietary intervention or supplementation of these micronutrients can increase the secretion of many of these nutrients in breast milk and improve infant's nutritional status.

In general, milk production is most affected by the maternal intake of water-soluble vitamins, less influenced by the intake of fat-soluble vitamins, and relatively unaffected by maternal mineral intake or status.

REFERENCES

1. Park K. Preventive medicine in obstetrics, pediatrics and geriatrics In: *Park's Textbook of Preventive and Social Medicine*, 21st edn. Jabalpur: Banarsidas Bhanot 2011: 383-437.
2. Bhargava SK, Dadhich JP. Maternal nutrition and fetal outcome in nutrition In: Sachdeva HPS, Choudhury P (eds): *Nutrition in Children: Developing Country Concerns*. New Delhi: BI 1994: 34-45.
3. ICMR. *Recommended Dietary Intakes for Indians*. New Delhi: ICMR 1990.
4. Naeye RL. Maternal nutrition and fetal growth. *Nutr Rev* 1974; 32: 241-243.
5. Shah D, Sachdev HPS. Maternal nutrients and fetal outcome. *Indian J Pediatr* 2004; 71: 985-990.
6. Bhargava SK, Bhargava V, Kumari S, Madhavan S, Ghosh S. Birthweight, gestational age and maternal factors in low birthweight babies. *Indian Pediatr* 1973; 10: 161-166.
7. Naeye R. Maternal body weight and pregnancy outcome. *Am J Clin Nutr* 1990; 52: 273-279.
8. Devi RR, Agarwal KN. Maternal nutrition and fetal outcome. *Indian J Pediatr* 1984; 51: 443-449.
9. Sethi GR, Sachdev HPS, Puri RK. Women's health and fetal outcome. *Indian Pediatr* 1991; 28: 1379-1392.
10. Kramer MS. Determinants of low birthweight: Methodological assessment and meta-analysis. *Bull World Health Organ* 1987; 65: 663-737.
11. Neel NR, Alveraz JO. Maternal risk factors for low birthweight and intrauterine growth retardation in a Guatemalan population. *Bull Pan Am Health Organ* 1991; 25: 152-165.
12. Martorell R, Gonzalez-Cossio T. Maternal nutrition and birthweight. *Yearbook Phys Anthropol* 1987; 30: 195-220.
13. Galloway R, Anderson MA. Pregnancy nutrition status and its impact on birthweight *SCN News* 1994; 11: 6-10.
14. Rush D. Maternal nutrition and perinatal survival. *J Health Popul Nutr* 2001; 19: S217-S264.
15. Ostria TS. Maternal nutrition, infant health, and subsequent fertility. *Philipp J Nutr* 1982 ; 35: 106-111.
16. Habicht JP, Yarbrough C, Lechtig A, Klein RE. Relationship of birthweight, maternal nutrition and infant mortality. *Nutr Rep Int* 1973; 7: 533-546.
17. Yashodhara P, Ramaraju LA, Raman L. Trace elements in pregnancy 1. *Copper and Zinc. Nutr Res* 1994; 11: 15-21.
18. Leeal R, Veena S. Nutrition during pregnancy and lactation In: Bamji MS, Rao NP, Reddy V (eds): *Textbook of Human Nutrition*. New Delhi: Oxford and IBH 2002: 509-517.
19. Costello A M de L, Osrin D. Micronutrient status during pregnancy and outcomes for newborn infants in developing countries. *J Nutr* 2003; 133 (5 S-II): 1757S-1764S.
20. Katz J, West K, Khatry S, Pradhan E, LeClerq S, Christian P, *et al*. Maternal low-dose vitamin A or beta-carotene supplementation has no effect on fetal loss and early infant mortality: A randomized cluster trial in Nepal. *Am J Clin Nutr* 2000; 71: 1570-1576.
21. Fall CHD, Yajnik CS, Rao S, Davies AA, Brown N, Farrant HJW. Micronutrients and fetal growth. *J Nutr* 2003; 133(5 supple2): 1747S-1756S.
22. Dancis J, Wilson D, Hoskins IA, Levitz M. Placental transfer of thiamine in the human subject: *In vitro* perfusion studies and maternal-cord plasma concentrations. *Am J Obstet Gynecol* 1998;159: 1435-1439.
23. Dancis J, Lehanka J, Levitz M. Transfer of riboflavin across the human placenta. *Pediatr Res* 1985;19: 1143-1146.
24. Bamji MS. Enzymatic evaluation of thiamine, riboflavin and pyridoxine status of parturient women and their newborn infants. *Br J Nutr* 1985;35:259-265.
25. Reddy VA, Bates CJ, Goh SG, Rowland MG, Greenwood AM, Greenwood B, Paul AA. Riboflavin, folate and vitamin C status of Gambian women during pregnancy: A Comparison between urban and rural communities. *R Soc Trop Med Hyg* 1987;81:1033-1037.
26. Ramsay VP, Neumann C, Clerk V, Swendseid ME. Vitamin cofactor saturation indices for riboflavin, thiamin and pyridoxine in placental tissue of Kenyan women. *Am J Clin Nutr* 1983;37:969-973.
27. Chang SJ. Adequecy of maternal pyridoxine supplementation during pregnancy in relation to the vitamin B_6 status and growth of neonates at birth. *J Nutr Sci Vitaminol* 1999; 45: 449-458.
28. Mathews F, Yudkin P, Neil A. Influence of maternal nutrition of outcome of pregnancy: Prospective cohort study. *BMJ* 1999;112:206-211.
29. Doyle W, Crawford MA, Wynn MA, Wynn SW. The association between diet and birth dimensions. *J Nutr Med* 1990;1:17.
30. MRC Vitamin Research Group. Prevention of neural tube defects: Results of Medical Research Council vitamin study. *Lancet* 1991;338:131-137.
31. Iyengar L. Effect of folic acid supplementation on birthweights of infants. *Am J Obstet Gynecol* 1975;122:332-336.

32. Baumslag N. Reduction of incidence of prematurity by folic acid supplementation in pregnancy. *BMJ* 1970;1:16-17.
33. Zhou LM, Yang WW, Hua JZ, Deng CQ, Tao Xslotzfus R. Relation of Hemoglobin measured at different times in pregnancy to preterm and low birthweight in Shanghai, China. *Am J Epidemiol* 1998;148:998-1006.
34. Steer P, Alam MA, Wadsworth J, Welch A. Relation between maternal hemoglobin concentration and birthweight in different ethnic groups. *BMJ* 1995;310:489-491.
35. Lewis RM, James LA, Zhang J, Byrne CD, Hales CN. Effects of maternal iron restriction in rat on hypoxia-induced gene expression and fetal metabolic levels. *Br J Nutr* 2001;85: 193-201.
36. Rasmussen KM. Is there a causal relationship between iron deficiecy anemia and weight at birth, length of gestation and perinatal mortality? *J Nutr* 2001;131:590S-603S.
37. Scholl TO, Hediger ML. Anemia and iron deficiency anemia: Compilation of data on pregnancy outcome. *Am J Clin Nutr* 1984;59:492S-501S.
38. Chaoki ML, Benmiloud M. Prevention of iodine deficiency disorders by oral administration of lipiodol during pregnancy. *Eur J Endocrinol* 1994;130:547-551.
39. King J. Determinants of maternal zinc status during pregnancy. *Am J Clin Nutr* 2000;71: S1334-S1343.
40. Shah D, Sachdev HPS. Effect of gestational zinc deficiency on pregnancy outcomes: Summary of observation studies and zinc supplementation trials. *Br J Nutr* 2001;85 (Supple 2): S101-S108.
41. Goldenberg RL, Tamura T, Neggers YH, Copper RL, Johnston KE, DuBard MB, Hauth MD. Effect of zinc supplementation on pregnancy outcome. *JAMA* 1995; 274: 463-468.
42. Sibai BM, Villar MA, Bray EA. Magnesium supplementation during pregnancy: Adouble blind randomized controlled clinical trial. *J Obstet Gynecol* 1989;161:115-119.
43. Pathak P, Kapil U. Role of trace elements zinc, copper and magnesium during pregnancy and its outcome. *Indian J Pediatr* 2004; 71: 1003-1005.
44. Morten MS, Elwood PC, Abernethy M.Trace elements in water and congenital malformation of the central nervous system in South Wales. *Br J Prev Soc Med* 1976;36:36-39.
45. WHO. *Prevalence of Anemia in Women. A Tabulation of Available Information*. 2nd edn. Geneva: WHO 1992.
46. Anand S, Mittal R, Bhargava U, Vir SC. Copper status of Indian pregnant women of low socio economic group and its effect on the outcome of pregnancy. *Int J Vietnam Nutr Res* 1981;51:410-415.
47. Gopalan C. Low birthweight In: *Nutrition Research in South East Asia*. New Delhi, World Health Organization / SEARO;1994:13-31.
48. Kusin JA, Kardjati S, Hout Kooper JM, Renquist UH. Energy supplementation during pregnancy and post-natal growth. *Lancet* 1992;340:623-626.
49. Kardjati S. Energy supplementation in the last trimester of pregnancy in east Java: I. Effect on birthweight. *Brit J Obstet Gynaecol* 1988;95:783-794.
50. Elizabeth KE. Normal growth of children. In: *Nutrition and Child Development*, 2nd edn. Hyderabad: Para as 2000;237-253.
51. Wu G, Bazer FW, Cudd TA, Meininger CJ, Spencer TE. Maternal nutrition and fetal development. *J Nutr* 2004 ; 134:2169-2172.
52. Godfrey KM, Barker DJ. Maternal nutrition in relation to fetal and placental growth. *Eur J Obstet Gynecol Reprod Biol* 1995;61:15-22.
53. Kusin JA, Kardjati S, Renqvist U, Goei K. Reproduction and Maternal malnutrition in Madura, Indonesia. *Trop Geogr Med* 1992;44:248-255.
54. Newnham JP, Moss TJ, Nitsos I, Sloboda DM, Challis JR. Nutrition and the early origin of adult disease. *Asia Pac J Clin Nutr* 2002; 11 Supple 3:S537-S542.
55. Bhargava SK, Singh KK, Saxena BN. A National Collaborative Study of Identification of High Risk Families, Mothers and Outcome of their Offsprings, With Particular Reference to the Problem of Maternal Nutrition, Low Birthweight, Perinatal and Infant Morbidity and mortality in Rural and Urban Slum Communities. ICMR Task Force Study. New Delhi: Indian Council of Medical Research 1990.
56. Abrams B, Parker J. Maternal weight gain in women with good pregnancy outcome. *Obstet Gynecol* 1990;76:1-7.
57. Allen H. Maternal micronutrient malnutrition: Effects on breast milk and infant nutrition, and priorities for intervention. *SCN News* 1994;21-24.
58. Singh T, Gupte S. Community Pediatrics. In: Gupte S (ed). *The Short Textbook of Pediatrics*, 11th edn. New Delhi: Jaypee 2009; 78-96.
59. Government of India. *National Child Survival and Safe Motherhood Program. Progressive Interventions*. New Delhi: MCH Division, Ministry of Health and Family Welfare, 1994.
60. Hoffman SL. Maternal malnutrition and breast feeding. Is there really a choice for policy makers? *J Trop Pediatr* 1991;37:19-22.
61. Singh M. Maternal disorders and fetal outcome In: *Care of the Newborn*, 5th edn. New Delhi: Sagar 1999:71-80. *See* RAP Com Care.

PP Maiya • BP Karunakara

5 Nutrition and Growth

INTRODUCTION

Growth and development are continuous processes which begin at conception and end at maturity. They have a pattern throughout childhood and adolescence. During this process, any obstacle can result in aberration in growth and development. Many factors (antenatal, natal and postnatal) affect growth and development of the child. These factors may be genetic, demographic, environmental, physical, biological, emotional, social and cultural. All said and done, role of nutrition remains paramount in growth and development during childhood and adolescence.

India has diverse agro-climatic regions and ethnic multiplicities. Sociocultural practices, lifestyles and eating habits vary not only between states, but also between the districts within a state. Rural India needs more attention as 98% of geographical area of India and 72.9% of India's population occupy rural area spreading over 6 lakh villages. As per the report of National Nutrition Monitoring Bureau and National Institute of Nutrition, nearly 43.8% children suffer from moderate degrees of protein-energy malnutrition (PEM), 8.7% suffer from extreme forms of malnutrition and only 9.9% of the children are normal.[1] In India, malnutrition is the direct cause of death of 500,000 children every year. An estimated 450 million adult women in developing countries are stunted as a result of childhood PEM which further has an adverse effect on the intrauterine as also the later growth of the baby.

This chapter is a spotlight on the impact of nutrition at all stages of growth and development in children with a special reference to maternal nutrition, relevance of breastfeeding on growth and development, adolescent nutrition and growth, growth monitoring and nutritional assessment.

NUTRITION

Importance of Nutrition During Childhood

Nutrients are essential for normal physiological activities and optimal growth and development.

Nutrients fall into 6 major categories: Water, carbohydrates, proteins, fats, vitamins and minerals. Nutrients are organic and inorganic complexes present in food.

1. Macronutrients: Proteins, fats and carbohydrates.
2. Micronutrients: Vitamins and minerals (trace elements).

Macronutrients

These are often called proximate principles because they form the main bulk of the food. In the Indian diet, they contribute to the total energy intake in the following proportions: Proteins (7 to 15%), fats (10 to 30%) and carbohydrates (65 to 80%).

Energy is essential for physical activity, thermogenesis, tissue maintenance and growth. Dietary carbohydrates, proteins and fats provide energy. The unit of energy is 1 kilocalorie (kcal/cal) commonly designated as calorie. The energy requirement depends upon the BMR and physical activity. BMR constitutes 50 to 60%, physical activity 30 to 40%, and thermogenesis 5 to 9% of total energy expenditure. Children less than 5 years require more energy dense diet with less complex carbohydrates and a greater proportion of energy derived from fat to ensure optimum growth.

Carbohydrates are the chief source of energy. There are 3 major types of carbohydrates: starch, sugar and fiber. They play an important role in infant and child nutrition as they spare proteins, thereby allowing utilization of proteins for growth and various repair processes. They are also used for energy in preference to fat (when sufficient carbohydrate is available in diet). They are therefore, said to possess antiketogenic properties. One gram of carbohydrate gives 4 kilocalories of energy. A deficient intake of carbohydrates may result in undernutrition, ketosis and constipation. Carbohydrate malnutrition/carbohydrate deprivation syndrome results from excessive intake of milk without added carbohydrates among 1 to 6-month-old infants in higher socio-economic group.

Fiber is an indigestible carbohydrate. There are 2 types of fibers; crude and dietary. Diet with adequate amount of fibers lower serum cholesterol. Very high fiber content may bind trace elements. Indian diets supply upto 40 g fiber per day. The suggested intake is 20 to 40 g per day or 200 to 300 mg/kg/day.

Proteins are essential components of every living cell and are necessary for numerous biological activities. An adequate amount of proteins is essential to maintain nitrogen balance in the body. Protein intake is particularly important in childhood where rapid growth requires amino acids to provide the building blocks for new muscles and other structural proteins. Meat and meat products provide higher proteins than cereal products. Protein yields 4 kcal/g. Out of 24 amino acids needed by body, 9 are essential amino acids (leucine, isoleucine, lysine, methionine, phenylalanine, valine, tryptophan, threonine and histidine). Adequate protein intake is particularly important during periods of growth or recovery from disease. Biologically complete protein contains all the essential aminoacids in amounts corresponding to human needs. Animal proteins are biologically complete compared to vegetable proteins. Egg protein is best among food protein and used in nutrition studies as a reference protein. Cereal proteins are deficient in methionine and lysine, pulse proteins are deficient in methionine. Hence, these are called "limiting amino acids". Arginine, cysteine and taurine are essential for low birthweight babies. Protein requirement decreases with age from the maximum requirement of 4g/kg during neonatal and early infancy to 1g/kg in adults.

Fats are one of the major energy sources with an energy density of 9 kcals/g. Fats are essential for the formation of membranes and neural tissues. Dietary fats are mostly triglycerides containing a wide variety of fatty acids. Fats from animal products contain mainly saturated fatty acids and fat from plants and fish tend to contain mono and polyunsaturated fatty acids. High saturated fat diets have been implicated in the development of coronary artery disease in adults, whereas diets high in polyunsaturated and monounsaturated fats protect against coronary artery disease. Children below 5 years of age with increased energy requirement should consume more fat containing foods to meet their energy requirement. Children older than 5 years and adolescents should adopt a diet with similar fat that is recommended for adults. Essential fatty acids like linoleic and L-linolenic acid are very essential for growth and development in children. They are precursors of phospholipids, prostaglandins, thromboxane, leukotriens, arachidonic acid, eicosapentanoic acid and decosahexanoic acids (DHA). DHA is a major constituent of developing brain. Many infant formulae do not contain DHA. The membrane phospholipids in the brain of infants whose intake of DHA is deficient have substituted saturated fatty acids for DHA. This substitution is likely to change the functional characteristic of the neural cells. Deficiency of fats causes arrest of growth and underweight in babies, pale constipated stools and skin changes.

Micronutrients

The nutrients, which are required in small quantities for carrying out the biological functions at optimum level are called micronutrients. They are not synthesized by the body in adequate amounts and, hence, should be provided in the diet. With the progressive elimination of energy-protein deficits in the diets of children, micronutrient deficiencies could emerge as the major bottleneck to growth. Micronutrient includes vitamins and minerals.

Vitamins are one among the 6 categories of essential nutrients. There are 2 groups of vitamins: fat soluble vitamins (A,D,E,K) and water-soluble vitamins (B group and C).

Vitamins are essential for the maintenance of good health. The deficiency of vitamins sometimes lead to specific diseases like night blindness and corneal xerosis (vitamin A deficiency), rickets (vitamin D deficiency), hemorrhagic disease of the newborn (vitamin K deficiency), megaloblastic anemia (folic acid and vitamin B_{12} deficiency), scurvy (vitamin C deficiency), etc.[2-5]

Minerals are also known as trace elements because they are mineral elements present in the body in small amounts. Iron, iodine and calcium have been known for many years to be dietary essentials. Others like zinc, selenium, magnesium, copper, fluorine have been detected and established recently. Deficiencies of these can cause various deficiency states like osteoporosis/rickets (vitamin D and calcium deficiency), anemia (iron deficiency), goiter (iodine deficiency), growth failure, skin changes (zinc deficiency), Keshan's disease (selenium deficiency), etc.[2,6,7] The factors responsible for micronutrient deficiencies are: deficient intake, faulty absorption, increased loss, greater demand and poor utilization.

IMPACT OF NUTRITION ON GROWTH AND DEVELOPMENT

Growth of IUGR Babies

The causes of intrauterine growth retardation (IUGR) are multiple. Placental insufficiency can significantly affect the nutritional supply to the fetus and result in intrauterine malnutrition. Antenatal malnutrition is an important cause of IUGR in developing and underdeveloped countries. Children who suffer from IUGR can have significant problems in growth and development following birth. The growth of these children is subnormal to a great extent.[6,8,9] However, an asymmetric IUGR baby who becomes growth retarded during the third trimester of pregnancy can retain his potential for postnatal growth and an appropriate nutrition can result in normal growth. The catch-up growth can be improved with good nutrition in these children. Postnatally, these malnourished babies continue to suffer in their growth and development. IUGR and poor nutrition during the first 3 years of life are important causes of stunting in the adults. The IUGR children are at an increased risk for cognitive deficits that undermine their academic performance during school age, adolescence and adulthood. Associated nutritional deficiencies and environmental factors also contribute to their poor performances.

Growth of Premature and Small for Gestational Age (SGA) Babies

For a child to become the same size as his or her full-term peers, growth has got to be faster than usual. This is called "catch-up growth" and is also defined as growth velocity (cm/year) greater than the median for chronologic age and gender.[6,8] In full-term babies, the catch-up growth is about 200 g/week after the first 10 days of life. In preterm, the catch-up growth can be upto 10 times for the age or upto 5 times for the length. The preterm baby is expected to grow at par with the intrauterine growth or as per the corrected age. About 85% of premature infants have catch-up growth and they land on the regular growth chart by two years of age. The bottom-line is that catch-up growth can continue into adolescence and the majority of tiny premature infants should be normal-sized adults.

Small for gestational age infants whose birthweight and length are 2 SD below mean for gestational age and very premature appropriate for gestational age infant/very low birthweight /sick preterm, exhibit early postnatal growth failure and may have a longer period of spontaneous catch-up growth.

Delay in Catch-up Growth

Some of the common reasons for delay in catch-up growth include: Initial growth of the child being far below the growth chart and, hence, takes a long time to have catch-up growth. Associated conditions like bronchopulmonary dysplasia, cerebral palsy and other illnesses increase the nutritional requirements. The poor appetite of these children is another contributing factor.

Among children who are born SGA and do not achieve catch-up growth by 2 years of age, the relative risk of short stature at 18 years of age is 5.2 for those with low birthweight and 7.1 for those with low birth length. A child who has not caught up by 2 to 3 years of age or in whom there is no evidence of continuing catch-up growth should be evaluated in details. Some studies have shown that impaired pancreatic exocrine function is associated with intrauterine malnutrition and hence supplementation with **nucleotides** (trophic effects) in formula feeds improves catch-up growth in SGA infants.

BREASTFEEDING AND GROWTH

Breastfeeding on demand remains the ideal form of feeding for both term and preterm babies. Human milk provides optimum nutritional needs for growth and development. The first 4 to 6 months are a period of very rapid growth, particularly for the brain.[10] Breast milk supports neurological development by providing amino acids (cysteine and taurine) and long-chain polyunsaturated fatty acids (decosahexanoic acid—DHA 22:6N-3 and arachidonic acid—AA 20:44-6) which promote faster development, maturation and myelination of human brain.[11,12] Premature infants lack in adequate quantity of DHA and AA and, hence, are more in need of breast milk. They are benefited more in terms of faster retinal maturation and rapid cortical brain development. Breast milk contains antibodies, anti-infective agents, anti-inflammatory agents, growth factors, enzymes, hormones and immunoglobulins which have an important role to play in boosting up immune function along with other nutritional benefits to infants.

Breastfeeding is strongly advocated for physiological, psychological and normal emotional development. Breastfed babies grow slower and leaner than formula-fed infants and need supplementation with iron and other minerals in infancy.[13] The superior cognitive development, absence of any features and consequences of lower weight gain and lower morbidity among breastfed infants suggest that growth pattern of breastfed babies is the *biological norm*.[14-20] Some of the studies found that continued breastfeeding beyond 1 to 2 years has beneficial effect on growth and development.[2, 21]

NUTRITION AND ADOLESCENT GROWTH

Adolescent growth proceeds at an astonishing pace. The relative amount of physical growth that occurs during the adolescent years is second only to the relative amount seen during the first year of life. It is a time of intense physical, psychosocial and cognitive development (growth spurt). Increased nutritional needs at this juncture is due to the fact that in addition to attaining sexual maturation, adolescents gain upto 50% of their adult weight, more than 20% of their adult height and 50% of their adult's skeletal mass during this period.[22-24] Calories, proteins, vitamins and minerals (particularly iron and calcium) requirements are maximal during this period. The need of these nutrients varies between the adolescents depending on their growth rate, degree of maturation and activity level. The world's adolescent population—1,200 million persons between 10 to 19 years, or about 19% of the total population–faces a series of serious nutritional challenges not only affecting their growth and development but also their livelihood as adults.

Malnutrition among adolescent girls in Southeast Asia is exceptionally large and complex problem. Studies have shown that age at onset of peak height velocity and menarchial age is delayed by 1 to 2 years in rural adolescent girls in comparison to urban affluent adolescents.

The main nutrition problems include undernutrition (stunting and thinness), partial catch-up growth, iron, iodine, vitamin A, calcium, zinc and folate deficiencies. Continuation of growth at later age coupled with early age of marriage has increased the risk for pregnancy wastages and IUGR babies in rural adolescent girls.

Physical inactivity in affluent adolescents play a prime role in development of overweight, obesity and also in development of chronic diseases such as heart disease, cancers, diabetes, hypertension and bowel problems in later life. Current recommendations is to give optimum nutrition and aim at gaining healthy weight and to be physically active for at least 30 to 60 minutes per day (for 5 or more days a week) along with right lifestyle choices for normal adolescent growth.

ASSESSMENT OF NUTRITIONAL STATUS

The nutritional assessment is a process of assessing the nutritional status of an individual. It helps in finding whether the nutrition of an individual is normal or abnormal and also in identifying the nutritional abnormalities like undernutrition and overnutrition. It also helps in early identification of malnutrition (both undernutrition and overnutrition) and in instituting appropriate measures to correct the abnormalities.[23-25] At individual level, it helps in identifying an individual's nutritional status and his requirements. At the community level, it helps in identifying the prevalance of malnutrition, its causative factors and the measures warranted for its reduction.

Table 5.1 lists various methods of assessing nutritional status.

Table 5.1: Methods of assessing nutritional status

1. Clinical examination
2. Nutritional anthropometry
3. Biochemical evaluation
4. Assessment of dietary intake
5. Vital statistics
6. Epidemiological studies

For assessing growth, we need nutritional anthropometry, skinfold thickness and muscle mass (for tissue growth), bone age, dental age and biochemical and histological means.

Nutritional Anthropometry

It is the science that deals with the measurement of size, shape, weight and proportions of human body (*anthrop* – biological study, *anthropod – apes,* metron – to measure). For day-to-day work, it is a simple and useful tool.

Weight

This is the most frequently-used and important anthropometric measurement.

Gadgets used for weighing include beam balance (Table 5.2), a spring balance (Table 5.3), and electronic weighing machines.

Table 5.2: Beam balance

Type	*Advantages*	*Disadvantages*
Platform scale (for older children)	Accurate measurement upto 100 g	Expensive; needs carrying
Platfom scale (for infants)	Accurate measurement upto 10 g	Expensive
Bar weight scale (Tansi scale)	Do	Do

Table 5.3: Spring balance

Type	*Advantages*	*Disadvantages*
Salter weighing scale	Easy to carry and use	Variable accuracy, frequent calibration
Bathroom scale	Do	Unreliable in children
UNICEF scale model 890	Uses solar energy; can weigh infants and small children with mother	Not medically calibrated; variations over 100g; infant's weight should be at least 2 kg.

Electronic weighing scales for infants and children have the following features:

Here, we propose to deal with the clinical examination and anthropometry in some details.

Clinical Examination

The identification of symptoms and signs on clinical examination is helpful in determining nutritional status of an individual. Some of these signs are specific whereas others are non-specific with doubtful value. Clinical signs like anasarca, apathy and wasting are classical signs of PEM. Hair changes, various skin changes, pallor, angular stomatitis and Bitot's spots too are quite specific signs of malnutrition.

The drawback of clinical signs is that malnutrition cannot be quantified on their strength only. Moreover, some deficiencies may not be accompanied by clinical signs, particularly in early stage. Therefore, nutritional status cannot be assessed on the basis of mere clinical sign.

Capacity = 20 kg

Resolution = 5 gm/ ± 10 gm

Accuracy = ± 5 gm/ ± 10 gm
Baby pan = Size = 470 mm × 250 mm
Operating voltage = 220 volts +/- 10% AC.

Electronic weighing scales accuracy for infants (+/-1 to 5 gm) and for children (+/- 10 gm).

The weighing scales must be checked for accuracy using known weight from time to time.

Weight recording is essential for assessing the growth of the child and his/her nutritional status, important for planning the diet, for follow-up of child, especially while recuperating from an illness or during nutritional rehabilitation. Record weight during every examination and if child is on treatment with drugs, to calculate the right dose of the drugs to be given.

Height/Length

Length

Until 24 or 36 months of age—length in recumbency is measured using an Infantometer and the length is recorded, in centimetres upto one decimal point. Both 'crown heel and crown rump' length can be measured.

a. **Infantometer: Method:**
   1. Make the baby lie down on measuring board of infantometer. Fix the head firmly to head board with head of the baby in **Frankfurt plane** (i.e., vertex-looks upwards outercanthi of an eye in same horizontal plane as external auditory meatus) with no gap between head and the head board.
   2. With the help of a trained person, knees, should be extended fully to touch the measuring board.
   3. Foot piece made to slide along the measuring board till it touches flushes/touches against the sole of the baby.
   4. Measure length upto the nearest 0.1 cm.

b. **Mat type Infantometer:** Also called *carpet type infantometer,* marked mats are spread over examination table. Then, length is recorded.

c. **Stadiometer:** After the age of 2 years, standing height is recorded by a stadiometer (with the head held in the Frankfurt plane). Both sitting and standing heights are measured.

d. **Detectoscale:** Detecto weighing scales fixed with anthropometric rods are in common use.

e. **Scale marked on wall:** A commonly-employed method.

f. **Stanley-Mabo "Microtoise":** It is the best instrument for stature measurement. It has to be fixed on a straight wall precisely 2.00 m above a flat floor.

g. **WHO Scale-Anthropometer:** Specialized wooden device used for length measurement under 2 years of age.

h. **Prematometer:** It is for measuring supine length of premature babies.

Method of Measuring Standing Height

1. The child should remove his/her shoes/socks.
2. Stand on the flat surface of stadiometer.
3. Stand straight with arms relaxed by his/her sides.
4. Ankles and knees together.
5. Heels, buttocks and shoulder should touch the wall.
6. Head positioned in Frankfurt's line (i.e, outer canthus of eye should be in the same horizontal plane as the external auditory meatus).
7. Should be asked to relax with deep breath taking in and out.
8. With help of a measuring stick, vertex flush touched and height recorded.
9. If the scale marked on wall, use a hardbound book to flush/touch vertex instead of stick.

Method of Recording Sitting Height

It is defined as the distance from the highest point of the head in the sagittal plane to the surface on which the child is seated.

A. Make him/her sit on the flat surface of stadiometer.
B. The back should be a straight, thighs horizontal and comfortably positioned.
C. The feet should be supported on the footboard and hands should rest comfortably on the subject's lap.
D. Outer canthus of eye should be on the same horizontal plane as the external auditory meatus.
E. Bring the headboard down with measuring stick flush/touch the vertex and measure the sitting height.

Sitting height and crown rump length are useful in assessing growth of a child.

< 2 years—crown rump length is taken.

>2 years—sitting height is taken.

Instruments used is stadiometer or Harpenden's anthropometers.

Uses of Measuring Height

- Height of a child is basically an indicator of his past nutritional status.
- It is relatively insensitive to rapid changes in nutritional status.
- It is a good indicator of the chronicity of any debilitating illness.
- Equipments to measure are expensive and skill is required for measurement.
- Slowing of rate of growth cannot be demonstrated in a period much less than 6 months.
- In areas, where more children with malnutrition are present, most frequent measurement of accurate length/height is difficult.

Indices Associated with Height

Height for age

Severe stunting < 85% of reference.

Stunting 85-90% of reference.

There are two ways of classifying nutritional status according to weight for height and height for age (Tables 5.4 and 5.5):

Table 5.4: Classification of nutritional status in terms of percentage parameter

Height for age	*Weight for height*	*Degree of wasting*
(Degree of stunting)	**> 80 percent**	**< 80 percent**
>90 percent	Well nourished	Wasted only
< 90 percent	Stunted only	Wasted and stunted

The cut offs using the new WHO recommendation would be Z scores < - 2 for both weight for height and height for age.

Table 5.5: Classification of nutritional status in terms of Z-score

Weight for height	*Height for age*	*Inference*
> 2 SD	> 2 SD	Normal
< 2 SD	> 2 SD	Wasted
> 2 SD	< 2 SD	Stunted
< 2 SD	< 2 SD	Wasted and stunted

Weight for Height: $\frac{\text{Wt. of child}}{\text{Wt. for ht. of the child}} \times 100$

> 90%—Normal

< 90%—PEM

> 120-130—Obesity.

Rao's Index/Body Mass Index

Weight/Height^2:

> 0.0015—Normal

0.0013 to 0.0015—Moderate PEM

< 0.0013 – Severe PEM.

Dugdale's Index:

Wt/Ht$^{1.6}$: > 0.79 = Normal nutrition.

< 0.79 = Malnutrition.

Head Circumference (HC)

The size of the head is a good indicator of the past and current malnutrition during fetal life and early childhood. Any abnormality in the head circumference should alert the pediatrician, as it has important diagnostic significance in the first few years of life.

Method: With the help of a non-stretchable plastic/steel tape: measure the occipito frontal head circumference from external occipital protuberance to the glabella.

Other Indices using Head Circumference are:

Kanawati Index: Constant for children between 4 months and 4 years irrespective of sex.

Midarm circumference/head circumference: N > 0.32

Mild PEM = 0.28–0.32

Mod PEM = 0.25 – 0.28

Severe PEM = < 0.25

Advantage: Corresponds to Gomez classification

Mild 0.28–0.32 = Grade I PEM

Mod. 0.25–0.28 = Grade II PEM

Severe < 0.25 = Grade III PEM.

Chest Circumference (CC)

Method: With the help of non-stretchable tape, chest circumference is measured at the level of nipples, midway between inspiration and expiration. Upto the age of 5 years, it is measured in recumbancy position and then in standing position.

Inference: In infant, CC is less than HC by about 2.5 cm. In undernutrition: CC < HC (even beyond 1½ years). In well-nourished children**:** CC > HC (even before 1 year).

Table 5.6: Head and chest circumferences relationship at different ages

Age	*Chest circumference*
At Birth	33 cm; HC > CC
9 months to 1 year	HC = CC
After 1 year	CC > HC

Midarm Circumference (MAC)

As the name indicates, it is the measurement of circumference of the arm at the midpoint between the acromion and olecranon with the arm hanging by the side of the body and recorded to the nearest 0.1 cm. It can be confidently measured with a special slotted "insertion" tape which can be purchased from UNICEF.

Importance: It is useful for detecting malnutrition in young children in the community (especially between 1-4 years). It is especially a useful screening procedure in rural areas to identify "at risk" children.

MAC is constant between 1-5 years of age (partially age dependent).

Values: 13.5 – 17 cm= Normal.

12.5–13.5 cm= mild malnutrition (at risk).

< 12.5 cm= moderate to severe malnutrition.

Advantages: Simple, cheap and easy method for any one to measure—irrespective of literacy status.

Disadvantage: Difficult/erroneous in a kwashiorkor child (because of edema).

Indices used with MAC are:

- Shakir tape
- Quac stick
- Kanawati index
- Bangle test.

Arm Span

It is the distance between the tips of the middle fingers with both arms held wide open, i.e., spread apart.

In young children: It is 1-2 cms less than the length/height.

After 10 years: It is 1-2 cm more than the height.

Arm span is increased in Marfan's syndrome and homocystinuria.

Skinfold Thickness

It is the measurement of subcutaneous fat taken by measuring a fold of skin running parallel to the length of the arm over the triceps muscle midway between the acromion and the olecranon.

It is used for estimating percentage of body fat.

Instruments used: Harpenden's callipers, Ross adipometer (plastic callipers).

Technique

1. Flex child's right arm to 90 degree at elbow, mark midpoint on posterior aspect of the arm.
2. Allow arm to hang freely; grasp 1 cm above midpoint a fold of skin between thumb and forefinger and pull this fold away from underlying muscle.
3. Place caliper jaw over skinfold at midpoint mark and apply pressure with thumb.
4. Read to the nearest 1.0 mm, after applying pressure for 2-3 seconds.
5. Repeat measurements until repeat values agree within 1 mm.

Inference: Skinfold thickness is an index of total body fat.

Arm circumference is an indirect measure of total muscle mass.

Sites to measure skinfold thickness: Triceps, subscapular, suprailiac, and abdomen or upper thigh with special callipers.

Inference: <60% = Severe malnutrition

60-80% = Moderate malnutrition

80-90% = Mild malnutrition

90-100% = Normal malnutrition.

These are no standard reference data. Hence, skinfold is used for routine screening procedure in well childcare; but not in follow-up of actual obesity/malnourished children.

Table 5.7 gives skinfold measurement in various age groups.

Table 5.7: Skinfold thickness (at triceps) in various age groups

	Measurement (mm ± SD)	
Age	*Male*	*Female*
5 years	7.56 ± 2.94	9.56 ± 1.57
10 years	9.50 ± 3.69	11.50 ± 3.58
15 years	9.03 ± 3.07	14.08 ± 4.47
18 years	9.32 ± 4.76	13.46 ± 4.36

Newer Anthropometry Measurements

- Thigh circumference.
- Calf circumference.
- Foot length.

Thigh and Calf Circumference

These, at the maximum point, vary depending upon the birthweight of the infant. It is useful to find out indirectly whether the newborn baby is weighing > 2.5 kg or < 2.5 kg.

Calf circumference	<10 cm	<2.5 kg
MAC	<9.3 cm	<2.5 kg
Thigh circumference	<14.9 cm	<2.5 kg

Foot Length

It is measured from tip of the heel to the tip of the great toe/2nd toe. Values vary with weight of newborn and gestation.

1500 g: <6.5 cm foot length.

Newborn (>2.5 kg): >7.3 cm foot length.

Age-independent Anthropometric Indicators

1. **Bangle Method**
   It consults in slipping a bangle with an inner diameter of 4 cm up the forearm. If it crosses the elbow the child is malnourished. Basically, this is a midarm circumference. Simple to perform.
   Disadvantage: It is quite unreliable and is less sensitive as elbow circumference represents the thickness of the bone.
2. **Shakir's Tape**
   This is a plastic tape with colored zones: Green, yellow and red representing > 13.5 cm, 12.5-13.5 cm and <12.5 cm respectively to measure MAC (midarm circumference).
3. **Quac Stick**
   It is the short name for Quacker arm circumference stick. It is a rod with 2 sets of markings, one indicating the height and the other, the MAC (mid-arm circumference) for the corresponding height. The arm circumference is measured and the stick is placed behind the standing child. If the height is more than the expected height for the measured arm circumference, the child is considered malnourished.
4. **Modified Quac Stick**
   This utilizes rod that is colored green, yellow and red, representing normal nutritional status, borderline and severe PEM respectively.

5. **MAC to HC (MH) ratio (Kanawati Index)**
   0.28 to 0.314 = mild PEM
   0.25 to 0.279 = moderate PEM
   <0.249 = severe PEM
6. **HC to CC Ratio**
   > 1 = Normal
   < 1 = PEM (in children above 9 months of age).
7. **MAC to Height Ratio**
   < 0.29 = Severe PEM
   0.32-0.33 = Normal
8. **Rao and Singh's Weight/Height^2 Ratio**
   Ratio > 0.0015 = Normal
   0.0013-0.0015 = Moderate PEM
   < 0.0013 = Severe PEM
9. **Ponderal Index**
   Weight (g)/ Height (cm)^3 Ratio
   < 2.0 = Asymmetrical IUGR
   2.0-2.5 = Borderline PEM
   > 2.0 = Symmetrical IUGR
   < 2.0 = Severe PEM >2.5 = Term AGA.
10. **Body Mass Index (BMI)**

$$\text{BMI} = \frac{\text{Weight (kg)}}{\text{Height 2 (Metres)}} = -\text{Kg/met}^2$$

(Same as Quetlet's Index but values are in SI Units)

BMI	18.5–220	=	Normal
	13.0–15.0	=	Moderate malnutrition
	<13.0	=	Severe malnutrition
	> 22.0	=	Overweight
	> 25.0	=	Obesity

11. **Dughdale's Weight/Height^3 Ratio**
    > 0.79 = Normal nutrition
    < 0.79 = Malnutrition
12. **Quetlet's Index**
    Weight (kg) × 100/Height (cm)^2
    Values 0.14-0.16 = Normal
    < 0.14 = Gross malnutrition
13. **Mid-arm Muscle Circumference**
    MAMC = MAC – π × triceps skinfold thickness.
14. **The Nabarrow's Thinness Chart**
    It is a graphic chart that represents the expected weight for height has been prepared by Save the Children's Fund. It shows the grades of malnutrition in different color zones (upper and lower red, yellow, green). It is easy for health worker to assess the nutritional status.
    Method: Child is made to stand against the column on the chart for the recorded weight of the child.
    If child is in:
    Lower red zone: Thin (Wasted) Help him quickly.
    Yellow zone: Thin Watch him regularly.
    Green: Well nourished.

Wasting, Stunting Classification (Table 5.8)

$$\frac{\text{Height \%}}{\text{Weight \%}} = \frac{\text{Weight of child}}{\text{Weight of normal child at same height}} \times 100$$

$$\frac{\text{Height \%}}{\text{Age \%}} = \frac{\text{Height of the child}}{\text{Height of a normal child at same age}} \times 100$$

Table 5.8: Stunting and wasting of height at different nutritional status

Nutritional status	*Stunting (% of Height/Age)*	*Wasting (% of Weight/Height)*
Normal	>95	>90
Mildly impaired	87.5-95	80-90
Moderately impaired	80-87.5	70-80
Severely impaired	<80	<70

GROWTH MONITORING

Growth monitoring aims at detecting abnormal growth. This is followed by nutritional or social intervention or further investigations for serious diseases. Although it has been universally practised, its benefits and implications have not been well-studied. Recently, there has been increased interest in this aspect and planned studies have been done to identify the usefulness of routine growth monitoring.

What is Growth Monitoring?

Growth monitoring consists of routine measurements to detect abnormal growth, combined with necessary action when an abnormal growth is detected. It aims to improve nutrition, reduce the risk of death or inadequate nutrition, help educate parents and lead to early referral for conditions manifested as growth disorders.

Benefits of Growth Monitoring

1. It helps in knowing growth status of children and growth velocity.
2. It indicates whether growth is normal or abnormal.
3. Abnormal growth indicates need for evaluating the child for possible causes.
4. It aims at detecting and intervening in malnutrition, thereby reducing the risk of death.
5. It can be part of health promotion, to discuss feeding, hygiene, and other aspects of the child's health and behavior.
6. It can be used to reassure parents about their child's growth, and convince them about the value of good nutrition.

GROWTH CHART

The growth/road to health chart is a visible display of the child's physical growth and development. It is designed primarily for the longitudinal follow-up (growth monitoring of a child so that changes overtime can be interpreted). It was first designed by David Morley and later modified by World Health Organization (WHO).

A growth chart is basically a graph on which a child's weight is shown in different ages. There are many types of growth charts, but most of them have the same basic features. The horizontal lines in this chart represent weight (kg) and the vertical lines represent age in months. Across the graph are printed growth reference lines. These lines give the general direction of growth in healthy children. They are not the target for the growth of all children. If child's weight is much below these growth reference lines, there is some reason for concern, but it is the direction or angle of a child's own growth line that is much more significant than weight recorded below the lower reference line. Different charts use different reference curves.

Uses of Growth Chart

1. For growth monitoring and promotion.
2. To make growth a tangible, visible attribute.
3. Diagnostic tool: For identification of high-risk children, early identification of malnutrition before clinical features become apparent.
4. Tool for action: It helps the health workers to make necessary early interventions and early referrals.
5. Educational tool: Because of its visual character, the mother can be educated in the care of her own child and encouraged her for active participation in growth monitoring of her child.
6. Planning and policy-making: By grading malnutrition, it provides an objective basis for planning and policy-making in relation to child health care at the local and central levels.
7. Evaluation: It provides a good method to evaluate the effectiveness of the corrective measures and the impact of programs of special intervention for improving child's growth and development.
8. Tool for teaching: The importance of adequate feeding by illustrating the adverse effects during various negative events, e.g., infection, maternal deprivation, seasonal scarcity, etc.

   Growth chart has been described as a "passport" to child health care.

Types of Growth Chart

UNICEF Growth Chart (Rainbow Chart)

With the cooperation of the government, NGOs and bilateral and multilateral agencies, UNICEF has commissioned growth monitoring test and cards. These cards were designed after a discussion between health workers and mothers and these help to link the direction of growth and health promotion behaviors. This card is to be filled by the worker in the mother's presence and is given to mothers for retention following interpretation and discussion about the child's health. The vertical dimensions increasing with 100 grams graduations are depicted by small circles or bubbles, those marking 1000 gram divisions have slightly larger bubbles. Hence, a series of rainbow-colored growth channels. Similar percentile lines on standard pediatric growth charts justify the name "rainbow chart". Here the range is limited to 36 months in order to attract attention to growth at the earliest vulnerable age.

NCHS Growth Chart

National Centre for Health Statistics Growth charts have 7 percentile curves: 5th, 10th, 25th, 50th, 75th, 90th and 95th percentile curves.

Limitations of NCHS Charts

a. NCHS data are representative of a population of well-nourished and healthy children (so do not match nutritional distribution of birthweight).
b. Less appropriate for adolescence.
c. NCHS curves may indicate poor or excessive growth when a child is growing normally, but happens to be a late or early maturer.

Advantages of NCHS Charts

a. Facilitate assessment of growth over time.
b. Specialized chart available for various conditions including Down's syndrome, Turner's syndrome and Klinefelter's syndrome.

Centre for Disease Control (CDC) Growth Charts

CDC growth charts are improvements over the 1977 NCHS charts. The chart represents a cross-section of children who live in the United States. Unlike the 1977 NCHS charts, the CDC 2000 growth charts are based on the current mix of breastfed and formula fed infants in United States.[26] As it is not well-known that breastfed and formula fed infants grow differently, CDC-2000 growth charts can be used to assess the growth of breastfed and formula fed infants differently. However, the data on the growth of breastfed infants is still not completely satisfactory as the adequate data do not exist for exclusively or predominantly breastfed infants. The prepubescent weight-for-stature charts are stopped at the age of 10 for girls and 11 for boys. In 2000 CDC revision, the BMI chart is available for children and adolescents 2-20 years of age. BMI is recommended for screening overweight children and adolescents.

Growth Chart Recommended by the Government of India

The growth chart recommended by the Government of India has 4 reference curves:

1. The topmost curve corresponds to 80% of the median weight (50th percentile of WHO reference standard), which represents the level of optimum growth.
2. The second line represents 70% of the median weight (3rd percentile which is approximately equivalent to 2 standard deviations below the median which is the conventional lower limits of normal range).
3. Third and fourth lines represent 60 and 50% of median weight.

Four degrees of malnutrition can be known through this chart:

First degree: If the child's weight is between 80 and 70% lines (mild malnutrition).

Second degree: If the child's weight is between 70 and 60% lines (moderate malnutrition).

Third degree: If weight is below 60% line (severe malnutrition).

Fourth degree: Below 50% (profound malnutrition).

Growth Chart Used in Integrated Child Development Service (ICDS) Scheme

It contains 3 reference lines in addition to the standard (median) representing 80, 60 and 50%.

Indian Academy of Pediatrics (IAP) Growth Card

Based on NCHS standards, it has additional parameters such as immunization, and developmental assessment using Trivandrum Developmental Scale.

New (2006) WHO Growth Charts

Classically, WHO growth charts have 2 reference curves. The upper reference curve represents the median (50th percentile) for boys (slightly higher than that for girls) and lower reference curve, the third percentile for girls (slightly lower than that for boys). Thus, the chart can be used for both sexes.

The space between the 2 growth curves is called the "road to health". This will include the zone of normality for most populations. Space is also provided on growth chart for recording and presenting information on the following: identification and registration, birth date and weight, chronological age, history of sibling health, immunization, introduction of supplementary foods, episodes of sickness, child spacing, and regions for special care. It is the direction of growth that is more important than the position of the dots on the line. Flattening or falling of the weight curve signals growth failure which is the earliest sign of PEM. The objective in childcare is to keep the child's growth above 3rd percentile.

WHO had previously adopted Centers for Disease Control and Prevention (CDC) and modified 1977 National Center for Health Statistics (NCHS) growth charts for international reference.

Later, however, realizing the drawbacks of CDC/NCHS growth charts and need for a better growth charts for international reference, WHO in 2006 released growth chart for preschool children. Unlike 1977 NCHS or 2000 CDC curves, the new WHO growth charts are based on breastfed infants and contain data from study centers in 6 representative countries, including India. Today, these are the most acceptable growth curves for international use and comparison.

To have a normal or optimum growth and development of children, strategies and program need to be implemented right from maternal nutrition to nutrition in infancy, childhood and adolescence, bearing in mind age-appropriate needs. Unless nutritional requirement is taken care of at all these levels, we cannot expect normal or optimum growth and development of our infants, children and adolescents.

Figures 5.1 to 5.3 show the three major types of growth charts.

REFERENCES

1. Vashisht RN, Krishnan K, Devlal S. Physical growth and nutritional status of Garhwali girls. *Indian J Pediatr* 2005;72: 573-578.
2. Grummer-Strawn LM. Does prolonged breastfeeding impair child growth? A critical review. *Pediatrics* 1993;91:766- 771.
3. Elizabath K.E. Vitamins minerals and micronutrients. In: Elizabath KE (ed) *Nutrition and Child Development,* 2nd edn. Hyderabad: Paras 2004;86-114.
4. Von Schenck V, Bender-Gotze C and Koletzko B. Persistence of neurological damage induced by dietary vitamin B_{12} deficiency in infancy. *Arch Dis Child* 1997; 77: 137-139.
5. Graham SM, Arvela OM, Wise GA. Long-term neurological consequences of nutritional vitamin B_{12} deficiency in infants. *J Pediatr* 1992; 121: 710-714.
6. Osendarp SJM, Van Raaij JMA, Darmastadt GL, *et al.* Zinc supplementation during pregnancy and effect on growth and morbidity in low birthweight infants: A randomized placebo controlled trial. *Lancet* 2001; 357:1080-1085.
7. Imeta M, West CE, Haider J, *et al.* Zinc Supplementation and stunted infants in Ethiopia: A randomized controlled trial. *Lancet* 2000;355:2021-2026.
8. Black MM, Sazawal S, Black RE, Khosla S, Kumar J and Menon V. Cognitive and motor development among small for gestational age infants: Impact of Zinc supplementation, birthweight and care giving practice. *Pediatrics* 2004;113:1297-1305.
9. Bhatia BD, Bhargava V, Chatterjee M, Kota VLN, Singh LI and Jain NP. Studies on fetal growth patterns: Intrauterine growth percentiled for single ton live-born babies. *Indian Pediatr* 1981;18:647-653.
10. Reynolds A. Breastfeeding and brain development. *Pediatr Clin North Am* 1999; 26:159-172.
11. Uauy RD, Birch DG, Birch EF, *et al.* Effects of dietary omega-3 fatty acids on retinal function of very low birthweight neonates. *Pediatr Res* 1990;28:485-492.

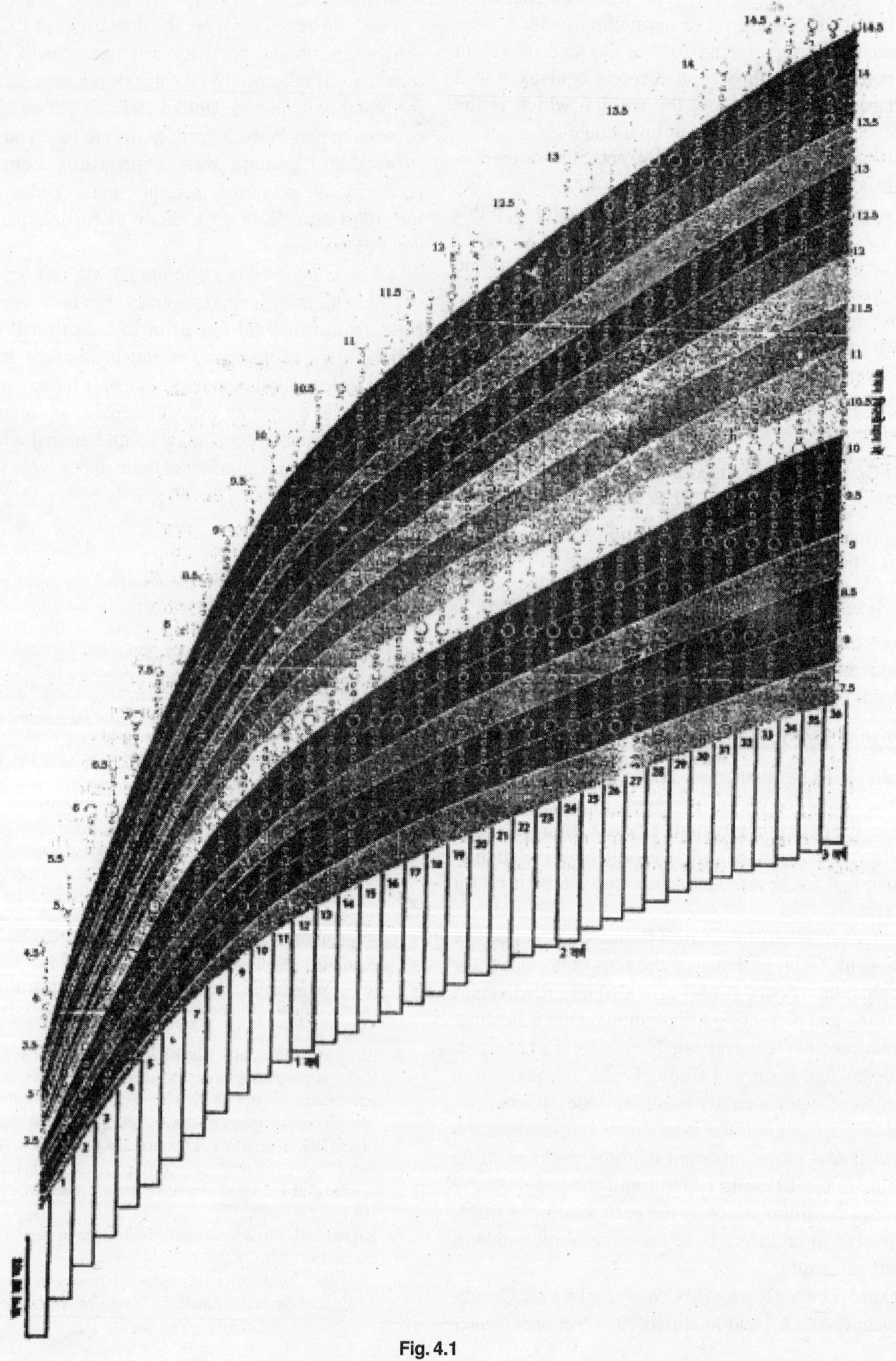

Fig. 4.1

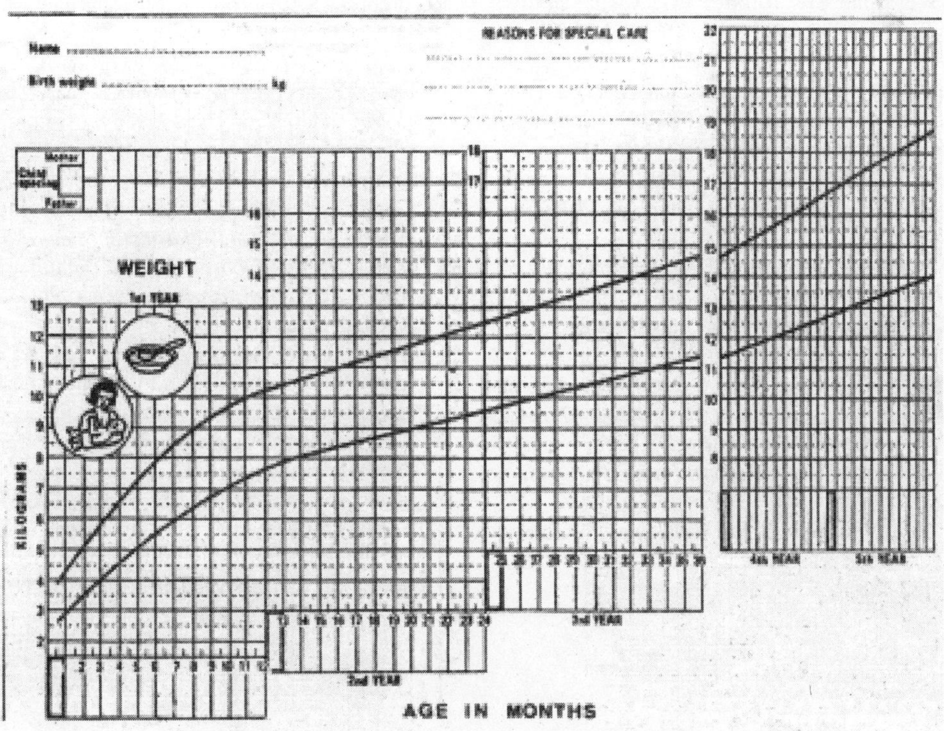

Fig. 4.2: The WHO prototype growth chart

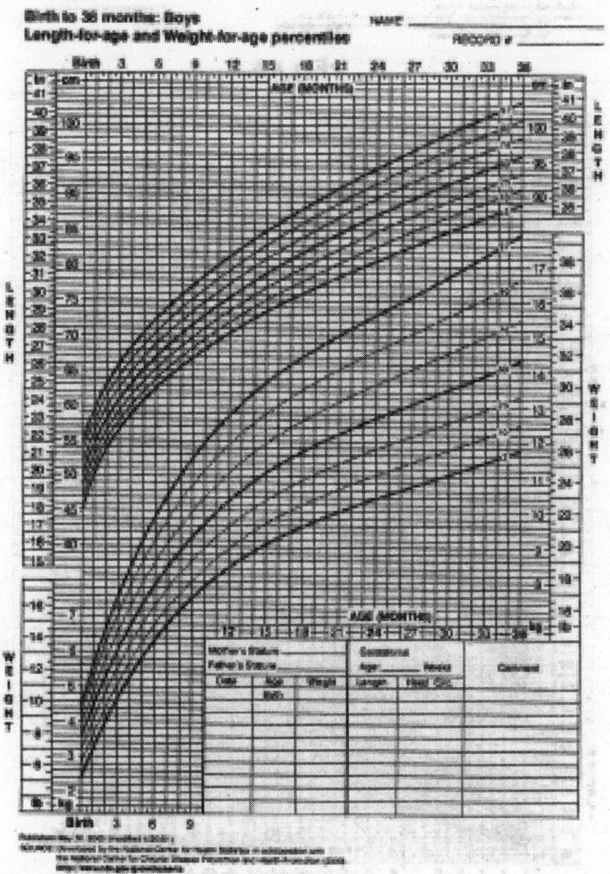

Fig. 4.3

12. Carlson SE, Werkman SH, Rhodes PG. Visual acuity development in healthy preterm infants: Effects of marine oil supplementation. *Am J Clin Nutr* 1993;58:35-42.
13. Dewey KG, Heinig MJ, Nommsen LA and Lonnerdal B. Breast-fed infants are leaner than formula-fed infants at 1 year of age: The DARLING study. *J Clin Nutr* 1993; 57: 140-145.
14. Buttle NF, Garza C, Smith O and Nichols BL. Human milk intake and growth in exclusively breast-fed infants. *J Pediatr* 1984;104:187-195.
15. Dewey KG, Heinig MJ, Nommsen LA, Peerson JM and Lonnerdal B. Growth of breastfed and formula fed infants from 0-18 months: The DARLING study *Pediatrics* 1992; 89: 1035-1041.
16. Dewey KG. Nutrition, growth and complementary feeding of the breastfed infant. *Pediatr Clin North Am* 2001; 48:87-104.
17. Anderson JW, Johnstone BM and Remkey DT. Breastfeeding and cognitive development: A meta-analysis. *Am J Clin Nutr* 1999; 70:525-535.
18. Angelson NK, Vik T, Jacobsen G and Bakketeig LS. Breast-feeding and congnitive development at 1 and 5 years. *Arch Dis Child* 2001; 85:183-188.
19. Jacobson SW, Jacobson JL. Breastfeeding and intelligence. *Lancet* 1992;339:926-931.
20. Jacobson SW, Chiodo LM, Jacobson JL. Breastfeeding effects on intelligence quotient in 4 and 11 years old children. *Pediatrics* 1999; 103:e71-75.
21. Poivanetti Y. Breastfeeding beyond 12 months: A historical perspective. *Pediatr Clin North Am* 1999;26:199-206.
22. Aneja S. Nutritional concerns in adolescence. In: Gupte S (ed) *Recent Advances in Pediatrics (Special Vol 6: Gastroenterology, Hepatology and Nutrition)*. New Delhi: Jaypee 2000; 519- 530.
23. Brook CGD. *Growth Assessment in Childhood and Adolescence*. Oxford: Blackwell 1982.
24. Agarwal K.N, Saxena A, Bansal AK, Agarwal DK, Physical growth assessment in Adolescence, *Indian Pediatr* 2001; 38:1217-1235.
25. Ghosh S. *Nutrition and Child Care: A Practical Guide*, 2nd edn. New Delhi: Jaypee 2004.
26. Ogden CL, Kuczmarski RJ, Flegal KM, Mei Z, Guo S, *et al.* Centers for Disease Control and Prevention 2000 growth charts for the United States. Improvements to the 1977 national center for health statistics version. *Pediatrics* 2002; 109:45-60.

Suraj Gupte

6 New (2006-07) WHO Child Growth Standards and Charts

INTRODUCTION

Growth is an essential expression of health. It is also a way to measure efforts designed to reduce child mortality and disease.[1,2]

Basic growth assessment involves measuring a child's weight and length or height and comparing these measurements to growth standards.

The purpose is to determine whether a child is growing normally or has a growth problem or trend towards a growth problem that should be addressed.

Understandably, growth assessments that are not supported by appropriate response programs are not effective in improving child health.

The norms of growth are determined from cross-sectional or longitudinal studies in large populations. These may be:

1. *International growth standards*: Useful for making intercountry comparisons and for research purposes.
2. *Country-specific growth standards*: Useful for assessment of growth/nutritional status of individual children.[3,4]

Growth norms may be represented in the form of graphics (growth chart) or tables. A growth chart consists of a series of percentile curves which depict the distribution of certain measurements of the body.

Today, it stands well-accepted that all children have same genetic potential/especially in early years (say 5 years), and their growth is more influenced by nutrition, illness and environment rather than by heredity. Furthermore, growth of children of affluent groups in developing countries compares favorably with that of children in the developed countries. This fact had led World Health Organization (WHO) to recommend use of data collected from North American children as the single international reference standard to replace the earlier Harvard data. These data were popularly referred to as National Center of Health Statistics (NCHS) data. Following further revision in 2000, the standards circulated by the Centers for Disease Control and Prevention (CDC) – precisely, the CDC Growth Charts and CDC Growth Tables were in use.[1,5]

Not satisfied with these standards, in 2006 and 2007, WHO released new growth standards in two installments. These new standards, based on anthropometric studies on breastfed children from 6 representative countries are expected to replace all previous standards globally.[6-8]

HISTORICAL BACKGROUND

Harvard Standard

For quite a few decades, Harvard data were accorded the status of international reference standard and were widely employed despite their limitations.

NCHS Standard

The National Center for Health Statistics (NCHS), USA, is credited for producing the well-known 1977 growth charts.[5] With the adoption of these charts by the WHO and its recommendation to regard it as a single international standard, these earned international status and were widely used. Following this, the Harvard standards became obsolete. This recommendation was based on two counts:

- The observation that all children have the same genetic potential especially in early childhood, and their growth is more influenced by nutrition, illness and environment rather than by heredity.
- It has been convincingly demonstrated that the growth of well-nourished children in the developing countries compares favorably with that of the developed world's children.

Across the world, therefore, the old Harvard standards stood replaced by the NCHS standards.

NCHS-CDC Standard

Later, NCHS and Center for Disease Control (CDC) revised the 1977 norms to make them more valuable for the professionals. Termed simply 2000 CDS growth charts, these were accepted as the most appropriate international growth reference in the given circumstances.

The 2000 CDC growth charts consisted of 16 charts, eight for either sex plus two new BMI for age charts.[5]

Criticism of NCHS-CDC Standards

In view of the importance of normal growth as a summary indicator for health, WHO established a working group to examine issues related to anthropometry. The working group concluded that the NCHS references and its variations being used in countries around the globe were fraught with numerous technical inadequacies. These technical fallacies were pinned down to the following:

- The data for development of these standards was collected from predominantly formula-fed infants who resided in a restricted geographic area in USA and were of relatively high socio-economic background. This approach was widely inconsistent with the multiple health benefits associated with breastfeeding.
- The measurements from the sample were taken only once in three months and the analytical methods available at the time were inadequate for the task and were likely to depict inappropriately the pattern of growth and variability of normal growth. The measurements at three monthly intervals are inadequate to capture the dynamic pattern of growth in the first six months of life.

The argument was that these shortcomings caused mischaracterization of the shape of the curve particularly during the first six months.

Convinced by the inadequacy of the NCHC-CDC growth standards, WHO set out on a huge international project to collect anthropometric data on breastfed children from six representative countries, including India.

2006-07 WHO GROWTH STANDARDS[6-8]

WHO Reference 2006 Growth Charts

As pointed out earlier, in response to the findings and recommendations WHO succeeded in developing new growth references. The new WHO Growth standards were officially released on 27th April, 2006. These charts depicted the growth of children from birth to 5 years who had been raised in six different countries (Brazil, Ghana, India, Norway, Oman and USA) according to recommended nutritional and health practices.

The optimal growth displayed in these WHO growth charts represents the prescribed gold standard for children's growth or the way all healthy children should grow.

Breastfed infants were used as the normative model for growth and development so that the growth patterns aligns with current recommended feeding practices.

The WHO charts address the growth of a multi-ethnic international population.

These standards also provide a wider range of available charts, allowing more detailed assessment of growth parameters when necessary. Equally importantly, they emphasize the use of BMI-for-age as the index of weight relative to height starting at 2 years of age.

WHO Reference 2007 Growth Charts

A year later i.e. in 2007, the WHO also released charts for monitoring the growth of older children and adolescents. These charts had been updated and improved to pointedly address the growing epidemic of childhood obesity in 5-19 years age group.

Thus, the new WHO Growth Standards differed from earlier growth charts in a number of innovative ways (Box 6.1)

Box 6.1: Major innovative improvements in the new WHO growth standards

1. The curves are drawn from a sample of children residing in six different countries around the globe, allowing the development of a truly international standard which is in contrast to the previously used international references based on children residing in one particular country.
2. A key characteristic of the new standard is that it establishes breastfeeding as the biological norm and the breastfed infant as the standard for measuring healthy growth. Previous reference charts were based on the growth of random mixture of breast fed and artificially fed children.
3. For the first time, they describe "how children should grow", which is a prescriptive approach, not just descriptive. These charts show that all children across all regions can attain a similar standard of height and weight and development with correct feeding practices, good health care and a healthy environment. It is a more pro-active way of measuring and evaluating child growth, setting out normative conditions and evaluating children and populations against standards.
4. The development for the first time of standardized BMI charts for infants to five years of age is a major innovation in assessing healthy weights of children.
5. Additionally the development of "Windows of Achievements" for six key motor development milestones will provide a unique link between physical growth and mental development.
6. There are separate charts available for boys and girls.

CONTROVERSY ABOUT NATIONAL STANDARD VS INTERNATIONAL STANDARD

The question whether the developing countries should use international growth standards or develop their own standards for comparison has been considerably debated. According to the protagonists of a single international standard, it argued that a single reference standard gives uniform and comparable data. By deliberately adopting the lower standard that fails to reflect the full genetic potential for growth, the very purpose of growth monitoring is defeated.

Then, there are protagonists favoring every country/ region having its local data for future comparisons. In India, the available data from Indian Council of Medical Research (ICMR) have been criticized for two major snags. Firstly, growth velocity has not been taken into consideration since these are based on cross-sectional rather than longitudinal studies. Secondly, growth potential is underestimated since half of the population studied was of low socioeconomic status. At one stage, Indian Academy too favored having our own growth standards. Nevertheless, its call was to use international standard until India's own dependable standard become available.

It has been argued that since the average stature of Asian children fits about the 25th centile of the NCHS standards, there is need for availability of local standards that are based on well-nourished children and that are periodically upgraded.[6,7]

From time to time, attempts were made to generate reference standard based on information on Indian children, including the ICMR data. These were, however, not found quite acceptable.

The Indian Academy of Pediatrics, therefore, recommended that, until acceptable Indian data become available, we should continue referring to the international standard for comparison. To begin with Harvard data, then NCHS data and later CDC data have been in use in India as well. Now that the new WHO growth standards are available since 2006-07, we in India too are expected to use these standards.

SPECIAL USEFULNESS OF WHO 2006 GROWTH STANDARDS

Research Opportunity

The availability of the WHO standards has created an opportunity and a need for new methodological and operational research in the domain of growth and nutrition. In the transitional period researchers may take the opportunity to use and compare various indices and indicators, even if such comparisons are not the primary aim of the research. Infant body composition studies using dual energy X-ray absorptiometry (DEXA) scanning may provide the opportunity of including MUAC, TST and SSST measurements so as to enable the validation of indices based on these measurements.[1] In due course, the exact need and methods for the re-analysis of older scientific data will become progressively clearer. There may be room for meta-analyses of older articles addressing major issues in nutritional anthropometry.[9]

Conduct of Research Studies

The impact of the WHO growth standards on research is likely to extend well beyond issues of use and usefulness of anthropometry as a public health or clinical tool.[1, 2] The importance of MGRS, on which the new standards are based, may also reside in the area of growth research methodology.

Training and Standardization

An extensive review of literature shows that growth studies in the past have employed particularly refined and well-described anthropometric methods and have introduced a number of useful tools that are of potential interest to researchers.[1,9] For example, portable light-weight stadiometers have been developed specifically for this study and have already found other users worldwide. An anthropometry training video has been developed showing the detailed measurement techniques. High levels of standardization were achieved in MGRS, and the accuracy of the final measurement values used for the construction of the growth charts was enhanced by averaging independent duplicate measurement values taken by two different observers.

When scoring an individual measurement using the international standards, the validity of the resulting Z-score will be optimal only if the techniques used to take the measurements were the same as those used to construct the standards themselves.

That is why it is highly recommended that researchers to:

- Use instruments of similar quality;
- Apply the same measurement standardization protocols; and
- Take the average of independent replicate measurements as the final values for analysis.

These recommendations mainly concern the desired level of standardization in clinical–epidemiological growth studies. A similar level of standardization is not very likely to be attainable in primary health care settings.

Data Management and Analysis

The WHO growth standards are useful for designing range and consistency checks for data entry in virtually all research using anthropometry in under-5s.[1] This is a potential contribution to data quality in particular and the quality of growth and nutrition research in general.

What is noteworthy, the WHO has developed macros that enable Z-scores in research datasets to be calculated easily. These tools are available for a variety of statistical packages and are intended to replace the software that was used in conjunction with the old NCHS references.

A NOTE OF CRITICAL APPRAISAL

The 2006-07 WHO growth standards are in for a word of caution. It has been argued that these may translate into the fact that more children can be treated at an earlier stage of the disease, leading to a gain in public health impact achieved.[1,9]

Undoubtedly, this is very true. However, for this to happen:

- Policy-makers must be fully aware of the varied effects, and possible side-effects of the change.
- They must ensure adequate resources to increase supply of treatment for severe acute malnutrition (SAM) strategies and practicalities for feeding programs.
- The roll-out of the WHO growth standards must be harmonized.
- Immediate efforts should prioritize roll-out of effective evidence-based community programs.

This needs to be clearly understood that horizontal health system approaches (undoubtedly, with extensive local integration with existing services), take extra time initially. Nevertheless, these often pay off in the long run. Once treatment supply increases, coping with extra demand becomes somewhat easy.[10]

In conclusion, it is suremised that the introduction of the WHO growth standards shall have wide implications for growth and nutrition research. As the researchers make the transition to using the new standards, re-evaluate results of past approaches, and explore the uses and functional validity for etiology, diagnosis, and prognosis of the standards, including for indices that were not available earlier, the full scope of this effect will become apparent.

Acknowledgements: Thanks are due to the WHO for permission to incorporate its two sets of growth charts released in 2006 and 2007, respectively. Thanks are also due to the Director, Principal and Medical Superintendent, Narayana Medical College and Hospitals for providing motivation and encouragement to complete this chapter for the book, ***Pediatric Nutrition***.

REFERENCES

1. Becker E. *Growth charts:From A-Z.* London: Smith and Smith 2008.
2. Gupte S, Gomez EM. Growth and development. In: Gupte S (ed) *The Short Textbook of Pediatrics,* 11th edn. New Delhi: Jaypee 2004:25-39.
3. Banerjee B. Growth and development from birth to puberty. In: Gupte S, Gupte SB (eds): *Recent Advances in Pediatrics (Special Vol 20: Nutrition, Growth and Development).* New Delhi: Jaypee 2009: 207-262.
4. Banerjee B. Growth and development during adolescence. In: Gupte S, Gupte SB (eds): *Recent Advances in Pediatrics (Special Vol. 17: Adolescence).* New Delhi: Jaypee 2006:18-37.
5. Hamill PVV, Drizd TA, Johnson CL. NCHS growth curves for children birth–18 years. Vital and Health Statistics Series 11, No 165. Hyattsville: National Center for Health Statistics, US Department of Health and Human Services 1977.
6. World Health Organization. *WHO Child Growth Standards: Methods and Development. Length/height-for-age, Weight-for-age, Weight-for-length, Weight-for-height and Body Mass Index-for-age.* Geneva: WHO 2006:18-37.
7. World Health Organization. *WHO Child Growth Standards: Methods and Development. Head Circumference-for-age, Arm circumference-for-age,Triceps Skinfold-for age and Subscapular Skinfold-for-age.* Geneva: WHO 2007.
8. Onyango AW, de Onis M, Caroli M, Shah U, Sguassero Y, Redondo N. Field-testing the WHO child growth standards in four countries. *J Nutr* 2007;137:149-152.
9. Kinsley S, Yasmeen A. WHO growth standards: A critical note. *Eur J Gr Dev* 2011; 3:132-138.
10. Kinsley S. A review of WHO 2006 standards. *Nutr Health* 2010;12:8-12.

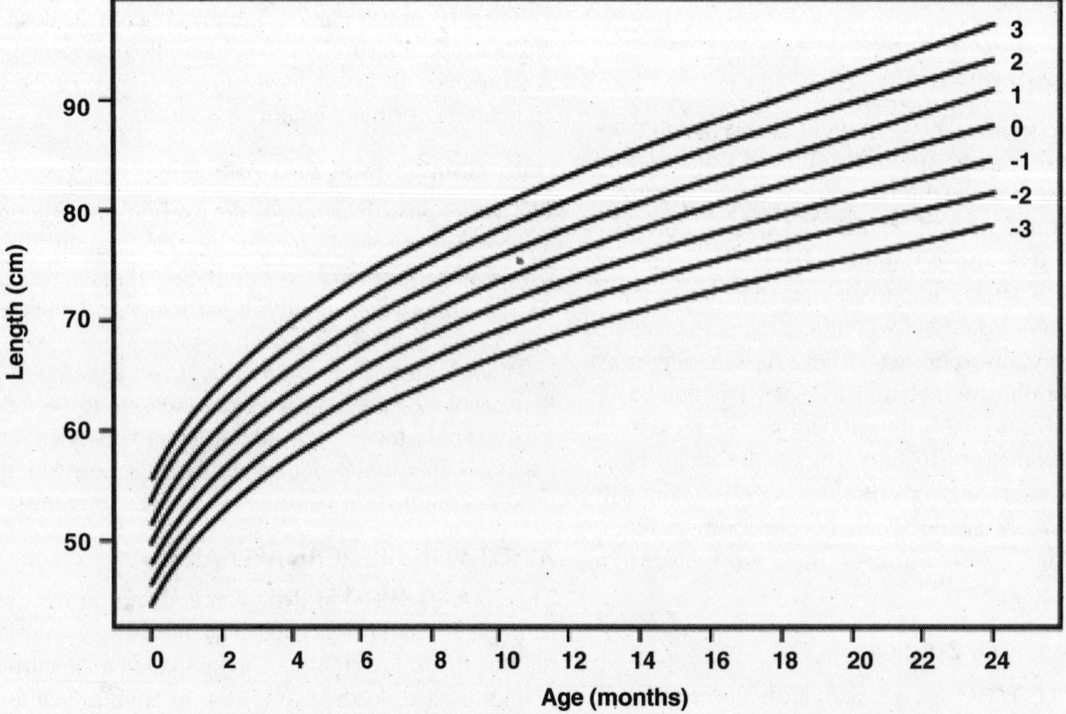

Fig. 6.1: WHO length-for-age z-scores for boys from birth to 24 months

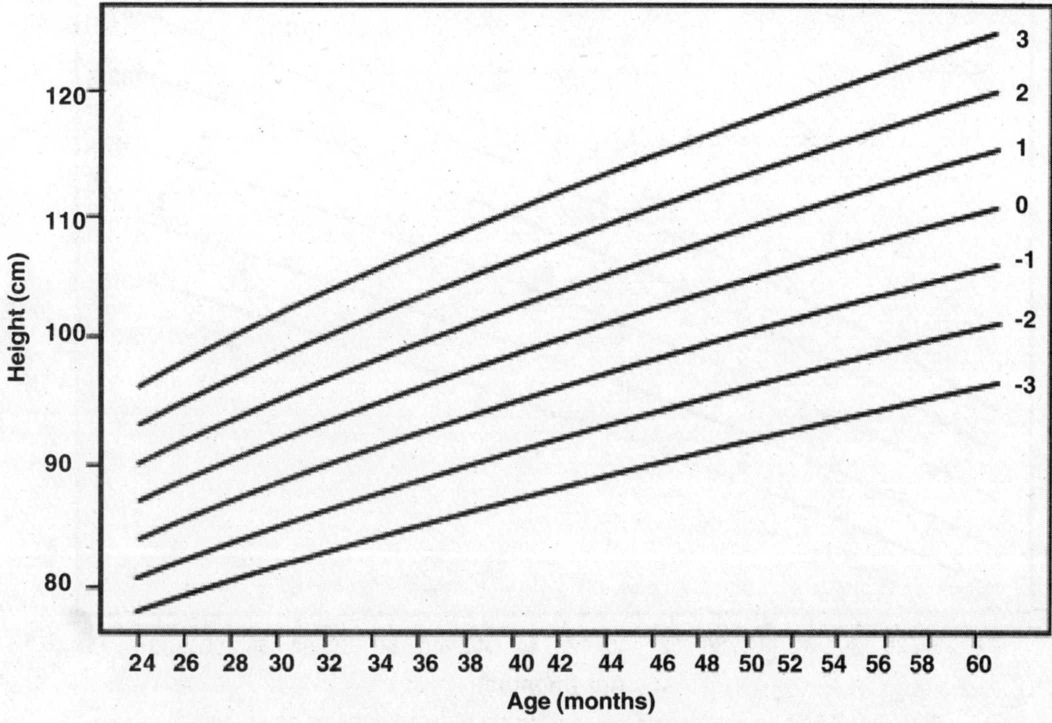

Fig. 6.2: WHO height-for-age z-scores for boys from 24 to 60 months

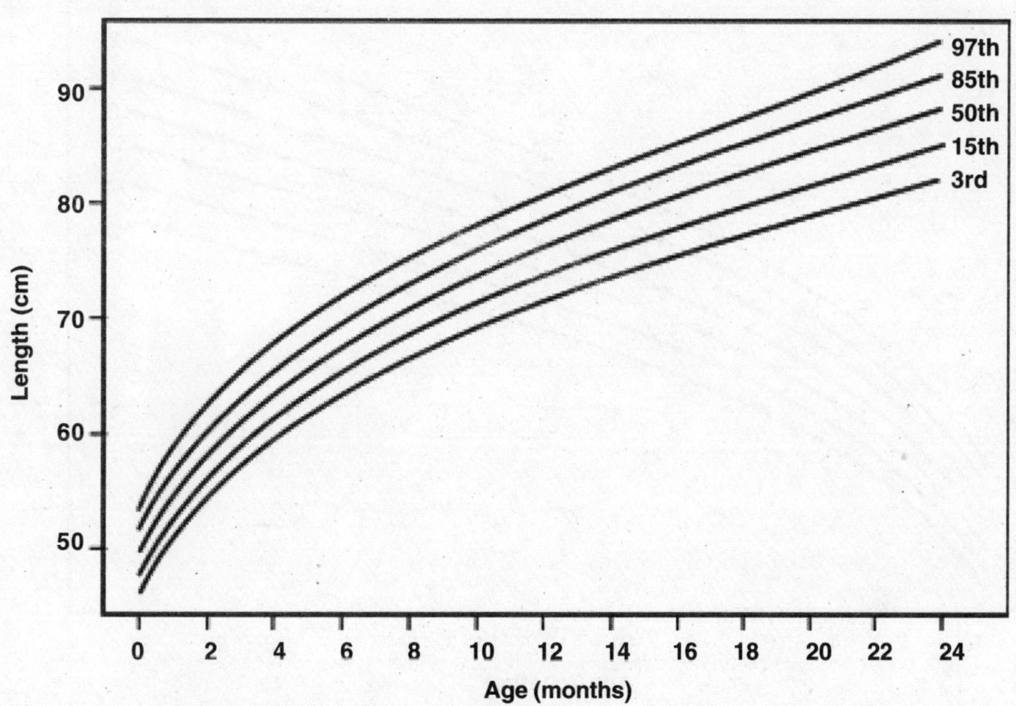

Fig. 6.3: WHO length-for-age percentiles for boys from birth to 24 months

Section 2

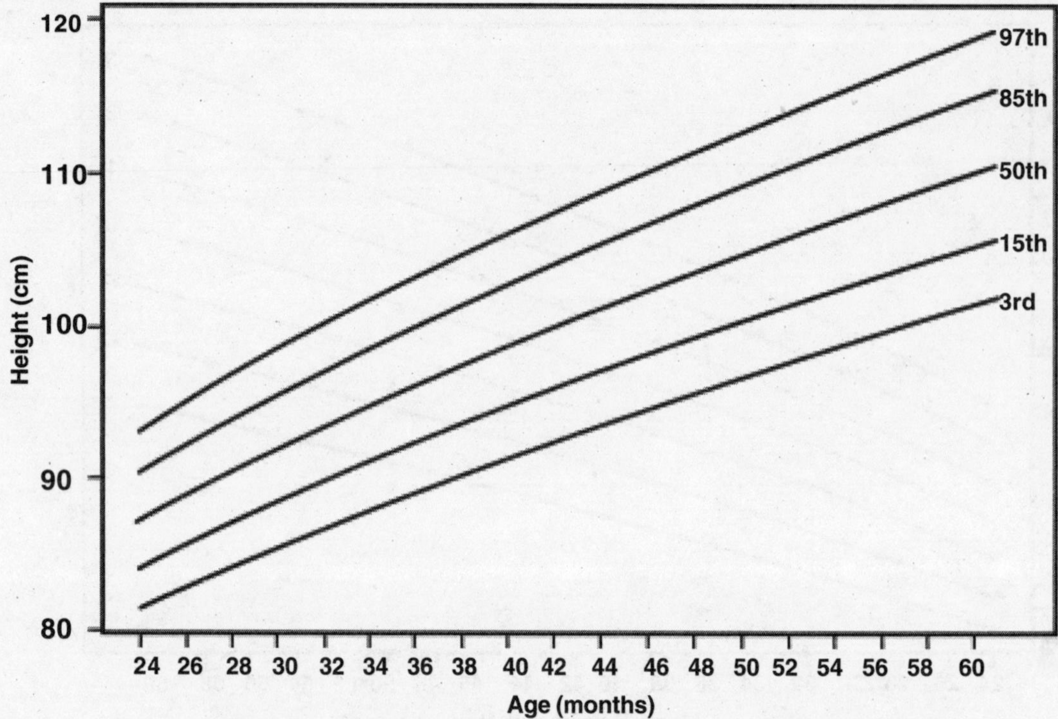

Fig. 6.4: WHO height-for-age percentiles for boys from 24 to 60 months

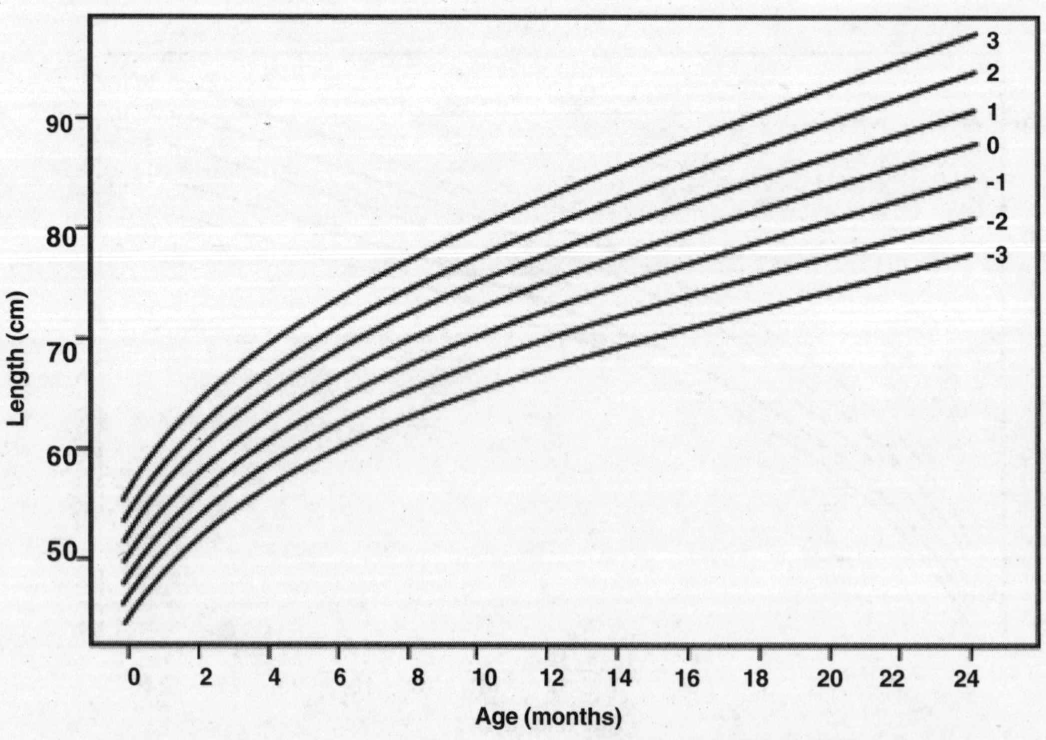

Fig. 6.5: WHO length-for-age z-scores for girls from birth to 24 months

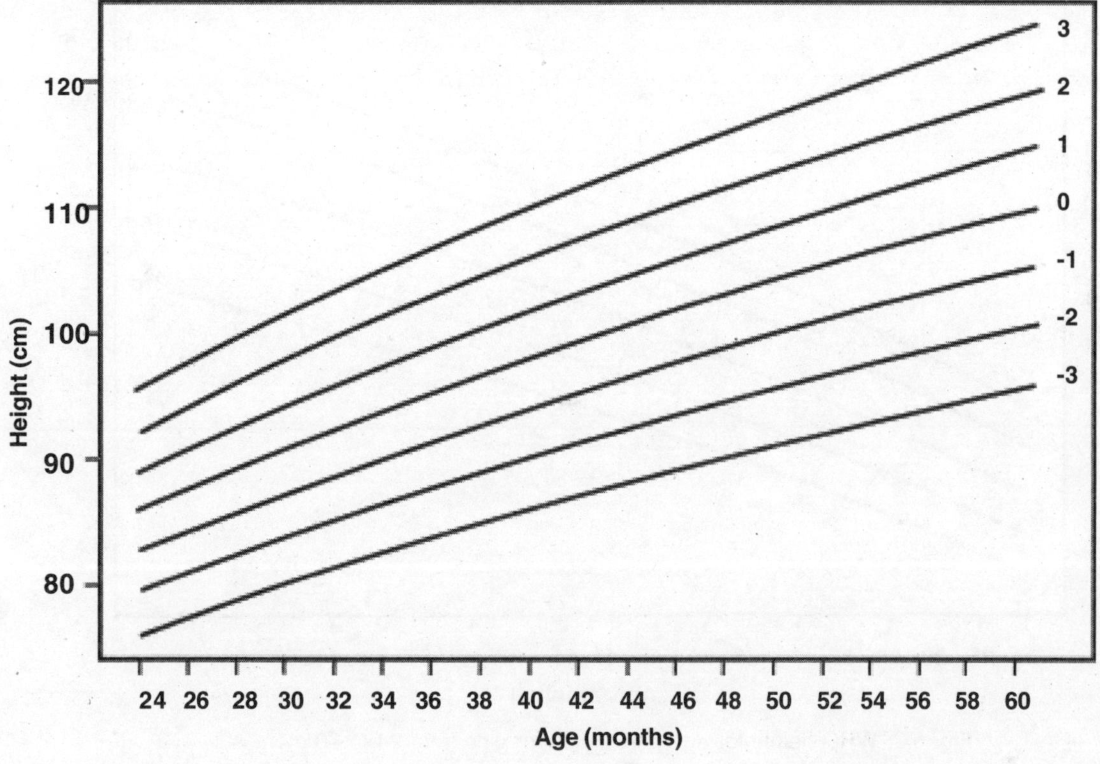

Fig. 6.6: WHO height-for-age z-scores for girls from 24 to 60 months

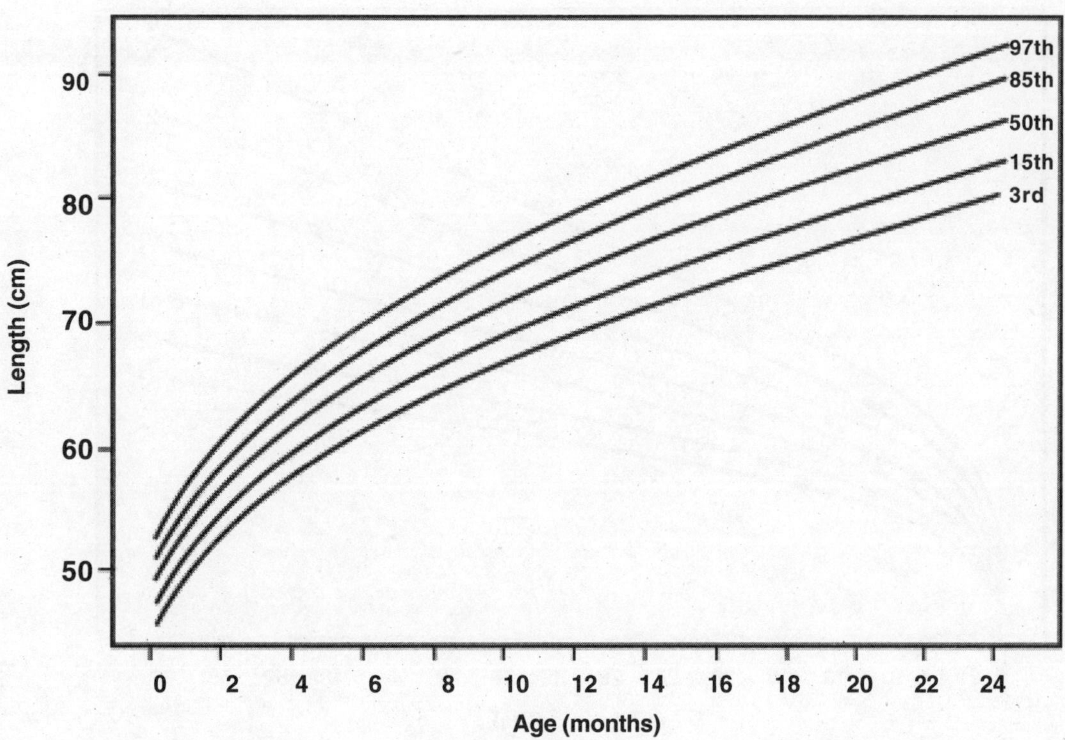

Fig. 6.7: WHO length-for-age percentiles for girls from birth to 24 months

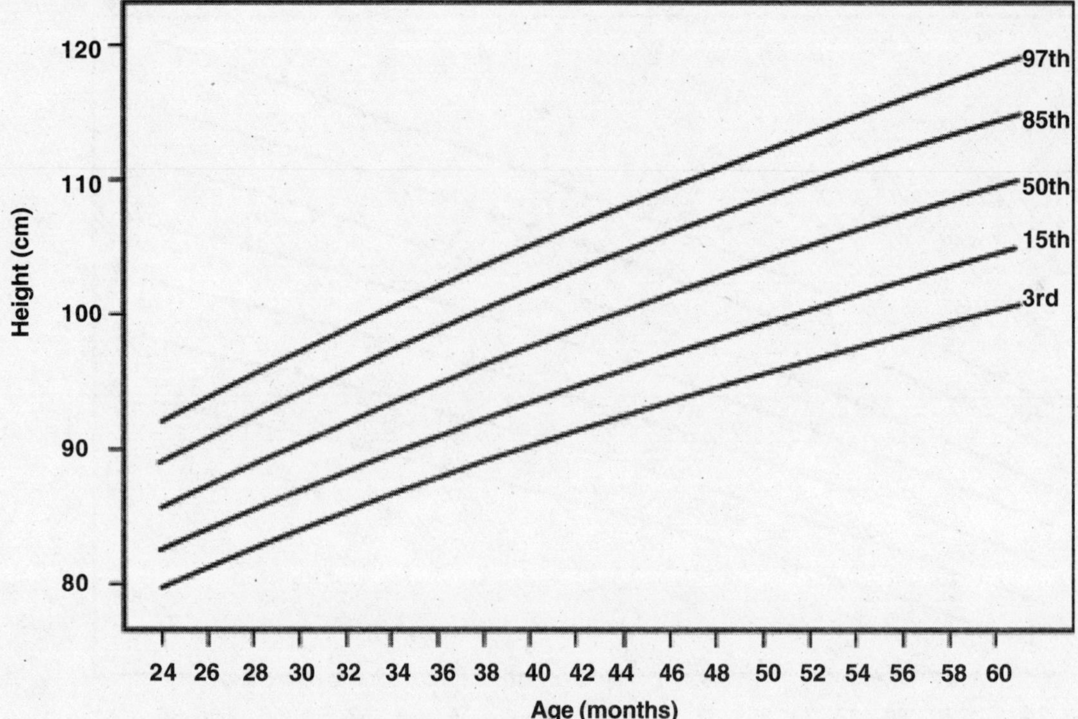

Fig. 6.8: WHO height-for-age percentiles for girls from 24 to 60 months

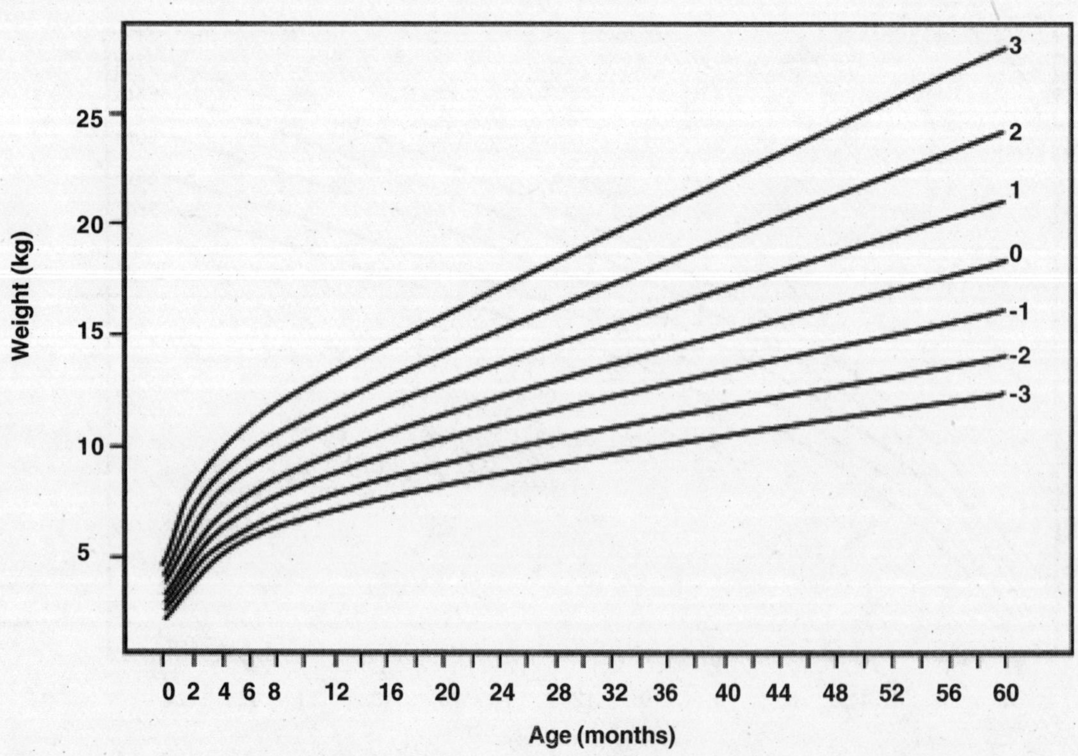

Fig. 6.9: WHO weight-for-age z-scores for boys from birth to 60 months

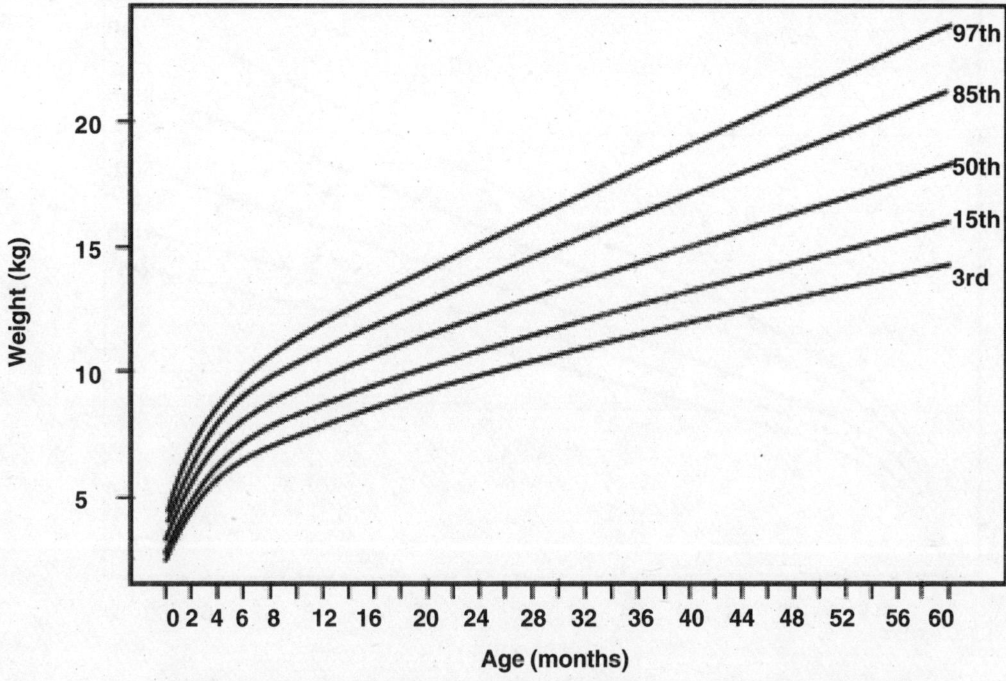

Fig. 6.10: WHO weight-for-age percentiles for boys from birth to 60 months

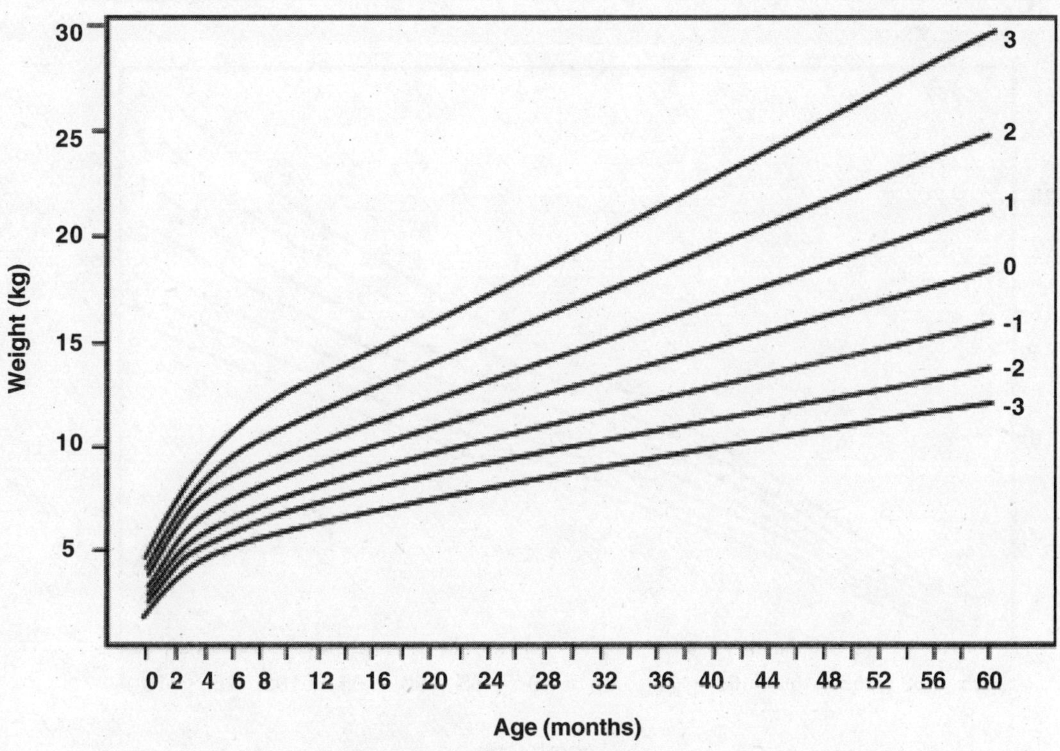

Fig. 6.11: WHO weight-for-age z-scores for girls from birth to 60 months

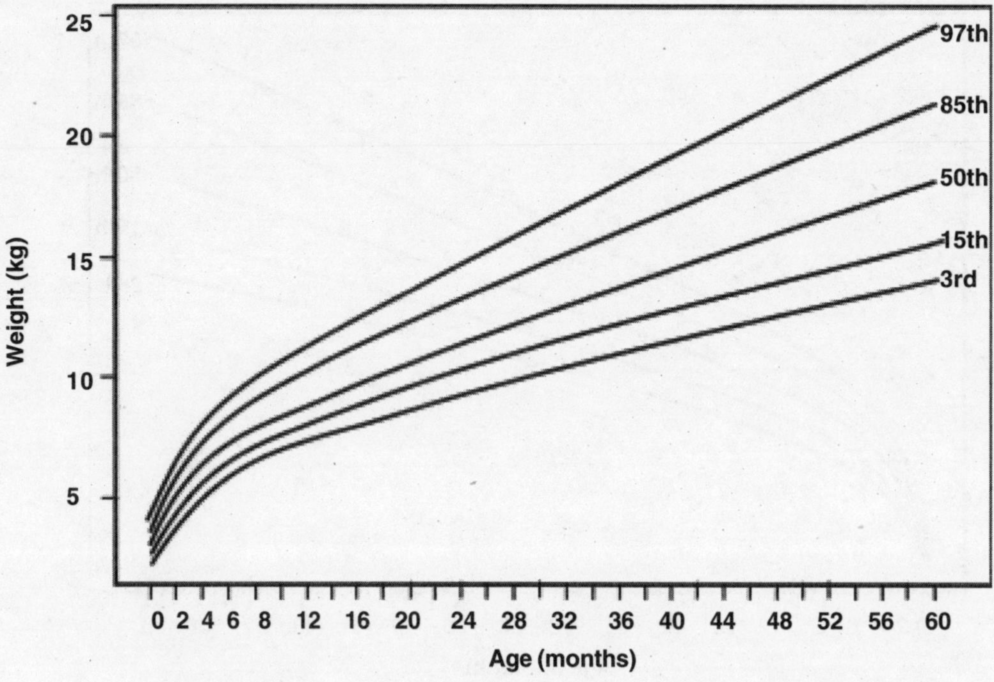

Fig. 6.12: WHO weight-for-age percentiles for girls from birth to 60 months

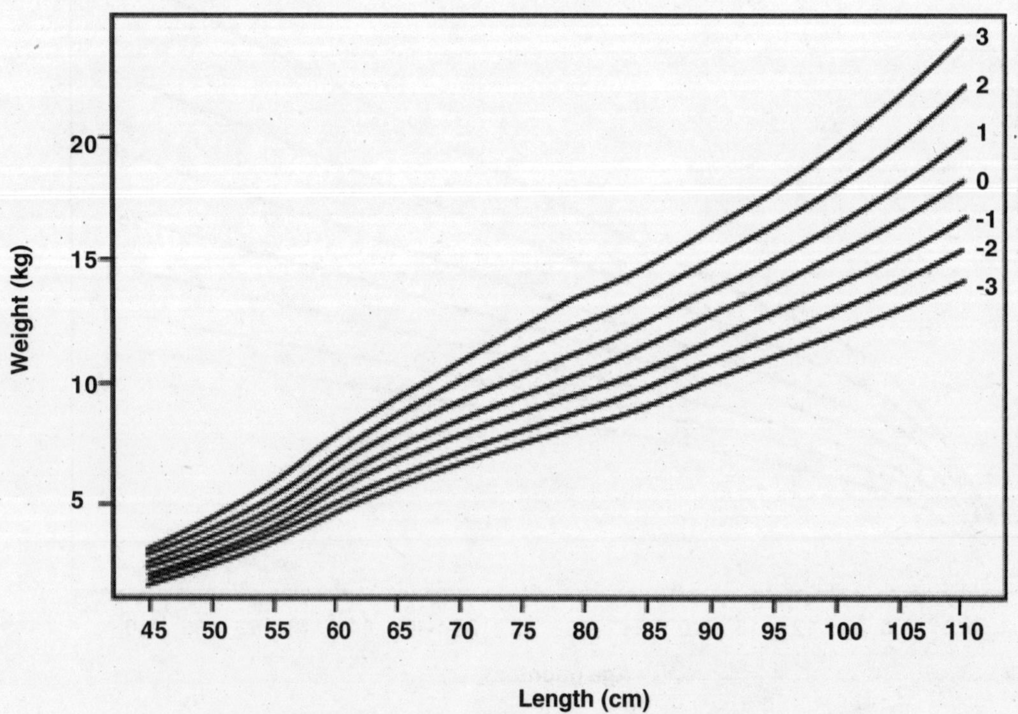

Fig. 6.13: WHO weight-for-length z-scores for boys from 45 to 110 cm

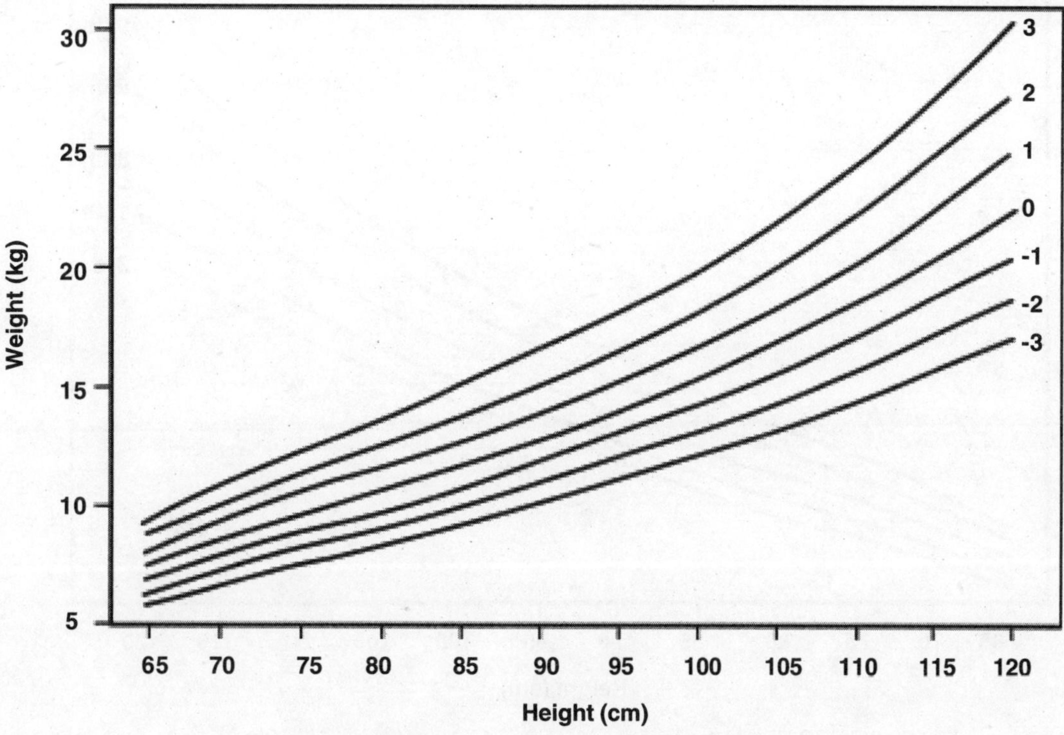

Fig. 6.14: WHO weight-for-height z-scores for boys from 65 to 120 cm

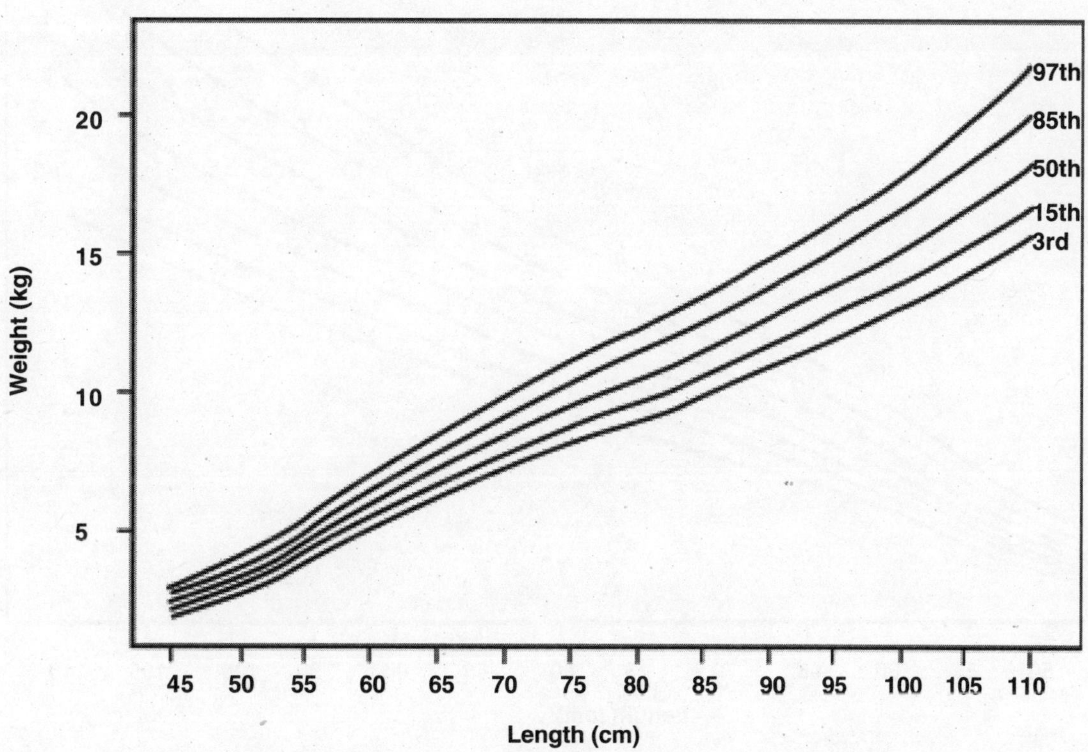

Fig. 6.15: WHO weight-for-length percentiles for boys from 45 to 110 cm

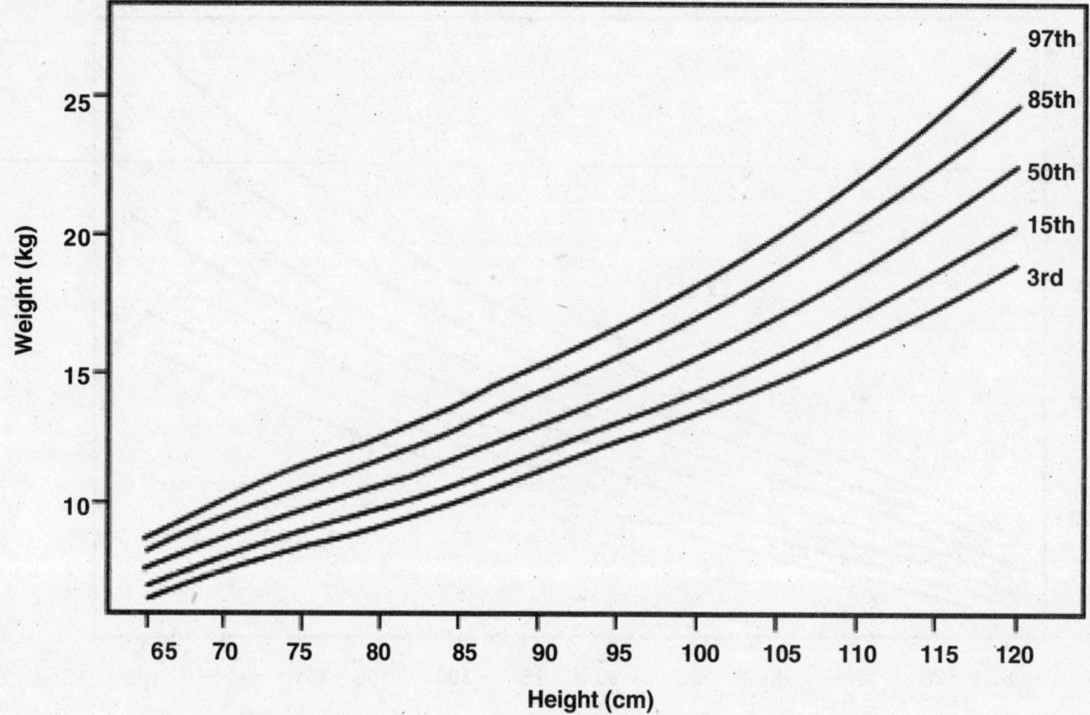

Fig. 6.16: WHO weight-for-height percentiles for boys from 65 to 120 cm

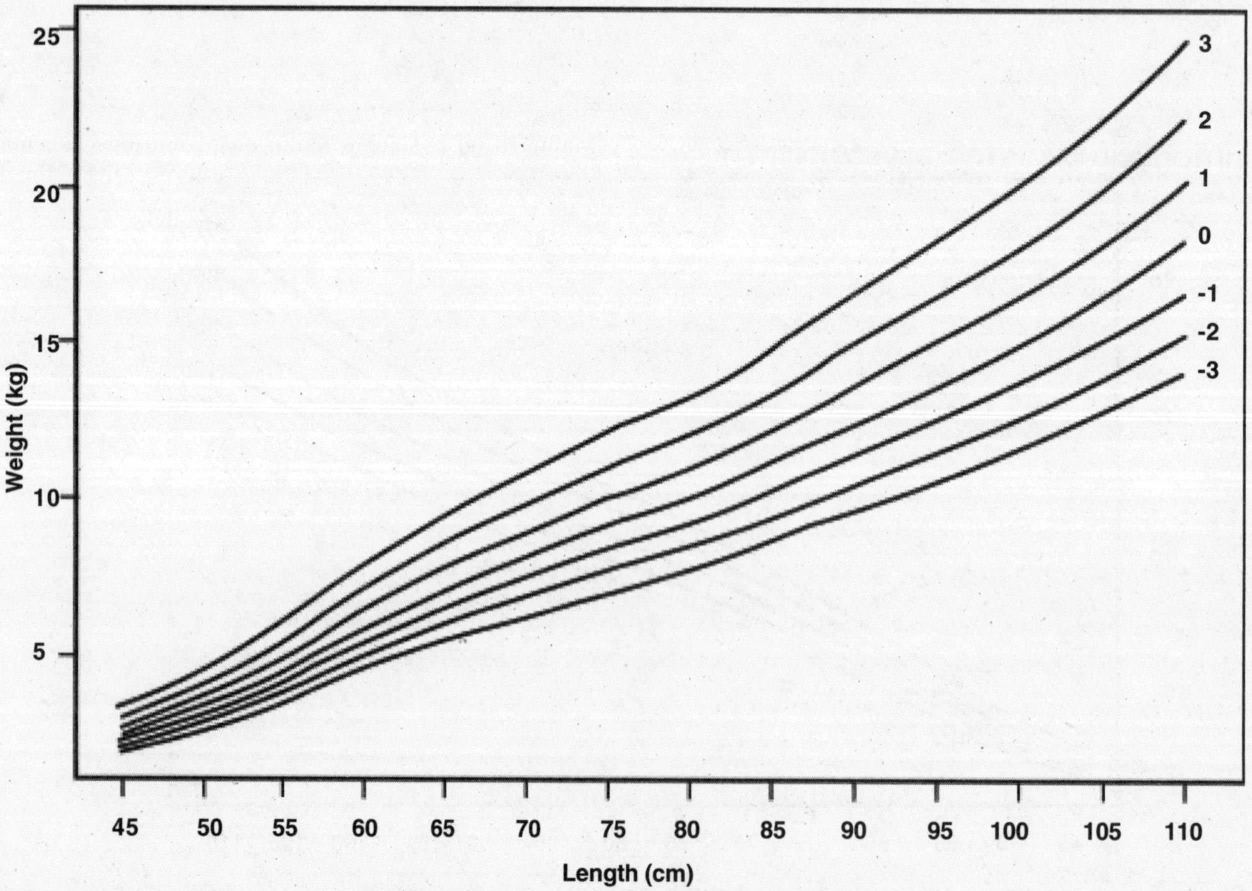

Fig. 6.17: WHO weight-for-length z-scores for girls

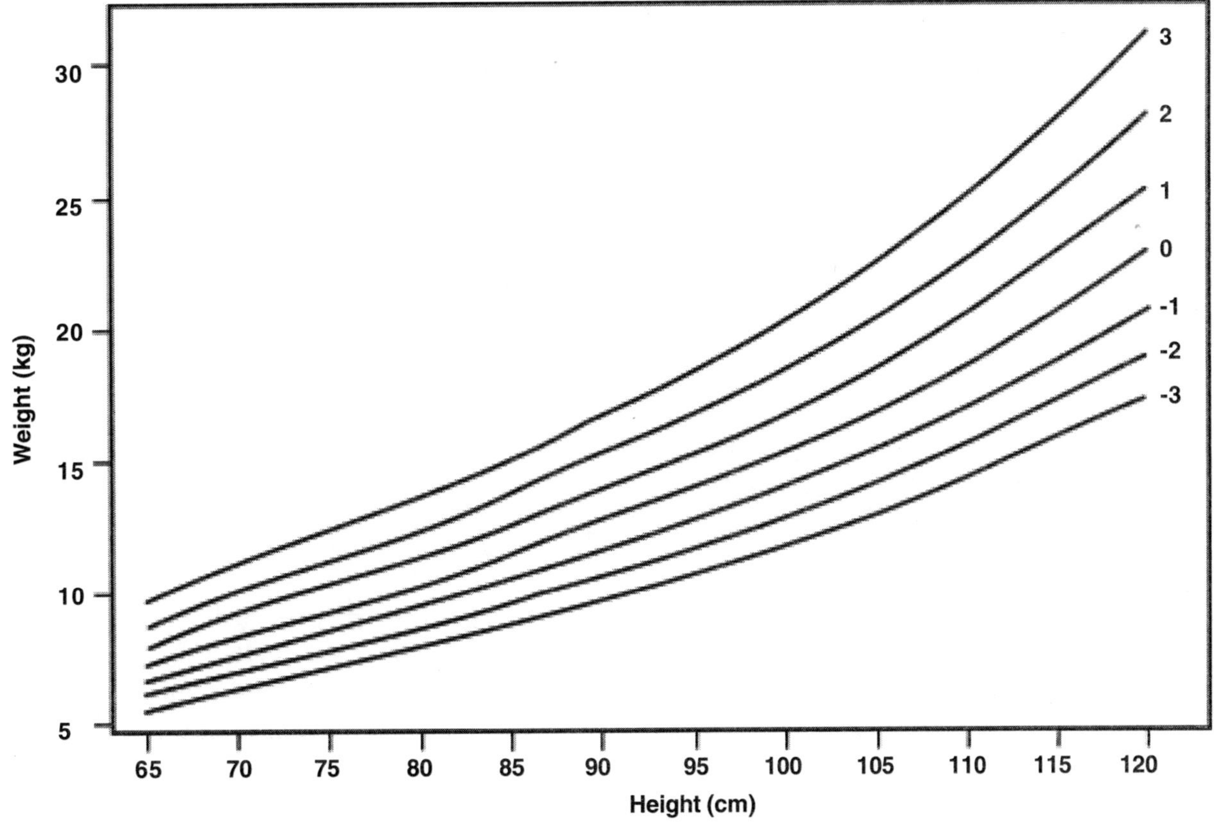

Fig. 6.18: WHO weight-for-height z-scores for girls

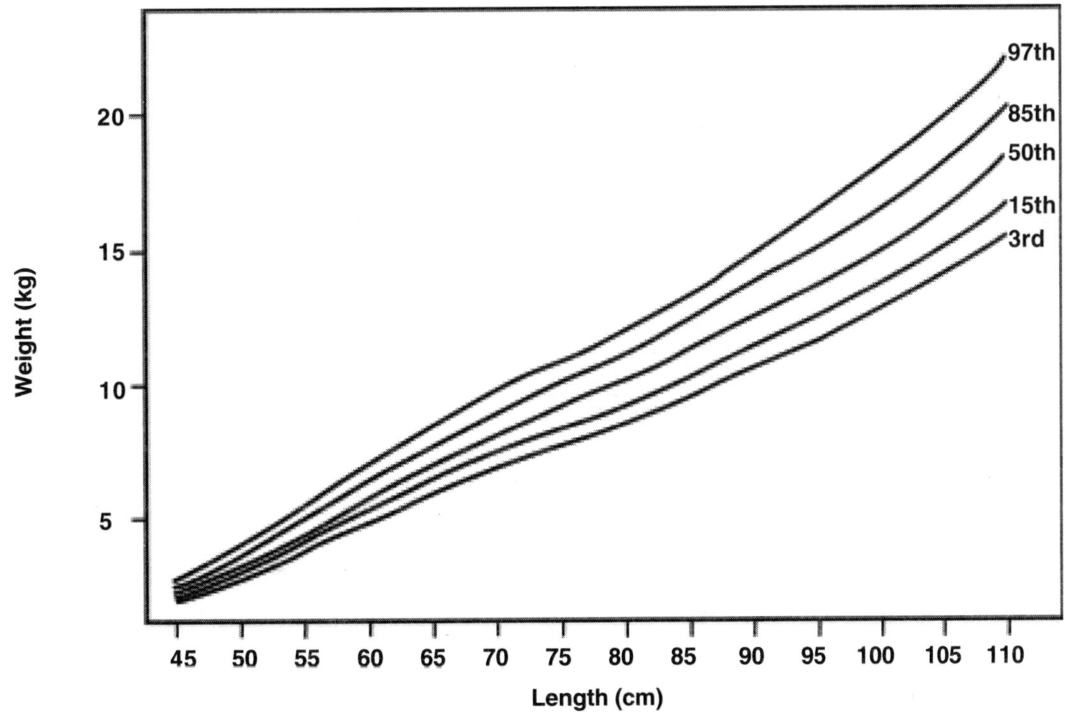

Fig. 6.19: WHO weight-for-length percentiles for girls

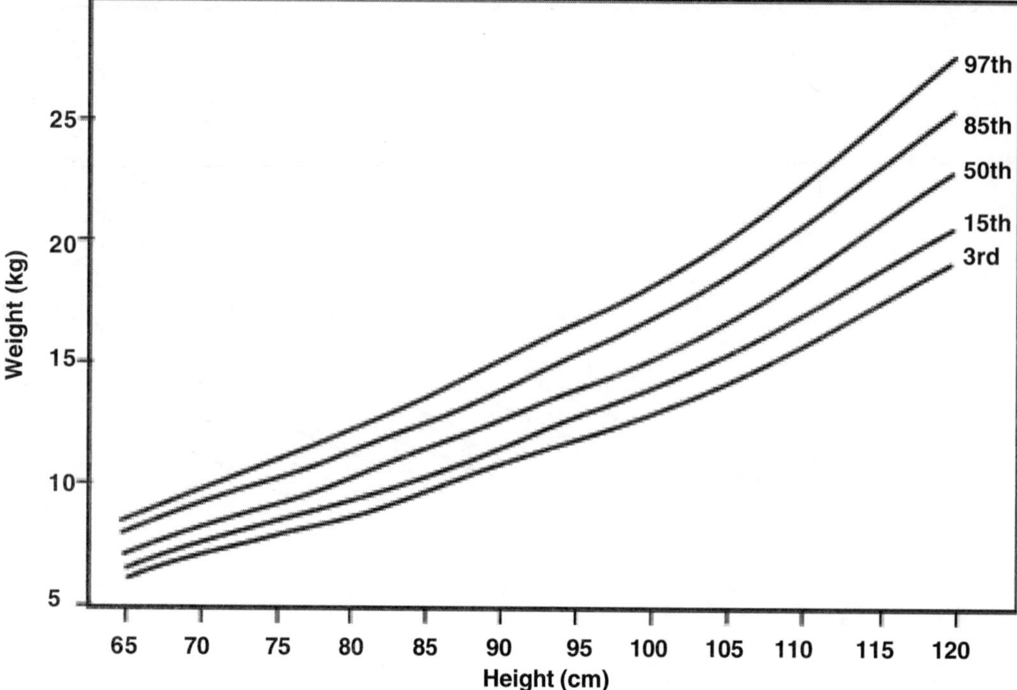

Fig. 6.20: WHO weight-for-height percentiles for girls

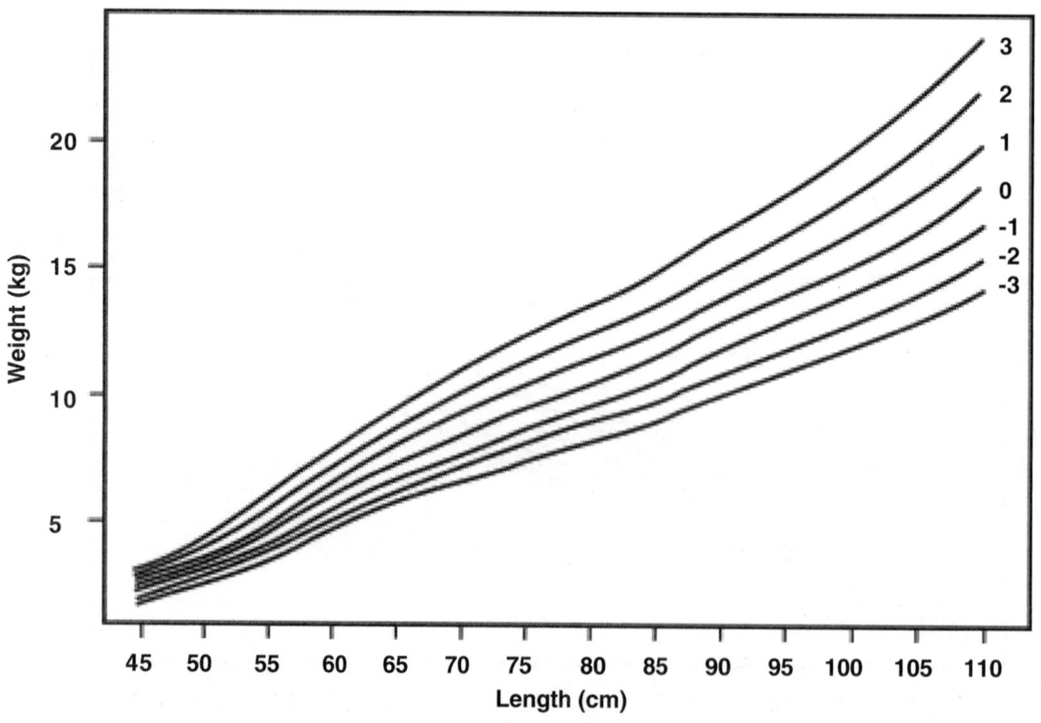

Fig. 6.21: WHO weight-for-length z-scores for boys from 45 to 110 cm

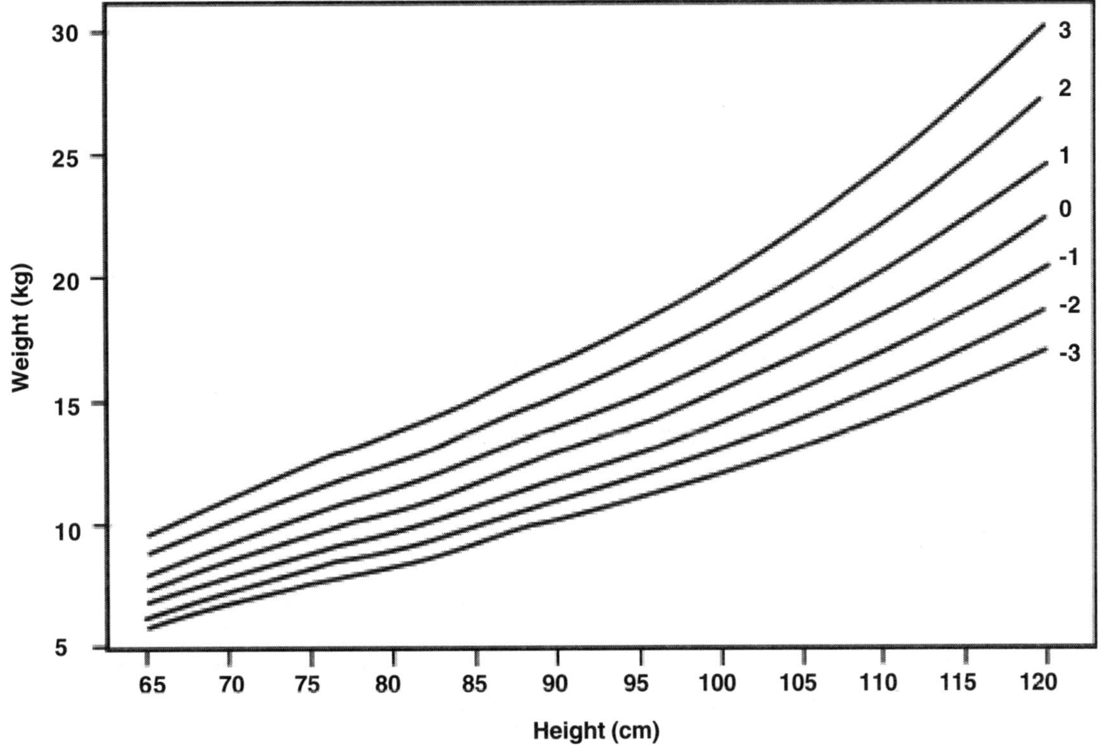

Fig. 6.22: WHO weight-for-height z-scores for boys from 65 to 120 cm

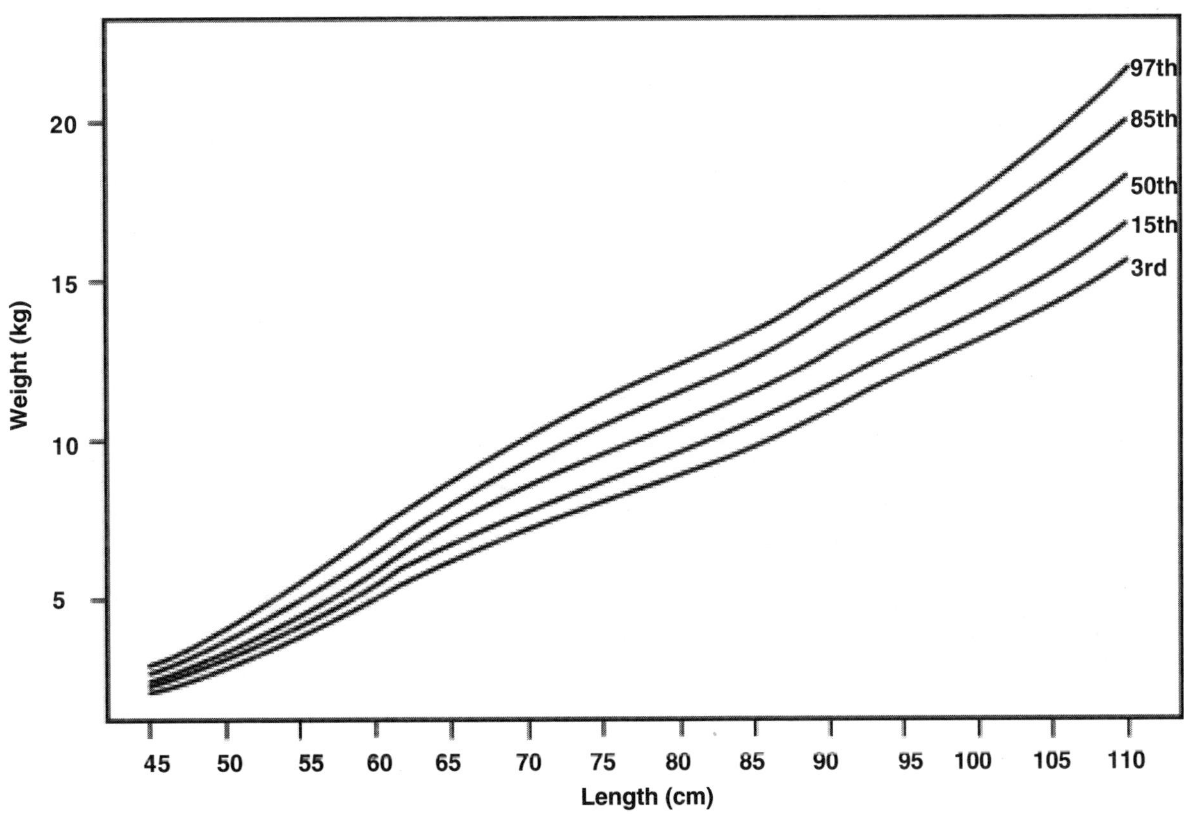

Fig. 6.23: WHO weight-for-length percentiles for boys from 45 to 110 cm

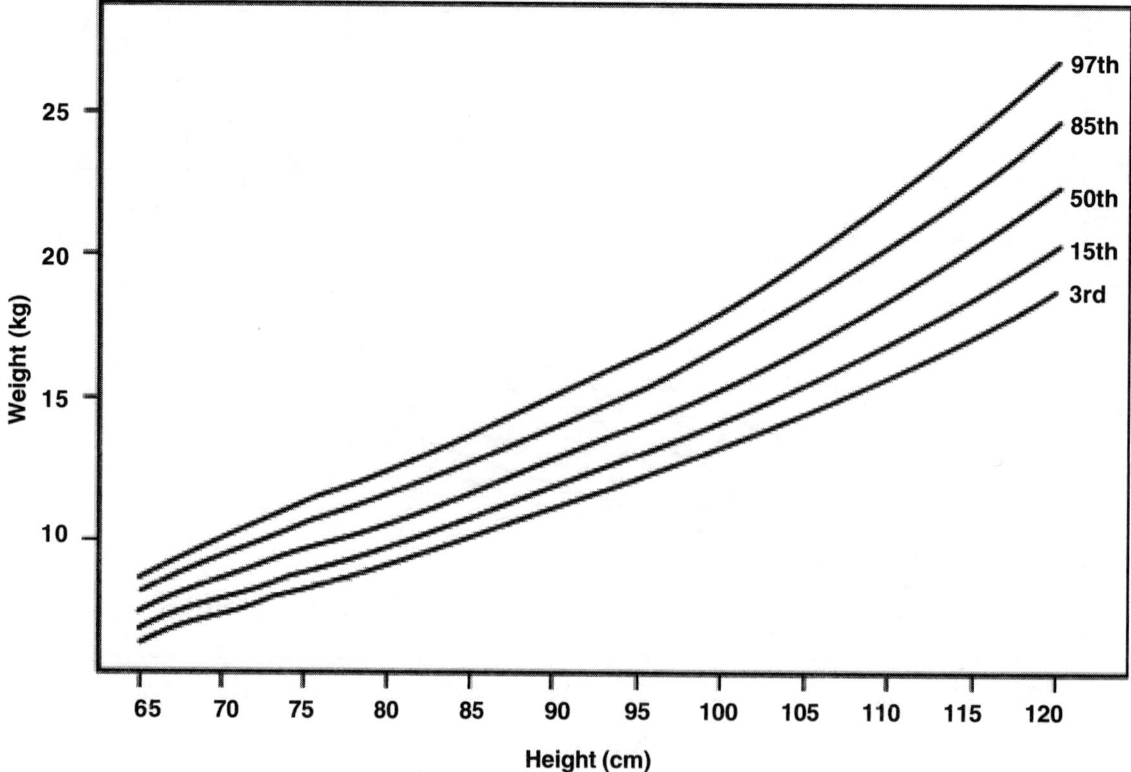

Fig. 6.24: WHO weight-for-height percentiles for boys from 65 to 120 cm

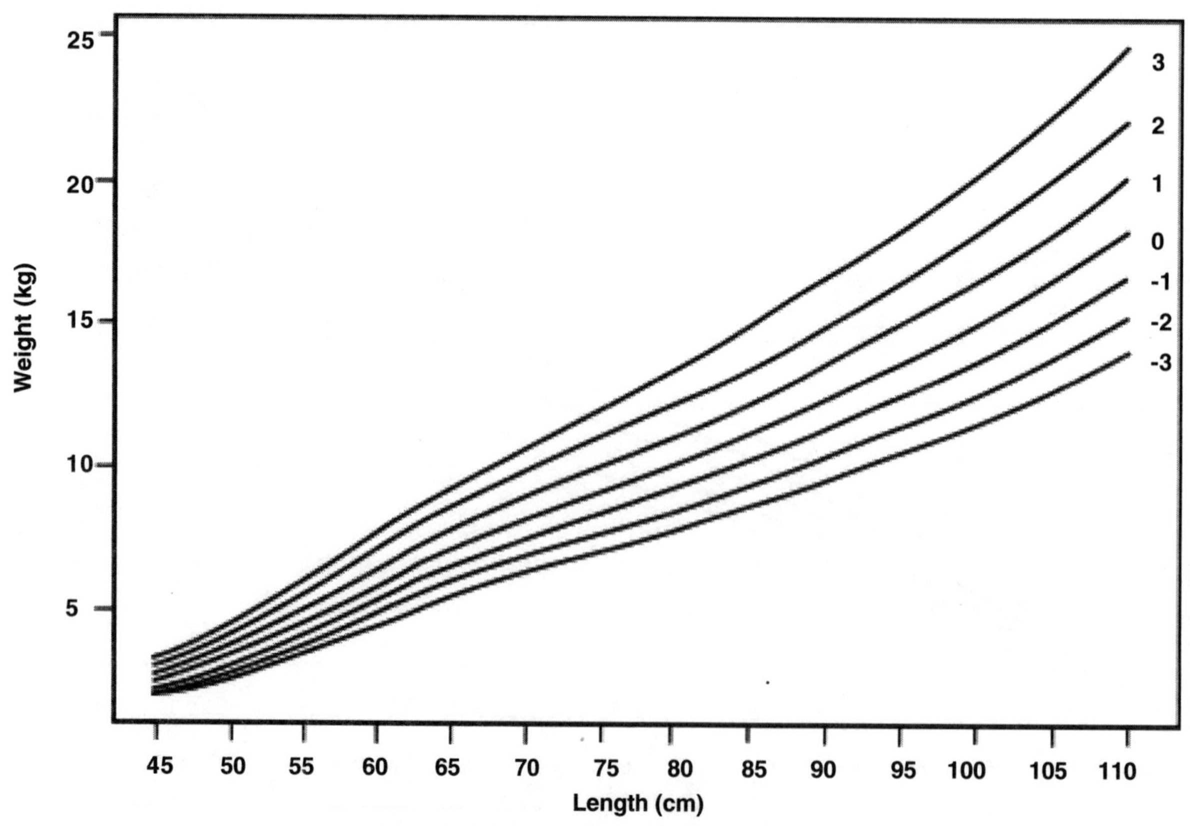

Fig. 6.25: WHO weight-for-length z-scores for girls

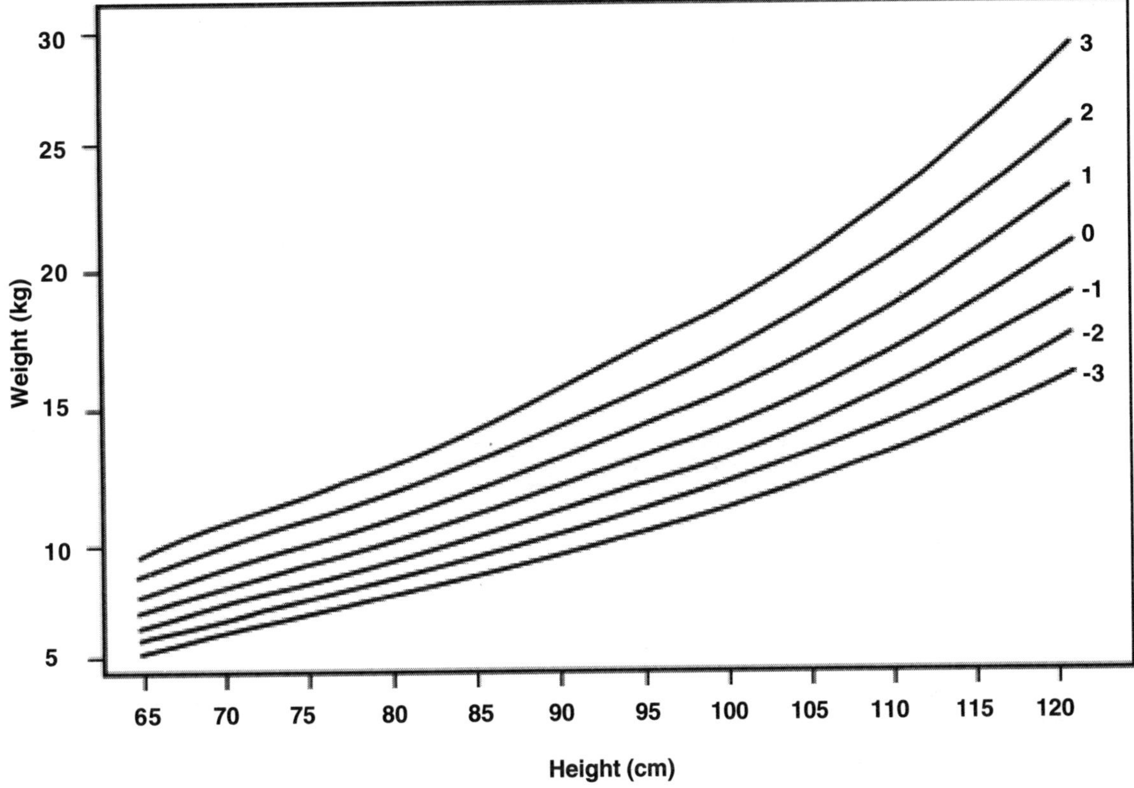

Fig. 6.26: WHO weight-for-height z-scores for girls

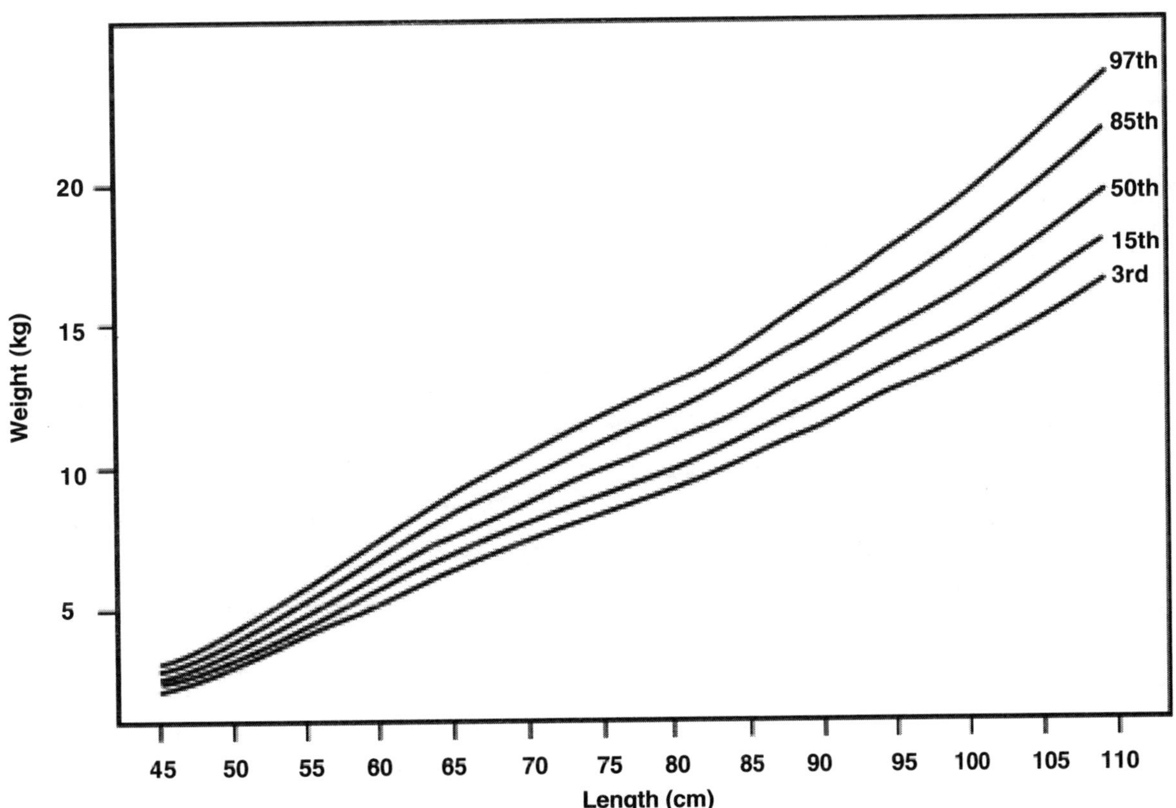

Fig. 6.27: WHO weight-for-length percentiles for girls

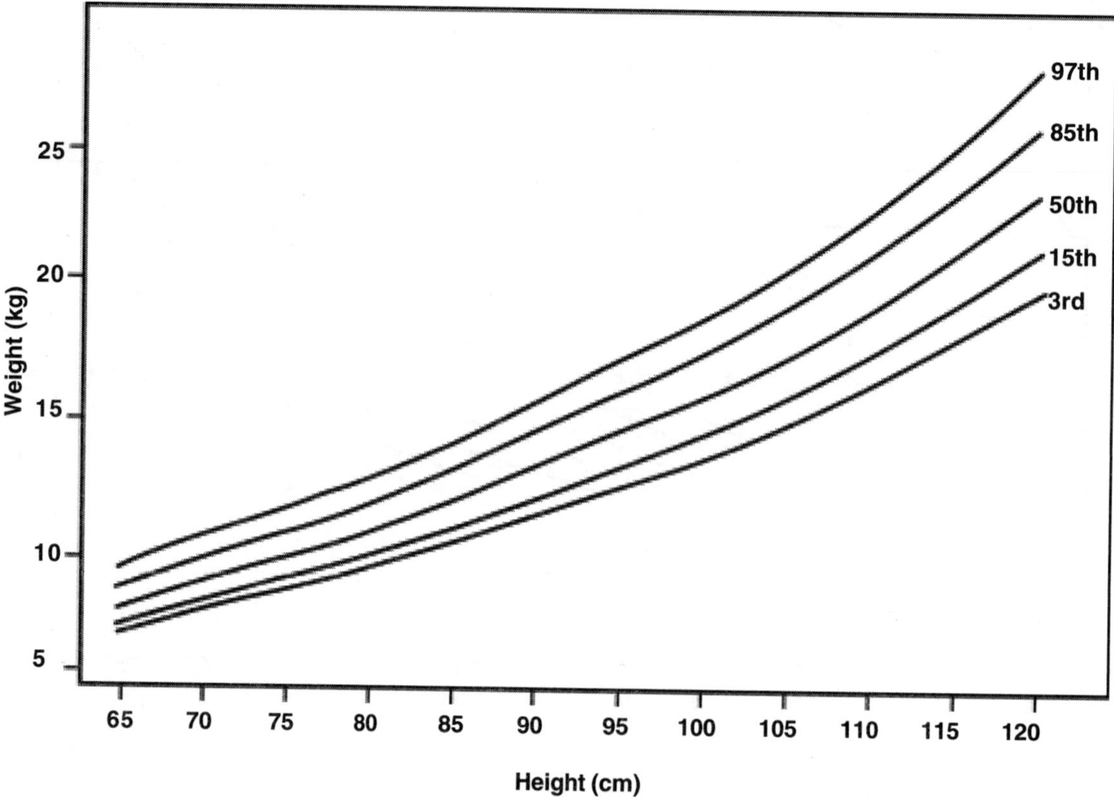

Fig. 6.28: WHO weight-for-height percentiles for girls

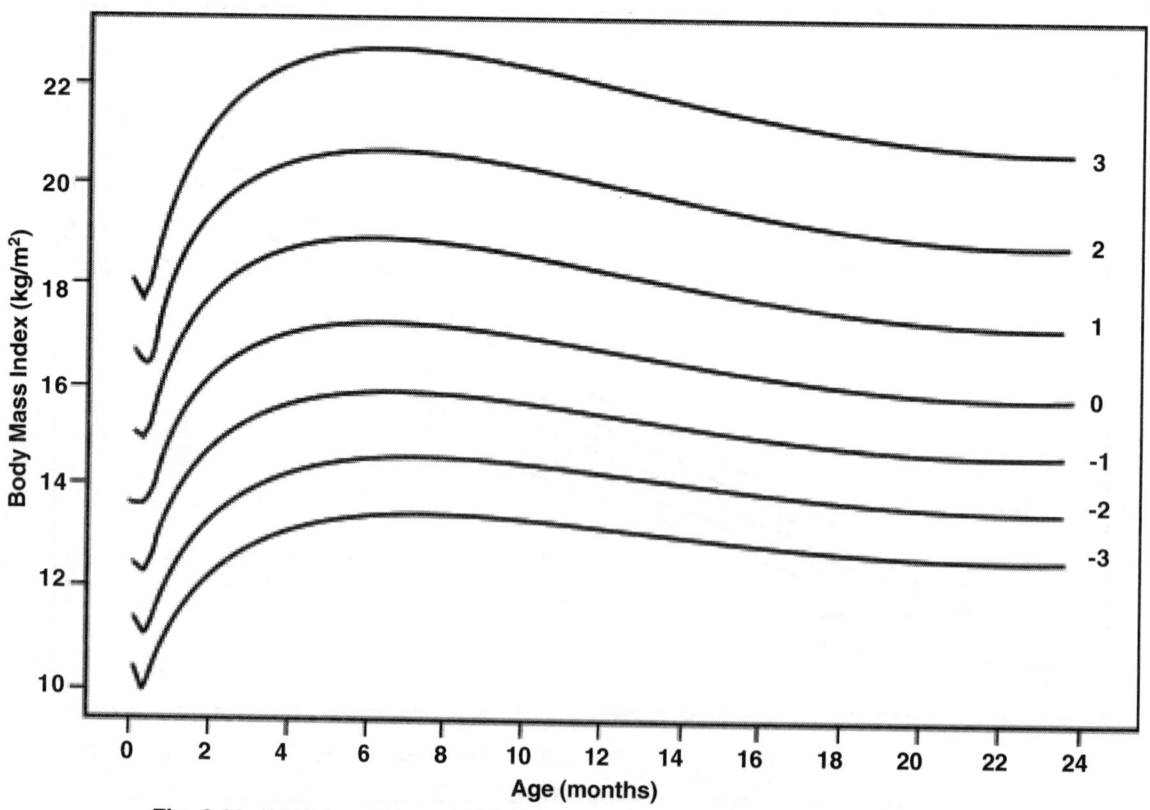

Fig. 6.29: WHO length-based BMI-for-age z-scores for boys from birth to 24 months

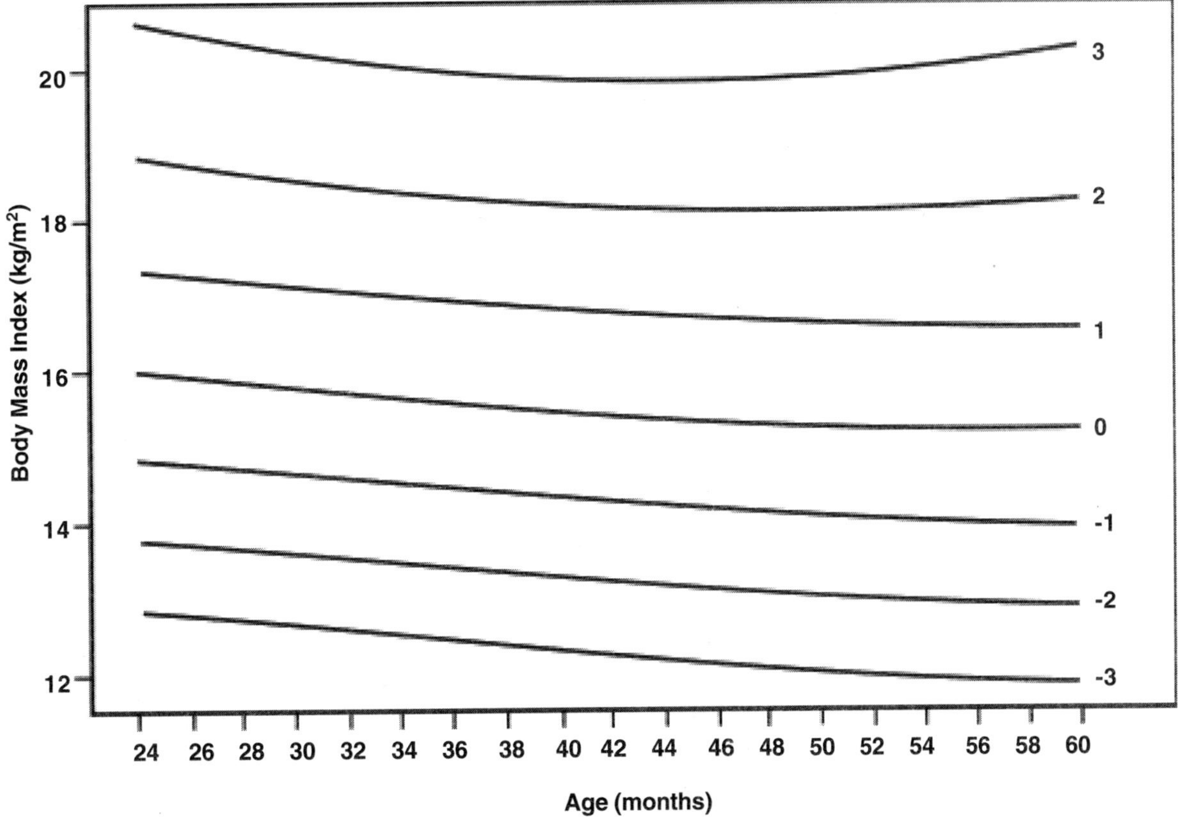

Fig. 6.30: WHO height-based BMI-for-age z-scores for boys from 24 to 60 months

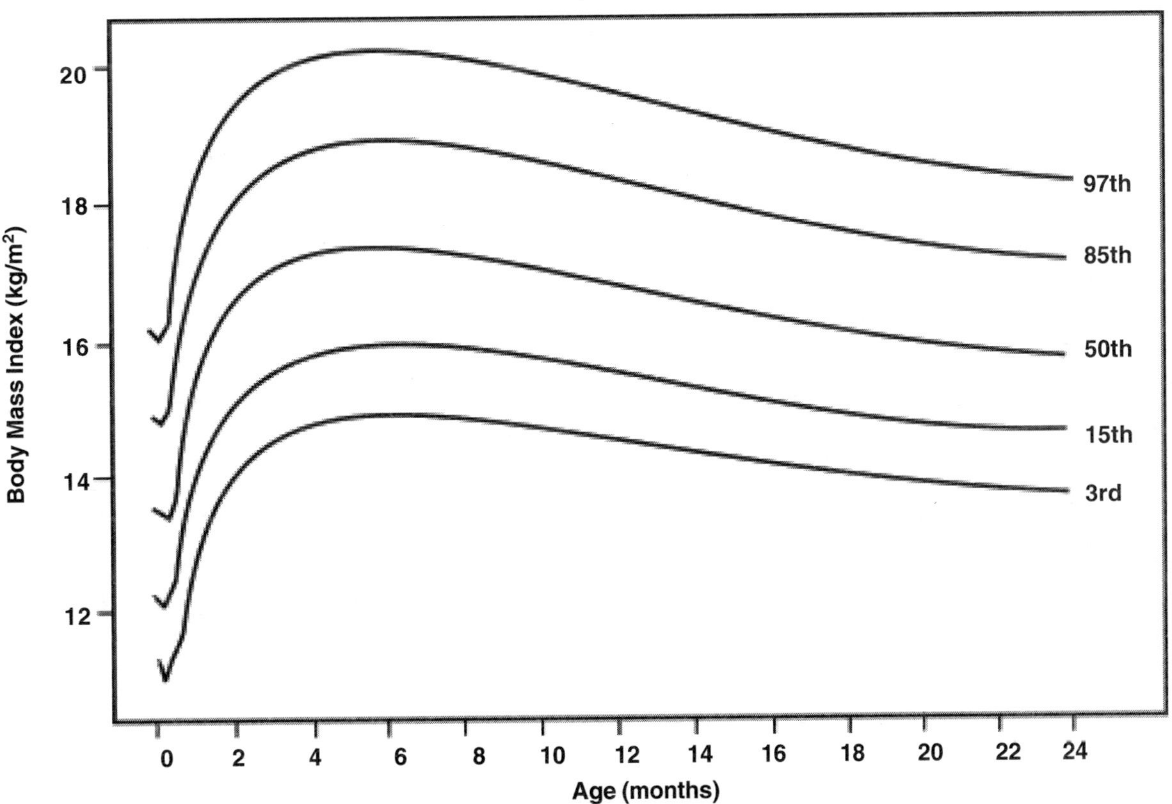

Fig. 6.31: WHO length-based BMI-for-age percentiles for boys from birth to 24 months

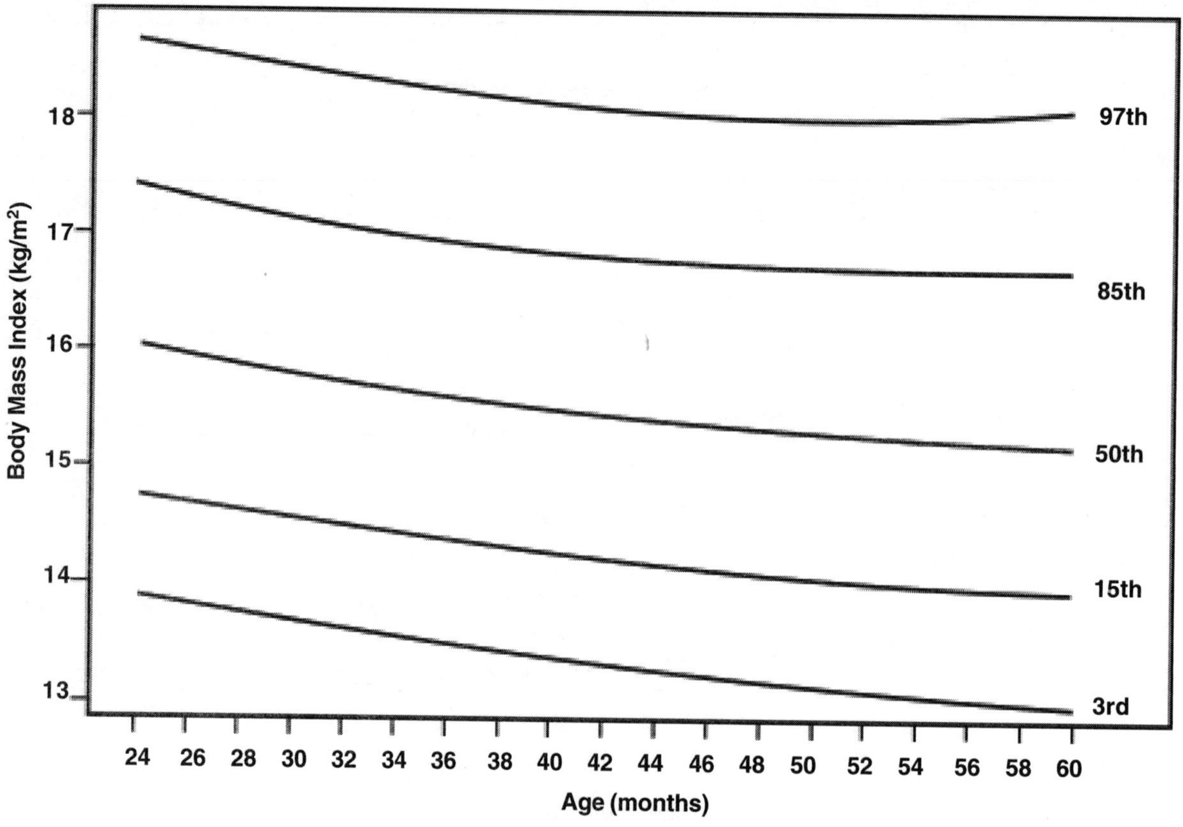

Fig. 6.32: WHO height-based BMI-for-age percentiles for boys from 24 to 60 months

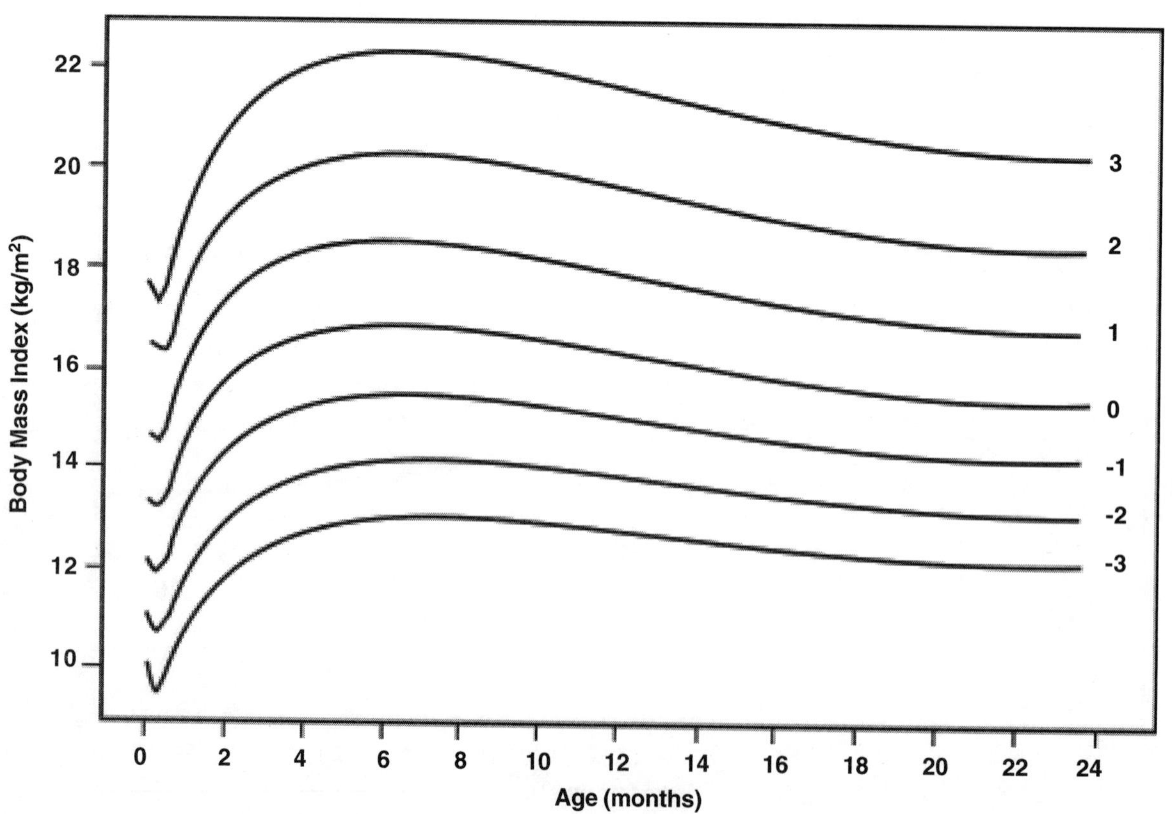

Fig. 6.33: WHO length-based BMI-for-age z-scores for girls from birth to 24 months

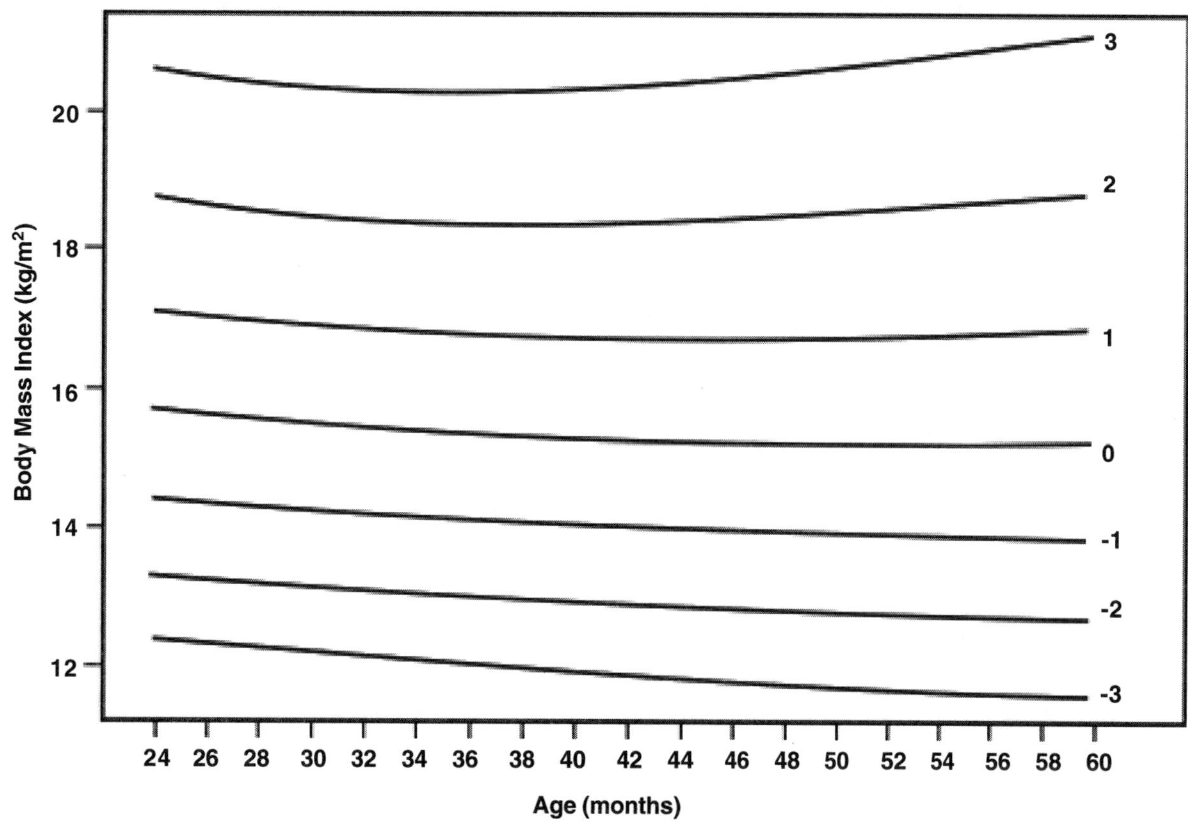

Fig. 6.34: WHO height-based BMI-for-age z-scores for girls from 24 to 60 months

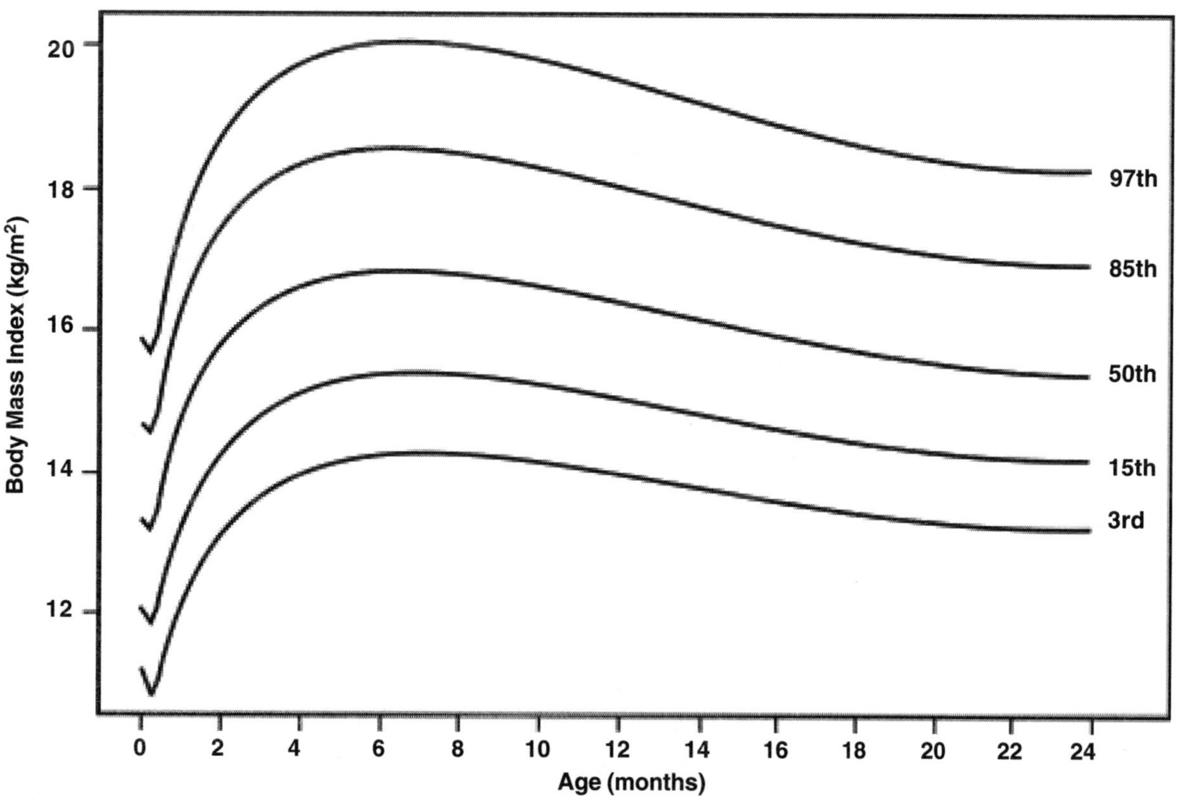

Fig. 6.35: WHO length-based BMI-for-age percentiles for girls from birth to 24 months

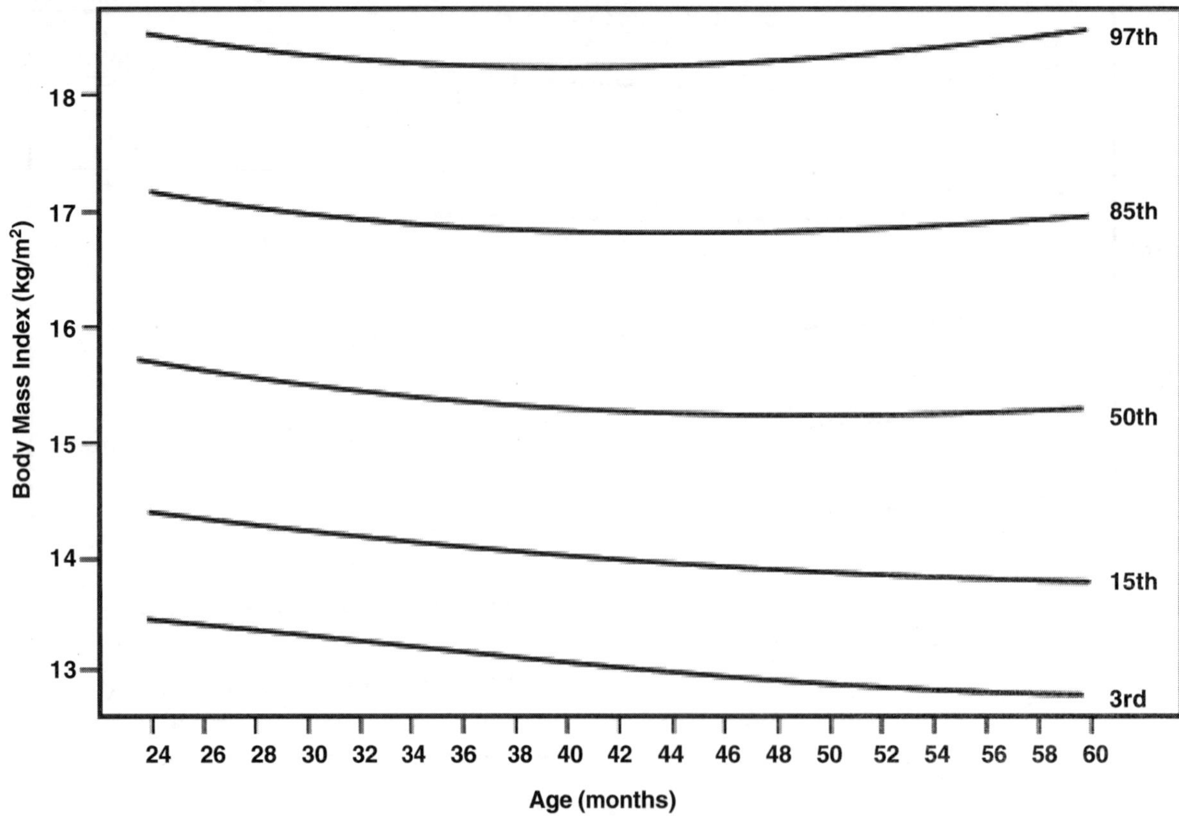

Fig. 6.36: WHO height-based BMI-for-age percentiles for girls from 24 to 60 months

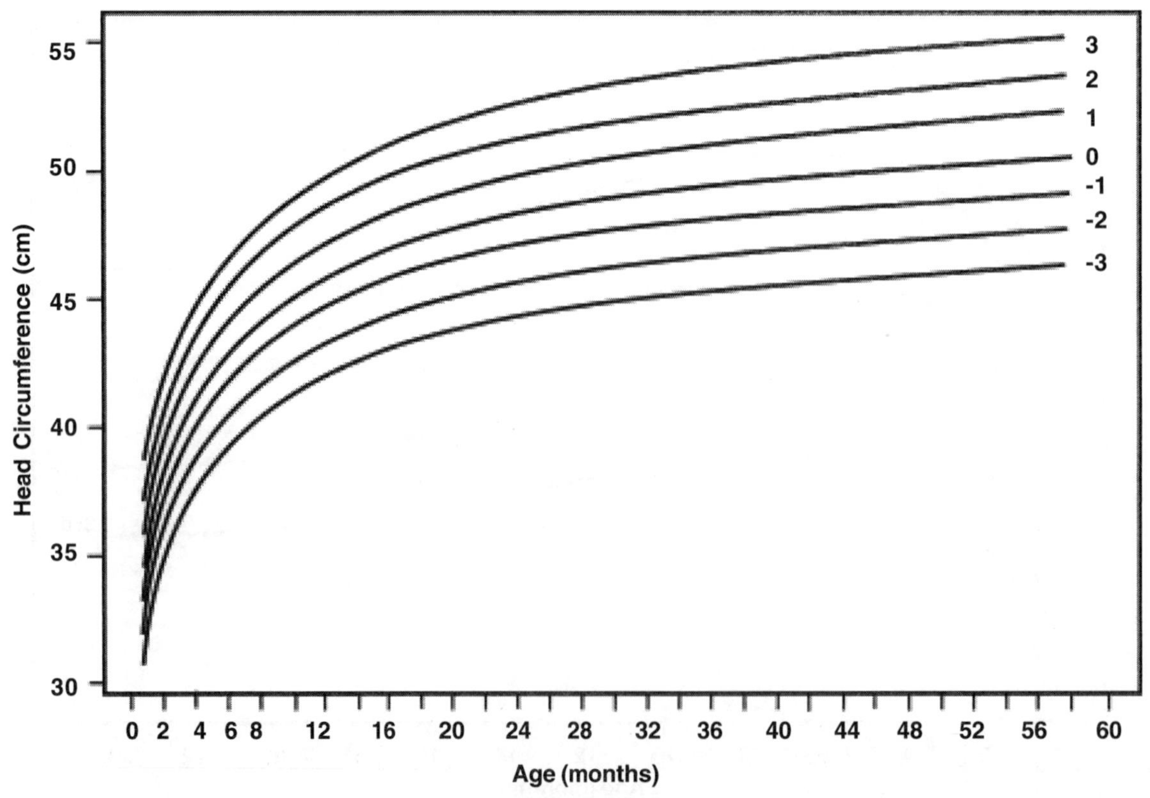

Fig. 6.37: WHO head circumference-for-age z-scores for boys from birth to 60 months

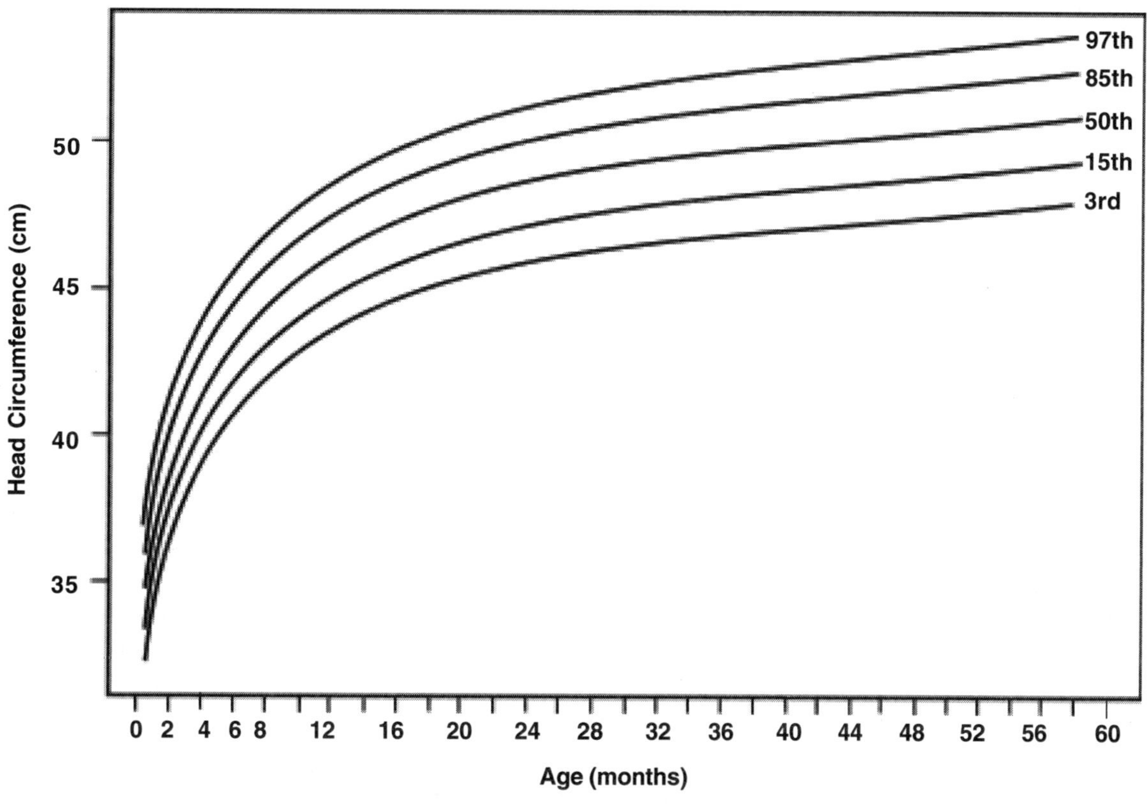

Fig. 6.38: WHO head circumference -for-age percentiles for boys from birth to 60 months

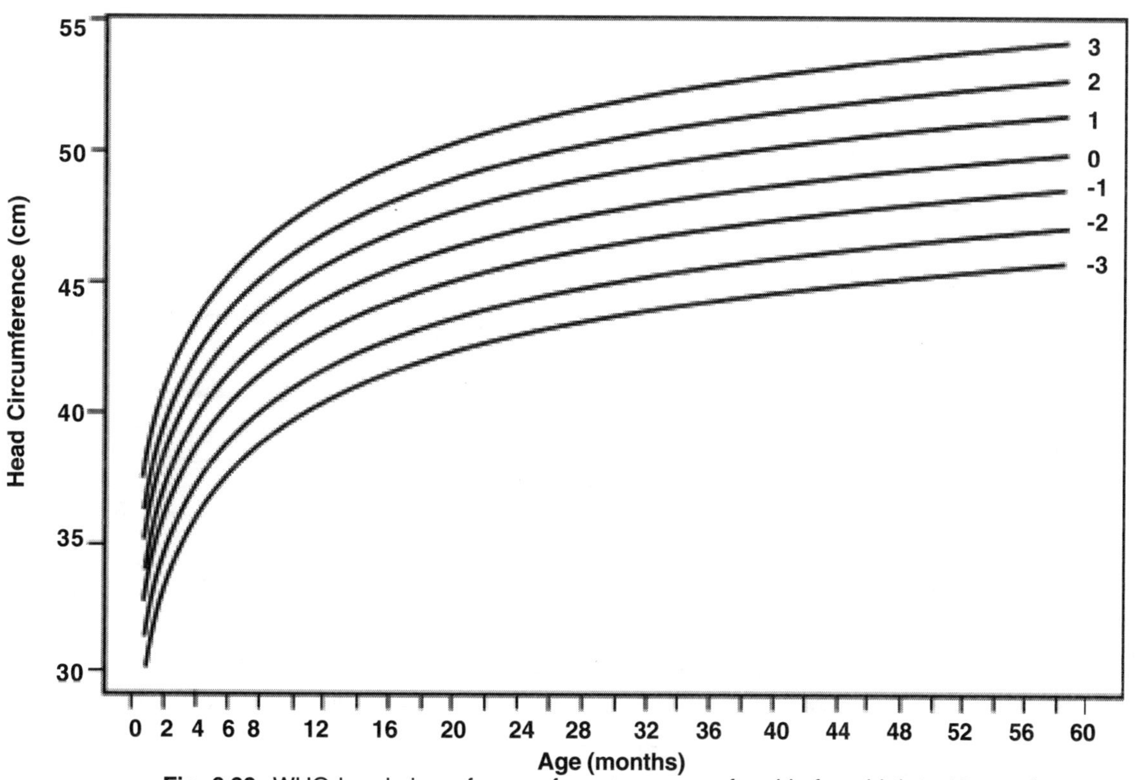

Fig. 6.39: WHO head circumference-for-age z-scores for girls from birth to 60 months

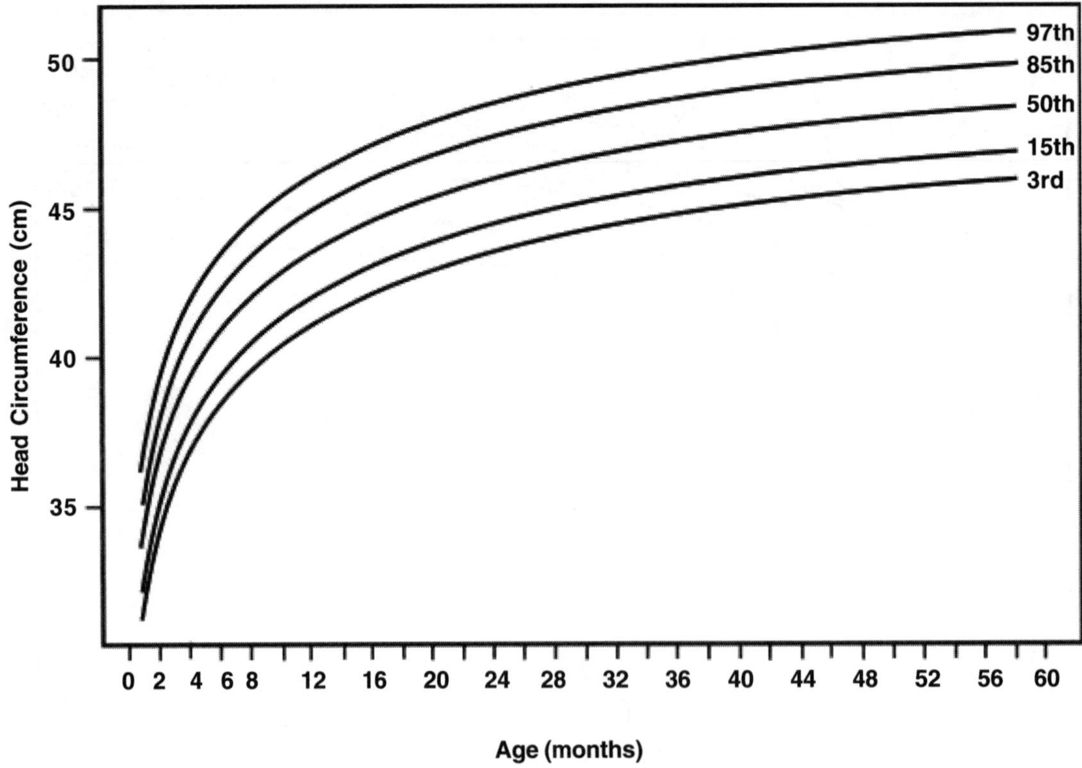

Fig. 6.40: WHO head circumference-for-age percentiles for girls from birth to 60 months

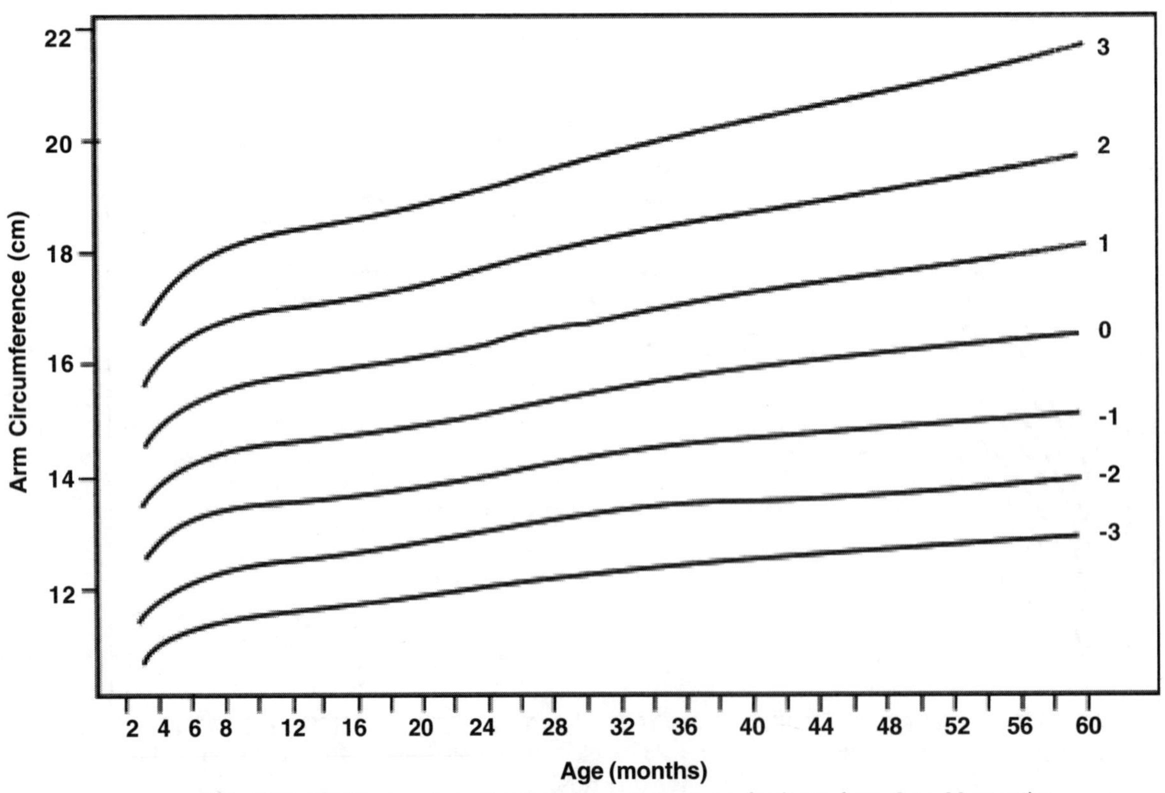

Fig. 6.41: WHO arm circumference-for-age z-scores for boys from 3 to 60 months

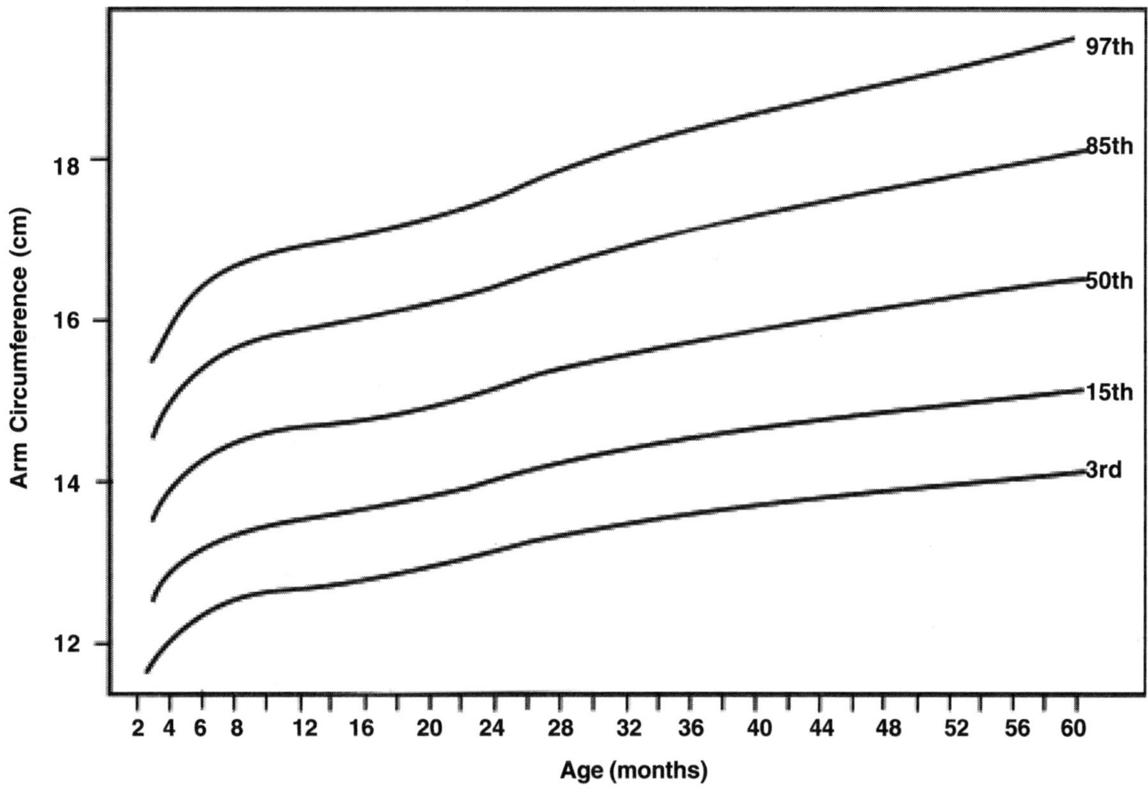

Fig. 42: WHO arm circumference-for-age percentiles for boys from 3 to 60 months

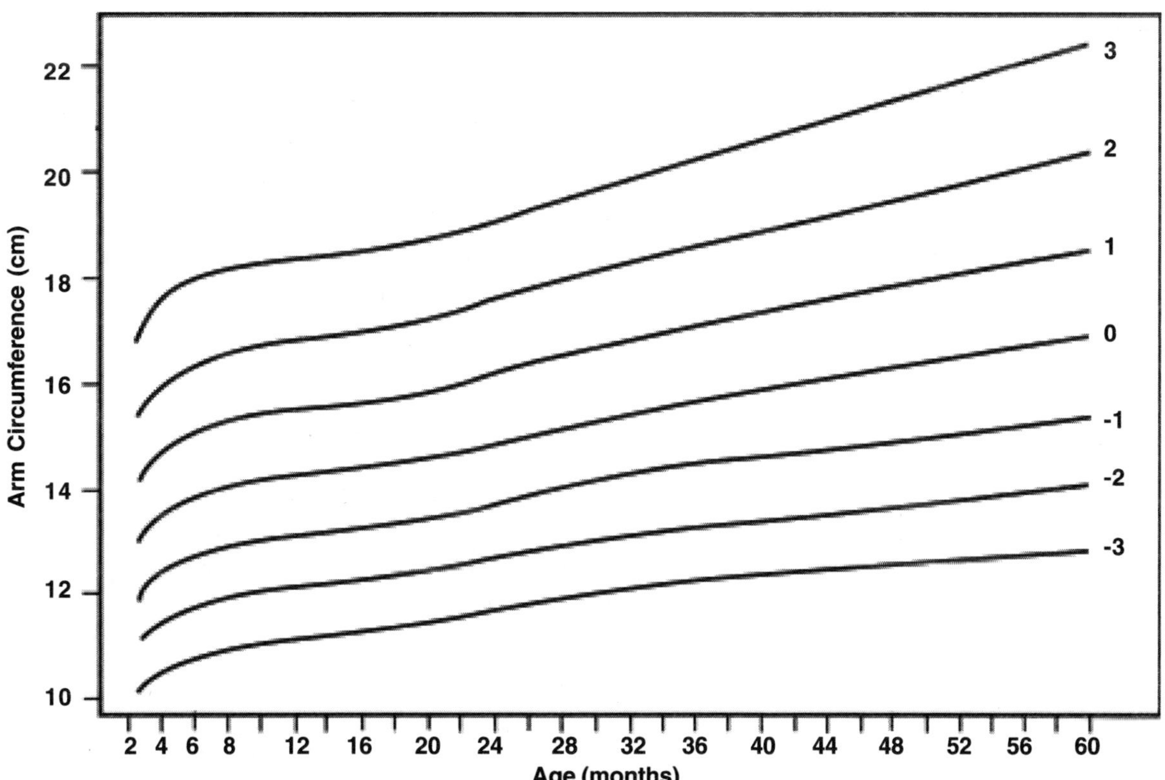

Fig. 6.43: WHO arm circumference-for-age z-scores for girls from 3 to 60 months

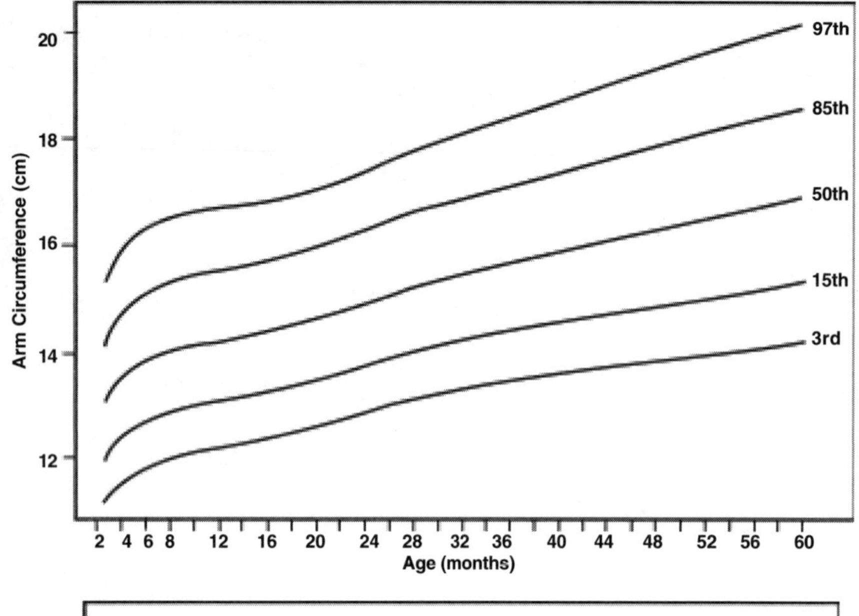

Fig. 6.44: WHO arm circumference-for-age percentiles for girls from 3 to 60 months

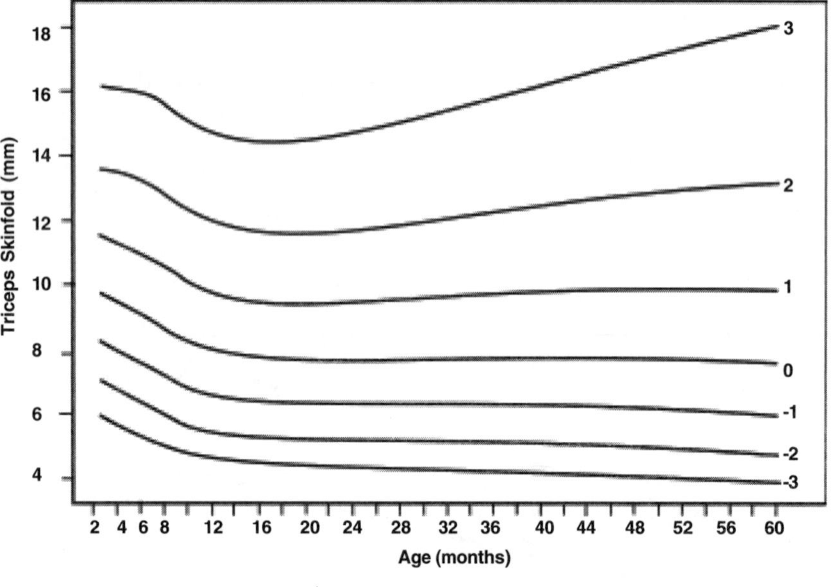

Fig. 6.45: WHO triceps skinfold-for-age z-scores for boys from 3 to 60 months

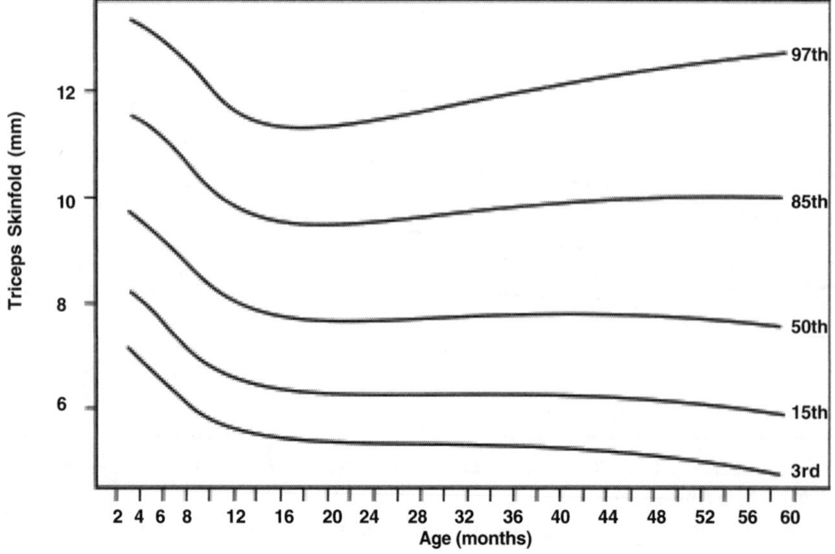

Fig. 6.46: WHO triceps skinfold-for-age percentiles for boys from 3 to 60 months

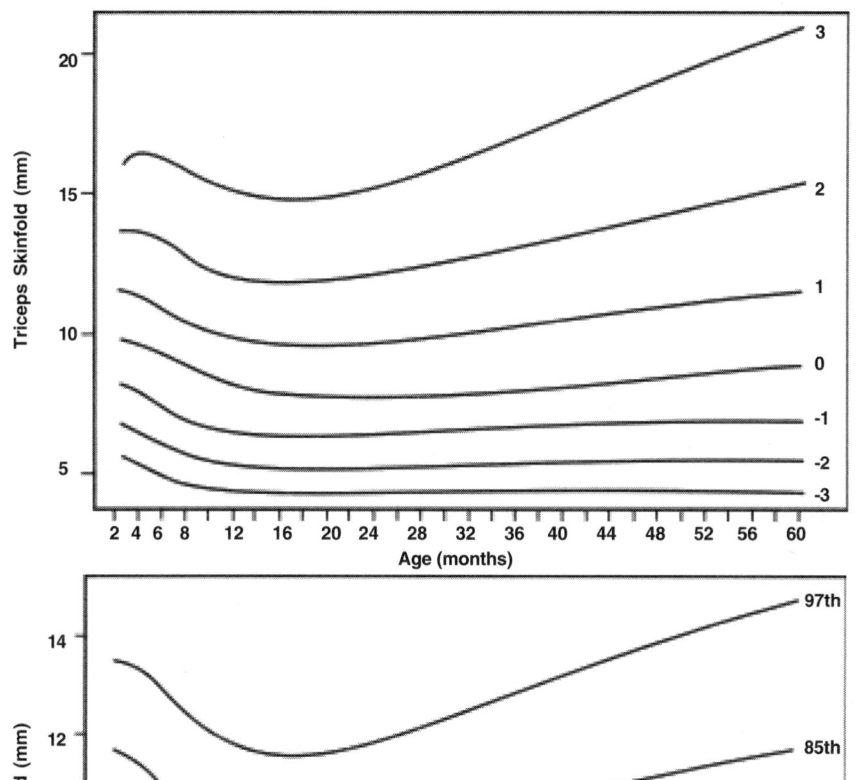

Fig. 6.47: WHO triceps skinfold-for-age z-scores for girls from 3 to 60 months

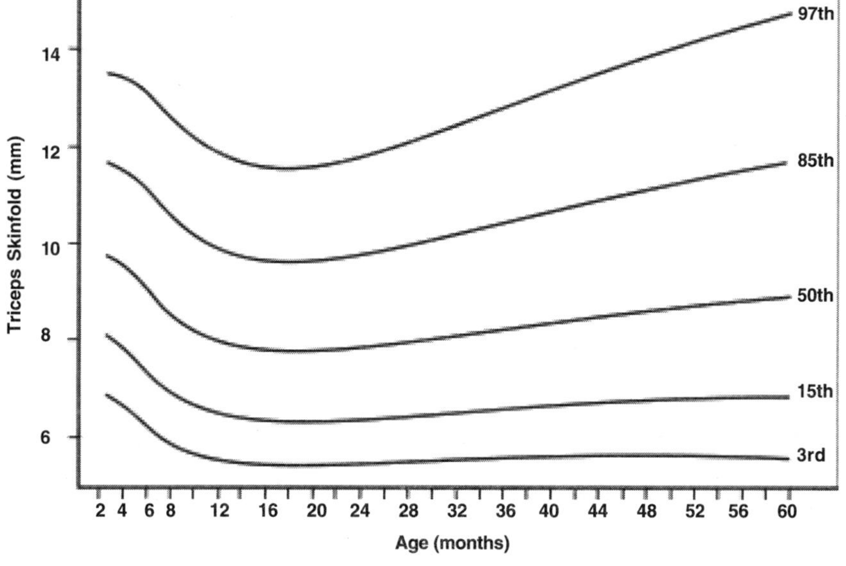

Fig. 6.48: WHO triceps skinfold-for-age percentiles for girls from 3 to 60 months

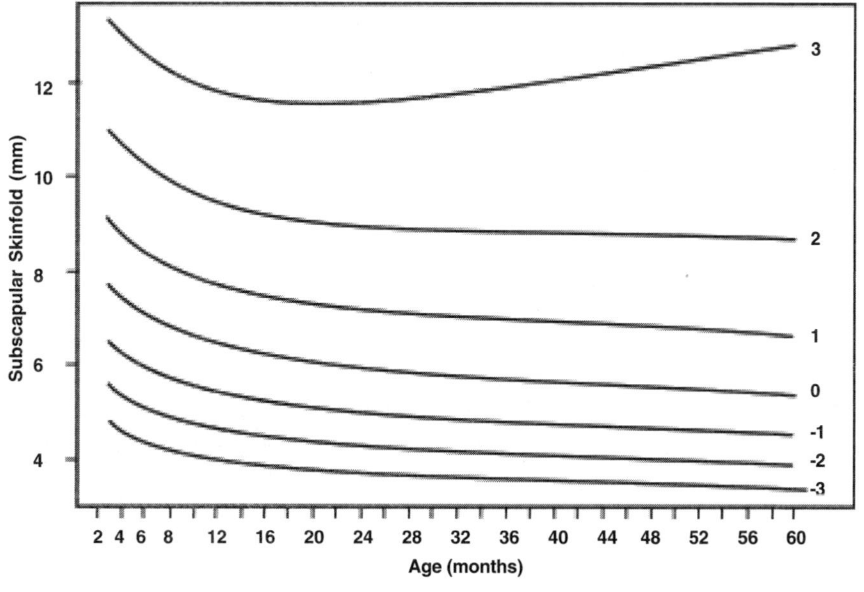

Fig. 6.49: WHO subscapular skinfold-for-age z-scores for boys from 3 to 60 months

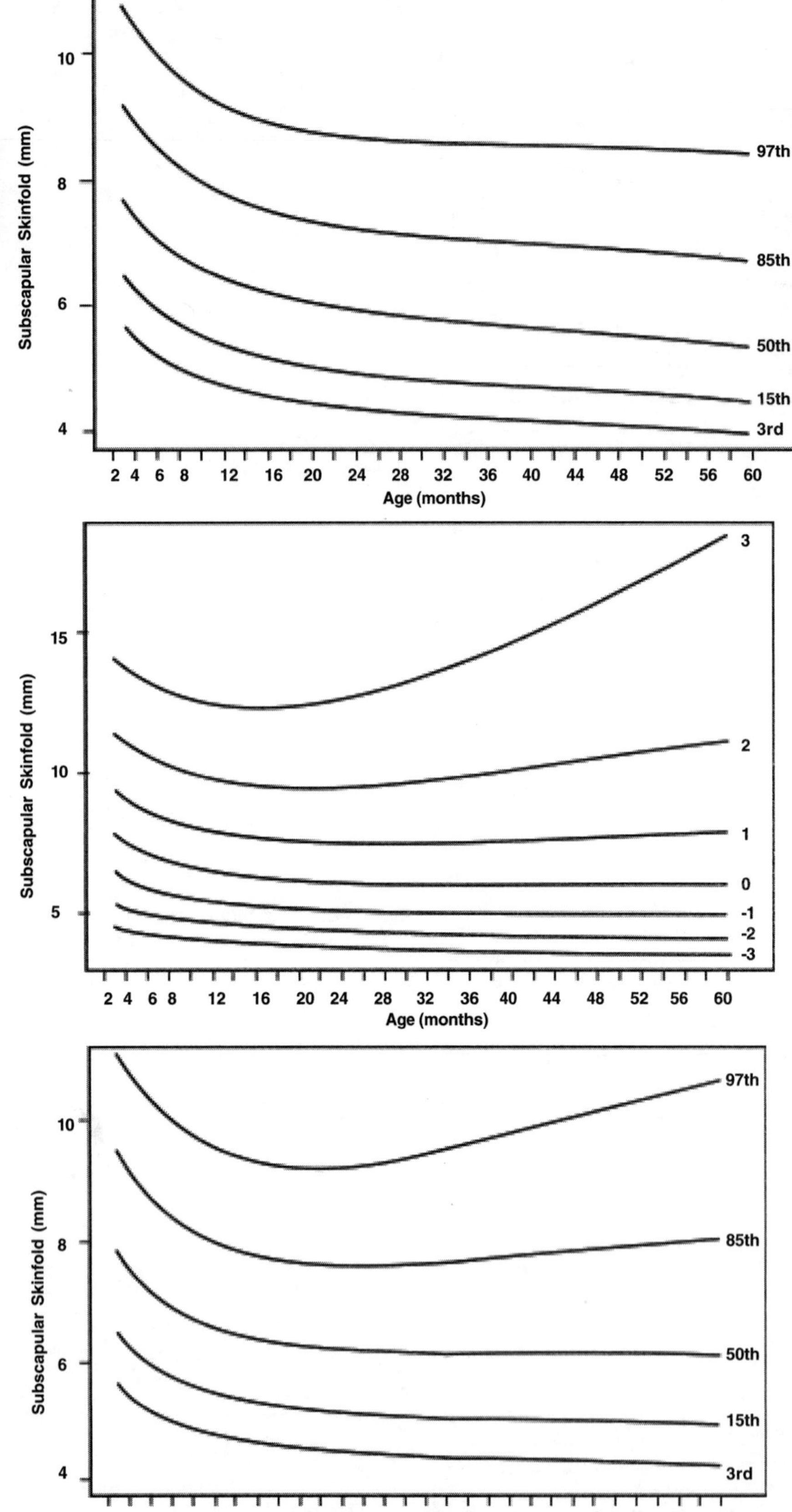

Fig. 6.50: WHO subscapular skinfold-for-age percentiles for boys from 3 to 60 months

Fig. 6.51: WHO subscapular skinfold-for-age z-scores for girls from 3 to 60 months

Fig. 6.52: WHO subscapular skinfold-for-age percentiles for girls from 3 to 60 months

NC Prajapati

7 Nutrition and Cognitive Development

INTRODUCTION

The semantic, *cognitive development*, covers human perception, thinking and learning. In addition to the genes and the environment, nutrition plays a great role in ones cognitive development. Nutrition affects cognitive development of a child right from the intrauterine life. Thereafter, nutrition during the early years of child's life has been linked with the performance in later years of life. During schooling and adolescence too, nutrition has been found to play a very important role in the cognitive development. The present review discusses some of the major research findings linking nutrition and cognitive development.

COGNITION AND COGNITIVE DEVELOPMENT[1-2]

Cognition and cognitive processes are described as higher mental functions and include perception, discovery, recognition, imaging, judging, memorizing, thinking and speech. Just like knowledge, cognition refers to a human activity, which is intellectual and communicable.

We learn about our world through listening, observing, copying and experimenting. The learning starts immediately after birth, the child is the active participant in learning process through reaching and grasping objects, copying sounds and actions etc. Piaget, a Swiss psychologist proposed a comprehensive theory about cognitive development as early as 1929. His theory states that cognitive development is the result of interaction between the individual and environment. These views still remain as the most useful account of cognitive development despite several criticisms.

Cognitive assessment can be done using several checklists, IQ tests, developmental scales and tests of specific cognitive skills. Many of these tests used for assessment in developing countries are based on western tests and have been modified, adapted and standardized using local norms. They, therefore have certain limitations when drawing conclusions out of them.

UNDERNUTRITION AND COGNITIVE DEVELOPMENT[3-9]

Nutrition is important for the survival and functioning of the body. Good nutrition in addition to promoting proper growth also provides first line of defense against several childhood diseases. It also improves their ability to learn, communicate, think analytically, socialize effectively and adapt to new environments and people. As regards cognitive development, "when there isn't enough food, the body has to make a decision about how to invest the limited foodstuffs available". Survival comes first, growth comes second. In this nutritional triage, the body seems obliged to rank learning last—"Better to be stupid and alive than smart and dead".

Malnutrition is state wherein adapt nutrients are not delivered to the cells to provide the substrate for optimal functioning. Malnutrition includes both under-nutrition and over-nutrition but in children under-nutrition is a major problem.

Undernutrition affects the physical dimensions of the body as well as the psychosocial development. It adversely influences various biochemical and physiological functions of the body and through them the functions of the brain. The relationship between malnutrition and psychological development was recognized as early as 1955 by Jelliffe.[3] The studies, thereafter, on the subject also indicated that persistent malnutrition in children was associated with low IQ and behavioral and psychological problems. Nutrition alone is probably not responsible because, these problems though reversible to a great extent with nutritional rehabilitation, are also influenced by parental and socio-economic factors.[4-7]

There are three theories associating growth and genetic potential. Primary or secondary deprivations of food or nutrients lead to decrement in growth. This growth decrement could also be associated with functional impairment.

Deprivation Theory

According to the deprivation theory, everyone is born with a genetically determined potential growth curve. If well-nourished, the child continues to grow along that curve. Anyone below the 'maximal' curve is malnourished and may show functional impairment.

Homeostatic Theory

It states that the genetic mechanism provides a potential growth space. A child grows within the boundaries of this space in response to nutritional and environmental experiences. There are, therefore, several bands or trajectories of growth curve rather than a single curve.

Third Theory

This theory states that genetic determination regulates the growth potential of an individual through homeostatic boundaries. An individual is healthy as long as he/she is within these homeostatic boundaries. Exceeding either way outside or the edges of the boundaries (i.e. over and under-nutrition); the system becomes unstable and detrimental to health and function. The maximum level compatible with homeostasis is as bad as minimum level.

Undernutrition in young children can have devastating and enduring effects. It can impede behavioral and cognitive development, educability, and reproductive health, thereby undermining future work productivity. As growth failure occurs mainly during the intrauterine period and in the first two years of life, undernutrition during this period of life will have more harmful effects.

Undernutrition can also cause physiological crippling in terms of low birth weight and retarded brain growth, thereby leading to developmental problems. Limited and abnormal interaction and lack of adequate stimulation for such physiologically crippled children might be other factors hampering healthy development. Malnutrition is also linked directly with childhood mortality as over half of child mortality in developing countries is attributed to malnutrition.

In chronically undernourished children body energy is first reserved for maintenance of critical organ function, second for growth, and last for social activity and cognitive development. As a result, undernourished children decrease their activity levels and become more apathetic. This in turn affects their social interactions, inquisitiveness, and overall cognitive functioning. Even nutritional deficiencies of a relatively short-term nature influence children's behavior, ability to concentrate, and to perform complex tasks.

In short, undernutrition can impair cognitive and behavioral development by:

- Delaying physical growth and motor development.
- General effects on cognitive development—lowering IQs (lower by 15 points or more in the severely malnourished).
- Increasing degree of behavioral problems and deficient social skills at school age, and
- Decreasing attention, learning, and educational achievement.

Much of the human research in this area has been conducted in developing countries where undernutrition is severe, manifested by two major syndromal states, namely kwashiorkor and marasmus. Scientific understanding of the nutrition-cognition relationship has evolved over time. Early studies on the relationship between nutritional deficits and brain function were guided by a "main effect" theory. This theory held that early exposure to a biological risk factor such as undernutrition during critical periods of brain growth could result in actual neurological trauma and permanent developmental abnormalities. The extent of neurological damage was thought to be directly related to the magnitude of undernutrition. Recent evidence indicates that malnutrition alone does not necessarily cause cognitive alterations. E.g. Children malnourished due to illness generally do not show developmental delays associated with their malnutrition, whereas such delays are evident among malnourished children living in poverty.

One school of thought believes that malnutrition alone does not cause irreversible damage to the brain. The long-term cognitive impairment is also not necessarily due to alteration of brain structure itself, although evidence is insufficient to rule out structural damage altogether.

Cognitive deficits related to undernutrition are now believed to result from complex interactions between environmental insults and undernutrition. The longer a child's nutritional, emotional and educational needs go unmet, the greater the overall cognitive deficits. Continuous low nutritional intake, usually affects psychological factors such as motivation, attentiveness and emotional expression. These in turn, may have a negative effect on critical developmental processes including parent-child interaction, attachment, and play and eventually learning. But unless major and irreparable physiological insult has occurred, improved nutrition and conditions in the social environment can modify the developmental effects of biological and social risk factors to which the child is exposed in early life.

In addition to favorable qualities in a child's environment, nutritional supplementation can modify and, in some instances rectify, cognitive impairment caused by earlier undernutrition. In general new research findings show that lack of sufficient food during childhood, even on a relatively mild basis, is far more serious than previously thought. It can produce cognitive impairments in children which may last a lifetime. But the evidence also suggests that adequate nutrition can prevent many of these undesirable outcomes, and is capable of modifying harm that actually has occurred.

NUTRIENTS RESPONSIBLE FOR COGNITIVE AND BEHAVIORAL IMPAIRMENTS[4-8]

Nutrient deficiencies tend to occur in combination. Isolating the specific contributions of single nutrient deficiency as the causative factor, is difficult to elicit and prove. Iodine and iron deficiencies have been extensively studied and concluded that both of these micronutrients are involved specifically in causing impairments.

Anemia is one of the most prevalent nutritional disorders in the world, affecting nearly one quarter of all low-income children. Recent research shows that iron deficiency anemia has an adverse effect on a child's ability to learn by influencing attention span and memory. This pervasive deficiency is now known to have a severe impact on cognitive development. Beyond its independent effect on cognitive development, iron deficiency anemia puts children at higher risk of lead poisoning. Scientific evidence shows that high lead levels result in neurodevelopmental disorders. Low-income children face a double jeopardy—they are more likely to be anemic and more likely to live in an environment where the risk of lead poisoning is high.

POVERTY, NUTRITION AND COGNITION[4,5]

Poverty, nutrition and cognition are closely linked. The primary factor associated with poor nutritional status is poverty. This is accompanied with inadequacy of family resources and a range of other environmental insults associated with poverty like poor housing, inadequate health care, unemployment and weakened family and community support systems. Interaction of these factors with undernutrition impedes a child's healthy development. The programmes aimed at protecting children's health and cognitive development therefore needs to be comprehensive. Addressing health care, or education, or housing or nutritional needs alone will not be of any help.

Undernutrition along with environmental factors associated with poverty can permanently retard physical growth, brain development, and cognitive functioning. Poor children who attend school hungry perform significantly below non-hungry low income peers on standardized test scores. There exists a strong association between family income and the growth and cognitive development of children. Improved nutrition and environmental conditions can modify the effects of early undernutrition.

MATERNAL UNDERNUTRITION, BREASTFEEDING AND COGNITIVE DEVELOPMENT[6-8]

Undernutrition begins to exact its toll even before the child is born. Pregnant women who are undernourished are more likely to have low birthweight babies. Along with other health risks that are common to low birthweight babies, these infants are more likely to suffer developmental delays. In the case of very low birthweight infants, permanent cognitive deficiencies associated with small head circumference may reflect diminished brain growth. When children reach school age, developmental delays associated with pre- and post-natal malnutrition often results in a greater need for costly special education services.

SCHOOL BREAKFAST AND LUNCH[6-9]

Undernourished children typically are fatigued and uninterested in their social environment. Compared with their well-nourished peers, they are less likely to establish relationships or explore and learn from their surroundings. Being more susceptible to illness (due to undernutrition) they are more likely to be absent from school.

Children who attend school hungry have diminished attention spans and are unable to perform tasks as well as their nourished peers. In these cases, the full value of the education provided is lost. The children must therefore be encouraged to take their breakfast and lunch regularly.

The Losses

Increasing independence and the development of social skills are central to a child's early development. When these activities are curtailed due to undernutrition, the child's overall cognitive development is threatened.

Effects of undernutrition cost far more than the diminished wellbeing of youngsters during childhood. It robs the children of their natural human potential and results in lost knowledge, brainpower and productivity for the nation. The longer and more severe the malnutrition, the greater are the likely loss and the greater is the cost to the country.

By virtue of chronic undernutrition, cognitive limitations and behavioral impairments educational experiences and later adult productive capacity are affected. These are the lifelong "lost opportunities".

Nutritionally-deprived children are unable to benefit fully from schooling. Poor performance early in school/dropping out of school in later years diminishes their potential as adults. The nation has to subsequently pay the cost indirectly through lost contributions, and directly through the provision of additional social welfare services.

INTERVENTIONS[6-9]

Undernutrition is preventable and its effects often modifiable. Nutrition and prenatal care for women reduces the incidence of low birthweight babies and subsequent developmental delays associated with that condition. Iron repletion therapy can reverse some of the effects of anemia on learning, attention and memory. And research consistently establishes that federal initiatives such as the School Breakfast Program and the Special Supplemental Food Program for Women, Infants and Children (WIC) have positive effects on the cognitive development of children. The benefits include higher performance on standardized tests, better school attendance, lowered incidence of anemia, and reduced need for costly special education.

For the nutritional management therefore the safest course for ensuring cognitive and behavioral development would be to meet all nutrient needs with natural or fortified foods prepared appropriately for young children. The benefits of breastfeeding are undoubted and must be considered and emphasized in fostering growth and development. Nutrition interventions must begin during pregnancy and specially cared for during first 2-3 years of life. For those who have suffered severe malnutrition considerable evidence indicates that substantial improvements can be achieved, even in them if appropriate steps are taken at a young age to satisfy nutritional and psychosocial needs. The longer the developmental delays remain uncorrected, the greater the chance of permanent effects. Long-term studies indicate that nutrition interventions in the first few years of life lead to measurable improvements in adolescence and adulthood.

Intervention programs to stimulate cognition have shown to improve cognition and physical growth both. The earlier these programs are started, the better are the results. Children who receive combined nutrition and stimulation programs perform better than those who receive either type of intervention alone. Iron repletion therapy can reduce some of the effects of anemia on learning, attention and memory. Supplemental feeding programs can help to offset threats posed to the child's capacity to learn and perform in school which result from inadequate nutrient intake. Once undernutrition occurs, its long-term effects may be reduced or eliminated by a combination of adequate food intake and environmental (home, school) support.

PARENTS ROLE

Mother should take adequate nutrition before and during pregnancy. She must continue the same during lactation period too. Once the child has arrived, the infant must receive adequate nutrition. They themselves should be good role models for their children. They should plan well balanced nutritious meals taking into considerations child's likes and dislikes, in order to develop good eating habits.

NUTRITION PROGRAMS FOR CHILDREN[7-9]

There are networks of nutrition programs that are developed with the underlying aim to protect all who are vulnerable to the harmful effects of undernutrition. In US the major nutrition programs targeted to children include Special Supplemental Food Program for Women, Infants and Children (WIC), School Breakfast, School Lunch, Summer Food Service Program, The Food Stamp Program, Child and Adult Care Food Program.

These programs safeguard the health of pregnant, postpartum and breastfeeding women, infants and children under five years of age. They have proven to be cost effective as demonstrated that by decreasing the number of low birthweight babies born and the need for medical aid, and the long-term benefits include protection of a child's cognitive development. The incidence of anemia has been found to decrease by these programs. The School Breakfast Program has demonstrated improvements in academic functioning among low-income elementary school children. Further it has led to reduced absence and tardiness rates.

COMBATING UNDERNUTRITION—INDIAN PROGRAMS[6,7]

In India malnutrition is a social disease of multifactorial etiology and would require actions at various levels in a coordinate manner.

a. Action at family level
   - Promotion of breastfeeding.
   - Correct infant and child rearing practices.
   - Integrated Management of Neonatal and Childhood Illnesses.
   - Nutritional attention to pregnant and lactating mothers (Nutritional supplementation, anemia prophylaxis, birth spacing).

b. Action at community level
   - Supplementary feeding programs.
   - Mid day school meals.
   - Applied nutrition program.

c. Action at national level
   - Supplementary feeding programs
   - Mid day school meals.
   - Environmental sanitation and education.
   - Population control.
   - Nutritional interventional programs.
   - Immunizations.

SUMMARY AND CONCLUSION

Inadequate nutrition harms the cognitive development of children in ways that may produce lasting damage. The damage can occur at all stages starting from conception. Undernutrition—even in its "milder" forms—during any period of childhood can have detrimental effects on the cognitive development of children and their later productivity as adults. It harms children silently. There is a need to recognize the hazards of this modifiable factor and take necessary measures.

REFERENCES

1. Borel MJ. Cognition. In: Eysenck HI, Arnold WJ, Meili R (eds): *Encyclopedia of Psychology*. London: Fontana 1975;177-178.

2. Grantham-McGregor SM. Assessments of the effects of nutrition on mental development and behavior in Jamaican studies. *Am J Clin Nutr* 1993; 57: 303S-309S.
3. Jelliffe DB. *Infant Malnutrition in the Subtropics and Tropics*. Geneva: World Health Organization 1955.
4. Martin SL, Ramey CT, Ramey S. The Prevention of intellectual impairment in children of impoverished families: Findings of a randomized trial of educational day care. *Am J Publ Health* 1990;80:844-847.
5. Pollitt E. Poverty and child development: Relevance of research in developing to the United States. *Child Develop* 1994;65:283-295.
6. Gupte S, Gomez EM. Protein-energy malnutrition. In: Gupte S (ed): *The Short Textbook of Pediatrics*, 11th edn. New Delhi: Jaypee 2004: 129-153.
7. Hendarto SK. Nutrition and developing brain. In: Gupte S (ed): *Recent Advances in Pediatrics*-2. New Delhi: Jaypee 1991:201-215.
8. Aggarwal KN. Nutritional needs. In: *Pediatrics and Neonatology*. New Delhi: Modern 2000:296-312.
9. Park K. Nutrition and health. In: *Park's Textbook of Preventive and Social Medicine*, 21st edn. Jabalpur: Banarsidas Bhanot 2005:438-487.

Harish Chellani • Sugandha Arya

8 Breastfeeding: The Supreme Gift

INTRODUCTION

It is a well-established fact that best milk for a neonate is the breast milk. It is estimated that over one million children die each year from diarrhea, respiratory and other infections because they are not adequately breastfed. The program for the control of diarrheal diseases has long recognised the need to promote breastfeeding to prevent diarrhea in young children. More recently, it has become clear that breastfeeding is important also in the management of diarrhea, to prevent dehydration, and to promote recovery.

This chapter deals with the:

- Advantages of breastfeeding,
- Breastfeeding technique,
- Common problems in breastfeeding, and
- Technique to express breast milk.

ADVANTAGES OF BREASTFEEDING

The advantages of breastfeeding are more than just the advantages of feeding a baby on breast milk. Breastfeeding protects the mother's health in several ways, and can benefit the whole family, emotionally and economically.

Advantages for the Baby

- It contains exactly the nutrients that a baby needs for optimum growth and development of a baby during the first six months. It has a high percentage of lactose and the galactose, an important component of galacto-cerebroside, which is essential for brain growth. It also facilitates absorption of calcium. It contains aminoacids like taurine and cysteine which are important neuro-transmitters. The fats are mostly polyunsaturated fatty acids, which are necessary for myelination of the central nervous system. Breast milk contains hormones and epidermal growth factors, which are necessary for the maturation of the intestinal tract.
- It is easily digested and efficiently used by the baby's body. The proteins of breast milk are mostly lactalbumin and lactoglobulin (more than 60%) that form a soft curd and easy to digest. The enzyme lipase in the breastmilk helps in the digestion of fats.
- It protects a baby against infections. Breast milk contains a number of protective factors, which include IgA, macrophages, lymphocytes, bifidus factor, unsaturated lactoferrin, lysozyme, complement and interferon etc. The baby who takes other foods before 6 months gets sick more often and has a bigger chance of getting infection such as diarrhea or pneumonia.[1] Breastfed babies are less likely to develop infections. A breastfed baby is 14.2 times less likely to die of diarrhea and 3.6 times less likely to die of respiratory infections. If every baby were exclusively breastfed from birth, about 1.5 million lives would be saved each year.[2]
- Other benefits for the baby: Breastfeeding protects against allergies, including asthma. It enhances emotional bonding between mother and baby. Studies have demonstrated that breastfed babies have a higher IQ and have less chance of developing hypertension, diabetes mellitus, coronary heart disease, appendicitis, liver disease and even cancer in later life.

Composition of the Breast Milk

The composition of breast milk is not always the same. It varies according to the age of the baby and from the beginning to the end of a feed. It also varies between feeds, and may be different at different times of the day.

Colostrum is the breast milk that women produce in the first few days after delivery. It is thick and yellowish in color. It contains more antibodies, white blood cells and other anti-infective proteins than mature milk. These anti-infective proteins and white cells provide the first immunization against the diseases that a baby meets after delivery. The antibodies probably also help to prevent a baby from developing allergies. Colostrum has a mild purgative effect, which helps to clear the baby's gut of meconium. This clears bilirubin from the gut and also helps to prevent jaundice (decreases enterohepatic circulation).

Mature milk: After a few days, colostrum changes into mature milk. This is larger amount of milk and the breasts feel full, hard and heavy during this milk. The mature milk consists of "Foremilk" which is bluish milk and is produced early in a feed, whereas "Hindmilk" is the whiter milk and is produced later in a feed. The extra fat in hindmilk makes it looks whiter than foremilk. This fat provides much of the energy of a breastfeed and satisfy the baby's satiety. The foremilk is produced in large amounts and it provides plenty of water, protein, lactose, and other nutrients. Because a baby gets larger amount of foremilk, he gets all the water that he needs from it. Babies in very hot and dry climates do not need other fluids if they breastfeed exclusively and on demand.[3,4] It is important to remember that baby must have both foremilk and hindmilk to get a complete "meal", and all the water that he needs. The breast milk contains the adequate amount of vitamins and minerals that a baby needs during first 6 months of life.

Advantages for the Mother

- Breastfeeding accelerates the process of involution of uterus, reducing chances of postpartum hemorrhage.
- It helps delaying the next pregnancy. It provides 98% protection against pregnancy if the baby is exclusively breastfed during first four months of life.
- It lowers the risk of breast and ovarian cancer in mother.
- It also decreases mother's workload involved in preparation of artificial feeds.

Advantages for the Family and the Society

- Breastfeeding is more economical than artificial feeding.
- It promotes family planning.
- Since it decreases the risk of infection in infants, the need for their hospitalization is also reduced. Hence it contributes to reduction in infant morbidity and mortality.

BREASTFEEDING PRACTICES TO BE RECOMMENDED

General

- Ensure exclusive breastfeeding during first 6 months of life.
- Start breastfeeding within ½ - 1 hour of birth. Most babies are ready to feed for the first time from 15-55 mins after birth.[5]
- Don't give baby ghutti, gripe water, honey, animal or powdered milk. Babies reduce breastfeeding if they get other foods.[6,7]
- Breastfeed day and night at least eight times or whenever he cries with hunger. Allow baby to feed at one breast till he leaves the nipple on his own. Then feed him at the other breast if he continues to be hungry.
- Give complementary foods from 6 months of age.
- Continue breastfeeding upto 2 years of age or beyond.

If the Mother is HIV Positive

The baby of a mother who is HIV positive has about 1 in 7 (15%) chance of getting the HIV infection through breastfeeding. The HIV positive mother faces a difficult situation because of the possible risk of transmission that breastfeeding carries.

The risk of HIV transmission through breastfeeding is less:

- If the baby breastfeeds exclusively.
- If the mother seeks immediate care for cracked nipples or breast infections.
- If the baby is breastfed for only a few months.
- If the mother and the baby are given anti-retroviral medications.

When resources are limited, feeding the newborn with breast milk substitutes may be riskier than breastfeeding by an HIV positive mother. Top feeding in low resource areas causes many infant deaths due to diarrhea, malnutrition and other infections. In ideal conditions, however, it is possible to successfully feed an infant with commercial formula, or animal milk, although this is not easy and may be expensive.

The World Health Organisation, the Joint United Nations Program on HIV/AIDS, and the United Nations Children's Fund recommend that a woman with HIV should be given all the information on the risks and benefits of the different feeding options and then support the woman's feeding choice.[8]

ANATOMY AND PHYSIOLOGY OF LACTATION

For a better understanding of breastfeeding practice, its technique and problems, it is important to know the relevant anatomy and physiology of breast.[11-13]

The breast consists of partly glandular tissue and partly supporting tissue and fat. Milk is secreted by the gland and travels through tubules, which drain, into lactiferous sinuses. The sinuses, which store small quantities of milk, lie below the areola. They open out on to the nipple through lactiferous ducts. The thin layer of muscle (myo-epithelium) surrounds each gland. The contraction of these muscles causes ejection of milk from the glands (Fig. 8.1).

Physiology of lactation is determined by two hormones, Prolactin and oxytocin, secreted in the mother and reflexes in the baby. Prolactin helps in milk production and oxytocin helps in ejection of milk.

a. **Prolactin reflex:** Prolactin is produced by the anterior pituitary gland, which is responsible for milk secretion by the mammary gland cells. The production of the hormone is stimulated when the baby sucks at the breast. When the baby sucks, the nerve endings in the nipple carry messages to the anterior pituitary, which in turn release prolactin. This hormone passes through the blood to the glands in the breast, promoting milk secretion.

Section 3

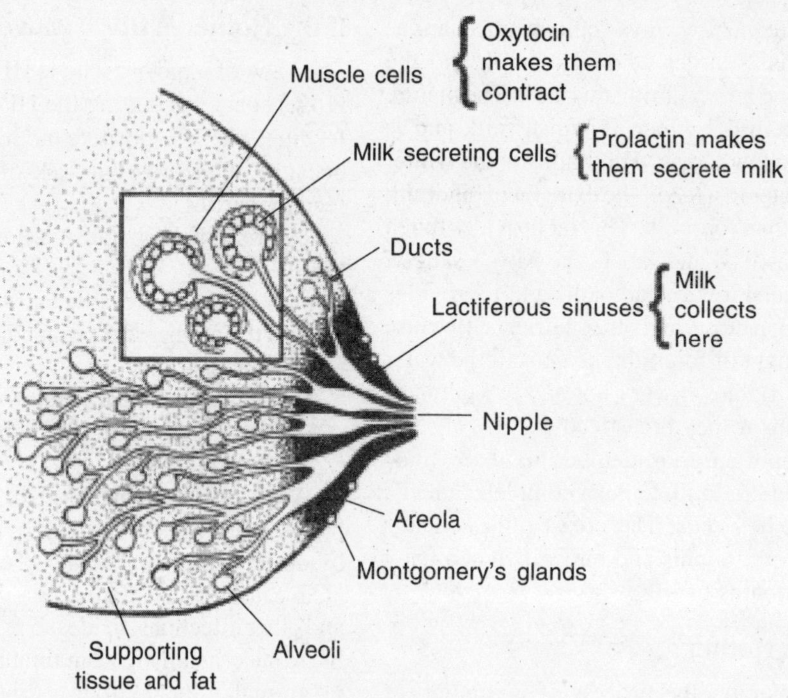

Fig. 8.1: Anatomy of the breast

This cycle from stimulation to secretion is called the prolactin reflex or the 'milk secretion reflex'. The more the baby sucks at the breast, the greater is the stimulus for milk production. The earlier the baby is put to the breast, the sooner the reflex is initiated. Most of the prolactin is in the blood about 30 minutes after the feed, so it makes the breast produce milk for the next feed. The greater is the demand for milk; larger is the volume of milk produced. It is therefore important for the mothers to feed baby early, frequently and ensure complete emptying of the breasts at each feed. Most women can produce more milk than their babies' need or take. If a mother has two babies, and they both suckle, then breasts make milk for two.

Some special things to remember about prolactin are:

- More prolactin is produced at night; so breastfeeding at night is especially helpful for keeping up the milk supply.
- Prolactin makes a mother feel relaxed, and sometimes sleepy; so usually rests well even if she breastfeeds at night (Fig. 8.2).

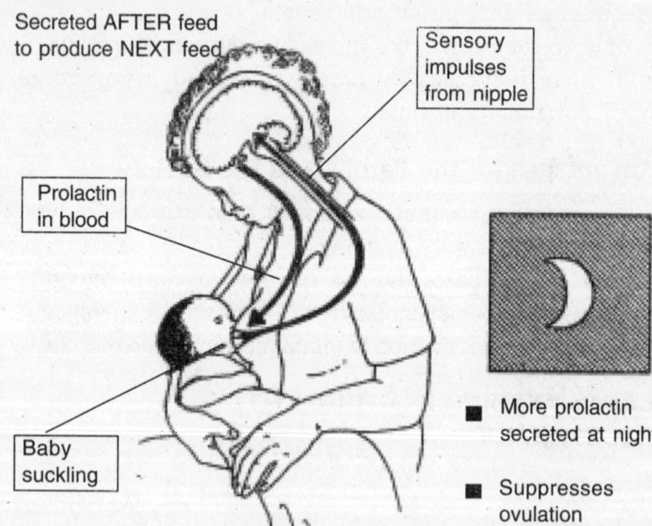

Fig. 8.2: Prolactin reflex

b. **Oxytocin reflex:** Oxytocin is a hormone produced by the posterior pituitary. It is responsible for the contraction of the myoepithelium around the glands leading to ejection of the milk from the glands into the lacteal sinuses and the lacteal ducts. This hormone is produced in response to stimulation of the nerve endings in the nipple by sucking as well as by the thought, sight or sound of the baby. Oxytocin is produced more quickly than prolactin. It makes the milk in the breast flow for the feed. Oxytocin can start working before a baby suckles, when a mother learns to expect a feed. Since this reflex is affected by the mother's emotions, a relaxed, confident, attitude helps this 'milk ejection reflex'. On the other hand, tension, pain and lack of confidence, hinders the milk flow. This stresses the importance of a kind and supportive person—professional health worker or a relative—to reassure the mother and help gain

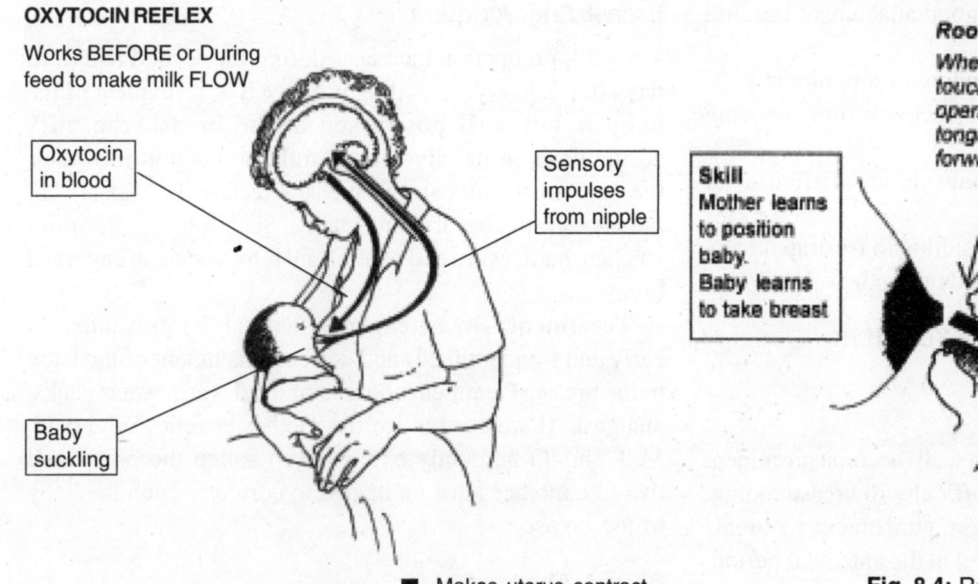

Fig. 8.3: Oxytocin reflex

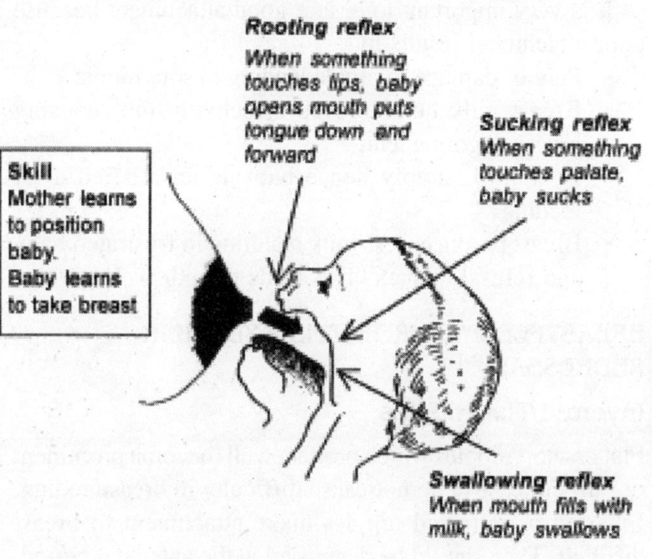

Fig. 8.4: Reflexes in the baby

confidence so that she can successfully breastfeed. Another important point about oxytocin is that it makes a mother's uterus contract after delivery. This helps to reduce bleeding, but it sometimes causes uterine pain and a rush of blood during a feed for the first few days (Fig. 8.3).

c. **Reflexes in the baby:** Rooting, sucking and swallowing reflexes help the baby to take the milk secreted from the breast. When something touches a baby's lip or cheek, he opens his mouth and may turn his head to find it. He puts his tongue down and forward. This is the "rooting" reflex. It should normally be the breast that he is "rooting" for. When something touches a baby's palate, he starts to suck it, and when his mouth fills with milk, he swallows. All these are reflexes, which happen automatically without the baby having to learn to do them (Fig. 8.4).

BREASTFEEDING TECHNIQUE

Breastfeeding is natural and most mothers take to it without any problem. There are many ways to breastfeed and each mother develops her own style to suit her baby. However, few mothers need some assistance in positioning the baby and attaching to breast. For a mother to produce enough milk, her baby must suckle often enough, and he must also suckle in the right way.

a. **Correct positioning** is important because it will ensure effective suckling and prevent sore nipples and breast engorgement. Proper position of the baby while breastfeeding involves:
   1. Supporting whole of baby's body.
   2. Keeping the head, neck and body of the baby in the same plane.
   3. Entire baby body should face the mother.
   4. Baby's abdomen should touch mother's abdomen (Fig. 8.5).

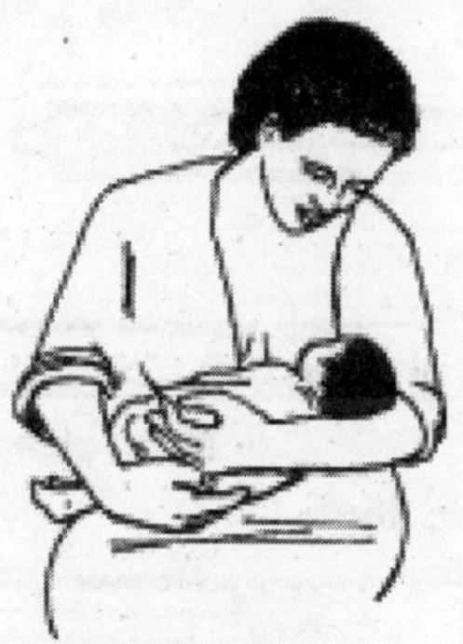

Fig. 8.5: Correct positioning

b. **Attachment of baby on mother's breast:** Four signs of good attachment are:
   1. Baby mouth wide open.
   2. Lower lip turned outwards.
   3. Baby's chin touches mother's breast.
   4. Majority of areola inside (Fig. 8.6).

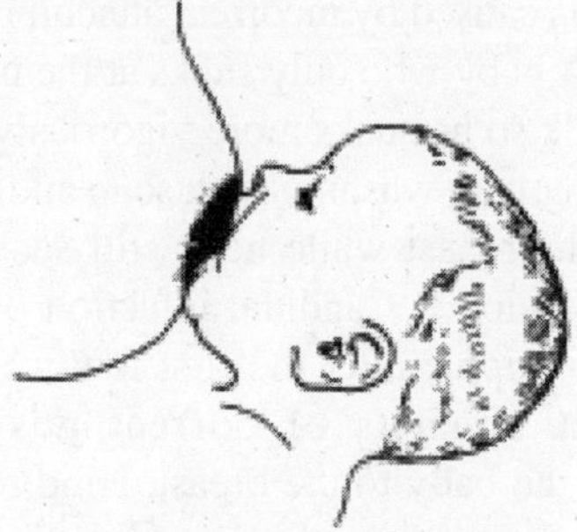

Fig. 8.6: Good attachment

It is very important to ensure good attachment because poor attachment results in:

- Pain or damage to nipple leading to sore nipple.
- Breast milk not removed effectively thus causing breast engorgement.
- Poor milk supply hence baby is unsatisfied after feeding.
- Breast produces less milk resulting in frustrated baby and refusal to suck. This leads to poor weight gain.

BREASTFEEDING PROBLEMS AND THEIR REDRESSAL[14-16]

Inverted/Flat Nipples

Flat or short nipples which protract well (become prominent or pull out easily) do not cause difficulty in breastfeeding. Inverted or retracted nipples make attachment to breast difficult. They should be diagnosed in the antenatal period. These mothers need additional support to feed their babies.

Treatment is started after birth of the baby. Nipple is manually stretched and rolled out several times a day. A plastic syringe is used to draw out the nipple and the baby is then put to the breast.

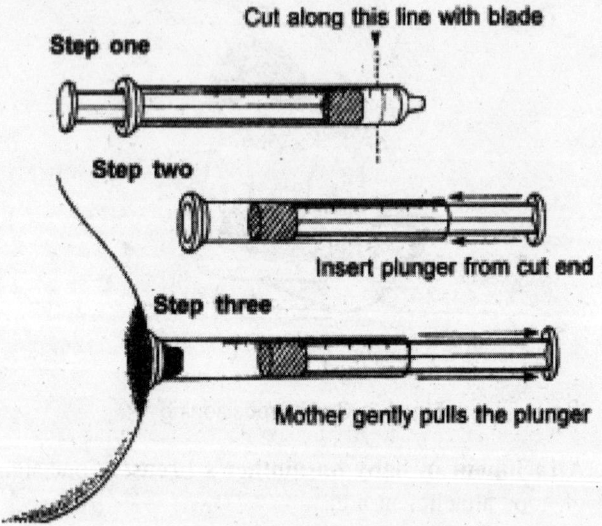

Fig. 8.7: Preparing and using a syringe for treatment of inverted nipples

Sore Nipple

A sore nipple is caused by incorrect attachment of the baby to the breast. A baby who only sucks at the nipple does not get enough milk so he sucks more vigorously resulting in a sore nipple. Frequent washing with soap and water, pulling the baby off the breast while he is still sucking may also result in a sore nipple. Candidal infection of the nipple is cause of a sore nipple after the first few weeks.

Treatment consists of correct positioning and attachment of the baby to the breast. Hind milk should be applied to the nipple after a feed and the nipples should be aired, to allow healing in between feeds.

Breast Engorgement

The milk production increases during the second and third day after delivery. If feeding is delayed or infrequent or the baby is not well positioned at the breast, the milk accumulates in the alveoli. As milk production increases, the amount of milk in the breast exceeds the capacity of the alveoli to store it comfortably. Such a breast becomes swollen, hard, warm and painful and is termed as an engorged breast.

Treatment: Breast engorgement can be prevented by early and frequent feeds and correct attachment of the baby to the breast. Treatment consists of local warm water packs, analgesic (Paracetamol) to the mother to relieve the pain. Milk should be gently expressed to soften the breast and then the mother must be helped to correctly latch the baby to the breast.

Breast Abscess

If a congested, engorged breast, an infected cracked nipple, or a blocked duct and mastitis are not treated in the early stages, then an infected breast segment may form a breast abscess. The mother may also have high grade fever and a raised blood count.

Treatment: Mother must be treated with analgesics and antibiotics. The abscess is to be incised and drained. Breastfeeding must be continued.

Not Enough Milk

Many mothers complain that they do not have enough milk. Reassurance is needed if baby is gaining weight adequately, passing urine at least 6 times/day and sleeps for 2-3 hrs after each feed.[9] Common causes of not enough milk include—not breastfeeding often enough, too short or hurried breastfeeds, poor suckling position, poor oxytocin reflex, breast engorgement or mastitis.

Treatment: If baby is not gaining weight adequately, ask the mother to feed the baby more frequently and feed especially during night. Make sure that attachment is proper. Any painful condition in mother such as sore nipple, mastitis should be taken care of. Back massages are especially useful for stimulating lactation.

EXPRESSION OF BREAST MILK[9, 10, 17, 18]

There are situations when it becomes mandatory or, at least desirable to resort to expression of breast milk. In olden times, it was usually recommended for relieving breast engorgement. Now it has turned out to be a valuable means of feeding working mothers' babies in their absence as also for feeding babies who cannot suckle well to tide over the difficult passing phase.

It is, therefore, useful for all mothers to know how to express and store their milk. Expression of breast milk is required in the following situations:

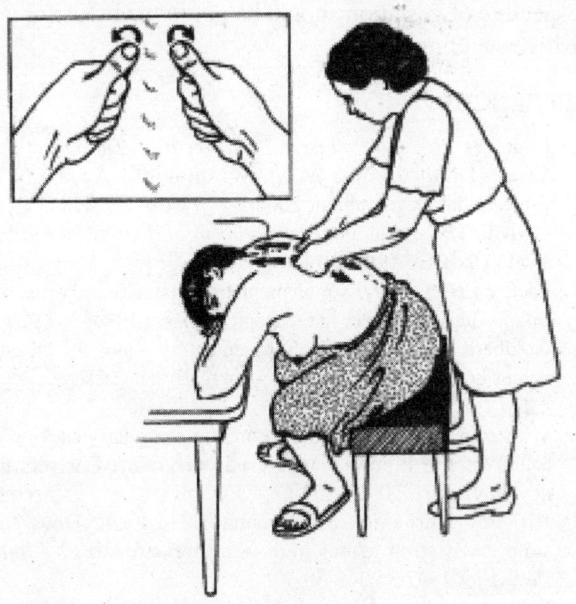

Fig. 8.8: Helper rubbing a mother's back to stimulate the oxytocin reflex

Indications

- To maintain milk production and for feeding the baby who is premature, low birth weight or sick and cannot breastfeed for some time.
- Working mothers, who plan to return to work can express the milk in advance and store it for exclusively breastfed babies.
- To relieve breast problem e.g. engorgement.

Technique of Expression

Teach the mother to:

- Wash her hands with soap and water thoroughly before expression.
- Sit or stand comfortably, and hold the clean container near her breast.
- Put the thumb on her breast above the nipple and areola, and her first finger on the breast below the nipple and areola, opposite the thumb. She supports the breast with her other fingers.
- Press her thumb and first finger slightly inwards towards the chest wall.
- Press her breast behind the nipple and areola between her finger and thumb. She must press in the lactiferous sinuses beneath the areola. Sometimes in a lactating breast it is possible to feel the sinuses. They are like peanuts. If she can feel them, she can press on them, press and release, press and release.

  This should not hurt—if it hurts the technique is wrong.

  At first no milk may come, but after pressing a few times, milk starts to drip out.
- Press the areola in the same way from the sides, to make sure that milk is expressed from all segments of the breast.
- Avoid rubbing or sliding her fingers along the skin. The movements of the fingers should be more like rolling.
- Avoid squeezing the nipple itself. Pressing or pulling the nipple cannot express milk.
- Express one breast for at least 3-5 minutes until the flow slows; then express the other side; and then repeat both sides. She can use either hand for either breast.

TO EXPRESS BREAST MILK BY

- Explain that to express breast milk adequately may take 20-30 minutes. Having the baby close or handling the baby before milk expression may help the mother to have a good let-down reflex. It is important not to try to express in a shorter time. To stimulate and maintain production one should express milk frequently—at least 8 times in 24 hours.

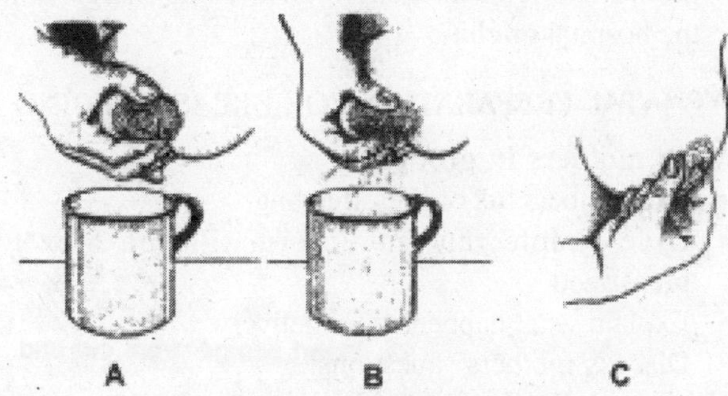

Fig. 8.9: Technique hand: (a) Place finger and thumb each side of the areola and press inwards towards the chest wall (b) Press behind the nipple and areola between your finger and thumb (c) Press from the sides to empty all segments

STORING EXPRESSED BREAST MILK

- Wash the container thoroughly with soap and water.
- Cover the container of expressed breast milk (EBM) with a clean cloth or a lid.
- EBM can be kept at room temperature (26°) for upto 6 hours,[1] or in the refrigerator (0-4°C) for upto 24–48 hours[2] and in the deep freeze (-20°) for upto 3 months.
- EBM stays in good condition longer than animal milk because of the protective substances it contains. It is not advisable to boil the EBM. If it needs to be warmed, place the container in a bowl of warm water.
- Gently shake the container to recombine the separated fat globules with the rest of the milk before feeding.
- Feed with cup or spoon or paladai, never feed with bottle.

THE TEN STEPS TO SUCCESSFUL BREASTFEEDING

Every facility providing maternity services and care for newborn infant should:

1. Have a written breastfeeding policy that is routinely communicated to all health care staff.
2. Train all health care staff in skills necessary to implement this policy.
3. Inform all pregnant women about benefits and management of breastfeeding.
4. Help mothers initiate breastfeeding within half hour of birth.
5. Show mothers how to breastfeed, and how to maintain lactation even if they are separated from their infants.
6. Give newborn infants no food or drink other than breast milk, unless medically indicated.
7. Practice rooming—in—allow mothers and infants to remain together—24 hours a day.
8. Encourage breastfeeding on demand.
9. Give no artificial teats or pacifiers (also called dummies or soothers) to breastfeeding infants.
10. Foster the establishment of breastfeeding support groups and refer mothers to them on discharge from the hospital or clinic.

ANTENATAL PREPARATION FOR BREASTFEEDING

a. **With mothers in groups:**
   - Explain benefits of breastfeeding.
   - Give simple relevant information on how to breastfeed.
   - Explain what happens after delivery.
   - Discuss mothers' questions.

b. **With each mother individually:**
   - Ask about previous breastfeeding experience.
   - Ask if she has any questions or worries.
   - Examine her breasts if she is worried about them.
   - Build her confidence, and explain that you will help her.

Feeding of Low Birth Weight Neonates

The low birth weight and preterm babies require higher calories and proteins. Milk of a mother who has delivered prematurely has a higher protein content and fulfills the requirement of her preterm baby. The higher level of immunoglobulins protects the baby from infections. Babies above 34 weeks of gestation can be breastfed. Babies between 32 to 34 weeks should be spoon-fed. All babies irrespective of gestation should be put to the breastfor non-nutritive suckling.

REFERENCES

1. Linkages Project. *Exclusive Breastfeeding. The Only Water SourceYoung Infants Need*. Washington: Academy For Educational Development 2002.
2. UNICEF. *Breastfeeding Foundation for a Healthy Future*. New York: UNICEF 1999.
3. Sachdev HPS. Water supplementation in exclusively breastfed infants during summer in the tropics. *Lancet* 1999; 337:929-33.
4. Goldberg NM, Adams E. Supplementary water for breastfed babies in a hot and dry climate—not really a necessity. *Arch Dis Child* 1983; 58:73-74.
5. Widstrom AM (1990). Short-term effects of early sucking and touch of the nipple on maternal behavior. Early human development 1990; 21:153-63.
6. Hill PD, Hurnenick SS, Brennan ML, *et al*. Does early supplementation affect long-term breastfeeding? *Clinical Pediatrics* 1997;36:345-50.
7. Enkin M, Keirse MJNC, Neilson J, *et al*. *A Guide to Effective Care in Pregnancy and Childbirth,* 3rd edn. Oxford: Oxford University Press 2000.
8. Guay LA and Ruff AJ (2001). HIV and Infant feeding. An ongoing challenge. *JAMA* 2001;286:2462-64.
9. Gupte S, Gomez EM. Infant feeding. In: Gupte S (ed) *The Short Textbook of Pediatrics*, 11th edn. New Delhi: Jaypee 2004:115-126.
10. Hathi GS, Bavdekar SV. Human lactation and breastfeeding management. In: Gupte S (ed) *Recent Advances in Pediatrics, Vol-3*. New Delhi: Jaypee 1993:3:11-34..
11. Jindal T, Chattree S. Anatomy and physiology of lactation. In: Anand RK, Kumta NB, Kushwaha KP, Gupta A (eds) *The Science of Infant Feeding*. New Delhi: Jaypee 2002:23-35.
12. Kulski JK, Hartmann PE. Changes in milk composition during the initiation of lactation. *Aust J Exp Biol Med Sci* 1981;59:231-237.
13. Helsing E, King FS. *Breastfeeding in Practice: A Manual for Health Workers*. Oxford: Oxford University Press 1982.
14. Banapurmath CR, Banapurmath S, Kesaree N. Breastfeeding problems. In: Anand RK, Kumta NB, Kushwaha KP, Gupta A (eds) *The Science of Infant Feeding*. New Delhi: Jaypee 2002:137-154.
15. Kearney MH, Cronnenwett LR, Barett JR. Breastfeeding problems in the first week postpartum. *Nursing Res* 1990; 39:91-95.
16. Gupte S, Smith R. *Infant Feeding*. New Delhi: Jaypee 1981.
17. Barger J and Bull PA. Comparison of the bacterial composition of breast milk stored at room temperature and stored in the refrigerator. *Int J Childbirth Educ* Year;2:29-30.
18. Report of the Adhoc Group on Infant feeding in Emergencies. *Infant Feeding in Emergencies: Policy, Strategy and Practice. Dublin*: Emergency Nutrition Network 1999.

Ravinder K Gupta • Ritu Gupta

9 Breastfeeding and Maternal Medication

INTRODUCTION

The right of child to be fed, nurtured and loved by the mother is the most ancient of all human rights recognized by all societies and cultures. Breastfeeding is an unequalled way of providing ideal food for the healthy growth and development of infants and has a unique biological and emotional influence in the health of both mother and child. Numerous advantages of breastfeeding over artificial milk have been documented and promotion of breastfeeding is justified on firm scientific grounds.[1-5]

As a rule, most drugs taken by a lactating mother are secreted in her milk. The decision to stop or withhold breastfeeding, especially in developing countries can have serious implications. The alternative to breast milk are all fought with dangers. Questions commonly arise regarding the safety of maternal medication 'during breastfeeding'.

A combination of the biological and chemical properties of the drug and the physiology of the mother and infant determine the safety of any individual medication. Consideration is given to the following factors in particular:

- Amount of drug that is found in breast milk.
- Half- life of the drug in the infant, and
- Biological effect of the drug on the infant.[5, 6]

DRUG PROPERTIES THAT AFFECT ENTRY INTO BREAST MILK

Molecular size, pH, pKa, lipid solubility, and protein-binding properties of the drug all affect the *M/P ratio*. The M/P ratio is defined as the relative concentration of the protein-free fraction of the drug in milk and maternal plasma. Small molecular size, slightly alkaline pH, non-ionization, high lipid solubility, and lack of binding to serum proteins all favor entry of a drug into breast milk. The half-life of the medication and frequency of drug administration are also important. The longer the cumulative time the drug is present in the maternal circulation, the greater is the opportunity for it to appear in breast milk.

Maternal Factors

The total maternal dose and mode of administration (intravenous versus oral) as well as maternal illness (particularly renal or liver impairment) can affect the persistence of the drug in the maternal circulation. Medications taken in the first few days postpartum are more likely to enter breast milk as the mammary alveolar epithelium does not fully mature until the end of the first postpartum week.

Infant Factors

The maturity of the infant is the primary factor determining the persistence of a drug in the infant's system. Preterm infants and term infants in the first month after birth metabolize drugs more slowly because of renal and hepatic immaturity. The total dose of drug that the infant is exposed to is determined by the volume of milk ingested (per kg of body weight) as well as frequency of feeding (or frequency of milk expression in the case of preterm infants).

DETERMINATION OF DRUG SAFETY DURING BREASTFEEDING

Ideally, direct measurements of the entry of a drug into breast milk, and the level and persistence of the drug in the breastfed infant, as well as experience with exposure of infants to the drug, are all used to make a judgment regarding drug safety. Unfortunately, this type of information is available for relatively few medications. In the absence of specific data, a judgment is made on the basis of both the known pharmacologic properties of the drug and the known or predicted affects of the drug on the developing infant. Clinicians providing advice to the nursing mother about the safety of a particular medication should bear in mind of the following points:[6,7]

- *Resources may differ in their judgment of a particular drug*. Information about some medications (especially newer ones) is in flux, and safety judgments may change over a relatively short period of time.

- *Safety of a drug in pregnancy is often not the same as the safety of the drug during breastfeeding***.** Occasionally a medication that is contraindicated in pregnancy (for example, warfarin or ibuprofen) is safe to use while breastfeeding.
- *Definitive date are not available for most medications or for specific clinical situations***.** There is a need for individualized clinical judgment in many cases, taking into account the available information, the need of the mother for the medication, and the risk to the infant of both exposure to the drug and of exposure to breast milk substitutes.

Section 3

While deciding about advisability of breastfeeding by a mother on a drug, other, questions that demand answers include:

- Whether the drug is absorbed through the infant's GI tract.
- Whether infant can detoxify and excrete it.
- Whether the drug can be given safely to an infant directly; and
- At what risk, and what dosages blood levels are safe.

VARIOUS CATEGORIZATIONS OF MATERNAL MEDICATION

Swedish Classification

A Swedish classification system for drug information regarding drug use during pregnancy and breastfeeding is devised by the National Swedish Board of Health. The system classifies drugs into the following four groups to describe drugs during lactation.[5,8]

Group I : Active ingredients do not enter the milk.

Group II : Active ingredients enter the milk but in such small amounts that there is no risk to the infant.

Group III : Active ingredients enter the milk in sufficient quantities to present a risk to the child even at therapeutic levels.

Group IV : Not known whether active ingredients enter the breast milk.

American Academy of Pediatrics (AAP) Classification

The American Academy of Pediatrics (AAP) has published a list which also has four categories:[5,9]

1. Drugs contraindicated during breastfeeding.
2. Drugs requiring temporary cessation of breastfeeding.
3. Drugs usually compatible with breastfeeding.
4. Food and environmental agents affecting breastfeeding.

Temporary cessation of breastfeeding is recommended if the mother is on metronidazole, or has been exposed to radioactive compounds like radioactive sodium, ^{67}(Ga) citrate or ^{99M}TC. Drugs like busulfan, chlorambucil, azathioprine, cisplatin, doxorubicin, methotrexate, ^{123}I, ^{125}I and ^{131}I do not appear in the AAP's list of contraindicated drugs because sufficient information about them is not available.

All antibiotics (with the possible exception of metronidazole), including antiviral and antifungal agents, can safely be given during lactation. Short-term narcotic use such as codeine, morphine and meperidine appears to be safe for the baby. Inhalation anesthetics present no hazard to the nursing infant. Lactating mothers who need surgery usually do not nurse for 12 to 24 hours. By this time, virtually all anesthetic agents disappear from the maternal blood. This is an opportunity for hospitals to encourage "reverse rooming-in"—a well baby with a sick mother. Occasional ingestion of an alcoholic beverage (beer, wine) is permissible. Caffeinated beverages are safe.[10] There seems to be some controversy regarding the use of aspirin in a nursing mother. AAP considers aspirin compatible with breastfeeding. In general, chemotherapeutic agents for cancer, antipsychotics, antidepressants and antianxiety drugs are considered unsafe.[10] Nursing may have to be interrupted for 1 to 14 days depending upon the radioactive compound used. Digoxin, all diuretics, calcium channel blockers and beta-blockers appear to be safe though a recent report implicating maternal exposure of atenolol for adverse reactions in infants has been published.[11,12]

American Academy of Pediatrics, Committee on Drugs (Transfer of Drugs and other Chemicals into Human Milk), has published the policy on medications and breastfeeding:[6,9]

- *Cytotoxic drugs* that may interfere with cellular metabolism of the nursing infant and are contraindicated during breastfeeding.
- *Drugs of abuse* for which adverse effects on the infant during breastfeeding have been reported and are contraindicated during breastfeeding.
- *Radioactive compounds* that require temporary cessation of breastfeeding.
- *Drugs for which the effect on nursing infants is unknown* but may be of concern.
- ***Drugs that have been associated with significant effect*** on some nursing infants and should be given to nursing mothers with caution.
- *Maternal medication* usually compatible with breastfeeding.
- *Food and environmental agent* effects on breastfeeding are also included in a separate evaluation.

Antiepileptic medications are excreted into breast milk to a variable degree. The ratio of drug concentration in breast milk relative to serum is 80% for ethosuximide, 40 to 60% for phenobarbital, 40% for carbamezepine, 15% for phenytoin and 5% for valproic acid. Given the overall benefits of breastfeeding and the lack of evidence for long-term harm to the infant by being exposed to antiepileptic drugs, mothers with epilepsy can be encouraged to breast feed. This should be reconsidered, however, if there is any evidence of drug effects on the infant, such as lethargy or poor feeding.[13]

In general, if a drug is used therapeutically in the neonatal period, there is no need to be concerned about its use in breastfeeding mothers. One should always look for safer alternatives and a mother taking medication should feed the baby just prior to drug dose and try to avoid nursing at times of peak drug levels.

Food and Drugs Administration Classification

The Food and Drugs Administration's Pregnancy Risk Categories for drugs are detailed as follows:[6]

1. **Category A:** Controlled studies in women fail to demonstrate a risk to the fetus.
2. **Category B:** Either animal-reproduction studies have not demonstrated a fetal risk or, if such a risk was found, it was not confirmed in later controlled studies in women.
3. **Category C:** Either studies in animals have revealed adverse effects on the fetus and there are not controlled studies in women, or studies in women and animals are not available. Drugs should be given only if the potential benefit justifies the potential risk to the fetus.
4. **Category D:** There is positive evidence of human fetal risk, but the benefits from use in pregnant women may be acceptable despite the risk (e.g., in a life-threatening situation or for a serious disease).
5. **Category X:** Studies in animals or human beings have demonstrated fetal abnormalities, and the risk of the use of the drug in pregnant women clearly outweighs any possible benefit.

MMM Classification

Medications in Mother's Milk (MMM) rating for drugs prescribed to lactating mothers.[6]

L1 : Safest.

L2 : Safer.

L3 : Moderately safe. Many drugs fall into this category, which is defined as follows : "There are no controlled studies in breastfeeding women, how- ever, the risk of untoward effects to a breastfed infants is possible, or controlled studies show only minimal, unthreatening effects. Drugs should be given only if the potential benefit justifies the risk to the infant."

L4 : Possibly hazardous.

L5 : Contraindicated.

USEFUL INFORMATION ON COMMON MEDICATIONS

Tables 9.1 to 9.8 provide information on medications commonly prescribed to breastfeeding women. They are organized by category the Food and Drug Administration Pregnancy Risk Category (PRC), A-D and X; American Academy of Pediatrics (AAP) rating (1-6, or NR=not reviewed), the Medications in Mother's Milk (MMM) rating (L1-L5).[6]

Table 9.1: Antibiotics

Medications	*PRC*	*AAP*	*MMM*
Acyclovir, Fluconazole, Ketoconazole	C	6	L2
Amikacin, Clarithromcin, Gentamicin, Griseofulvin, Imipenem-cilastatin, Itraconazole	C	NR	L2
Amoxicillin,Cephalosporins *List 1, Erythromcycin,	B	6	L1
Penicillin G	B	NR	L3
Amphotericin B, Methicillin			
Ampicillin, Augmentin, Floxacillin, Mupirocin, Nafcillin	B	NR	L1
Azithromycin, Famciclovir, Loracarbef, Piperacillin/Zosyn	B	NR	L2
Aztreonam, Cephalosporins +List 2, Nitrofurantoin	B	6	L2
Cefprozil,	C	6	L1
Ciprofloxacin	C	6	L4
Clindamycin	B	6	L3
Doxycycline, Minocycline	D	NR	L3
Isoniazid, Ofloxacin, Trimethoprim	C	6	L3
Kanamycin	D	6	L2
Metronidazole	B	4	L2
Norfloxacin, Sulfamethoxazole	C	NR	L3

AAP = American Academy of Pediatrics; MMM = Medications in Mother's Milk; NR = Not reviewed; PRC = Pregnancy risk category.

* List 1 : cefadroxil, cefazolin, cefoxitin, ceftazidime, cephalexin, cephapirin, cephradine.

\+ List 2 : cefaclor, cefdinir, ceftibulen, cefepime, cefixime, cefoperazone, cefotaxime, cefotetan, cefpodoxime, ceftriaxone, cefuroxime, cephalothin.

Table 9.2: Analgesics

Medications	*PRC*	*AAP*	*MMM*
Acetaminophen, Ibuprofen	B	6	L1
Aspirin	C/D	5	L3
Butorphanol, Fentanyl, Indomethacin, KetrolacMeperidine, Methadone, Morphine	B/D	6	L3
Codeine	C	6	L3
Hydrocodone, Nubain, Oxycodone	B	NR	L3
Hydromorphone	C	NR	L3

Table 9.3: Antihypertensive and cardiac medications

Medications	*PRC*	*AAP*	*MMM*
Amiodarone	C	4	L5
Atenolol	C	5	L3
Captopril	D	6	L4
Clonidine	C	NR	L3
Digoxin, Hydralazine, Labetalol, Methyldopa, Nifedipine, Procainamide	C	6	L2
Diltiazem, Propanolol	C	6	L3
Dopamine/dobutamine, Nimodipine	C	NR	L2
Enalapril	C/D	6	L4
Epinephrine	C	NR	L1
Flecainide	C	6	L4
Magnesium sulfate	B	6	L1

Table 9.4: Allergy and respiratory medications

Medications	PRC	AAP	MMM
Albuterol, Dextromethorphan	C	NR	L1
Beclomethasone, Diphenhydramine, Hydrocortisone (topical)	C	NR	L2
Betamethasone, Budesonide, Flunisolide, Phenylephrine	C	NR	L3
Cetrizine	B	NR	L2
Clemastine	C	5	L4
Cromolyn sodium	B	NR	L1
Fexofenadine, Pseudoephedrine, Theophylline	C	6	L3
Loratadine, Prednisone	B	6	L2
Methylprednisolone	C	6	L3
Montelukast	B	NR	L3

Table 9.5: Psychoactive medications

Medications	PRC	AAP	MMM
Alprazolam, Diazepam, Lorazepam, Midazolam	D	4	L3
Amitryptyline	D	4	L2
Bupropion, Fluoxetine (Prozac), Paroxetine (Paxil)	B	4	L3
Caffeine	B	6	L2
Carbamazepine	C	6	L2
Chloral hydrate	C	6	L3
Chlordiazepoxide, Oxazepam, Pentobarbital	D	NR	L3
Chlorpromazine, Clozapine	C	4	L3
Citalopram (Celexa), Clonazepam, Gabapentin, Methylphenidate (Retalin), Prochlorperazine	C	NR	L3
Clomipramine, Haloperidol	C	4	L2
Desipramine	C	4	L2
Lithium	D	5	L4
Phenobarbital	D	5	L3
Phenytoin, Valproic acid	D	6	L2
Sertraline (Zoloft)	B	4	L2

Table 9.6: Gastrointestinal medications

Medications	PRC	AAP	MMM
Bismuth Subsalicylate	C/D	4	L3
Cimetidine	B	6	L2
Docusate, Kaolin-pectin, Nizatidine, Omeprazole	C	NR	L2
Loperamide	B	6	L2
Metoclopramide	B	4	L2
Ondansetron, Ranitidine	B	NR	L2

AAP = American Academy of Pediatrics; MMM = Medications in Mother's Milk; NR = Not reviewed; PRC = Pregnancy risk category.

Since oral contraceptives reduce the milk production they should not be used by the lactating mother. Intrauterine contraceptive devices are the best choice. They can be fitted at 6 weeks postpartum. Most IUCDs are effective for upto three years. This offers an easy way of birth spacing.[14]

Table 9.7: Drugs that are contraindicated during breastfeeding along with their adverse effects

Drugs	Adverse effects on infant or on lactation
Anti-cancer drugs	Potential effect on growth or Carcinogenesis : possible bone Marrow suppression suppression
Radioactive pharmaceuticals (^{125}I, ^{131}I, Ga, ^{99M}Tc)	Radiation toxicity
Carbimazole/methimazole	Goitre, hypothyrodisim
Ergotamine	Vomiting, diarrhea, convulsions
Gold salts	Rash, nephritis, hepatitis
Pheninidione	Hemorrhagic diathesis
Bromocriptine	Suppression of lactation
Tetracycline	Teeth staining, bone changes
MAO inhibitor antidepressants (phenelzine)	Suppression of lactation, hypertensive crisis with tyramine exposure
Lithium	Hypotonia, cyanosis and other features of lithium toxicity syndrome

Table 9.8: Drugs that, though not contraindicated, should be avoided and alternative medication substituted for the reasons cited alongside

Drugs	Adverse effects on infant or on lactation
Indomethacin	Potentially large dose may be excreted, case Report of seizures
Phenylbutazone	Nephrotoxicity, bone marrow suppression
Ethambutol	Potential for ophthalmic toxicity
Hydroxychloroquine	Retinotoxicity
Quinidine	Optic neuritis, rash, anemia, ECG abnormalities.
Captopril	Insufficient information in neonates potentially toxic
Valproic acid	Insufficient information in neonates, potential For hepatitis, pancreatitis, bleeding tendency Sedation
Iodides	Allergic rash, goiter

REFERENCES

1. World Health Organization. *Indicators for Assessing Breastfeeding Practices. Report of an Informal Meeting, 11-12 June 1991.* Geneva: WHO: 1991.
2. Gupta R K, Gupta R, Infant feeding practices among rural mothers. *JK Sci* 2001;3;25-28.
3. Gupte S, Gomez EM. Infant feeding. In Gupte S (ed): *The Short Textbook of Pediatrics,* 10th edn. New Delhi: Jaypee 2004;113-124.
4. Heird C William. The feeding of infants and children. In : Behrman RE, Kliegman RM, Jenson HB (eds): *Nelson Textbook of Pediatrics,* 17th edn. Philadelphia: Saunders 2004: 157-160.
5. Hathi GS, Bavdekar SB. Human lactation and breastfeeding management. In: Gupte S (ed): *Recent Advances in Pediatrics,* Vol 3. New Delhi: Jaypee 1993;11-34.
6. Puopola MK. Maternal medication and breastfeeding. In Cloherty JP, Eichenwald EC, Stark A R (eds): *Manual of Neonatal Care,* 5th edn. Philadelphia: Lippincott Williams and Wilkins 2004;771-779.
7. Sureka VP, Sureka PR, Anand RK. Breastfeeding and drugs in human milk. *Indian Pediatr* 1989;26:373-378.

8. Bregkend F, Flodh H, Lundbor P. Drug use during pregnancy and breastfeeding. *Acta Obstet Gynecol Scand* 1984;126 (Suppl):118-130.
9. Committee on Drugs, American Academy of Pediatrics. The Transfer of drugs and other chemicals into human breat milk. *Pediatrics* 2001;108:776-789.
10. Berlin CM. Drugs and Chemicals. Exposure of the nursing mother. *Pediatr. Clin North Am* 1989;36:1089-1097.
11. Ehrenkraz RA, Ackerman BA, Hulse JD. Nifedipine transfer into human milk. *J Pediatr* 1989;114:478-480.
12. Schininmel MS, Eidelman AJ, Wilshanski MA. Toxic effects of Atenolol consumed during breastfeeding. *J Pediatr* 1989;Vol: 476-478.
13. Lowenstein DH. Seizures and epilepsy. In: Braunwald E, Kasper DL, Fauci SA, Longo DL, Jameson JL, Hauser SL (eds): *Harrison's Principles of Internal Medicine*,16th edn. New York: McGraw-Hill 2005;2372-2373.
14. Chetan R, Indirabai K. Breastfeeding promotion: Practical guidelines: In: Gupte S, Gupte SB (eds): *Recent Advances in Pediatrics, Vol. 3.* New Delhi: Jaypee 1993;51-62.

AK Patwari

10 Lactation Failure and Relactation

INTRODUCTION

Efforts for promotion of exclusive breastfeeding (BF) are primarily focused on initiating BF soon after birth. Lactation education in the antenatal period, discouraging prelacteal feeds, and rooming-in are some of the interventions which have proved to be successful world over for achieving this objective. Even with the initial success in starting BF, which is otherwise a cultural practice in India, the introduction of top feeds during or after neonatal period undermines these efforts at exclusive BF. It is a worldwide observation that even in societies where BF is still the norm, only a small proportion of infants are breastfed exclusively for more than a few weeks. Mothers often introduce complementary foods or drinks at an early age.[1] In India, proportion of exclusively breastfed infants has been observed to decline from 42 percent in first month to 20 percent by 4 months.[2] The reason for the partial or complete switch over to top milk is generally attributed to secretion of inadequate milk, which most of the times is a consequence rather than a cause.

LACTATION FAILURE

Lactation failure (LF) is believed to be the main reason for decline in exclusive BF in early infancy. LF may be partial or complete, and may pose as a critical problem soon after birth or later on after initial success with BF. There is no uniformly accepted definition of LF. It can be regarded as the "failure of the breast to produce adequate milk which manifests as failure to sustain growth in a normal infant within 2 standard deviations of the norm for the infant in the first 4 to 6 months of age". However, it needs to be realized that LF is usually not the cause, but a consequence of a number of factors which are responsible for introduction of top milk under the wrong notion of insufficient milk, or because of maternal-child separation, working mothers, sore/cracked nipples, etc.

Complete LF pertains to total absence of milk flow or secretion of only a few drops of milk following regular suckling for a period of at least 7 days.[3] When a mother, who is, otherwise, regularly breastfeeding her baby, complains of inadequate milkflow and the infant requires supplementation by artificial milk to sustain growth, it is termed as partial LF.

A number of causes have been attributed to failure of initiating BF in a newborn baby which include maternal, infant and other causes (Table 10.1). In mothers with complete LF right from the beginning of their puerperal period, one or more of these factors may be responsible. Some of these factors may also contribute to LF in the postpuerperal period.

Table 10.1: Causes of lactation failure

Maternal causes	*Infant causes*	*Other causes*
Lack of motivation	Infant's sickness	Prelacteal feeds
Maternal sickness	Prematurity	Misbeliefs and superstitions of mother/family
Breast conditions (short/long/inverted sore/cracked nipples)	Problems in suckling (nasal block, oral thrush, cleft palate, etc.)	Wrong advice by doctors/nurses
Painful swelling in the breasts (engorgement, mastitis, blocked duct, breast abscess)	Twins	Advice by relatives and friends
Previous unpleasant experience		Advertisement of commercial milk substitutes
Stress and anxiety		Cultural/religious practices/rituals (mahurat, 'aanchal kholna', 'than doi', etc.)
Obstetric problems (Cesarean section, infected stitches)		Mothers' concern for figure and shape
		Considered socially inconvenient

Lactation Failure in the Postpuerperal Period

Over the past two or three decades the period of exclusive BF is gradually diminishing. The underlying social reasons are many: mothers' involvement with work for monetary reasons, breakup of the joint family system, migration into urban areas and breakup of the support system not only in the family, but also in the community. This trend of 'social' progress is a serious threat to infants nutrition and survival.

Partial or complete LF in the postpuerperal period after initial successful BF is matter of great concern since it is not the failure to initiate but to sustain exclusive BF which is the major problem in these situations. By virtue of their initial successful experience, these mothers have already overcome several apprehensions and problems related to lack of knowledge and inexperience. These are the mothers who initially offer top feeds to their infants for one or the other reason, but gradually BF is replaced, partly or completely, over a period of time, depriving these infants of the full advantages of BF on one hand and exposing them to risk of artificial feeding, particularly if given by a bottle, on the other. Some of the common reasons given by mothers for supplementing top milk in this group are depicted in Table 10.2.

Table 10.2: Common reasons for supplementing top milk

- Insufficient breast milk
- Obstetric complications
- Sickness of the baby
- Twins
- Working mothers
- Family pressures
- Advertisement of milk substitutes

Not Enough Milk?

One of the most common reasons given by mothers all over the world for stopping BF or introducing complementary foods is their belief that they do not have enough breastmilk or the quality of their milk is poor.[4-9] Most of the Indian studies[10-14] have also reported inadequacy or failure to secrete breastmilk as the top most cause of LF. Lack of motivation has been identified as the primary reason for LF in these mothers.[15-16] Young mothers with lack of confidence, information and support are particularly vulnerable to wrong advice by health personnel[10,13,17] and by relatives and friends.[10,13] Commercial advertisement of milk substitutes is also an important hurdle in practising exclusive BF.[17]

It is a well-known fact that almost all mothers can produce enough breast milk for one or even two babies, provided the baby suckles effectively and breastfeeds as often as he or she wants. Even when a mother perceives her milk to be insufficient, her baby is usually getting the required amount of milk.[4] The amount of milk the breasts produce primarily depends upon the amount that the baby takes (it increases when the baby takes more) and is not significantly influenced by the diet of the mother. Although a good diet is important for the health of the mothers themselves, even women who are quite undernourished are capable of producing enough milk to breastfeed their babies. Uncommonly, poor mammary gland development or hormone disturbances may be responsible for poor milk secretion by the mother.[18]

Feeling of inadequacy of breast milk is more often conceptual than real. The main reason for an infant not getting enough milk is that the baby is not suckling enough, or is not suckling effectively. Indepth interviews of mothers have revealed that they attribute inadequacy of milk to anxiety because of family problems. Those who are fortunate enough to get support from their husbands can deal with anxiety successfully.[19] Apart from family support, which is essential to encourage all lactating mothers, professional help and support is a must for those who think they do not have enough breastmilk. There are hardly any support services for working mothers outside their homes. Invariably they do not get the desired help and support from the family or the health system when it is needed the most. This leads to introduction of topmilk/food earlier than necessary which further reduces the chances of frequent suckling. The eventual catastrophy is lactation failure and by that time there actually is a definite reduction of milk secretion due to less frequent suckling.

Working Women and Exclusive BF

The triple burden of women housekeeping, child bearing and rearing, and economic activity is well-known.[20] Most women participate in work, either at home or outside for wage or on family land. The heavy domestic work starts within a month of delivery.[21] Those who deliver in their natal home fare better. Time spent on work varies in different situations but on an average mothers spend 5-6 hours. Wage laborers spend less time in feeding and playing with their children. While other family members can compensate for other child rearing activities, the task of BF cannot be shared.[20] Thus, BF does suffer when the mother is away at work and it can only be compensated by feeding the baby at night. Lack of facilities at the working place like creches, attitude of the employers and the type of work she is expected to do are contributory factors.

Ignorance and Lack of Support

It is important to realize that some mothers have a genuine problem which warrants supplementation of milk or early introduction of solids. However, in most of the situations the reasons for supplementing top milk are simply related to ignorance rather than lack of motivation. Lack of confidence and family support make the situation even worse. Smith[22] did not show any significant correlation of

LF in postpuerperal period with the parity, literacy, pressure of domestic chores, professional work and even commercial advertisement on television and print media.[22] Even in Punjab where very few women work, the incidence of BF has fallen considerably.[23] It is generally observed that majority of the mothers who start top feeding their infants do so within the first month of infant's life. Therefore, in order to sustain exclusive BF during first 4 months, the first month of infant's life is the most critical time for frequent reassurance and support to the mother regarding the adequacy of her milk. However, some of the mothers may have genuine problem for which they may require a reasonably good professional support.

RELACTATION

Relactation is the resumption of BF following cessation or significant decrease in breast milk.[24] Establishment of adequate milk supply of a woman is possible if she has partial or complete LF ranging from few days to few months. Relactation also includes increasing an insufficient milk supply in partial LF.[25,26] Induced nonpuerperal lactation refers to establishing milk supply in a woman who has never been pregnant. This concept has practical importance in breastfeeding the adopted babies.[26-28]

Relactation attempts in primary as well as secondary LF can be extremely rewarding in promoting exclusive BF in early infancy. Results from India and abroad[14,29-35] have clearly shown this. Success of relactation significantly depends upon the presence and extent of some of the consequences of top feeding. Some of the common problems with which these mothers present apparently seem to be very difficult to manage and, therefore, may dampen the enthusiasm of the mother as well as the pediatrician to attempt relactation. Some of these problems include:

1. *Failure to secrete any milk:* Mothers with complete LF find it impossible to imagine that they can secrete milk since they do not have any milk secretion at all. This is, in fact, an ultimate consequence of not breastfeeding from the beginning or not breastfeeding for a prolonged period of time, and is not only a deterrent to relactation but can even result in discouragement and failure of these attempts because of other associated problems as discussed below.
2. *Badly fissured nipples:* Wrong positioning and faulty attachment of the areola by the baby is the commonest cause of badly fissured nipples. The painful experience of the mother due to sore nipples further discourages her to put her baby on the breast. Frustration of the baby at not getting milk from the 'dried up breast', which usually is the aftermath of replacing breast milk by top feeds, is another common cause of sore nipples inflicted by the hungry infant.
3. *Nipple confusion:* Infants of mothers with complete LF who are bottlefed experience this peculiar problem termed as 'nipple confusion'. This is because different technique is adopted by the infant while breastfeeding and when he is fed with a bottle, pacifiers, or nipple shield. It is important to know that BF involves coordinated movements of the baby's jaw and tongue, and by latching his mouth on to the breast which is stretched into a 'teat' and pressed up against his palate. Feeding from artificial nipples including pacifiers, on the other hand, requires a different technique since milk flows just by pressing the artificial nipple without any need for moving the jaw. This results in instant gratification with little effort. Therefore, most of the babies find it confusing to switch back and forth between the breast and artificial nipple, particularly when they are learning to breastfeed. When such babies who are used to artificial teats are put to breast by the mother/surrogate mother, they try to suckle in closed mouth position resulting in nipple suckling (as they do not attach their lips properly around the areola). This results in feeling of pain in the nipple by the mother and inadequate milk transfer. The outcome is unsuccessful lactation response leading to frustration to the baby and injury to the breasts.

In order to achieve successful results with relactation attempts, it is necessary to take care of the following problems:

Management of Maternal Conditions

Maternal conditions like septicemia, infected stitches, etc. as well as other infections like tuberculosis and hepatitis B should be managed appropriately.

Management of Painful Breast Conditions/ Complications

The underlying cause for most of the breast problems is the poor positioning of the baby at the breast. Painful experience while breastfeeding in these situations itself tends to interfere in proper positioning and suckling the baby for sufficient period of time. The result invariably is a vicious cycle which further discourages the mother to breastfeed. Unless painful conditions of the breast are taken care of and the local pain is relieved, no amount of motivation or education can ensure frequent suckling of the baby for the desired period of time. Therefore, it is necessary to provide her appropriate professional support to manage breast engorgement, cracked/sore nipples as per the recommended methods.[36] After relieving her pain, make her comfortable and relaxed, show her how to support her breast while breastfeeding explain or show her how to help the baby to attach and look for signs of good attachment.[36] If the attachment is not good, try again. Inverted nipples generally do not interfere in successful BF. However, if it is a cause of concern to the mother. The nipple can be pulled out using a disposable syringe technique.[37]

Management of Infants' Problem

It is imperative to ensure that the baby is fit to suckle at the breast. Acute infections particularly of the respiratory tract need to be managed appropriately.

Reestablishment of Lactation

Lactation management of mothers with partial LF is relatively easier since they are already breastfeeding their infants, though not adequately. The ultimate objective of complete restoration of BF in these mothers can be achieved by motivation, providing information, encouraging them to frequently breastfeed and by gradually reducing the amount of top milk. However, establishing lactation in a mother who has never lactated before or has complete LF is not only challenging but requires lot of patience and perseverance both by the mother as well as the physician. Even the earliest visible lactation response in complete LF in the form of appearance of few drops of milk may range from 2 to 10 days.[28,31,34,35] Therefore, it is essential that the health worker is mentally prepared for the anticipated problems and is well versed with essential skills to take care of them. Mothers also have to be involved in the entire intervention by giving them necessary information and provide the desired support throughout the period till normal BF is established. In order to assist a successful relactation, the following steps are useful:

i. *Motivation of the mother*: Allay her anxiety, educate her and explain the importance and advantages of exclusive BF.
ii. *Build her confidence and give her support:* This can be achieved by: (a) accepting what she thinks and feels, (b) recognizing and praising what she is doing right, (c) offering practical help, (d) giving a little, relevant information at a time in simple language, and (e) making suggestions, not commands.
iii. *Nipple stimulating exercises:* Mothers should be encouraged to do nipple stimulation exercises by nipple stroking, massaging the breast and rolling the nipple between thumb and the fingers.
iv. *Ensure frequent suckling*: Infant should be put to breast 8-10 times a day in proper position for 10-15 minutes on each breast.
v. *Drop and drip method*: If the baby does not suckle at the breast for a desired period of 10-15 minutes, some breast milk is expressed into a cup/topmilk in complete LF, which is then slowly dripped over the breast in drops. These drops slide down over the nipple and help the baby to suckle at the breast.[30,31,35]
vi. *Nursing supplementor:* Lact-aid supplementor is used as a means to induce a baby to suckle on an 'empty' breast if he refuses to do so without it.[13,27,31,32] This is particularly useful in infants with nipple confusion. This device consists of a fine tube (infant feeding tube) which acts as a drawing straw. The tube passes from a cup of milk to the baby's mouth. The end of the tube is placed along with mother's nipple so that the baby suckles at both the nipple and the tube at the same time. He gets the milk from the cup through the tube. His suckling stimulates the nipple and enhances the prolactin reflex and, thereby, increases the milk production.
vii. Adequate nutrition and rest to mother is equally important. Additional diet should be provided to mother if she is undernourished.
viii. Bottle feeding and pacifiers should be stopped immediately.

MONITORING OF LACTATION RESPONSE

In order to have an objective assessment of success of relactation, it is imperative to monitor the process of establishment of successful BF which may take few days to few weeks for achieving the desired goal of exclusive BF. In mothers with complete LF, the earliest response of successful lactation is feeling of tingling sensation in the breast while the baby is encouraged to suckle. It is difficult to evaluate this response objectively but, if one is able to develop a good rapport with the mother, most of them would describe this feeling. However, it would largely depend upon the motivation, physical and psychological state of the mother, and also on number and duration of sucklings and nipple confusion of the baby. Tingling sensation of the breast is usually followed by first milk secretion.

There are a number of parameters which can be helpful to know that the baby is getting adequate milk. If the baby passes colorless urine at least six times a day and sleeps for sufficient time following a feed, the intake of milk (breast/top) is considered adequate. For an objective evaluation of relactation, the following outcome variables need to be monitored.

Appearance of First Milk Secretion

The earliest indicator of relactation in complete LF is appearance of first milk secretion. This period is variable ranging from 2 to 10 days[28,31,34,35] depending upon the unique characteristics of each infant-mother first. Lack of motivation, anxiety and lack of physical rest to the mother and nipple confusion in bottlefed babies can adversely affect the outcome. Once positive response is observed, top milk supplements should be gradually reduced making sure that the mother suckles her infant more frequently in order to increase the secretion of milk, and the baby gains weight at least by 20 g/day.

Partial Restoration of Breastfeeding

Partial restoration of BF would imply that top milk supplementation is reduced by half (partial relactation). Time for partial restoration of BF is reported between 4-28 days with a mean (SD) of 11.89 (5.83) days.[31]

Complete Restoration of Breastfeeding

Relactation attempts can be considered successful if BF is restored fully with total elimination of top milk (complete relactation). Time taken for complete restoration of BF varies from 7 to 60 days with a mean (SD) of 32.50 (12.5) days.[31] Most of the mothers achieve complete relactation between 16-45 days.[28,31,34,35] Variations depend upon different characteristics of every mother-infant bonding. Generally, mothers with complete LF having breast problems like fissured/sore nipples take longer than those who have partial LF and are motivated and willing to cooperate. However, these problems do not seem to have any significant effect eventually on the ultimate outcome of partial or complete restoration of BF.[31]

Weight Gain of the Baby

Weight gain of the baby is a reliable indicator of adequacy of feeding. Appropriate measures (e.g. increasing intake, screening for infection, etc.) should be taken if a baby gains less than 140-150 g in a week. Generally, a successful response of relactation is evident by a steady reduction in amount of top milk consumed and an increase in weight of the infant.

INDUCED LACTATION

The Saga of Throgils, written in 13th century, which narrates the story of a motherless infant who was breastfed by his father until he was one year old,[26] may sound more like a fairy tale in the present times. But anthropologists have described that in the pre-industrialized societies, women who had not borne children were able to produce adequate milk to feed their infants after a few weeks of placing the suckling infant to their breasts.[38] There have been several reports of successful lactation by surrogate mothers in recent times,[27,28,35,39-41] though they may take longer (40-45 days) for establishment of exclusive BF.[35]

LACTAGOGUES AND RELACTATION

Metoclopramide is a dopamine antagonist and inhibits the secretion of prolactin inhibitory hormone from hypothalamus leading to increased prolactin level and, therefore, increased milk secretion. By virtue of its being a potent stimulator of prolactin release, various authors have used it as a potent lactation booster.[3,13,27] The drug although secreted into the breast milk, is considered safe even in premature children. However, most of the clinical trials of metoclopramide as a lactogogue were not controlled and the groups studied were not randomly selected limiting the widespread application of these results. A recent randomized controlled trial has not shown any beneficial effect of metoclopramide on any of the outcome variables of relactation.[31] Other lactogogues like high doses of nasal oxytocin,[25] chloropromazine,[25] sulpiride (a cogener of metoclopramide) and oral thyrotropin releasing hormone may help in initiating relactation but are not considered safe for the purpose.

It is the nature's gift to womanhood that physiology of the milk production and ejection is built into the human female endocrinal system. Therefore, there seems to be no reason for using any lactagogues for this purpose. However, the use of metoclopramide may perhaps be of value for indirect reasons:

- First, it may help in initiating the flow of prolactin, and, thus, possibly be an external pharmacological booster for a few days for what would anyhow result from the normal inherent reflex mechanisms.
- Secondly, it may be helpful in restoring the confidence of the mother, particularly in induced lactation.

Without disputing the pharmacological actions of lactagogues, it is prudent to say that for successful relactation all that is required is maximal prolactin secretion and an uninhibited let down reflex by stimulation of nipple which can be successfully achieved by repeated suckling at the breast, making sure that the baby is positioned correctly and the mother is mentally and physically comfortable.

REFERENCES

1. World Health Organization. *Not Enough Milk: Update*. Geneva: WHO (Division of Diarrheal and Acute Respiratory Disease Control) 1996.
2. Gupta A, Sobti J, Rohde JE. Infant feeding practices among patients of pediatricians and general practitioners. *Indian J Pediatr* 1992;59:193-196.
3. Rath BK, Ghai OP, Bhan MK. Metoclopramide in lactation failure. *Indian Pediatr* 1983; 20:341-344.
4. Hillervik-Lindquist C. Studies on preceived breast milk sufficiency—A prospective study in a group of Swedish women. *Acta Pediatr Scand* 1991;80:6-27.
5. Winikoff B, Catle MA, Laukaran VH. Feeding infants in four societies, causes and consequences of mothers' choice. London: Green Wood Press 1988.
6. Martines JC, Ashwroth A, Kirkwood B. Breastfeeding among the urban poor in southern Brazil—reasons for termination in the first 6 months of life. *Bull WHO* 1989; 67: 151-161.
7. Forman MR, Lewando-Hundt G, Graubard BI, *et al.* Factors influencing milk insufficiency and its long-term health effect—The Bedouin infant feeding study. *Int J Epidem* 1991;21:53-58.
8. Mukasa GK. A 12-month lactation clinical experience in Uganda. *J Trop Pediatr* 1992; 38: 78-82.

9. Segura-Millan S, Dewey KG, Perez Escamilla R. Factors associated with perceived insufficient milk in low-income urban population in Mexico. *J Nutr* 1994; 124: 202-212.
10. Kalra A, Kalra K, Daya RS. Breastfeeding in different residential, economic and educational groups. *Indian Pediatr* 1992; 19: 419-425.
11. Samal GC. Infant feeding and rearing practices in a rural community of Western Orissa. *J Pediatr* 1984; 21:214-215.
12. Anand RK. Maternity home practices and breastfeedings. Bombay: ACASH 1991.
13. Mathur GP, Chitranshi S, Mathur S, Singh SB, Bhalla M. Lactation failure. *Indian Pediatr* 1992; 29:1541-45.
14. Cameorn M, Hofvander Y. Manual of feeding infants and young children. London: Oxford University Press, 1983; 81-91.
15. Sjolin S, Hofvander Y, Hillervik C. Factors related to early termination of breastfeeding. *Acta Pediatr Scand* 1977;66: 505-511.
16. Bathija CG, Anand RK: Effects of perinatal motivation on breastfeeding in educated mothers. *Indian Pediatr* 1987;24: 933-937.
17. Shrivastava DK, Sahni OP, Kumar A: Infant feeding with commercial milk formula in an urban community of Central India. *Indian Pediatr* 1987;24: 889-894.
18. Neifert MR, Seacat JM, Jobe WE. Lactation failure due to insufficient glandular development of the breast. *Pediatrics* 1985;76:823-828.
19. Rahmatullah L. Breastfeeding in the low socioeconomic group:A matter for conern. *Indian J Pediatr* 1995; 62:128-130.
20. Ghosh S. Breastfeeding and Women's work. In Patwari AK, Sachdev HPS (eds): *Frontiers in Social Pediatrics.* New Delhi: Jaypee 1997.
21. Narayan R. At what cost? *Women's Multiple Roles and the Management of Breastfeeding*. Research report no. 2 MS Swaminathan Research Foundation, 1996.
22. Smith R. *Lactation Failure: Reality or Myth.* Ukison: London 2003.
23. Walia BNS, Gambhir SK, Swea SR, Chaoudhary S. Decline in breastfeeding practices in urban population of Chandigarh during a decade. *Indian Pediatr* 1987;24: 879-882.
24. Auerback KG, Avery JL. Relactation—A study of 36 cases. *Pediatrics* 1980; 65: 236-242.
25. Brown KH. Milk consumption and health status of exclusively breastfed infants in a warm climate. *J Pediatr* 1986;108:677-680.
26. Helsing E, King F. *Breastfeeding In Practice:A Manual For Health Workers*. London: Oxford University Press 1982.
27. Thearle MJ, Weissenberger R: Induced lactation in adoptive mothers. *Aust NZ J Obs Gynaecology* 1984;24:283-286.
28. Banapurmath CR, Banapurmath S S, Kesaree N. Successful induced Non-puerperal lactation in surrogate mothers. *Indian J Pediatr* 1993;60:639-643.
29. Auerback KG, Avery JL. Induced lactation. A study of adoptive nursing by 240 women. *Am J Dis Child* 1981;135:340-343.
30. Kesaree N. Drop and Drip method. *Indian Pediatr* 1993;30:277.
31. Seema, Patwari AK, Satyanarayana L. Relactation: An effective intervention to promote exclusive breastfeeding. *J Trop Pediatr* 1997;43:100-105.
32. King FS. Helping Mothers to Breast Feed. Nairobi: African Medical and Research Foundation, 1985.
33. Katherine C. How to help a woman to re-establish lactation. *Dialogue on Diarrhoea*, Issue 50, AHRTAG: London, 1992.
34. Chaturvedi P. Relactation. *Indian Pediatr* 1994;31:858-860.
35. Banapurmath CR, Banapurmath SC, Kesaree N. Initiation of relactation. *Indian Pediatr* 1993;30:1329-1332.
36. Gupta A. *Human Lactation Management Training*. New Delhi: Breastfeeding Promotion Network of India1994.
37. Kesaree N, Banapurmath CR, Banapurmath S, Shamanur K. Treatment of inverted nipples using a disposable syringe. *J Human Lact* 1993; 9:27-29.
38. Brown RE. Some nutritional considerations in times of major catastrophe. *Clin Pediatr* 1972;11:334-337.
39. Newton M. Breastfeeding by adoptive mother. *JAMA* 1970; 212:1967-1970.
40. Cohen R. Breastfeeding without pregnancy. *Pediatrics* 1971;48:996-997.
41. Chaturvedi P, Dubey AP. Induced nonpuerperal lactation. *Indian J Pediatr* 1985; 52:319-320.

Satish K Tiwari • Pratibha Kale • Samta Agarwal

11 Complementary Feeding

INTRODUCTION

The basic necessities of human life, like the "food, clothing, shelter, health care and love", are the same in all cultures. Yet, the infant caring practices and resources vary tremendously by culture in families and communities. There are many misconceptions and confusions regarding the dietary requirements in most communities.

Infant feeding is no exception to this. Inappropriate infant feeding practices re sult in feeding difficulties and malnutrition ultimately leading to increased mortality and morbidity in children. More than 2.4 million child deaths occur in India each year and two-thirds of these deaths are related to inappropriate infant feeding practices. Despite standard and optimal infant feeding (IF) recommendations depending upon cultural habits, locally available food etc., based on well researched studies, the problem of infant feeding still continues in the entire world. According to the WHO and UNICEF, poor infant feeding practices and their consequences are one of the world's major problems and a serious obstacle to social and economic development. Being, to a great extent, a man-made problem, it must be considered as a reproach to our science and technology and our social and economic structures, and a blot on our so-called development achievements. It is not only a problem of developing world; it occurs in many parts of the developed world as well.

Ideally, infant feeding compromises of exclusive breastfeeding for 6 months followed by sequential addition of semisolid and solid foods to complement [not replace] breast milk, till the child is gradually able to eat normal family food. Lack of confidence, widespread ignorance and misconceptions frequently result in improper management of infant feeding. Although effort has been made since long, yet infant feeding practices are far from satisfactory in many countries.[1] The timely complementary feeding (CF) rate for India, as a whole is only 31%. The timely CF rate varies substantially from state to state, ranging from 9% in Rajasthan to 69% in Kerala. In most of the states >50% of the children after 6-9 months are not receiving solid foods in addition to breast milk. For India as a whole, the bottle-feeding rate among infants below age of 12 months is14%. Goa by far has the highest bottle-feeding rate at 67%. These patterns of feeding are not simply the result of low income, low food availability in the household or lack of time for the mother. The low nutrient density and the poor quality of the foods, that complements the breastfeeding accounts for much of the nutritional deficiency.

WHEN TO START WEANING AND WHY

The Term "Weaning"

The concept of the word "weaning" has now changed to complementary feeding for the simple reason that, with the introduction of other nutritious food, breastfeeding needs to continue in the babies for a period of 2 years. As per the UNICEF, weaning is defined as "the systematic process of introduction of suitable food at the right time in addition to mother's milk in order to provide needed nutrients to the baby." Weaning is the second step for self-existence, the first being cutting of umbilical cord. The literal meaning of the term, *weaning,* is to "make free from the habit of breastfeeding or take the baby away from the breast and nourish by other means".

Development of Reflexes and Skills

The biting or 'munching' i.e. up and down movement of mandible appears around 5 months of age. The presence of gag reflex interferes with early introduction of semisolids and solids. This sensitivity diminishes around 7 months of age facilitating feeding of solid foods. The lateral movements of tongue which moves food gruel to molars develops by 8-12 months and full rotary chewing movements by 12-18 months.[2] The optimal age for introduction of complementary foods should be the time when breast milk alone fails to meet the nutritional requirements of the growing infants, so as to decrease the energy gap between demand

and actual availability. The concept of introduction of complementary feeding is at around 6 months of age and this is the ideal time for introduction of semisolids, as the baby becomes biologically fit and ready to accept complementary food. This is also the "sensitive period" for the infant to learn swallowing.[3] If introduction of semisolids and solids are delayed and the stimulus for the "chewing development" is not applied at appropriate age then the child may enter "critical period" after which the infant will always be a poor chewer and will be poor in eating solids later. The other reasons for complementary feeding at this age are:

1. At this age complementary feeds doesn't replace breast milk intake.
2. The risk of introduction of infection by unhygienic feeding overweighs the energy and nutrient supply. Early weaning results in high risk for diarrhea and respiratory infections.
3. Develops head control and also has hand to mouth coordination.
4. Starts enjoying mouthing and biting.
5. Intestinal amylase matures and gut becomes ready to accept cereals and pulses.
6. Gums harden prior to tooth eruption and baby enjoys gumming semisolids.
7. Tendency to push solids out of mouth decreases.

The dilemma regarding the age (especially between 4 to 6 months of age) when complementary feeds should first be given to exclusive breast fed infants living in poverty has been referred to as the "weaning dilemma".[4,5]

Pancreatic amylase is not adequately secreted until an infant is 6 months old and hence may lead to limitation of starch absorption. Similarly decreased rate of bile acid synthesis is likely to interfere in solubilization of long-chain dietary fatty acids.[6]

The Honduras study[7] also indicates that there is no caloric advantage of introducing complementary foods at 4 months instead of 6 months of age. The complementary foods introduced at 4 months merely displaced breast milk without a net increase in caloric consumption.

Delayed introduction of complementary foods to exclusively breast fed infants living in poverty carries the risk of compromised nutritional status leading to under nutrition, if the quality and quantity of breast milk from malnourished mothers is inadequate to supply their nutritional requirements. Ghosh[8] has argued that, the high rates of PEM in India are not primarily caused by poverty; rather, the behaviors of delayed initiation of breastfeeding, early introduction of water/liquids and delay in CF results in a period of "perpetual hunger for the child". This is "because the child was dependent on someone else for feeding and this person did not have the knowledge, awareness or time regarding how much food the child needed and how often." Concurrent with this is the other aspect in which introduction of complementary food carries the risk of diarrheal infection from contamination as well as uncertain benefits because of the poor nutritional quality of weaning foods available to such families. However the decision in an individual infant regarding the age for starting complementary food should be guided by the growth performance and subjective appearance of good/faltering growth by an experienced person, if periodic weighing is not feasible.

In many families, introduction of semisolid food is associated with a religious ceremony commonly known as 'Anna Prashna'.[9] In some communities it takes place around 6 months but in others performed only at the age of 1 year. In such cases, weaning gets delayed to 1 year.[10] It has to be emphasized to the mothers that delayed weaning causes malnutrition and hence this ritual should be performed early—if at all it is compulsory. A late age of weaning seems to contribute to the problem of malnutrition as observed in studies by Gupte and Sharma[10] and Sharif *et al.*[11]

Weaning should, however, be considered to start early i.e. before the age of 6 months in circumstances like:

1. Babies having growth faltering.
2. Babies on top milk since birth due to some reason like babies of sero-positive mothers or when top milk has been supplemented with breast milk due to decreased maternal lactation.
3. Low birth weight babies those born prematurely.

A proper time to start weaning is to be emphasized very strongly. Notably, the mean age of introduction of semisolids was 10 to 13 months (SD 4 months); only 13.9% were weaned before 6 months of age while in one third it was delayed till more than one year of age in a study by Kumar *et al.*[12]

WHICH FOODS SHOULD BE USED AS WEANING FOODS

Lot many myth and food fads among mothers and child's grandparents when it comes to the introduction of complementary foods are prevalent. There is a great reluctance in giving semisolids and only the water off the top of solids such as dal and vegetables is offered in small quantities. Before advising about the type of weaning food, certain factors need to be considered. They are:

1. Easy availability of the food.
2. Simple method to prepare and time taken to prepare/cook should be considered.
3. The cost, which the parents have to incur for the food, depending upon the socioeconomic status.
4. Traditionally and culturally acceptable and locally available weaning food by the family. Prefer the regular family food rather than cooking special food.
5. Nutritive value of the food as per the requirement of growing infant. Soft and easy to eat.

6. Physiologically suitable, easily digestible and nourishing.
7. Consider taste and palatability.
8. Clean and safe.

Use of Staple Food as Basic Weaning

Different cereals form staple diet in various parts of India and rice, wheat, maize, ragi etc. can be used. Porridges made from these cereals in water or milk is good weaning food for the babies. Some oil and sugar can be added to increase the caloric density.

Several kinds of legumes, which can be used, are lentils, bengal grams, black gram, rajma etc, which are rich in protein content i.e. upto 20-25%. They are also good sources of vitamins and minerals.

Cereal and pulses combination should be used as cereals lack lysine and pulses lack methionine (limiting amino acids).

Use of Non-Vegetarian Food

Vegetable proteins alone do not provide essential amino acids in a balanced proportion as compared to animal protein. Addition of proteins of animal origin such as egg or meat will help to make up the deficiency of limiting amino acids, methionine. But this has to be advised only if acceptable to family and mothers should not be stressed to start using this by promoting that they are very essential for the bay.

In fact there is nothing in modern nutrition science to suggest that meat intake is obligatory in order to ensure optimal nutrition.[13] It was recognized that even in totally vegetarian diets, containing a diversity of foods and plants sources, tended to complement one another in amino acid supply.[14] Vegetarians, who use eggs (ovovegetarians) or milk (lactovegetarians) have more choices for different preparations of a well balanced diet. Food of animal origin no doubt provides high quality proteins, vitamin B_{12} and iron.[15]

Milk and Milk Products

Cow's milk is one of the most accepted foods in any Indian society. In India cow is considered as god and cow's milk is considered almost equivalent to mother's milk in most of the traditional Indian families. Cow's milk is used as ritual or customary infant food in such families. But, the recent scientific studies have proved that the animal milk has many disadvantages:

i. It can result in milk protein allergy.
ii. Micro-hemorrhages or GIT bleeds increases prevalence and severity of iron deficiency anemia.
iii. It can result in constipation.

Several milk products can be used in addition to milk like–curd, cheese, khoya, yogurt, etc. which have good nutritive value. Curd has the same food value as milk. There are myths regarding the use of curds in babies of this age group as curd is considered to be cold food. But there is no harm in giving these foods to babies. However, curd being a fermented food is a rich source of lactobacillus, with more vitamin C content and increased digestibility value. The only advantage of animal milk is that it is an important source of reference protein and vitamin B_{12} for those individuals who are vegetarians. The important issue that arises is whether the animal milk is essential for the infant or not? Should we use milk or milk products in the diet of the child? The various advantages of curds includes:

a. Curd may be more palatable and acceptable to the children especially in form of 'lassi'.
b. It can be used in cases of lactose intolerance and other cases of diarrhea.
c. It provides the advantage of Lactobacillus i.e. probiotics.
d. It avoids the use of bottle (a potent "baby killer instrument" in any developing country), which can lead to development of "Bottle baby disease" (diarrhea, dehydration and malnutrition which is the result of unsafe bottlefeeding).

Even if milk and milk products are not added to infants weaning diet, they can thrive well on cereals, pulses and vegetables alone. Overemphasis on milk should be avoided—the child may not have appetite for anything else and may develop a distaste for milk.

The Hot and Cold Food

In many communities there are deep-rooted beliefs, taboos or misconceptions that some foods are cold or hot. The cold foods like; banana, curd, ice cream, sugars etc. are supposed to cause common cold, cough or pneumonia. As against this, it is believed that hot foods are responsible for diarrhea or indigestion to the child. The foods believed to be hot are groundnuts, jaggery, mango, papaya, til etc. Such beliefs can be overcome with patience, or alternatives can be suggested. No one food (except breast milk) is must for a child.[1]

There is no scientific literature to support this concept in modern medicine. Every individual has his own body constitution and body response. Some individuals may be allergic to some of the foods but the concept cannot be generalized. Some children may develop allergic reaction or malabsorption to certain foods but it doesn't mean that all other babies should be kept away from such foods. In today's technological age where most of the parents are educated, it is our responsibility to explain to them that there is no scientific basis for all such misconceptions. The earlier such misconceptions are removed from the society, lesser will be the problems in infant feeding.

Supplementation of Vegetables and Fruits: Is it Beneficial?

Vegetables are good sources of vitamins and minerals especially iron. Hence, when added to the weaning food, they increase the nutritive value of food. Cooked and mashed vegetables can be added to the food of the infants and vegetable soups can be given to infants if wished by mothers, but it does not have any special added benefit. Mashed fruits like banana, papaya, mango etc can be added if affordable by parents. Banana is an excellent food. It is available everywhere throughout the year, has a thick skin, which keeps it clean and safe and doesn't need cooking. It is not hard and fast that fruits should be given in early infancy, when weaning is started.

The calorie density of these weaning foods is low, though they are good source of vitamins and minerals. Among the general population, particularly the middle and low socio economic strata, there exist a thought that, fruits and vegetables are superior and good nutritive quality food. A lot of money is spent on grapes, mousambi and apples because of strong belief that they are nourishing fruits. These fruit juices are generally given in small volumes, not necessarily fresh, diluted with water and strained so that they neither provide adequate vitamins nor avoid constipation, and the only nutritive value is of the small amount of fructose they contain. These fruits are not good source of nutrition. In fact money spent on them can be utilized on more nutritious foods. Some 89.7% of mothers think that costly food like fruits are of great nutritional value according to a study by Sharma *et al.*[16] conducted in a rural community development block. Mothers use this costly food at the cost of deprivation of the basic weaning food, which is cheaper than fruits and vegetables. Hence, these foods should be avoided in poor, malnourished children as also those suspected to be moving in that direction. Such foods may be used in cases where there is possibility or tendency for obesity.

WAYS TO INCREASE THE ENERGY DENSITY OF WEANING FOODS

Role of Fat

Oils and fats can be added to weaning food as they increase the energy density and make food soft. Any cooking oil or ghee used in the house can serve this purpose. Fried foods can be used in comparison with roasted food in babies with growth faltering or who are malnourished, as they have high caloric value. Oily or fried food should be avoided only when we suspect or encounter obese infant. Optimal fat intake is essential for:

a. Increasing palatability of the food.
b. Increasing calorie density.
c. It is a source of essential fatty acids.
d. Increasing absorption of some of the vitamins and micronutrients.

Sugar/Jaggery can be used which also helps to make food sweet and more acceptable and palatable to the infant.

Modification in Nutritive Value of Weaning Food

Vitamin B-complex content, amylase content and the bulk on cooking of the weaning foods can be modified. The following methods also increase the digestibility of food:

1. *Amylase Rich Food (ARF):* The amylase rich food addresses the twin problems of dietary bulk and poor energy density of most weaning gruels.[17] It is nothing but germinated cereal flours, which are extremely rich in the enzyme alpha-amylase. It can permit the mother to mix in much more flour into the gruel and consequently make it high in energy density, yet low in viscosity and dietary bulk.
2. *Sprouting:* When cereals are sprouted, the bulk of it decrease on cooking and so the child accepts an increased amount of food, providing more calories. Sprouting also increases the vitamin B content of food and makes it amylase rich food. The other advantage include:
   a. Cheap cost.
   b. Widely known household technology.
   c. Small amount to be made intermittently.
   d. Can be made at home, community or commercial levels etc.
3. Soaking and **malting** increases the digestibility and vitamin (riboflavin and niacin) content of food. Malting also increases the iron content of food. Malting breaks down the starch in the grain and converts it into sugar.
4. **Fermentation** technologies have several advantages. It is low cost, is simple, doesn't need fuel, the soured products prevents bacterial contamination, more palatable, many anti-nutritional factors are minimized, viscosity is lowered, digestibility is increased, fresh preparation can be kept without refrigeration for reuse for several hours even in hot and humid condition. Fermentation also reduces the amount of phytates and increases the absorption of some of the nutrients.

HOME-MADE/HOME AVAILABLE WEANING FOODS

Commercially available ready-made tinned foods have no distinct advantages over home-made food. Nevertheless, a notion does exist among mothers that the tinned foods are better, superior and more nutritious than home-made food for their babies. Existence of this notion is very harmful for mothers who belong to the middle or low socio-economic strata as they use this food at a cost, unaffordable to them. Here starts the process of use of diluted weaning food, so that the tin lasts for a longer time and the child falls prey to the pit of malnutrition. ICMR study[13] found, high intake of heavy metals by infants on commercial formulas. These formula foods also contain organochlorine pesticides in significant quantities. This is because these formulas are prepared from animal milk, which is rich in these chemicals due to its high fat content, and use of pesticides around cattle-sheds, and in fodder. Commercial foods interfere with improvement in efficiency of chewing solid family foods. Moreover, they are monotonous foods and interfere with development of taste of polytexture family foods. As against this, home-made food gives repeated exposure to sweetened or salty foods and changing the variety of foods also helps in development of food preferences and food intake.

Facilitating availability of readymade foods like biscuits, bread, pastry, cheese, butter etc. at home is advisable. These home available foods can be used at odd times like night or when fresh cooking is not possible due to some reason or during travelling.

HIV AND COMPLEMENTARY FEEDING

The emergence of HIV in last few decades has increased the mortality and morbidity manifolds especially if it is associated with malnutrition and inappropriate infant feeding practices. The mother has to chose and decide whether she wants to breastfed her newborn or not? If she decides for replacement feeding, she should have access to safer alternatives which provides all the nutrients as per the babies' needs.[19] The replacement feeding must be **s**afe, **s**ustainable, **a**cceptable, **f**easible and **a**ffordable. Mother should receive the necessary information and counselling required for making a fully informed choice regarding the practices of infant feeding and giving them full support in their choice. Minimize the risk misuse and spillover of infant formula among women who are uninfected or whose HIV status is unknown. In case she decides for artificial feeding, the important issues that arises include:

- When to start complementary feeding with solids/semisolids.
- Should she continue "exclusive formula feeding" or "exclusive animal milk" for six months?
- Can we go for early introduction of semisolids/solids in such situation?

We have already discussed that the ideal age for introducing semisolids and solids is around six months.[17,18] But in past, many of us were advising it around four months. Infant's interest in solid increases at about 4 months of age. Before, the development of a coordinated swallowing, the tongue thrust is upwards and outwards to express the milk from the nipple instead of backward motion, which propels the solid towards the esophageal inlet. It has been observed that a baby shows preferences for sweet and salty foods around one month of age.[20] Though the concentrations of pancreatic lipase, amylase and trypsin are considerably low during early months of infancy than during later childhood, the absorption of most cooked starch is almost complete and that of fat is little affected.[21, 22] Acid secretion is low at birth but increases dramatically by 24 hours. Acid and pepsin secretion peaks during the first 10 days and decreases from 10-30th days after birth. The intrinsic factor secretion rises slowly during the first two weeks of life. Even if cereals/pulses are given around 3-4 months, the infant's digestive system is going to digest most of the carbohydrate or proteins. Even premature infants usually tolerate lactose-containing formulae because of carbohydrate salvage by colonic bacteria. Protein digestion and absorption is efficient even in pre-term infants. The human gut is capable of absorbing antigenic intact proteins during the first few weeks of life because of "leaky" junctions between enterocytes.[23] This may result later on in food and microbe induced symptoms. So it is important to decide if in HIV positive mother we should continue animal milk and expose the baby to animal protein or shall we prefer cereals, pulses or fruits containing protein of vegetarian or plant origin.

The conclusions drawn are thus conflicting and confusing. Replacement feeding of young babies with non-human milk and other foods may be hazardous in poverty-stricken population.

WEANING IN SOME SPECIFIC DISEASE SITUATIONS

Introduction of solids and semisolids has got to be modified if the infant is suffering from some specific metabolic disorders.[15] Such infants may need restricted, eliminated or modified diet and co-factor therapy.

A. Carbohydrate disorders like galactosemia needs exclusion of milk and milk containing products. Soya milk or rice gruels may be used in such babies. Infants with fructosemia shall have fructose and sucrose restricted diet. Foods rich in protein are acceptable and allowed. In glycogen storage disorders, foods containing galactose and fructose should be avoided. Small frequent feed, rich in proteins may be used in these infants.
B. In disorders of protein and amino acid metabolisms reduction in protein may be needed. Rigorous dietary controls and careful monitoring of amino acid levels should be done in such infants. The diet should mainly consist of carbohydrate for sufficient calories.
C. Fat malabsorption may occur during early infancy due to cystic fibrosis or pancreatic insufficiency. Such babies are to be supplemented with medium chain triglycerides, lipase enzyme and pancreatic enzymes.
D. In babies with celiac disease, wheat, rye and barley are to be restricted in the weaning foods.
E. In cases of severe and primary lactose intolerance milk and milk containing foods are to be avoided.

Food Allergy/Food Additive

The "allergic march" refers to a sequence of events that is seen from fetal life to adulthood, and consists of sensitization to foods, gastrointestinal symptoms, eczema, wheezing and asthma, and hay fever.[24] Some babies may be allergic to cow's milk protein specially beta lacto-globulin which is mostly allergenic. Soya protein allergy may develop as a cross-reacting response in infants with proven cows milk allergy. Infants with severe allergy to milk can be given extensively hydrolyzed formulas. Soy formulas are also helpful but one runs the risk of subsequent development of allergy to soy in as many as 45% of patients. The other highly allergenic foods are dairy products, eggs, peanuts etc. Egg white is a potent allergen in some infants and it is important to remember that egg yolk is not allergen. Food additives may evoke an allergic response if artificially available foods are used during weaning. Citrus fruits may aggravate a hyperactive airway disease if infants are prone for it. It would be prudent to consider active measures for the prevention of food hypersensitivity and allergic disease.[25]

Food Fadism and Nutrition Quackery

These are the unusual patterns of food behaviors that are promoted or adopted by its adherents. It is claimed that a particular food or nutrient has a specific therapeutic value, can cure disease, or has only positive effects. Their protagonists down play or totally ignore any negative or side-effects. They may claim that dietary supplements have special value and are routinely needed. Food fadism or nutrition quackery causes harm in many ways e.g:

- The costs and expenses are increased.
- Treatments or advice may be delayed.
- Psychological harms result in many unfounded beliefs.[26]

How Much and How Many Times Feeding is Sufficient?

To accustom the baby to weaning food requires time and is a job of patience, as the child takes his own time to get fed. Mealtimes should be pleasant and forceful feeding must not be practised. The child should be active and encouraged to eat by social interaction, favourite foods, different foods, talking, patience and attention. Force must not be used in feeding under any circumstances. Start with single, low viscous food and gradually increase the viscosity, texture of food. If a particular food is refused consistently, don't offer it again for a few days but try something different. During the initial part of weaning, a small amount of food is to be given 2-3 times a day and then slowly increased to 4-5 times a day. Feeding frequency is an important factor that affects a child's nutritional status. Given their small stomach sizes, young children need to be fed frequently to ensure adequate food intake. Complementary feeds may be given before, after or with breastfeeds as they don't influence 24 hours breast milk intake and total energy intake. The order in which these foods are introduced probably is not crucial, but only one new food should be introduced at a time, and additional new food should be spaced by at least 3-4 days to allow detection of any adverse reaction or acceptance.[27] It is important to recognize that no single rule applies to all infants. Each infant follows his or her own schedule of maturation, and there is a wide variation from one infant to another. Remember, the babies, may be more hungry on some day than other days. Infant and child may be erratic eaters and this may be a worry for the parents. There may also be tendency to eat only a limited variety of foods during a meal. Parents should be encouraged to view nutritional intake over several days and not be overly concerned about individual meals. Remember, there are many foods to choose from and just as grown-ups have their likes and dislikes, a baby is also entitled to her preferences. The greater the variety of foods a baby is offered, the better the chances that her nutritional needs will be met. Transitional complementary food should be prepared from family food to help development of taste for the family foods. To avoid monotony change the food recipes, taste and flavors. Encourage 'family pot feeding'. A caring environment contributes to better nutrition and development of the child. A child who is talked to and fed in a pleasant environment eats more and grows and develops better.

Types of Complementary Foods

The complementary foods can be divided into different (**3 "A"s**) groups as per their availability and nutritional advantages:

Appropriate (First Line) Weaning Food

These includes fresh home-made, locally available, culturally acceptable, hygienically prepared, energy dense and cost-effective foods like.

a. Combination of cereals and pulses (khichadi, dal-rice etc.), porridge, suji, dalia, kheer, khaman dhokla, idli, dosa, ragi, rice preparations etc. in any form fortified with sugar and oil or fried.
b. Mashed banana, sweet potato and potato.
c. Milk added to cereals preparations.
d. Sprouted legumes, nuts, dry fruits etc. depending upon the affordability.

Acceptable (Second Line) Weaning Foods

These includes home available foods like (a) breads, cakes, pastry, biscuits, cheese, ice cream etc. (b) caloric dense fruits etc.

3 Avoidable (Third Line) Weaning Foods

These includes foods like

a. Commercially available artificial foods or tinned foods.
b. Fast food or junk food.
c. Low caloric fruits juices, soups.
d. Repeatedly fried foods containing trans fatty acids (which predispose to obesity, atherosclerosis, cardiac and neurological problems in future life).

Preparation, Storage and Hygiene

Maximum incidence of diarrhea has been reported during the weaning phase.[28] The presence of *E. coli* in almost all types of weaning food samples has been reported.[29] So proper preparation, storage and hygiene of weaning food is important, as a compromise here may predispose the child to infection and subsequent hazards. Education of care-giver and food handler in food hygiene and preparation is important. Following measures should be taken:

- Hands should be washed with soap before handling and preparing the food.
- Before feeding also, mother should wash the hands properly.
- Clean and washed utensils should be used.
- Food must be properly covered.
- Fresh food must be cooked whenever possible.
- Cooked foods should not be stored for prolonged periods or refrigerated.

Strategies Applied to Improve Weaning Practices

Infant feeding policy has been endorsed by the Indian Academy of Pediatrics and, as per the guidelines on infant feeding, by the Food and Nutrition Board, Department of Women and Child Development, Government of India known as "Policy on Infant Feeding". The Government of India adopted the National Nutrition Policy in 1993 in view of the widespread malnutrition and its effect on health and survival of the population. A National Plan of Action on nutrition was developed in 1995 and the National Nutrition Goals for the year 2000 were identified.

Some of the strategies are:

A. Appropriate infant feeding practices which include:
   - Breastfeeding exclusively for six months.
   - Addition of semisolids and solids foods after six months of age.

B. Operational guidelines for promotion of proper infant feeding which includes:
   - Thorough Child Survival and Safe Motherhood and other Developmental programs for women and children.
   - Institutional promotion of appropriate breastfeeding through Baby-friendly Hospital Initiative etc.

NUTRITION EDUCATION ABOUT WEANING

Lack of awareness of the nutritional quality of the foods, irrational beliefs about certain foods and cultural taboos about feeding contributes to development of PEM. People should be educated about the quality, quantity, acceptability and availability of low cost foods.

Nutritional planning involves a political commitment by the government in developing a nutritional policy and long-term planning to improve feeding practices. A well planned, strategies may be permanent and more rewarding. The feeding practices that are satisfying and comfortable to both the mother and the child are crucial for the emotional development and adequate feeding. The maternal feelings are readily transmitted to the infant and are major determinant of the settings in which feeding takes place. We will need to conceptualize the multiple tasks of child feeding and development from the perspective of the family and to empower them to provide the best possible care.[30]

A more effective approach is to identify and support good practices, rather than simply provide messages asking for change. Mother and family should be motivated, encouraged, educated and supported regarding proper IF practices so as to sustain and maintain infant health. Since fathers play a dominant role in the households, it is best to involve them in decision-making as well as participating in child feeding.

Infant feeding should be a part of comprehensive child-care, so child should be cared for all its health needs simultaneously. Appropriate nutritional practices play a pivotal role in determining health and development of children.

SUMMARY AND CONCLUSIONS

- Appropriate time for introducing semisolids and solids is after 6 months of age.
- The ideal food should be home-made, indigenous, hygienic, fresh, and caloric dense. A proper combination of cereals with pulse in any form acceptable to the baby is a gold standard for infant feeding.
- The feeding bottle as also only milk diet should be avoided. Milk may be added to cereals or fruits. Milk products may be easily acceptable and are better for the infant.
- The choice/taste of the infant is very important because it will help the feeding in a pleasant and enjoyable atmosphere.
- If a HIV-positive mother decides for replacement feeding, care must be taken that the feeding is safe, acceptable, feasible, affordable and sustainable. Avoid all possibilities of spillover of infant formula.
- Avoid misconceptions, taboos and food fadism.

REFERENCES

1. Anand RK. Feeding practices on infant and young children. In: Anand RK, Kumta NB, Kushwaha KP, Gupta A (eds): *The Science of Infant Feeding*. New Delhi: Jaypee 2002: 3-20.
2. Kushwaha KP. Complementary feeding of breastfed infants. In: Anand RK, Kumta NB, Kushwaha KP, Gupta A (eds): *The Science of Infant Feeding*. New Delhi: Jaypee 2002: 117-134.
3. Gupte S, Gomez EM. Infant feeding. In: Gupte S (ed): *The Short Textbook of Pediatrics*, 11th edn. New Delhi: Jaypee 2009:115-126.
4. Rowland MCM, Barrell RAE, Whitehead RG. The Weanling's dilemma: Bacterial contamination in traditional Cambian foods. *Lancet* 1978; 1: 136-138.

5. Lutter C. *Recommended Length of Exclusive Breast-feeding, Age of Introduction of Complementary Foods and the Weanling Dilemma*. Geneva: World Health Organization 1992.
6. Santosham M, Brown KH, Sack RB. Oral rehydration therapy and dietary therapy in acute childhood diarrhea. *Pediatr Rev* 1987;8:273-278.
7. Cohen RJ, Brown KH, Canahuati J. Rivera LL, Dewen KG. Effects of age of introduction. of complementary foods on infant breast milk intake, total energy intake and growth: A randomized intervention study in Honduras. *Lancet* 1994, 344:288-293.
8. Ghosh S. ICDS program: Need for reappraisal. *Indian Pediatr* 1997; 34: 911-918.
9. Sachdev HPS. Infant feeding: Major practical considerations. In: Sachdev HPS, Choudhary P (eds): *Nutrition in Children: Developing Country Concerns*. New Delhi: BI Publications 1994: 79-128.
10. Gupte S, Sharma A. Changing trends in KAPs in relation to infant feeding in north India. *Asian Bull Nutr* 1985;5:124-129.
11. Sharrif A, Farsana C. Breastfeeding practices, beliefs and taboos in Karnataka. *Indian J Social Work* 1990,31:141-148.
12. Kumar S, Nath LM, Reddaiah VP. Supplementary feeding pattern in children living in a resettlement colony. *Indian Pediatr* 1992; 29; 219-222.
13. Gopalan S, Puri RK, Sachdev HPS. Adequacy of vegetarian diets for optimal nutrition of mother and child. *Indian Pediatr* 1993; 30; 1379-1386.
14. World Health Organization. *Diet, Nutrition and the Prevention of Chronic Diseases*. WHO Techn Report Series 797, 1991.
15. Ghosh S. Starting of other family foods. In: *Nutrition and Child Care: A Practical Guide*. New Delhi, Jaypee 1997:96-107.
16. Sharma KP, Thakur AK. Maternal beliefs regarding diet during common illness. *Indian Pediatr* 1995,32:909-910.
17. Gopaldas T. Technologies to improve weaning foods in developing countries. In: Sachdev HPS, Choudhary P (eds): *Nutrition in Children: Developing Country Concerns*. New Delhi: B I Publications 1994: 129-134.
18. Gupte S. Food contamination and the child. *Proceedings International Workshop on Food Contamination and Adulteration*, Bangkok 2003. Abstract IWFC/Ped-5.
19. NACO, IAPO, UNICEF, WHO. *Manual for Management of HIV/AIDS in Children*. New Delhi: NACO, IAPO, WHO, UNICEF 2004-05.
20. Wyellie R. Clinical manifestations of gastrointestinal diseases. In Behrman RE, Kliegman RM, Jenson HB (eds): *Nelson Textbook of Pediatrics*,17th edn. Philadelphia: Saunders 2004;1197-1198.
21. Zoppi G, Andreotti G, Pajno Ferrara F, Njai DM, Gaburro D. Exocrine pancreatic function in premature and full term neonates. *Pediatr Res* 1972;6:880-886.
22. Watkins JB. Bile acid metabolism and fat absorption in newborn infants. *Pediatr Clin N Am* 2004;21; 501-512.
23. Wyellie R. Normal development, structure and functions of stomach and intestines. In Behrman RE, Kliegman RM, Jenson HB (eds): *Nelson Textbook of Pediatrics*,17th edn.Philadelphia: Saunders 2004: 1228-1229.
24. Chandra RK, Gill B, Kumari S. Food allergy and atopic disease. *Crit Rev Allergy Immunol* 1995; 13: 293-334.
25. Chandra RK. Food hypersensitivity and allergic diseases: A new threat in India. *Indian Pediatr* 2003; 40: 99-101.
26. Leleiko N, Cewin C. Nutrition deficiency states. In Rudolph AM, Hoffman J, Rudolph CD (eds): *Rudolph's Pediatrics*, 20th edn. Stanford: Prentice Hall International/Appleton and Lange 1996:1015-1017.
27. Leleiko N, Cewin C. Nutrition deficiency states. In Rudolph AM, Hoffman J, Rudolph CD editors; Rudolph's Pediatrics 20th edition Prentice Hall International, Appleton and Lange, Stamford, Connecticut; 1996;1015-1017.
28. Heird WC. The feeding of infants and children. In Behrman RE, Kliegman RM, Jenson HB (eds): *Nelson Textbook of Pediatrics*, 17th edn. Philadelphia: Saunders 2004:157-167.
29. Brit B, Kaurany M, Milter JW. A pilot research for environmental diarrheal disease in young children in Panama. *Environm Child Health* 1973;19:282-287.
30. Shah PR, Patel HH. Bacteriological studies of weaning food in relation to acute diarrhea in children. *Indian J Microbiol* 1989,29:165-168.

Suraj Gupte • Javed Chowdhary • EM Gomez

12 Low Birthweight Infants: Overview

INTRODUCTION

According to the World Health Organization (WHO), low birthweight infants (< 2500 g weight at birth), constitute 17% of all live births globally.[1] As high as 95% of these babies are born in developing countries, South Asia leading the tally. In India, as high as 25-30% of babies are LBW, a reflection of the poor health status, especially nutrition, of the mothers and insufficient antenatal care for variable reasons.

LBW is a predominant factor for high perinatal and infant mortality and morbidity. Infant mortality in LBW is 20 times higher than in good-weight infants. According to an estimate, 50% of all perinatal deaths and 33% of infant deaths are due to LBW. Protein-energy malnutrition and superadded infection are chiefly responsible for this state of affairs. Not just that! There is in all probability a high incidence of mental subnormality in the survivors. Understandably, therefore, LBW in India is by and large a reflection of intrauterine growth retardation (IUGR), carrying serious implications for

- Short-term in relation to postnatal growth and development in infancy, and
- Long-term in relation to risk of developing degenerative disease (e.g. diabetes, coronary heart disease, hypertension, stroke) in adulthood.

According to Gopalan,[2, 3] LBW, for India and other developing countries, is a major public health problem that should concern not just the obstetrician and neonatologist alone but also the large body of health professionals and policy-makers. He has, in fact, made out a strong case for viewing LBW deliveries as an index of our public health in general and of maternal health in particular and argued for according it nearly as much significance and importance as infant mortality rate (IMR).[4] He has further warned against complacency on attaining fall in infant mortality and improvement in child survival data which must not be considered as an indicator of child health/nutrition. Survival of LBW infants without ensuring their health and nutrition is likely to further expand the pool of substandard survivors, eroding the quality of human resources and development.

DEFINITION

By international definition, an LBW infant is a baby less than 2500 g at birth, regardless of the gestational age, the measurement being taken within the first hour of life before significant postnatal weight loss has occurred. Though, from time to time, an argument has been put forward for bringing down the upper cutoff point from 2500 g to 2000 g for developing word,[5] the controversy has now by and large died down. Today, therefore, the WHO's definition should be considered valid globally.

CLASSIFICATION

A. Based on Birthweight

- Simply low birthweight (SLBW): Birthweight 1800 to 2500 g.
- Quite low birthweight (QLBW): Birthweight 1500-1800 g.
- Very low birthweight (VLBW): Birthweight between 1000 to 1500 g.
- Extremely low birthweight" (ELBW): Birthweight between 500 to 1000g.
- Micropreemie: Birthweight < 500 g birthweight.

B. Based on Gestation Period

Two types are recognized:

- Preterm LBW, and
- Small for gestational age (SGA) or small for dates (SFD) LBW.

Occasionally, an LBW infant may be both preterm and SGA (SFD).

Preterm LBW Baby

This is the predominant type of LBW infants in the developed countries.

The causes include:

- Multiple births.
- Acute maternal infections.

- Strenuous physical work.
- Hypertension.
- Idiopathic.

Such a baby is born <37 weeks of gestation. His weight, length and development is usually in keeping with the duration of gestation.

Following good neonatal care, the preterm baby catches up growth, reaching normal size and performance by 2-3 years of age.

Prevention lies in good antenatal care, screening, treatment of hypertension and discouragement of teenage pregnancy.

SGA (SFD)-LBW Baby

Such a baby suffers from intrauterine growth retardation, weighing <10th percentile for gestational age. He may be born at term or prematurely. In the developing world, this is the predominant type of LBW seen. Three types are recognized: malnourished, hypoplastic and mixed.

1. *Malnourished:* The baby appears marasmic, long and thin, skin losing its normal elasticity and hanging in folds over the buttocks. Internal organs with the exception of brain are shrunk. Head circumference remains nearly normal, usually 3 cm in excess of chest circumference. Ponderal index is <2.5. Since cell number is not affected, these infants are responsive to nutritional rehabilitation. Ponderal index is calculated by dividing weight in kg by length in cm^3 and then multiplying by 100. Normal is over 2.5. In malnourished LBW infants it is reduced.
2. *Hypoplastic:* Such a baby is proportionally small in all parameters. Since cell population is reduced, growth potential is considerably affected, resulting in permanent retardation in physical and mental growth. Incidence of accompanying congenital malformations is high.
3. *Mixed:* The baby neither appears malnourished as in type I nor hypoplastic as in type II. Reduction in cell size as well as number is characteristic of this type of IUGR.

MAGNITUDE

Though all reports show that the overwhelming proportion of LBW infants in India is of the SGA (SFD) type, wide variation in the relative incidence is reported from various parts of the country. In north India, data gathered from different states show that 70-90% LBW infants are of SGA type, only 10-30% being of preterm type. A study conducted in New Delhi as far back as 1993 recorded only 12-15% of LBW infants with birthweight between 2000-2500 g were preterm, the remaining 85-88 being full-term SGA babies.[6]

ETIOLOGY[1, 7-10]

Maternal Malnutrition

Food deprivation, particularly during the last weeks of pregnancy in a mother who is already undernourished (weight <40 kg, height < 145 cm) is the cause. There is evidence that food supplementation in pregnancy considerably reduces the incidence of IUGR.

Intrauterine Infections

Such intrauterine infections as toxoplasmosis, cytomegalovirus disease, rubella, herpes, syphilis may exert their adverse influence early in embryonic life, causing hypoplastic type of IUGR. There is now evidence of a link between delivery of LBW infants and presence of vaginal mycoplasma or other infectious agents during pregnancy. In a controlled trial in Boston, erythromycin administered to pregnant women at risk resulted in a dramatic and unprecedented increase in the mean infant birthweight and a 3-fold decline in the LBW infants.

Placental Dysfunction

Such maternal problems as toxemias of pregnancy and hypertension may be responsible for placental dysfunction and IUGR.

Multiple Pregnancy

It is an established fact that, after 35 weeks of gestation, the mother becomes incapable of providing adequate nourishment to more than one fetus.

Maternal Diseases

Chronic maternal diseases such as heart disease, tuberculosis, renal disease, bronchial asthma, etc. are likely to cause IUGR.

Teenage Pregnancy

Teenage pregnancy predisposes the immature mother to such risks as toxemia, postpartum hemorrhage, postpartum infection, stillborn infant and LBW infant.

Genetic/Chromosomal Disorders

Certain genetic disorders (say short-limbed dwarfism) and chromosomal disorders (say Turner syndrome, trisomies) exert their adverse influence early during gestation, reducing both cell number and cell size. The result is hypoplastic IUGR with reduced growth potentials.

Miscellaneous

Narcotic addiction, teratogenic agents, tobacco smoking, high altitude, irradiation, pregnancy-out-of-wedlock contribute to LBW.

HANDICAPS/RISKS

Preterm LBW Infants

1. Asphyxia.
2. Apneic spells.

3. Respiratory distress syndrome (hyaline membrane disease).
4. Hypothermia.
5. Poor coordination in suckling and swallowing.
6. Intraventricular hemorrhage.
7. Hypoglycemia.
8. Metabolic acidosis.
9. Hyperbilirubinemia.
10. Sepsis.
11. Retinopathy of prematurity from hyperoxia due to unmonitored oxygen therapy.

SGA (SFD) LBW Infants

1. Aspiration of meconium, amniotic fluid or vernix caseosa, causing respiratory distress.
2. Asphyxia from cerebral anoxia.
3. Fetal hypoxia/death from placental dysfunction.
4. Symptomatic hypoglycemia due to insufficient glycogen stores.
5. Neonatal sepsis.
6. Polycythemia from chronic hypoxia.
7. Pulmonary hemorrhage.
8. Congenital malformations.
9. Poor temperature regulation, usually hypothermia, due to inadequacy of brown fat stores.
10. Permanent retardation in linear growth and psychomotor development.

MANAGEMENT

Delivery

It is desirable that delivery of the mother expected to give birth to an LBW infant is conducted in a hospital or a well-equipped center with facilities for neonatal resuscitation.

Care of the Baby

Weight 1800 g and above

Good nursing care is good enough for a vast majority of these babies. These babies can be managed at domiciliary level under supervision. Special attention needs to be paid to maintenance of their body temperature and feeding to prevent hypoglycemia.

Weight < 1800 kg

First class modern neonatal care, usually in a NICU until weight reaches 2 kg. The components of intensive care are:

- ***Thermal Care***: It is advisable to keep the baby in a thermoneutral environment, ensuring that his body temperature is maintained at 36.5°C.[10] To achieve this, the following measures are recommended:
- Placement in a prewarmed incubator or an open-care system.
- Covering of the baby with cotton, cellophane or thin transparent plastic sheet.
- Application of oil or liquid paraffin on baby's skin.
- Partial kangaroo-mother-care for preventing hypothermia, facilitate breastfeeding and promote bonding between the mother and the infant.
- ***Feeding and Nutritional Supplementation***: This is discussed in details in the subsequent Chapter. Unless the baby is <1200 g weight, < 30 weeks gestation or seriously sick with birth asphyxia, RDS, septicemia, seizures, apneic spells, etc. (needing intravenous fluids), attempt should be to provide enteral nutrition. Even in former categories, enteral feeding with expressed breast milk (EBM) should be started as soon as baby's condition improves and gradually increased in quantity while IV fluid are being accordingly reduced.

At 2 weeks of age, a human milk fortifier may be added to EBM for providing extra protein, energy and micronutrients.

Again at 2 weeks, multivitamin (including folic acid) drops should be introduced.

At about 4-8 weeks, low-dose (2-3 mg/kg/day) iron supplementation should be started.

Vitamin E, calcium and phosphorus supplementation is also recommended.

- ***Prevention of infection:*** High index of suspicion, early detection and prompt treatment of nosocomial infection are important for survival of the baby. Even more importantly, all attempts should be made to prevent occurrence of infection by such measures as minimal handling and vigilance on procedures.
- ***Oxygen therapy:*** Oxygen therapy should be only when indicated (SaO_2 > 90%), at lowest ambient concentration and for minimal period (withdrawn with SaO_2 < 85%).
- ***Phototherapy:*** Preterm LBW infants are prone to develop bilirubin encephalopathy at relatively lower serum bilirubin levels. Early phototherapy in jaundiced babies is, therefore, advisable.
- ***Immunization: All* LBW infants, unless they are critically sick, need to be vaccinated on the same lines as normal weight infants.**

PROGNOSIS AND FUTURE IMPACT

LBW infants account for 75-80% of deaths during neonatal period and 50% deaths in infancy.

Table 12.1 lists the major causes of death in LBW.

Table 12.1: Major causes of death in LBW

- Hypothermia
- Atelectasis
- Malnutrition
- Pulmonary hemorrhage
- Infections e.g. pneumonia, septicemia
- Intracranial bleeding

The survivors are prone to:

- Subnormal growth and development, even upto adult age.
- Lower levels of mental development. There is high incidence of learning disabilities, language disorders, attention deficit and hyperactivity, behavioral problems, etc.
- Neurologic handicap in the form of cerebral palsy, mental retardation, seizures, microcephaly, hydrocephalus, deafness, ROP ending up with blindness, etc.
- Six times greater chance of developing diabetes mellitus.
- Vulnerability to develop hypertension and degenerative cardiovascular disease in later life.

PREVENTION

Worldwide, there is now a growing realization that treatment of LBW is an expensive and cumbersome affair. Logically, therefore, the stress needs to be on its prevention.

Female Literacy and Formal Education

A well-informed, educated mother is likely to have better health before and during pregnancy, avoids harmful agents and influences during pregnancy and shows better reproductive performance and outcome. Education and training of traditional birth attendants (TBAs) or ensure adequate care of mothers during pregnancy and their referral to a nearby health center is also important. Teenage pregnancy should be discouraged.

Maternal Health Status

Adequate nutrition of the female throughout childhood and adolescence is a very effective way of ensuring good health status of the pregnant women, provided that the so-called "previous nutritional status" is maintained by continued good nourishment and freedom from medical ailments.

Antenatal Care

Birthweight is directly proportional to the number of antenatal checkups. Early detection of high-risk factors such as intrauterine infections, hypertension, toxemias of pregnancy, and timely intervention can prevent occurrence of IUGR.

Girl Child Nutrition

It is important to provide optimal nutrition to the girl child throughout life-cycle.[10] Else, she is likely to grow into a weakling as a woman. Such a small woman is set to give birth to an LBW baby. This way, the vicious cycle of LBW gets perpetuated. It is tough to break it.

Avoidance of Early Marriage and Teenage Pregnancy

India always had the dubious distinction of high incidence of child marriage and teenage pregnancy. It was expected that with increasing literacy and enlightenment, this malady would die down in due course. Now, the problem has got compounded as a result of western influences, resulting in increasing incidence of premarital sex even amongst the informed teenagers and, subsequent to that high incidence of these pregnancies in these irresponsible adolescents. The outcome of these pregnancies is often LBW.

REFERENCES

1. Park K. Preventive medicine in obstetrics, pediatrics and geriatrics. In: *Park's Textbook of Preventive and Social Medicine*, 18th edn. Jabalpur: Banarsidas Bhanot 2005;383-437.
2. Gopalan C. The changing profile of undernutrition in India. *Bull Nutr Found India* 1991;12:1-4.
3. Gopalan C. Women and nutrition in India: Some practical considerations. *Bull Nutr Found India* 1989;10:1-4.
4. Gopalan C. Low birthweights: Significance and implications. In: Sachdev HPS, Choudhury P (eds) *Nutrition in Children: Developing Country Concerns.* New Delhi: BI 1994:1-33.
5. Sur D. Low birthweight and associated morbidities. In: *Recent Advances in Pediatrics (Special Vol 11: Community Pediatrics).* New Delhi: Jaypee 2002;395-403.
6. Bhargava SK, Iyer PU, Nafda S, Dutta V, Ramji S, Sachdev HPS. Perspectives in low birthweight: Survival and outcome. In: Bhargava SK, Chhaparwal BC, Guha DK, Iyer PU (eds) *Proceedings of 3rd, 4th and 5th Annual Conventions of the National Neonatology Forum.* Indore: Organizing Committee 1985:44-52.
7. Gupte S, Gomez EM. Infant feeding. In: Gupte S (ed) *The Short Textbook of Pediatrics*, 11th edn. New Delhi: Jaypee 2009;115-126.
8. Vani S, Chowdhary J, Gupte S. Neonatology. In: Gupte S (ed) *The Short Textbook of Pediatrics*, 11th edn. New Delhi: Jaypee 2009;185-244.
9. Gupte S, Sahni AK. Adolescence. In: Gupte S (ed) *The Short Textbook of Pediatrics*, 11th edn. New Delhi: Jaypee 2009:6071.
10. Singh M. *Care of the Newborn*, 6th edn. New Delhi: Sagar 2004.

Suraj Gupte • Mohinder Pal • Stephen Abil

13 Feeding of the Low Birthweight Infants

INTRODUCTION

The LBW infant is known to suffer from one or the other feeding problem as a result of:[1-3]

- Need for a higher food intake compared to the normal infant in order to make up the deficit in weight.
- High frequency of suckling difficulties.
- Incoordination between suckling and swallowing.
- Abdominal distention as he is not capable of holding a large feed in his stomach.
- Regurgitation since the cardioesophageal sphincter is lax.
- Poor tolerance for saturated fatty acids.

Notably most of the problems are secondary to immaturity of the gastrointestinal system.

NUTRITIONAL NEEDS OF THE LBW INFANT[3-7]

According to estimates, the LBW infant requires on an average 140 (120-150) kcal/kg/day.

Understandably, about 200 ml of milk is required to meet this demand. Attempts to attain this target right at the outset often prove futile since the infant is simply unable to cope with this much feed. A realistic and practical approach is to aim at achieving this target by second week.

As regards protein, 4-6 g/kg/day is good enough. An intake outside this range is not in the interest of the infant. Higher intake may cause retention of fluid and solute as also high blood urea on account of renal immaturity. Rapid weight gain occurring in this situation is not in the interest of the baby. Low protein intake may cause hypoproteinemic edema and poor weight gain, further worsening the baby's nutritional status.

Over and above this, the infant also needs vitamin K at birth, and multivitamins (especially vitamins A, C, D and E), iron and folic acid, calcium, phosphorus, etc. subsequently.

Early feeding is the current recommendation—within 6-12 hours. Most centers give the first feed at about 3 hours of age. The risk of aspiration in early feeding can be minimized with careful supervision and vigilance.

Risks of delayed feeding include icterus, hypoglycemia, metabolic acidosis, metabolic acidosis and brain damage.

METHOD OF FEEDING/PROVIDING NUTRITION

Broad guidelines for fluids and nutrition of LBW infants are given in Table 13.1.

Table 13.1: Broad guidelines for providing fluids and nutrition to LBW babies

Time after birth	*Categories of LBW neonates*			
	< 1000 g	*< 1200 g /<30 wks*	*1200-1800 g/30-34 wks*	*>1800 g/>34 wks*
Initial	PN	IV fluids; may try gavage feeding if not sick	Gavage	Breast, may try "katori-spoon" feed
After 1-3 days	PN	Gavage	Katori-spoon	Breast
Later (2-4 wks)	BF	Katori-spoon	Breast	Breast
After some more time (2-4 wks)	BF	Breast	Breast	Breast

Note:

1. For gavage and katori-spoon feeds, use EBM only, starting with small volume and gradually building it up.
2. When the baby is on gavage or katori-spoon feed, he should be put on the breast before every feed. Though the baby may not obtain much feed, he learns sucking and stimulate lactation.
3. While shifting the baby from one mode to the other, care should be exercised to give the new mode for only some of the feeds and thereafter building up gradually.
4. Feeding of every LBW baby need to be individualized.

Breastfeeding

Many LBW infants, especially those weighing > 1800 g, are strong enough to suckle well from the breast. This should be encouraged. However, care should be exercised to safeguard against distention of abdomen. This is best achieved though small feeds at frequent intervals.

Breastfeeding should be considered as the preferred choice enteral feeding for all LBW babies. When it is not workable for some reason, gavage feeding (tube feeding) should be the choice, employing mother's own expressed milk. There is sufficient evidence that necrotizing enterocolitis is far less in LBW infants fed mother's milk than those on artificial feed. Further, LBW infants on own mother's milk are known to grow faster than those on another woman's milk.

Alternative Methods of Milk Feeding

Gavage (Tube) Feeding

It is needed in:

- LBW infants weighing < 1200 g or < 30 weeks gestation after initial stabilization with IV fluids.
- LBW infants weighing 1200-1800 g or < 34 weeks gestation.

Other indications of tube feeding are:

- Baby getting tired quickly.
- Baby taking > 20 min to finish the feed.

For LBW infants, recommended size of the tube is No. 6 FG (French gauge) and No 4 FG in case of complicating respiratory difficulty. On an average about 16-17 cm of tube is needed to reach the stomach from the gum margin. In a given situation, the tube may be measured from the tip of the nose to the ear lobe and further to the ansiform cartilage. The measurement should be marked of the tube per se.

In case tube feeding is required for a short period, it may be passed through the mouth. For this purpose, the wet tube is placed along the side of the tongue and then into the pharynx. The head-end of the baby needs to be raised.

If tube feeding is needed for several days, it should be passed through the nasal route into the esophagus and stomach. It should be kept in place.

Once the tube has been passed—irrespective of the route—its position should be confirmed. To do this, gentle aspiration is required. The gastric fluid is usually colorless and acidic in reaction. If aspiration is difficult, some air may be injected and its entry into the stomach verified by auscultating the epigastric region.

Intermittent Feeding: The outer end of the tube is attached to a syringe (20 ml) containing milk. It is important to bear in mind that milk should not be pushed, if safety is needed. Instead it should be allowed to trickle by gravity. The time taken by each feed nearly varies from 10 to 20 minutes, depending upon the size of the feed. This is about the time taken by an ordinary feed as well.

At the end of the feed, a few ml of plain water should be pushed to rinse the tube.

If the tube is to be removed, it should be pinched so that no fluid trickles into the trachea as the end reaches past the larynx.

Continuous Feeding (Intragastric Drip): Continuous milk drip has now won pride of the place in the feeding of LBW babies. Its advantages are many, e.g.:

1. Allows high milk intake.
2. Weight gain is more.
3. Less risk of regurgitation.
4. Less risk of aspiration into the lungs.
5. Less risk of hypoglycemia.
6. Nursing time is cut.
7. Minimal handling of the infant.

The technique of introduction of the tube into the stomach is same as in case of intermittent feeding. The outer end of tube is, however, attached to the intravenous set containing milk.

As in intermittent feeding, infants' head should remain slightly raised. His position should be supine.

The tube should be changed every third day. It should be aspirated thrice daily. The bottle requires to be changed every 12 hours and the giving set every 24 hours.

Table 13.2 gives details about intermittent and continuous feeding.

Table 13.2: Gavage (tube) feeding of the LBW infant

Schedule	*Indication*	*Milk/kg/day*									
		Day 1	*2*	*3*	*4*	*5*	*6*	*7*	*8*	*9*	*10*
Fast schedule	1. SFD 2. S bilirubin below 10 mg %	20	40	60	100	120	150				
Slow schedule	1. Infants < 30 weeks Gestation 2. Abdominal distention. Seizures, apneic attacks, Cyanosis following feeding Or congenital heart disease	15	30	35	60	75	90	105	120	135	150

Section 4

"Palady"/"Katori-spoon" Feeding

The fact that even LBW neonates of 30-32 weeks gestation are good at swallowing even though their sucking may not be upto the mark forms the guiding principle of feeding by a "palady" or "katori and spoon".

In case of the "palady", the tapering snout is placed at the angle of the mouth. Then, milk is allowed to trickle slowly. The infant manages to swallow it without sucking. Repeat until the required quantity has been fed. It is good to be slow and patient, to avoid spilling of the feed.

In case of "katori and spoon", required quantity of EBM is taken in a clean medium-sized katori (or a cup). Spoon is filled with milk and placed over the lips at the corner of the mouth. Milk starts flowing into the mouth while the infant actively swallows it. Repeat the process until the calculated quantity has been fed. Avoid spillage.

It is possible to find the quantity that has been spilled by wighing the napkin around baby's neck before and after the feeding.

Expressed Breast Milk (EBM)

EBM should be first choice. Milk of the LBW baby's milk provides higher protein and calories. It is, therefore, not only species-specific but also baby specific on account of its best suitability for the infant.

Expression of milk can be carried out by mother's attendant though mother herself is the best for this purpose. The choice about the manual expression or the use of a breast pump is influenced by the existing circumstances as well as mother's attitude. Table 13.3 gives the schedule for expression of breast milk.

Table 13.3: Breast milk expression

First 24 hours	Twice, 2 min at each breast
Second 24 hours	Thrice, 3 min at each breast
Third 24 hours	Four times, 4 min at each breast
Fourth day and onward	Five or 6 times, 5-10 times at each breast

Expression of milk must be done in a safe and clean manner. The concept of human milk banking now gaining popularity in the European countries poses several difficulties in the developing countries because of unfavorable climate, ignorance, illiteracy, impracticability of monitoring of each sample before administration and holder pasteurization. Nevertheless, in view of the greater need for human milk for the LBW infants, the need for modified human milk banking cannot be denied.

Expressed milk provides adequate amount of protein, energy, vitamins and copper and nearly adequate amounts of zinc, iron and magnesium which, however, are needed in yet greater measure by the LBW baby. It is poor in calcium and phosphorus. Supplementation with these nutrients is, therefore important in the care and feeding of LBW infants.

In case enough EBM from the biologic mother is not readily available, it may be collected from another lactating healthy mother.

Resort to top milk is indicated only in case of lactation failure despite best of efforts at relactation. It should be for a short period only and breastfeeding resumed as soon as possible.

Nutritional Supplements

Preterm human milk, though superior to pooled term milk, is deficient in iron, calcium, phosphorus, zinc and copper.[8] It provides more proteins and energy but the preterm LBW infant needs yet more of these. EBM, therefore, works better when supplemented with human milk fortifier or individual nutrients. At present, the only available HMF is Lactodex-HMF (Raptakos-Brett).

Human Milk Fortifiers: At 2 weeks of age, human milk fortifier may be added to EBM for providing extra protein, energy and micronutrients. The dose is 2 g of Lactodex-HMF for 50 ml of EBM. The resultant fortified EBM provides additional 0.2 g protein, 0.19 g fat, 1.2 g CHO plus calcium, phosphorus, vitamins, minerals and trace elements.

Vitamin K: Right at birth, 1 mg vitamin K should be given intramuscully.

Multivitamin Drops: Again at 2 weeks, multivitamin (including folic acid) drops should be introduced.

Iron: At about 4-8 weeks, low-dose (2-3 mg/kg/day) iron supplementation should be started.

Vitamin E, calcium and phosphorus: Supplementation with these micronutrients is recommended, especially in case of VLBW.

Intravenous (Central) Feeding

First 2 Days

For LBW of SGA (SFD) type, 90-100 ml/ kg of 5-10 % glucose is recommended. For LBW of short gestation type, 60-70 ml/kg of 5-10 % glucose suffices.

Later

Since the LBW needs extra sodium and potassium, N/5 saline with 15% potassium chloride (1 ml added to 100 ml infusate) should replace the 5-10% glucose after 2 days. The readymade Isolyte-P serves well as an alternative.

Parenteral Nutrition[9,10]

It may become mandatory to resort to parenteral nutrition in the following life-threatening situations in which enteral feeding has failed to establish or central feeding is not possible for prolonged periods:

- ELBW babies (<1000 g).
- LBW babies unlikely to attain full enteral nutrition by day 5 for some associated problem such as intractable diarrhea, necrotizing enterocolitis, surgically correctable GI anomaly (omphalocele, gastroschisis, tracheo-

esophageal fistula, malrotation with volvus, diaphragmatic hernia, etc.), extensive bowel resection.

This regimen provides adequate fluids and electrolytes, energy (from glucose, protein and lipids), amino acids and vitamins and micronutrients for sustained growth of the LBW babies. With this method, providing around 100 kcal/kg/24 hours, a weight gain of 15 g/kg/24 hours is likely to be attained in the first week.

Parenteral nutrition may be carried out employing an indwelling central venous catheter (per cutaneous or surgically-placed) or through a peripheral vein.

It is important to be vigilant about the complications, both catheter-related and metabolic (Table 13.4).

Table 13.4: Complications of parenteral nutrition and remedial measures

Complication	*Action Recommended*
Catheter-related Complications	Meticulous catheter care
Sepsis/septicemia (usually from coagulasenegative staphylococcus)	• Aseptic preparation of the infusate • Appropriate antibiotics • Removal of line if sepsis persists
Thrombosis	
Extravasation of fluid	
Accidental dislodgement of catheter	
Metabolic Complications	Biochemical and physiologic monitoring
Hyperglycemia	
Azotemia	
Nephrocalcinosis	
Hyperlipidemia	
Hypoxemia	
Hyperammonemia	
Cholestatic jaundice	
Liver disease	
Metabolic bone disease	

For details on Parenteral nutrition readers are referred to Chapter 65.

Nonnutritive Suckling

When the LBW infant is being kept on IV fluid or tube feeding, he may be given experience of suckling by providing opportunity to suckle the empty breast. This experience stands him in good stead later at the time of transition to nutritive suckling.

REFERENCES

1. Park K. Preventive medicine in obstetrics, pediatrics and geriatrics. In: *Park's Textbook of Preventive and Social Medicine*, 21st edn. Jabalpur: Bhanot 2011;383-437.
2. Gupte S, Vani S. Pediatric nutritional requirements. In: Gupte S (ed) *The Short Textbook of Pediatrics*, 11th edn. New Delhi: Jaypee 2009;109-113.
3. Gupte S, Gomez EM. Infant feeding. In: Gupte S (ed) *The Short Textbook of Pediatrics*, 10th edn. New Delhi: Jaypee 2004;115-126.
4. Vani S, Chowdhary J, Gupte S. Neonatology. In: Gupte S (ed) *The Short Textbook of Pediatrics*, 11th edn. New Delhi: Jaypee 2009;185-244.
5. Mathur NB. Feeding of low birthweight infants. In: Anand RK, Kumta NB, Kushwaha KP, Gupta A (eds): *The Science of Infant Feeding*. New Delhi: Jaypee Brothers 2002; 81-89.
6. Irani SF, Gupta G, Verma R. Controversies in feeding of low birthweight neonates. In: Gupte S, Gupte SB (eds): *Recent Advances in Pediatrics* (Special Vol. 5: Neonatology, Vol. 2). New Delhi: Jaypee 2000;184-191.
7. Hathi GS, Bavdekar SB. Human lactation and breastfeeding management. In: Gupte S, Gupte SB (eds): *Recent Advances in Pediatrics, Vol. 3*. New Delhi: Jaypee 1993;11-34.
8. Saili A, Nangia S, Guha DK. Feeding and nutrition. In: Guha DK, Saili A, Bhat S, Shenoi A (eds): *Guha's Neonatology: Principles and Practice*. New Delhi: Jaypee 2005;580-611.
9. Gaur A. Nutrition of the sick neonate. In: Gupte S (ed) *Textbook of Neonatal Emergencies*. New Delhi: Peepee 2006;340-353.
10. Nair PMC. Parenteral nutrition in the neonates. In: Gupte S (ed) *Textbook of Neonatal Emergencies*. New Delhi: Peepee 2006;354-359.

JP Dadhich

14 Fortification of Breast Milk

INTRODUCTION

Survival of low birthweight babies has improved over the period of last few decades. The nutritional management plays a large role in their immediate survival and subsequent growth and development.[1] While evaluating the nutritional needs and recommended intakes by an LBW infant, most of the authorities use criteria based on intrauterine growth rates, body composition and factorial assessment of nutrition accretion. These criteria may not constitute an ideal method for such a calculation.[2, 3] The American Academy of Pediatrics (AAP) recommends the optimal diet for premature infants as the one that supports growth at intrauterine rates without imposing stress on the infant's immature metabolic and excretory functions.[4] Recent AAP guidelines say that hospitals and physicians should recommend human milk for premature and other high-risk infants either by direct breastfeeding and/or using the mother's own expressed milk.[5]

GOALS OF NUTRITION IN LBW

The goals of low birthweight infant's nutrition include:
1. Short-term growth.
2. Prevention of neonatal morbidity.[6]
3. Long-term outcomes.

Short-term Growth

Pre-term infant fed pre-term milk demonstrate increase in weight, length and head circumference as well as retention rates of various nutrients comparable to those for the fetus of similar post-conception age. The pre-term infant's own mother's milk produced during early postpartum period offers nutritional advantage because of:

1. Higher protein content.
2. Higher electrolyte concentrations.[1, 7-9]
3. Better absorption.

Fat absorption in pre-term babies, fed their own mother's milk is significantly higher than in a similar group of infants fed cow's milk formula. Long chain polyunsaturated fatty acids (LCPUFAs), which are important for mental and visual development, are higher in human milk.[10, 11]

Preventing Neonatal Morbidity

Several studies have reported a reduced incidence of necrotizing enterocolitis (NE), the devastating acute inflammatory disease, in pre-term infants fed mother's milk in comparison to formula milk.[12-14] The reasons for protective role of human milk in the NEC is unclear but quantity of host defense factors in pre-term milk are greater than in term milk.[15]

In another report, the disease seemed to be less severe and the prevalence of intestinal perforation was lower during the course of the disease in infants who received human milk before diagnosis compared with formula, 7% v/s 39%, respectively.[16]

Clinical studies in nurseries worldwide have suggested a decreased rate of various infections in premature infants fed human milk compared with those fed infant formula.[14,17]

Use of human milk can justifiably be adopted as an important healthcare intervention in neonatal units.

Long-term Outcome

Studies now have also suggested a relationship between early diet and development of hypertension, hyper-cholesterolemia and ischemic heart disease.[1] The receipt of unfortified human milk during hospitalization has been associated with greater intellectual performances score at 7.5 to 8.0 years of age compared with the receipt of formula in former premature infants.[18] Premature infant fed donor human milk had advantages in psychomotor development at 18 months of age compared with infants fed pre-term formula.[19]

FORTIFICATION OF HUMAN MILK

Although breast milk has been shown to be of great advantages in preterm infants. The beneficial effects generally relate to improvements in host defense, digestion and absorption of nutrients, neurodevelopment, gastrointestinal function, as well as psychological effects on the mother.[20, 21] Human milk is suitable to meet many needs of premature infants. However, exclusive feeding of unfortified human milk has been associated with poorer rates of growth and nutritional deficits during and beyond the period of hospitalization.[20, 22] The goal for nutritional support is to meet the intrauterine rates of growth and nutrient retention. Nutrient supplementation is necessary to optimize the use of human milk in the feeding of premature infants.[23] Supplementation of human milk with multi-component fortifiers is associated with short-term increases in weight gain, linear and head growth. There is no effect on serum alkaline phosphates levels. It is not clear if there is an effect on bone mineral content. Nitrogen retention and blood urea levels appear to be increased. There are insufficient data to evaluate long-term neurodevelopmental and growth outcomes, although there appears to be no effect on growth beyond one year of life.[24]

A number of reports have been published by international organizations dealing specially with the nutritional requirements of low birthweight babies.[4, 25, 26] The European Society for Pediatric Gastroenterology and Nutrition (ESPGAN) provided a comprehensive report based on available literature on the LBW infant's requirement for each nutrient.[25] Still, specific recommendations for SGA neonates who constitute the bulk of LBW infants in developing countries are lacking.

The initial growth rate and accretion rates of nitrogen, fat, sodium potassium and chloride in pre-term infants fed pre-term milk have been shown to be close to that reported for the *in utero* fetus of comparable gestational age.[27, 28] If given in sufficiently large volume (180ml/kg/d), the energy content of human milk is sufficiently great to enable nearly all low birthweight infants to gain weight at intrauterine rates (approximately 15 g/kg/d).[29] The protein content is suboptimal especially for very low birthweight infants resulting in lower serum albumin and transthyretin levels.[30]

Mother's own milk can be supplemented by combining with a commercially prepared fortifier to provide increased protein, energy and minerals. Human milk fortifiers available in international market contain similar amounts of protein, energy, calcium and phosphorous. The differences relate to the type of protein and the amounts of lactose, sodium and vitamins. In general infants with a birthweight less than 1500g and less than 30 weeks gestation will benefit from addition of fortifier, which should be continued till the infant is put on breastfeeding. Breast milk fortification is often commenced at half strength for 2 days and if tolerated full strength supplementation is introduced.[31]

Safety Concerns of Human Milk Fortifier (HMF)

The safety and benefit associated with routinely adding "fortifiers" to human milk is still open to question. Human milk fortifier (HMF) has been available in India since late nineties but its safety and efficacy has still not been established.[32] Some genuine concerns have been voiced in various studies.

Increased Osmolality of Breast Milk

Higher than expected increase in osmolality results from breakdown of maltodextrin present in HMF, by breast milk amylase. The polysaccharides are broken down into smaller molecules by the amylase enzyme resulting in a higher number of osmotically active molecules. Bacterial degradation of constituents as a possible mechanism for unexpected increase in osmolality seemed improbable since there was no late rise in osmolality (Table 14.1). Osmolality is a critical determinant of feed tolerance. Milk fortification results in significant increase in osmolality.[32, 33] Cochrane meta-analysis has shown an increased tendency for feed intolerance with fortified milk. An association between hyper-osmolar feeds (400 mOsm/kg) and necrotizing enterocolitis has also been reported.

Table 14.1: Osmolality of breast milk[32]

Ingredients	*Breast milk*	*Breast milk + HMF (4 gm/100 ml)*
Calories	65	78
Proteins (g)	1.6	2.0
Carbohydrates (g)	7.0	9.4
Fats (g)	4.0	4.2
Calcium (mg)	40.0	140.0
Phosphorus (mg)	20.0	70.0
Vitamin A (IU)	250	1700
Vitamin D (IU)	2.5	500
Sodium (mEq)	0.8	1.6
Osmolality at 20 minutes (mOsm/kg)	302.3±1.82	392.9±3.01
Osmolality after 6 hours (mOsm/kg)	301±1.75	393.3±3.0

Neonatal Sepsis

In a study, total bacterial colony counts (TBCC) in milk stored at refrigerator temperature for 0, 24, 48, and 72 hours were significantly greater in fortified vs unfortified milk. Both increased similarly with storage. Osmolality was greater in fortified than unfortified milk. Both demonstrated a rise by approximately 4% with storage.[34] In the only large published intention-to-treat study, babies who received liquid fortifier were at increased risk of sepsis showed no short or long-term growth advantage.[35]

There have recently been a number of reports of significant *Enterobacter Sakazakaii* infections including sepsis, meningitis and necrotising enterocolitis in the neonates associated with powdered milk formula products. Powdered formula products are not sterile. Although, there has not been any report of infection due to the powdered HMF till now; many NICUs in US are using liquid fortifiers instead of powdered product. There has been concerns that nutritional additives to the human milk may alter its complex system of anti-infective properties.[36]

GUIDELINES FOR THE USE OF HUMAN MILK FORTIFIER[21, 37]

1. Although no data exist to conclude exactly which infants should receive fortified human milk, the general consensus is that all pre-term infants with a birthweight below 1500 g would benefit from the additional fortification
2. Human milk fortifier should be initiated when the infant is tolerating breast milk feeds of about 220-240 ml/kg/ day and not gaining weight for three consecutive days.
3. HMF is available in India as a two-gram pack, which is to be added to 50 ml of human milk. It provides additional 0.2 g protein, 0.19 g fat, 1.2 g CHO and significant amount of calcium, phosphorus, vitamins minerals and trace elements.
4. Infants who have shown tolerance to breast milk + HMF feeds and were then made NPO should be restarted on breast milk + HMF feeds.
5. Indications for using concentrated breast milk feeds in infants who are already tolerating full feeds with HMF include:
   - Fluid restriction < 140 ml/kg.
   - Poor weight gain (<10-15 g/kg/d) on 120 kcal/kg of breast milk + HMF.
   - Metabolic bone disease (alkaline phosphates > 600 U/L) with poor bone mineralization on X-ray requiring increased intakes of calcium and phosphorus.

SUMMARY AND CONCLUSIONS

Based on presently available evidence, human milk fortifier may be used in pre-term, low birthweight babies as per weight criteria mentioned in this communication. However, there is need to develop safer preparations of HMF, which can provide additional nutrients in VLBW infants without compromising survival. Procurement of expressed breast milk to supplement the HMF is also very vital. Mothers of NICU babies are already under tremendous stress, which compromises their ability to supply adequate breast milk. One should be very cautious while talking about supplementing nutrients to mother's milk since this may further decrease mother's confidence and, hence, production of milk. This should also be emphasized that after a certain period of supplementation, her milk alone will be sufficient for the baby.

REFERENCES

1. Gross SJ, Slagle TA. Feeding the low birthweight infant. *Clin Perinatol* 1993;20:193-209.
2. The low birthweight infant. *WHO Bulletin* 1989;67:68-84.
3. Gross SJ, David RJ, Bauman L, Tomarelli RM. Nutritional composition of milk produced by mothers delivering preterm. *J Pediatr* 1989;96:641-644.
4. American Academy of Pediatrics Committee on Nutrition: Nutritional needs of Low birthweight infants. *Pediatrics* 1985; 75:976-986.
5. American Academy of Pediatrics. Policy statement on breast-feeding and the use of human milk. *Pediatrics* 2005;115:496-506.
6. Dadhich JP. Nutrition of the low birthweight. *Bull Nat Neonatal Forum*. 1997;11:42-44.
7. Anderson GH, Atkinson SA, Bryan MH. Energy and macro-nutrient content of human milk during early lactation from mothers giving birth prematurely and at term. *Am J Clin Nutr* 1981;34:258-265.
8. Paul VK, Singh M, Srivastava LM. Macronutrient and energy content of breast milk of mothers delivering prematurely. *Indian J Pediatr* 1997;64:379-382.
9. Chessex P. Quality of growth in premature infants fed their own mother's milk. *J Pediatr* 1983;102:107-111.
10. Chappell JE, Clandinin MT, Kearney-Volpe C *et al.* Fatty acid balance studies in premature infants fed human milk or formula: Effect of calcium supplementation. *J Pediatr* 1986;108:439-447.
11. Wholtil HA, Van Beusekom CM, Siemensma AD *et al.* Erythrocyte and plasma cholesterol ester long chain poly-unsaturated fatty acids of LBW babies fed pre-term formula with and without ribonucleotides: Comparison with human milk. *Am J Clin Nutr* 1995;62:943-949.
12. Lucas A, Cole TJ. Breast milk and neonatal necrotizing enterocolitis. *Lancet* 1990;336:1519-1523.
13. Eibl MM, Wolf HM, Furnkrarz *et al.* Prevention of necrotizing enterocolitis in low birthweight infants by Ig A -Ig G feeding. *N Engl J Med* 1988;319:1-7.
14. Narayanan I, Prakash K, Gujral VV. The value of human milk in the prevention of infection in the high-risk LBW infants. *J Pediatr* 1981;99:496-498.
15. Jain N, Mathur NB, Sharma VK *et al.* Cellular composition including lymphocyte subsets in pre-term and full term human colostrums and milk. *Acta Pediatr Scand* 1991;80:395-399.
16. Covert RF, Barman N, Domanico RS *et al.* Prior enteral nutrition with human milk protects against intestinal perforation in infants who develops necrotizing enterocolitis. *Pediatr Res* 1995;37:305.
17. Schanler RJ. Suitability of human milk for the low birthweight infants. *Clin Perinatol* 1995;22:207-221.
18. Lucas A, Morley R, Cole TJ *et al.* Breast milk and subsequent intelligence quotient in children born pre-term. *Lancet* 1992; 339:261.
19. Lucas A, Morley R, Cole TJ *et al.* A randomized multi-center study of human milk versus formula and later development in pre-term infants. *Arch Dis Child* 1994;70:F141-F146.
20. Schanler RJ. The use of human milk for premature infants. *Pediatr Clin North Am* 2001;48:207-219.

21. Schanler RJ. Human milk fortification for premature infants. *Am J Clin Nutr* 1996;64:249-250s.
22. Kashyap S, Schulze KF, Forsyth M, Dell RB, Ramakrishnan R, Heird WC. Growth, nutrient retention, and metabolic response of low birthweight infants fed supplemented and unsupplemented pre-term human milk. *Am J Clin Nutr* 1990;52:254-262.
23. Porcelli P, Schanler RJ, Greer F, *et al.* Growth in human milk-fed very low birthweight infants receiving a new human milk fortifier. *Ann Nutr Metab* 2000;44:2.
24. Kuschel CA, Harding JE. Multicomponent fortified human milk for promoting growth in pre-term infants. *The Cochrane Library,* Issue 2,2005.
25. Committee on nutrition of pre-term infants, European society of pediatric gastroenterology and nutrition: Nutrition and feeding of pre-term infants. *Acta Pediatr Scand* 1987;336:1-14.
26. Nutrition committee, Canadian pediatric society: Nutrient needs and feeding of premature infants. *Can Med Assoc J* 1995;152: 1765-85.
27. Atkinson SA, Bryan MH, Anderson GH. Human milk feeding in premature infants: Protein, Fat and Carbohydrate balances in the first two weeks of life. *J Pediatr* 1981;99:617-624.
28. Hawthorne KM, Griffin IJ, Abrams SA. Current issues in nutritional management of very low birthweight infants *Minerva Pediatr* 2004;56:359-372.
29. Ziegler EE, O'Donnell AM, Nelson SE, Fomon SJ. Body composition of the reference fetus. *Growth* 1976;40:329.
30. Brooke OG, Onubogu O, Heath R, Carter ND. Human milk and pre-term formula compared for effects on growth and metabolism. *Arch Dis Child* 1987;62:917.
31. www.netswic.org.au/nets/handbook/about.cfm.
32. Agarwal R, Singal A, Aggarwal R, Deorari AK, Paul VK. Effect of Fortification with Human Milk Fortifier (HMF) and other Fortifying Agents on the Osmolality of pre-term Breast Milk. *Indian Pediatr* 2004;63:63-67.
33. Curtis MD, Candusso M, Pieltain C, Rigo J. Effect of fortification on the osmolality of human milk. *Arch Dis Child Fetal Neonatal Ed* 1999;81:F141-F143.
34. Maria AL Jocson, Edward O. Mason, and Richard J. Schanler. The effects of nutrient fortification and varying storage conditions on host defense properties of human milk. *Pediatrics* 1997;100:240-243.
35. Williams AF. Early enteral feeding of the pre-term infant. *Arch Dis Child Fetal Neonatal Ed* 2000;83:F219-F220.
36. Kathleen A, Marinelli, Hamelin K. Breastfeeding and the use of human milk in the neonatal intensive care unit. In: Macdonald MG, Mullet MD, Seshia MMK (eds): *Avery's Neonatology: Pathopysiology and Management of the Newborn*, 6th edn. Philadelphia. Lippincott Williams and Wilkins 2005;414-444.
37. http://www.vh.org/pediatric/provider/pediatrics/iowaneonatologyhandbook/feeding/guidelines humanmilk fortifier.html.

Deonath Mahto • B Vishnu Bhat

15 Immunology of Malnutrition

INTRODUCTION

The term, *immunity,* is derived from the Latin word "immunis", meaning exemption from a duty or punishment. Biologically, immunity means the ability of an organism to resist a particular infection. The cells and molecules responsible for immunity constitute the immune system and comprises about 2% of body weight. Cells which participate in immune responses are collected together in the lymphoid organs viz: thymus, spleen, lymph nodes and peyer's patches.[1] These cells give rise to two types of immunity.

1. Innate immunity.
2. Adaptive immunity.

Innate Immunity

It is most primitive, non specific and weak form of immune response. Innate immunity consists of mechanisms that exist before infection, are capable of rapid responses to microbes, and react in essentially the same way to repeated infections.[2] It provides the first line of defense against invasion by microorganisms.[3] The principal components of innate immunity are:

1. Physical and chemical barriers (epithelium and antimicrobial substances produced at epithelial surfaces).
2. Phagocytic cells (neutrophils, macrophages) and natural killer (NK) cells.
3. Blood proteins, including the complement and other mediators of inflammation.
4. Cytokines.

Mechanism of Innate Immunity

When a pathogen comes in contact with body, initial noninflammatory reaction occurs that depends on the body's static defenses, such as skin, gastric pH and lysozyme in specialized body fluids (tear, saliva and mucous). If pathogens breach these outer defenses, an acute local inflammation occurs, which promotes the migration of phagocytes and plasma proteins into the infected tissues.[3]

Among the phagocytic cells, neutrophil represents a prototypic phagocytic cell in the host defense that can respond rapidly to infection.[4] Neutrophils use adhesion molecules, together with chemoattractants, to move to a site of infection.[5,6] On arrival these mobile phagocytic cells are programmed to engulf and destroy infecting organisms. This process is markedly enhanced by specific antibody of the IgG class and certain complement components (e.g. C_3) on the surface of the antigen (microorganism).[2] These proteins serve as opsonins by acting as a 'bridge' between the microbe and specific receptors on the surface of the neutrophil. Oposonins facilitate phagocytosis. Neutrophil products (e.g. H_2O_2, superoxide, proteases, phospholipases and defensin) then are released into the intracellular compartment to destroy the microorganism.[7]

Adaptive Immunity

In contrast to innate immunity, adaptive immunity is more highly evolved form of defense mechanism and is stimulated by exposure to infectious agents or other foreign material. The adaptive response is slower to develop than innate response, but is more powerful.[3] The characteristics of adaptive immunity are 'specificity' for distinct macromolecules and ability to 'remember' and respond more vigorously to repeated exposures to the same microbe.[2]

The components of adaptive immunity are lymphocytes and their products, antigen presenting cells and complement. There are two broad classes of lymphocytes—T-lymphocytes (T-cells) and B-lymphocytes (B-cells).

T-cells develop from self renewing progenitors that migrate from the bone marrow to become situated in thymus.[8,9] In the thymus, they express antigen receptors—T-cell receptors (TCR) and co-receptors (CD_4 or CD_8) and are selected to recognize peptides displayed by major histocompatibility complex (MHC) molecules and reach functional competence.

B-cells mature in the bone marrow where they express antigen receptors (IgM and IgD) and become functionally competent.[2] B-cell antigen receptor is similar in structure to secreted antibody.[10]

Types

There are two types of adaptive immunity.

1. Cell mediated immunity (CMI).
2. Humoral immunity.

Cell-mediated Immunity

Cell-mediated immunity is the mechanism of defense against intracellular pathogens that are either engulfed by phagocytic cells or infected non-phagocytic cells. This form of immunity is mediated by T-lymphocytes.

Humoral Immunity

Humoral immunity is the mechanism of defense against extra cellular pathogens. It is mediated by antibodies produced by B-lymphocytes. Each B-lymphocyte synthesizes antibodies with one antigen binding specificity.[11]

Induction of Adaptive Immunity

All adaptive immune responses are initiated in peripheral lymphoid tissues such as lymph nodes spleen and the cutaneous and mucosal immune system. CD_4^+ T cells recognize antigens of phagocytosed pathogens and activate the phagocytes to destroy the pathogens by secreting cytokines mainly interferon -γ (IFN-γ) and tumor necrosis factor (TNF). CD_8^+ T cells recognize the antigens of pathogens in the cytosol of cells and kill the infected cells to eradicate the infection by secreting granule protein and expressing surface molecules.

B-lymphocytes are activated by protein antigens with signals provided by CD_4^+ T cells or by non-protein antigens without T cell help. The activated B-cells differentiate into plasma cells which in turn form specific antibodies. The secreted antibodies neutralize or eliminate the pathogen by various mechanisms.[2]

EFFECTS OF MALNUTRITION ON IMMUNE FUNCTION

Poor nutrition compromises immune function. Protein energy malnutrition (PEM) is a major cause of immunodeficiency in children. Immunologic manifestations of severe PEM are broad which include lymphoid tissue atrophy with lymphopenia, abnormally low CMI and humoral immunity. As a result, PEM is associated with a high incidence of morbidity and mortality from infection.[12,13]

One of the immunosuppressive mechanisms of malnutrition is inhibition of the activation of T-lymphocytes. The voltage dependent potassium channels K(V) are vital for the activation of T-lymphocytes. In severe malnutrition there is diminution in K^+ conductance due to alteration in K(V) channels leading to inhibition of activation of T-lymphocytes.[14]

Ozkan H. *et al.* (1993) observed that PEM was associated with increased plasma immune globulin levels and complement deficiency. In addition, CD_4+ and CD_8+ T-cells levels were depressed. Chronic infections or decrease in T-suppressor cells were suggested to be responsible for the elevation of antibodies.[15] Unlike the immune deficiencies observed in severe PEM, moderate calorie deprivation is associated with increased T-cell function.[16-18] Deficiency in protein and energy may be accompanied by other nutrient deficiency also.

EFFECT OF OTHER NUTRIENTS ON IMMUNE SYSTEM

Lipids

Dietary lipids have an important influence on cell function. Studies on experimental animals demonstrated associations between increasing consumption of dietary fats and immunosuppression.[12,13] Essential fatty acid (EFA) deficiency causes altered macrophage function.[19,20]

Vitamins

Vitamins are important factors in a variety of metabolic processes like gene transcription, enzymatic reactions and redox reactions.

Vitamin A: Vitamin A maintains the epithelial integrity and the production of mucosal secretions. Vitamin A deficiency is associated with increased morbidity and mortality, most likely because of increased severity of infections.[21] Some of the immunologic abnormalities that follow Vitamin A deficiency include leukopenia (except polymarphonuclear leukocytes, which may increase), hypocomplementia, impaired T-cell function and reduced weight of lymphoid organs, decreased antigen specific IgG responses, generalized hyper globulinemas.[22,23] Excess vitamin A increases antibody and cell-mediated immune responses: stimulates Kupffer cells.[24]

***Vitamin D*:** Vitamin D has both stimulatory and suppressive effects on immune responses. It stimulates maturation of myelomonocytic cells to more differentiated monocytes and macrophages.[23] 1, 25 dihydroxycholecalciferol stimulates the innate immunity but inhibits acquired immunity by down regulating MHC molecule expression required for antigen presentation.[25]

***Vitamin E*:** Vitamin E acts as a free radical scavenger and limits cells membrane peroxidation.[26] Vitamin E deficiency is relatively rare. Experimentally induced deficiency leads to depressed leukocyte proliferation, decreased chemotaxis and phagocytois by polymorphonuclear leukocytes and macrophages. While vitamin E supplementation increases lymphocyte proliferation, antibody levels, IL-2 and phagocytosis.[23]

***Vitamin K*:** There is no evidence that vitamin K influences the immune system.

Water-soluble Vitamins: Among the water soluble vitamins, deficiencies of pyridoxine (vitamin B_6) pantothenic acid and folic acid cause impairments in both cell mediated and humoral immunity. Thiamin deficiency leads to premature thymic atrophy, decreased antibody responses and reduced polymorphonuclear mobility.[23] Vitamin C enhances bacterial phagocytosis by macrophages, but there is no evidence that it has a role in specific immunity.[1]

Minerals and Trace Elements

Many minerals and trace elements are required for adequate immune responsiveness. Deficiencies of iron, calcium, magnesium, manganese, zinc, copper, selenium, cadmium, chromium and iodine causes depression in the immunity in experimental animals.[1] Among various minerals and trace elements, zinc, iron, copper and selenium have significant effect on the immune system.

***Zinc*:** Zinc ions are key structural components of a large number of proteins.[27] Zinc induces secretion of thymulin from cultured human thymic epithelial cells.[28] Hence zinc deficiency may cause numerous irregularities in the immune system. The immunologic consequences of Zn deficiency are low thymic weight and T-cell defects.[12,13,29] B-cell functions are relatively spared.

Iron: Iron deficiency anemia is common in India. Iron deficiency with or without anemia results in impaired immune function.[1] The changes in immune function following iron deficiency include lymphoid tissue atrophy, impaired neutrophil and macrophage cytotoxic activity, decrease in T-cell number, cytokine release and antibody production.[23]

***Copper*:** Copper is involved in complement functions, cell membrane integrity and immunoglobulin structure.[23] Copper deficiency may lead to impaired phagocyte function, decrease T-cell number and activities, IL-2 production and increased B-cell number.[12,30,31]

Selenium: Selenium is an essential component of glutathione peroxidase. Glutathione peroxidase in association with vitamin E, prevents peroxidation of cellular and membrane lipids.[13,32] Excess H_2O_2 produced by phagocytes is neutralized by phagocyte produced glutathione peroxidase, thus prevent auto-oxidation and damage to surrounding tissue during immune and inflammatory processes.[23]

Malnutrition is very common in developing countries and affects the immune system adversely. Abnormalities in the immune response in severely malnourished children could account for the increased incidence of infection, mortality and morbidity among them.

Section 5

REFERENCES

1. Seth V, Jain Y, Kabra S. Immunology of malnutrition. In: Gupte S (ed) Recent Advances in Pediatrics (Special Vol 1: Nutrition, Growth and Development. New Delhi: Jaypee 1997;240-260.
2. Abbas AK, Lichtman AH, Pober JS. *Cellular and Molecular Immunology*, 4th edn. Philadelphia, WB Saunders 2000.
3. Strohl W.A., Rouse H, Fisher B.D. *Lipincott's Illustrated Reviews: Microbiology*, Baltimore, Lippincott, Williams and Wilkins 2001.
4. Yong KD, Hill HR. Neutrophil function disorders: Pathophysiology, therapy and prevention. *J Pediatr* 1991;119:343-354.
5. Etzioni A: Adhesionmolecules: Their role in health and disease. *Pediatr Res* 1996;39:191-198.
6. Springer TA: Traffic signals for lymphocyte recruitment and leukocyte emigration: The multistep paradigm. *Cell* 1994;76:301-314.
7. Fleisher TA, Blessing JJH. Immune function. *Pediatr Clin North Am* 2000;47:6, 1197- 1208.
8. Kisielow P, Von Boetmer H. Development and selection of T cells: Facts and puzzles. *Adv Immunol* 1995;58:87-209.
9. Jameson SC, Hogquist KA, Bevan MJ, Positive selection of thymocytes. *Annu Rev Immunol*, 1995;13:93-126.
10. De Franco AL. Transmembrane signalling by antigen receptors of B and T lymphocytes. *Curr Opin Cell Biol* 1995;7:163-175.
11. Klinman NR, Selection in the expression of functionally distinct B cell subsets. *Curr Opin Immunol* 1994;6:420-424.
12. Newberne PM, Locniskar M: Nutrition and Immune Status. In: Rowland II(ed): *Nutrition, Toxicity and Cancer.* Boca Raton: CRC 1991.
13. Myrvik QN. Immunology and nutrition. In: Shils ME, Olson JA, Shike M (eds*): Modern Nutrition in Health and Disease*, 8th edn. Philadelphia: Lea and Febiger, 1994.
14. Fernandez RG, Leehan JA, Pastrana RF, Muniz RO. *Clin Diagn Lab Immunol* 2005,12: 7, 808-813.
15. Ozkan H, Olgun N, Sesmaz E, *et al*. Nutrition, immunity and infections: T-lymphocyte subpopulations in protein-energy malnutrition. *J Tro Pediat* 1993;39:257-260.
16. Cooper WC, Good RA, Mariani T. Effects of protein insufficiency on immune responsiveness. *Am J Clin Nutr* 1974;27:647-664.
17. Jose DG, Good RA. Absence of enhancing antibody in cell mediated immunity to tumour heterografts in protein deficient rats. *Nature* 1971;231:323-325.
18. Kramer TR, Good RA: Increased in vitro cell mediated immunity in protein-malnourished guinea pigs. *Clin Immunol Immunopathol*, 1978;11:212-228.
19. Lefkowith JB, Morrison A, Lee V, *et al*. Manipulation of the acute inflammatory response by dietary polyunsaturated fatty acid modulation. *J Immunol*, 1990;145:1523-1529.
20. Lefkowith JB, Rogers M, Lenmartz MR, *et al*. Essential fatty acid deficiency impairs macrophage spreading and adherence: Role of arachidonate in cell adhesion. *J Biol chem* 1991; 266: 1071-1076.
21. Ross AC, Hammerling UG. Retinoids and the immune system. In sporn MB, Roberts AB, Goodman DS (eds): *The Retinoids: Biology, Chemistry and Medicine*, 2nd edn. New York: Raven Press 1994.

22. Cantorna MT, Nashold FE, Hayes CE, Vitamin A deficiency results in a priming environment conducive for Th1 cell development. *Eur J Immunol* 1995; 25: 1673-1679.
23. Yoshida S. H, Keen CL, Ansai AA, Gershwin ME. Nutrition and the immune system. In: Shils ME, Olson JA, Shike M, Ross AC (eds): *Modern Nutrition in Health and Disease*, 9th edn. Philadalphia: Lippincott Williams and Wilkins 1999.
24. Watson RR, Earnest DL, Prabhala RH. Retinoids, carotenoids and macrophage activation. In: Cunningham–Rundles Se (ed): *Nutrient Modulation of the Immune Response*. New York: Marcel Dekker, 1993.
25. Tokuda N, Levy RB, 1,25 dihydroxy vitamin D3 stimulates phagocytosis but suppresses HLA-DR and CD13 antigen expression in human mononuclear phagocytes. *Proc Soc Exp Biol Med* 1996;211:244-250.
26. Meydani SN, Blumberg JB, Vitamin E and the immune response. In: Cunningham–Rundles S (ed): *Nutrient Modulation of the Immune Response*. New York: Marcel Dekker, 1993.
27. Berg JM, Shi Y. The galvanization of biology: A growing appreciation for the roles of zinc. *Science* 1996;271:1081-1085.
28. Saha AR, Hadden EM, Hadden JW, Zinc induces thymulin secretion from human thymic epithelial cells *in vitro* and augments splenocyte and thymocyte responses in vivo. *Int J Immunopharmacol* 1995;17:729-733.
29. Vruwink KG, Keen CL, Gershwin ME, *et al*. The effect of experimental zinc deficiency on development of the immune system. In:Cunningham–Rundles S, (ed): *Nutrient Modulation of the Immune Response*. New York: Marcel Dekker 1993.
30. Kramer TR, Johnson WT. Copper and immunity. In: Curringham–Rundles S (ed): *Nutrient Modulation of the Immune Response*. New York: Marcel Dekker 1993.
31. O'Dell BL. Interleukin-2 production is altered by copper deficiency. *Nutrn Rev* 1993;51: 307-309.
32. Kuvibidila S, Yu L, Ode D, *et al*. The immune response in protein—energy malnutrition and single nutrient deficiencies. In: Klurfield DM (ed): *Nutrition and Immunology*. New York: Plenum Press 1993.

B Adhisivam • B Vishnu Bhat

16 Malnutrition and Infection

INTRODUCTION

Good nutrition is the cornerstone for survival, health and development for current and succeeding generations. Well-nourished children perform better in school, grow into healthy adults and, in turn, give their children a better start in life. Well-nourished women face fewer risks during pregnancy and childbirth, and their children set off on firmer developmental paths, both physically and mentally.

Malnutrition is implicated in more than half of all child deaths worldwide. Malnourished children have lowered resistance to infection. They are more likely to die from common childhood ailments like diarrheal diseases and respiratory infections. For those who manage to survive, frequent illness saps their nutritional status, locking them into a vicious cycle of recurring sickness and faltering growth.

The 1968 WHO monograph entitled *Interactions of Nutrition* suggested for the first time that the relation between infection and malnutrition is synergistic.[1] The monograph brought together extensive evidence for both the adverse effect of infections on nutritional status and the increased susceptibility to infection of malnourished individuals. Its thesis was that each worsened the other and that the biological effects of malnutrition and infection combined were greater than the sum of the two for this reason.

Infections, no matter how mild, have adverse effects on nutritional status. The significance of these effects depends on the previous nutritional status of the individual, the nature and duration of the infection, and the diet during the recovery period. Conversely, almost any nutrient deficiency, if sufficiently severe, will impair resistance to infection. Measles was more severe in poorly nourished Guatemalan children than those in Rochester.[2] Scrimshaw *et al.* have proved the association between moderate to severe malnutrition among village children and a history of prior episodes of an infectious disease.[3] Kwashiorkor was almost always precipitated by one or more prior infections.[4] Diarrhea was so common among malnourished children that it was the most important precipitating factor.[5] However, measles, chicken pox, whooping cough, German measles and even skin infections were commonly implicated.[6] Recognition of the synergistic relationship between nutrition and infection influences most public health interventions to prevent malnutrition.

THE VICIOUS CYCLE OF MALNUTRITION AND INFECTION

According to Scrimshaw *et al.* the relationship between infection and malnutrition is bidirectional (Fig. 16.1). Infection adversely affects nutritional status through reductions in dietary intake and intestinal absorption, increased catabolism and sequestration of nutrients that are required for tissue synthesis and growth. On the other hand, malnutrition can predispose to infection because of its negative impact on the barrier protection afforded by the skin and mucous membranes and by inducing alterations in host immune function.[1]

NUTRITIONAL IMPACT OF DIARRHEA

A number of field studies conducted during the 1970s and 1980s concluded that one-fourth to one-third component

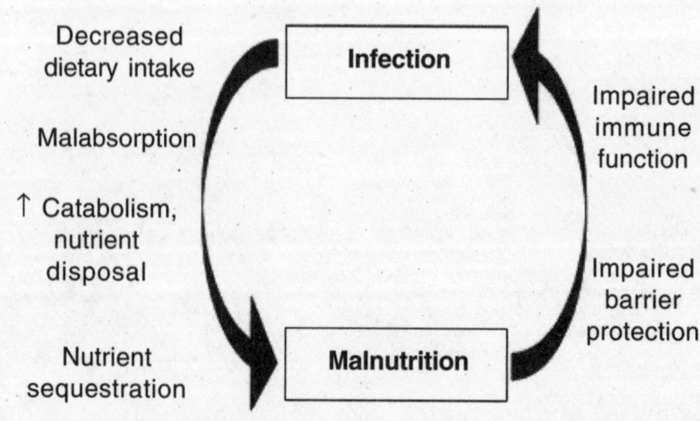

Fig. 16.1: Relationship between nutrition and infection

of the observed growth failure was attributable to enteric infections. The groups in Guatemala and Bangladesh proceeded to explore the mechanisms whereby diarrhea causes growth failure, focusing on dietary intake and intestinal malabsorption. Martorell *et al.*[7] reported that fully weaned Guatemalan children reduced their energy intake by 30% during acute infections, whereas Brown *et al.*[8] found that Bangladeshi children who were still breastfeeding reduced their intakes by only about 7%, suggesting that breastfeeding may protect against diarrhea-induced reductions in intake. Rowland *et al.*[9] concluded that exclusive breastfeeding prevents the adverse nutritional consequences of diarrhea. Lutter *et al.*[10] found that the usual diet also influenced the growth response to diarrhea in older children. Castillo-Duran *et al.*[11] assessed trace element balance during and after acute diarrhea, noting a negative balance of zinc during the early phase of illness.

MICRONUTRIENTS AND INFECTION

Nutrients enhance or depress immune function depending on the nutrient and level of its intake. Protein-energy malnutrition and vitamin A deficiency are strongly associated with impaired immunity and infectious disease. Multiple large field studies of vitamin A supplementation in different populations around the world demonstrated a marked decrease in childhood mortality attributed to all causes compared to those who were not supplemented. The essential role vitamin A plays in infection and maintenance of mucosal surfaces has long been known. Recent evidence shows that T-cell subpopulations, cytokines and antibody subclasses are all affected by vitamin A. Vitamin A-deficient experimental animals have decreased thymus and spleen sizes. Reduced natural killer cell activity, lower production of interferon, impaired delayed cutaneous hypersensitivity, less effective fixed fat macrophage activity, and lower lymphocyte response to stimulation by mitogens. Phagocytic activity may also be affected.[12]

Iron deficiency is the most widespread nutrient deficiency in the world today and in field studies is consistently associated with increased morbidity from infectious diseases. Moreover iron supplementation of iron-deficient populations results in decreased frequency of infectious episodes. Mechanisms clearly identified are impaired phagocytic killing power. Less response to lymphocyte stimulation, fewer natural killer cells associated with reduced interferon production, and depressed delayed cutaneous hypersensitivity.[12]

In animal studies supplementation with vitamin E protects against infection and is linked to stimulatory effects on the immune system. In man vitamin E and other anti-oxidants increase the number of CD4+ cells. Deficiency of pyridoxine induces atrophy of lymphoid organs, marked reduction in lymphocyte numbers, impairs antibody responses and IL-2 production. Dietary copper is important in the prevention of infection in some animal species and T-cell function is defective under deficiency states due to an inability to produce IL-2. Selenium has been linked to viral infection, enhanced T-cell functions and TNF beta induced increase in natural killer cell activity.

Iron and zinc are essential for the function of a number of metalloenzymes required for nucleic acid synthesis and cell replication. Without the ability to make new DNA and RNA for cell division the host response sputters, and this is clearly documented in a variety of in vitro studies. It has been more difficult to demonstrate these effects in vivo in humans, and the clinical importance of zinc and iron deficiency remains in doubt.

Current Perspectives

It is now recognized that specific defense mechanisms influenced by nutritional status include interference not only with the production of humoral antibodies and the bacteriocidal capacity of phagocytes but also with mucosal secretory antibodies, cell-mediated immunity, complement formation, numbers of thymus-dependent T-lymphocytes and T-cell subsets (helper, suppressor-cytotoxic, natural killer cells, etc.), the complement system and more. The neutrophile is seen as a complex of antimicrobial systems, all of which are potentially affected by malnutrition. They include both oxygen-dependent systems, such as those responsible for the respiratory burst, and oxygen-independent systems such as cationic proteins, lactoferrin, lysozymes, hydrolases and proteases. Essentially all these forms of immunity have been shown to be affected by nutrient deficiencies and these immune responses are not specific to a single nutrient.[12]

EFFECT OF NUTRITION AND INFECTION ON MORTALITY

A 2-year study in four villages near Antigua, Guatemala, compared the cause of deaths in infants and children under 15 years of age. It revealed that about one-third of the deaths were actually found to be associated entirely with the classical signs and symptoms of kwashiorkor.[13] Nutritional, respiratory and enteric disease each accounted for nearly 30% of the postneonatal deaths for which a cause could be identified and the remainder were ascribed to systemic infections, mainly whooping cough. This study concluded that after the neonatal period all of the deaths were attributable to the synergism between nutrition and infection.

Analysis of the death records of over 35,000 children under 5 years of age in 15 hospitals in Latin America[14] showed that nutritional deficiency was either the primary or the associated cause of most child deaths in at least 57% of cases. In some areas two-thirds of children had evidence of increased nutritional vulnerability to disease and death. This study concluded that the only way to measure the real magnitude of malnutrition as a health problem was the multiple causation approach. In industrialized countries particular attention must be paid to the nutrition of hospitalized patients since they are frequently debilitated by their primary disease, morbidity, and their nutritional status. Morbidity and mortality are increased by nosocomial infections to which the poorly nourished individual is more susceptible.

EVIDENCE FOR THE EFFECT OF IMPROVING NUTRITION ON INFECTION

Improving the nutritional status of underprivileged children lowers morbidity and mortality and improves growth impaired by infection. From 1959 to 1964, a study conducted in three Guatemalan villages to compare the effects of nutritional supplementation, excellent daily medical care with laboratory backup or a village in which there was no intervention directly affecting the children. There was lower prevalence of illness of children in the supplementary feeding village as compared with those in the village that received medical treatment but no nutritional supplement.[15]

There was a striking decrease in infectious disease morbidity in preschool children in a Mexican village when they were given a daily snack that included milk.[16] After the early months of breastfeeding when the infant is protected, supplemented children had fewer days of ill health and less severe infections. The effect was equally evident with regard to respiratory and diarrheal infection. Martorell *et al.*[17] showed the effect of supplementation on the growth response to diarrhea in children in two lowland Guatemalan villages, in which children were given a nutritious high protein supplement. The best growth was in children with low diarrheal prevalence, but supplementation improved growth even when diarrheal prevalence was high.

EFFECT OF INFECTION ON NUTRITIONAL STATUS

Acute and chronic infections may impair linear growth by causing micronutrient malnutrition. For example, diarrhea, acute respiratory infections and chicken pox have all been associated with the development of vitamin A deficiency. Micronutrient deficiencies may be produced by infectious diseases in one of the following five ways:

1. Decreasing food intake (anorexia).
2. Impairing nutrient absorption.
3. Causing direct micronutrient losses.
4. Increasing metabolic requirements or catabolic losses; and
5. Impairing transport to target tissues.

Both acute diarrhea, caused by bacteria, viruses and protozoa, and chronic intestinal helminth infections (e.g., caused by A. lumbricoides) can damage intestinal mucosal epithelial cells and thus impair absorption of both macro- and micronutrients. Even after nutrients are absorbed, they may still be lost as a result of infection with a number of pathogens that can cause direct nutrient loss, most commonly into the gut or urine. It appears that all febrile infections cause leakage of low molecular weight proteins into the urine. Although this phenomenon may cause some protein loss, one of the proteins lost may be retinol-binding protein, the serum transport protein for vitamin A. Thus vitamin A may be directly excreted into the urine with the losses increasing as the severity of infection increases.[12]

SUMMARY AND CONCLUSIONS

Applied research published since 1968 has confirmed the deleterious effect of infection on children's nutritional status and has produced new evidence in support of revised approaches to prevent and treat these infections. In particular, promotion of breastfeeding to prevent diarrhea and reduce its nutritional complications, continued feeding during illness and supplementation with selected micronutrients, both to prevent enteric infections and to reduce their severity, are all important nutritional aspects in the control of infections and their associated nutritional complications. Understanding the molecular and cellular immunological mechanisms involved in nutrient-immune interactions will increase our applications for nutrition of the immune system in health and in disease

REFERENCES

1. Scrimshaw NS, Taylor CE, Gordon AJ. *Interactions of Nutrition and Infection*. Geneva: World Health Organization 1968.
2. Gordon JE, Jansen AA, Ascoli W. Measles in rural Guatemala. *J Pediatr* 1965; 66:779-786.
3. Scrimshaw NS. Behar M. Protein malnutrition in young children. *Science* 1961;133:2039-2047.
4. Scrimshaw NS. Behar M, Viteri F, Arroyave G, Tejada C. Epidemiology and prevention of severe protein malnutrition (kwashiorkor) in Central America. *Am J Public Health* 1957; 47:53-62.
5. Salomon JB, Gordon JE. Scrimshaw NS. Studies of diarrheal disease in Central America: X. Associated chickenpox, diarrhea and kwashiorkor in a highland Guatemalan village. *Am J Trop Med Hyg* 1966;15: 997-1002.
6. Salomon JB, Mata LJ, Gordon, JE. Malnutrition and the common communicable diseases of childhood in rural Guatemala. *Am J Public Health* 1968; 58:505-516.
7. Martorell R, Yarbrough C. Klein RE. The impact of ordinary illnesses on the dietray intakes of malnourished children. *Am J Clin. Nutr* 1980; 33:345-350.
8. Brown KH, Black RE, Robertson AD. Becker S. Effects of season and illness on the dietary intake of weanlings during longitudinal studies in rural Bangladesh. *Am J Clin. Nutr* 1985; 41:343-355.
9. Rowland MG, Rowland SG, Cole TJ. Impact of infection on the growth of children from 0 to 2 years in an urban West African community. *Am J Clin Nutr* 1988; 47:134-138.

10. Lutter CK, Mora JO, Habicht JP, Rasmussen KM, Robson DS, Sellers SG. Nutritional supplementation: Effects on child stunting associated with diarrhea. *Am J Clin Nutr* 1989; 50:1-8.
11. Castillo-Duran C, Vial P, Uauy R. Trace mineral balance during acute diarrhea in infants. *J Pediatr* 1988; 113:452-457.
12. Scrimshaw NS, SanGiovanni JP. Synergism of nutrition, infection, and immunity: An overview. *Am J Clin Nutr* 1997; 66:464S-77S.
13. Behar M, Ascoli W, Scrimshaw NS. An investigation into the causes of death in children in four rural communities in Guatemala. *Bull World Health Organ* 1958; 19:1093-1102.
14. Puffer R, Serrano P. Patterns of Mortality in Latin American Children. Washington: Pan American Health Organization 1975.
15. Scrimshaw NS, Guzman MA. A comparison of supplementary feeding and medical care of preschool children in Guatemala, 1959-1964. In: Scrimshaw NS (ed): *Community-Based Longitudinal Nutrition and Health Studies: Classical Examples from Guatemala, Haiti and Mexico.* Boston: International Nutrition Foundation for Developing Countries (INFDC) 1995:1-28.
16. Chávez A, Martínez C, Soberanes B. The effect of malnutrition on human development: A 24-year study of well-nourished and malnourished children living in a poor Mexican village. In: Scrimshaw NS (eds): *Community-Based Longitudinal Nutrition and Health Studies: Classical Examples from Guatemala, Haiti and Mexico* . Boston: International Nutrition Foundation for Developing Countries (INFDC):1995:79-124.
17. Martorell R. The INCAP longitudinal study (1969-1977) and its follow-up (1988-1989); an overview of results. Scrimshaw NS eds. Community-Based Longitudinal Nutrition and Health Studies: Classical Examples from Guatemala, Haiti and Mexico 1995:124-142 International Nutrition Foundation for Developing Countries Boston, MA.

Sheffali Gulati • Lokesh Guglani

17 Nutrition, Malnutrition and Brain Development

INTRODUCTION

The influence of nutrition on children's long-term mental development and cognitive function is of great public health importance. During the early years of life when brain maturation is taking place, there are critical prenatal and postnatal windows during which nutrition could have lifetime consequences for the overall development. There have been recent evolutionary changes in the field of nutrition, which have clearly defined the role of early nutritional influences on brain development.

India, being the second most populous country in the world, has a total estimated child population of 400 million (aged 0-18 years).[1] According to latest UNICEF data, 47% of all under-five children in India are underweight (moderate to severe) and 16% show moderate to severe wasting whereas another 46% are moderately to severely stunted.[2] The overall Vitamin A supplementation coverage rate is 27% and the total percentage of households using iodized salt is still just 50%. The proportion of Low Birth Weight (LBW) babies remains high (30%) and the majority are due to intrauterine growth retardation, as against prematurity, which is the predominant cause in the developed countries. Thus for a major proportion of our child population, nutritional impairment begins at the very beginning of life and continues well into the early formative years of childhood. This has important consequences on the developing nervous system and its function and therefore affects overall mental development and cognitive function in later life.

This chapter discusses the scientific evidence available regarding the role of various nutrients on brain development and their long-term consequences.

EARLY BRAIN DEVELOPMENT AND PROGRAMMING

It is important to understand the process of ontogenesis of the brain and its cognitive function before we try to assess the effects of malnutrition in early years on brain development. This will not only facilitate the understanding of mechanisms of brain damage but also help to develop procedures to measure cerebral function and hence devise possible interventions to prevent them.

The first stage of development is the prenatal stage, which begins with the embryo getting organized into three layers of cells by 5th day of gestation. By the 4th week neuroectoderm is formed and forebrain development ensues from telencephalon impar. The Limbic system is derived from telencephalon semipar, and lays the foundation for the development of the supralimbic brain, which begins by 9th week. Myelinization of various brain parts proceeds throughout prenatal life well into postnatal life. The lateral lemniscus myelinization is completed by 30 weeks whereas that from the retina to the thalamus begins 3 weeks before birth. Hence the auditory information is received simultaneously with visual information after birth, which is fundamental for the acquisition of language. The subcortical associative fibers, which participate in the creation of cognition and of specialized memories, undergo myelinization over a brief period, in contrast to that of the intracortical neuropil, which occurs over years, if the brain remains in good health.[3]

A number of events in early life can influence brain development by either causing direct damage, or causing an insult during a critical period of growth of a somatic structure leading to impaired development, or causing its loss of function. Lucas has proposed the concept of "programming" whereby the programming stimuli exert long-term effects when applied at a critical or sensitive period.[4] So, 'nutritional programming' of the brain occurs in the intrauterine and well into postnatal life and may have long-term, irreversible, anatomic, biochemical and functional deficits which affect overall cognitive development.

GENE/NUTRIENT INTERACTIONS AND STRUCTURAL CNS DEVELOPMENT

Regulation of gene statement by nutrients can occur at multiple levels. The main sites for nutrient effects on gene statement are as follows[5]:

- Nutrients can bind to nutrient response elements in the DNA affecting gene transcription.
- Nutrients can interact with nuclear proteins that in turn act as transcription factors regulating gene statement.
- Nutrients can affect post transcriptional processing; mRNA transport, turnover and stability.
- Nutrients can modulate mRNA translation and protein synthesis rate.
- Nutrients can affect gene statement at the post-translational level by modifying the gene products formed.
- Nutrients can modify the turnover rates of proteins or enzyme activity level.

CRITICAL PERIOD OF BRAIN GROWTH

The critical period when the human brain is vulnerable to nutritional insults is uncertain. Animal experiments support that severe nutritional insult early in brain development can have a permanent adverse effect on cerebral structure and function. Periods of CNS growth spurt (15-20 weeks gestation, when neuronal multiplication is maximal; 30 weeks gestation till the first year, when glial division occurs) pose vulnerability to experimental nutritional deficiency.

EFFECT OF MALNUTRITION ON GROWTH OF BRAIN

The brain weight in all species, when plotted against age, follows a sigmoid curve. During 20-40 weeks gestation, both cerebrum and cerebellum show an exponential increase in weight, while the cerebellum multiplies its weight almost 12 times, the forebrain does so only five times. After birth, the growth process slows progressively in both, after 3 months in the cerebellum and 6 months in the cerebrum and process of myelination assumes significance.

A number of studies over the past few decades have evaluated the effects of early human malnutrition on development of the nervous system. A general reduction in energy and/or essential nutrient supply during the early part of life has effect on organ growth and its functional development. It specifically affects the brain by reducing cell replication cycles as the rate of DNA synthesis is slowed and there is a reduction in ganglioside content, which retards the process of dendritic branching and connection formation. Intrauterine and early post-natal malnutrition affects cell number, as measured by DNA content; and synaptic connectivity is affected if malnutrition occurs before the third year of life. Beyond this age, it may affect neurotransmitter levels in specific brain regions.[6] Significant reduction in cortical RNA suggest impairment in cell growth exceeds the reduction in cell number. Gangliosides and number of synapses in the cortex of undernourished rats are decreased. Serotonin, is increased, acetylcholine is unchanged and area-to-area variability exists in norepinephrine in experimental undernutrition.

The effects of malnutrition on the growing brain have been described on the basis of postmortem studies of infants who died of severe malnutrition. Besides overall growth retardation and atrophy, there is reduction of various parameters such as wet weight, dry weight, total protein, total RNA, cholesterol, Phospholipid, and total DNA content. In addition, there is a 15-20% reduction in total brain cell number. MRI studies have shown poor myelination of subcortical and periventricular white matter, thinning of corpus callosum, dilation of ventricles and gyral atrophy and poor development of hippocampus and cerebellum.[7] Table 17.1 lists some of the major neuropathologic abnormalities reported in experimental malnutrition.[8] Animals may recover from period of undernutrition as evidenced by some indices (Table 17.2).[8]

Table 17.1: Effects of malnutrition on the developing brain

Reduction in brain volume
Increased cell packing
Reduction in cortical dendritic spines
Decreased dendritic branching in cortex
Reduced number of cortical glial cells
Reduced number of cortical synapses
Reduced number of synaptic reactive zones
Sparing of cortical neurons
Disruption of cortical pyramidal cells
Decreases in width of cortical neurons

Table 17.2: Reversibility of brain lesions: Effects of restoring nutrition

Increase in brain weight and volume: "catch-up" head growth
Prolongation of period of mitotic activity
Prolongation of period of protein synthesis
Reversal of cell packing
Persistence of reduced myelination
Increase in number of mitochondria in neurons
Increase in synaptic density
Reduced cortical glial cell density
Persistence of reduced number of cortical dendrites and synaptic spines

The length of the insult during development is an important factor for permanency of effects. Physical growth also is decreased after long periods of kwashiorkor later in childhood. At age 1 year, premature infants who were malnourished *in utero*, born small for gestational age, and undernourished in early extra uterine life had smaller head circumferences and poorer performances on the Bayley Infant Development scales than did children of the same gestational age with normal birth weights who were undernourished in early extra uterine life. Combination of intrauterine and extra uterine malnutrition produces the greatest effect on brain weight, chemical composition and function.

Half the patients with severe protein-energy malnutrition have segmental demyelination of nerves. In severe and long-standing malnutrition an arrest in myelination of peripheral nerves occurs, with persistence of small myelinated fibers, striking failure of internodal elongation and a relative lack of the large myelinated fibers. Muscle pathology comprises obliteration of cross-striations, streaming of Z bands, increased interfibrillary spaces, mitrochondriomegaly and small-for-age fibers. Radioisotope assays reveal anomalous incorporation into various nerve and muscle constituents.

CLINICAL FEATURES

Apathy is the earliest and most constant neurological feature in moderate malnutrition. Mental changes have been reported in 87% of children hospitalized with protein-energy malnutrition, 77% had muscle wasting, 70% weakness, and 40% hyporeflexia. Hypotonia and reduced deep tendon reflexes are common, more marked in the lower extremities, and proximal musculature.[9] Intrauterine and early life under nutrition resulted in slower auditory and visual information processing between 11-14 years age when total premotor and motor reaction time was tested using audio-visual reaction time and electromyography (EMG). This indicates that early undernutrition affects perceptual and information processing abilities.[10]

"Soft" neurological signs, notably impaired fine motor coordination and choreoathetoid movements, are commoner in malnourished children. Chavez and Martinez reported neurological deficits in swift walking, balancing, one foot standing, tiptoe walking and jumping suggesting retarded cerebral maturation.[11] Shaffer *et al.* from Collaborative Perinatal Project reported soft neurological signs at 7 years among children with a lower birthweight relative to gestation,[12] Galler *et al.* demonstrated disappea–rance of soft signs after nutritional rehabilitation.[13]

Undernourished rural children between 10-12 years who suffered intrauterine malnutrition demonstrated a relative deficit on Wechsler memory scale, lower scores for abilities of mental control, logical memory, digit span, visual reproduction and associative learning.[14] Malnourished infants reveal cognitive inadequacies that result in delayed learning, particularly in reading and writing. Many studies have demonstrated that the postnatal influence on cognitive performance comes not from nutrition alone but from social stimulation. Children subjected to either nutritional or social stimulation, the effect becomes evident within 18 months. It is almost immediate when both interventions are made available to them. School children with early childhood malnutrition generally had poorer IQ levels, cognitive function, school achievement and greater behavioral problems than matched controls and, to a lesser extent, siblings. The disadvantages last at least until adolescence.

Head circumference, through variable, is often reduced but less affected than height and weight. The mean head circumference of malnourished children of either sex fell below the values for their well-nourished age matched controls. The significant reductions in head circumferences in these children may have serious implications for their future performance and achievement.

INVESTIGATIONS

Electroencephalography (EEG) demonstrates nonspecific abnormalities like diffuse slowing. Motor and sensory nerve conduction studies exhibit significant abnormalities. Nerve conduction times are significantly delayed in both the marasmic and the kwashiorkor forms of protein-energy malnutrition. The degree of delay correlates with the duration and the severity of protein-energy malnutrition, and is more marked in marasmus.[15] Young rhesus monkeys show myopathic EMG changes amendable to rehabilitation.

Hesse *et al.* examined the effects of chronic postnatal malnutrition on somatosensory evoked potentials. The mean central conduction time for the growth-stunted group was not different significantly from that of the control subjects suggesting appropriate myelination and fiber diameter. Somatosensory tracts may escape damage resulting from postnatal dietary deficiencies because myelination in these tracts is almost complete at birth.[16]

Durmaz *et al.* studied the brainstem auditory evoked potentials and flash visual evoked potentials in children with kwashiorkor, marasmus and healthy controls. Mean latency of the wave V and mean interpeak latencies of the waves I-V and the waves III-V in brainstem auditory evoked potentials were significantly different between the three groups, especially in kwashiorkor patients.[17] Chronic malnutrition revealed normal P3 latency with higher amplitudes of P2 and P3 consistent with compensatory phenomenon.

Neuroimaging demonstrates wide cortical sulci, cerebellar folia, and enlarged ventricles. These abnormalities resolve quickly with nutritional rehabilitation, suggesting that they represent ventricular dilatation and enlargement of sulci as a consequence of a decrease in plasma proteins and reduced colloid osmotic pressure. Age appropriate myelination has been reported even in children with severe kwashiorkor.[18]

MATERNAL NUTRITIONAL STATUS AND FETAL UNDERNUTRITION

Optimal fetal growth depends upon the uptake of adequate nutrients throughout pregnancy by the mother. Nutrients arriving at the placenta depend on the mother's intermediary metabolism and endocrine status; her partitioning of nutrients among storage, use and circulation; the capacity of circulating transport proteins; and cardiovascular adaptations to pregnancy, such as plasma volume expansion, which determine uterine blood flow. Thus fetal nutrition and development depends upon maternal nutritional status and the latter can influence the outcome of the pregnancy in more ways than one.[19]

Fetal undernutrition manifests as intrauterine growth retardation (IUGR) and it has its effects on various organ systems. Fetal growth is a dynamic process and birth weight is only a crude measure of that process, since it does not capture the effects of fetal undernutrition on body composition and development of specific tissues. Short-term consequences of IUGR include an increased risk of fetal, neonatal and infant death and impaired postnatal growth, immune function and intellectual development.[20] There are permanent changes in fetal structure and metabolism resulting from undernutrition during critical periods of early development and an inadequate supply of nutrients forces the fetus to adapt, down-regulate growth and prioritize the development of essential tissues. Adaptations include preferential blood flow to the brain and reduced flow to the abdominal viscera, altered body composition (reduced muscle mass) and reduced secretion of and sensitivity to the fetal growth hormones (insulin-like growth hormone and insulin). These adaptations enhance immediate survival but may carry a long-term price in terms of higher risk of cardiovascular disease and type-2 diabetes (the fetal origins of adult disease hypothesis—Barker Hypothesis).[21]

EFFECT OF MATERNAL NUTRITIONAL SUPPLEMENTATION

Pregnancy is associated with physiologic changes that result in increased plasma volume and red blood cells and decreased concentrations of circulating nutrient-binding proteins and micronutrients. These physiologic changes can be aggravated by pre-existing undernutrition, leading to various micronutrient deficiency states, such as anemia, that can have disastrous consequences for both mothers and newborn infants. Hence iron and folate supplementation are routinely prescribed during pregnancy but the role of multiple micronutrient prophylaxis in women of developing countries is debatable, considering the fact that even iron and folate supplementation is less than optimal and there are issues of cost-effectiveness at the public health level.[19]

Data on vitamin and mineral metabolism and requirements during pregnancy are scanty, and determining the consequences of apparently deficient or excessive intakes is not easy. Magnesium shows no gestational dependence until late pregnancy, when it declines continuously. Phosphorus remains constant because of maternal adaptation and copper increases in pregnancy. Calcium absorption increases early in pregnancy. At the same time, the protein-bound fraction of calcium in serum usually declines gradually throughout pregnancy, whereas the free ionic concentration remains relatively constant. The homeostatic control of ionic calcium is maintained by a complex interaction of vitamin D, parathyroid hormone and calcitonin.

Zinc declines progressively during pregnancy and a follow-up study of a supplementation trial of zinc in pregnant women in Bangladesh showed that even though it decreases the infants' infectious-disease-related morbidity, it does not seem to confer any benefit on the infants' mental development.[22] Blood vitamin A concentrations decline gradually in pregnancy because of hemodilution, and evidence exists that inadequate dietary vitamin A intake can also lower blood concentrations, although blood concentrations are difficult to interpret because they are not a good reflection of underlying status. The active metabolite of blood vitamin D (1,25-dihydroxycholecalciferol) increases in pregnancy whereas the inactive form (25-hydroxycholecalciferol) decreases. Vitamin E concentrations are known to increase during gestation, probably because of the hyperlipidemic state associated with pregnancy.

During pregnancy, serum vitamin C progressively decreases <50%, partly because of the extra uptake by the fetus and partly because of hemodilution. Plasma thiamine and riboflavin concentrations also decline during pregnancy. Evidence suggests that serum niacin concentrations decrease during pregnancy, whereas urinary excretion of niacin metabolites increases. Vitamin B-6 concentrations decline during pregnancy as a physiologic adjustment secondary to increased blood volume or as a result of increased requirements for active transport across the placenta. Folate concentrations may decline in pregnancy as a result of decreased intestinal absorption, inadequate intake, or increased demand. Serum vitamin B_{12} concentrations progressively decline during pregnancy, which may be independent of dietary intakes and may not represent decreased maternal stores or deficiency at the biochemical level. Biotin concentrations are significantly lower in pregnancy than in the nonpregnant, nonlactating state and decrease progressively throughout pregnancy. Pantothenic acid concentrations are thought to decline during pregnancy, returning to normal within 1 wk of delivery.[19]

The Pune Maternal Nutrition Study[23-26] was a prospective observational study of maternal diet and neonatal outcome carried out from 1994-1997 among women living in rural villages near Pune, Maharashtra. The mothers were short and thin (mean height and body mass index [BMI; expressed as kg/m2]: 152 cm and 18.1). Their main staple was millet roti (bread) eaten with dal (pulses) and vegetables, and there was a marked lack of day-to-day variety in the diet. Energy and protein intakes were low and did not increase during pregnancy (7.4 MJ and 45 g/d at 18 wk gestation). Intakes of nonvegetarian foods were also low. The most striking finding was that mothers with higher intakes of milk at 18 wk and of green leafy vegetables (GLVs) and fruits at 28 wk had larger infants. The trends were particularly strong for GLVs; women eating GLVs at least every alternate day had infants almost 200 g heavier than those who never ate them, and their odds ratio (OR) for low birth weight was 0.43 (95% confidence interval [CI]:20.12 to 0.99). Neonatal

Section 5

measurements were also related to maternal folate and vitamin C status, independent of food intakes. The trends for all birth measurements (with GLVs) and head circumference and placental weight (with fruit and milk) remained significant after adjustment for confounding factors that were carefully measured in this study, including maternal pre-pregnancy weight, weight gain during pregnancy, socioeconomic status and energy intakes. The study also showed effects of maternal workload on neonatal size. Higher total physical activity scores were associated with lower maternal weight gain, birth weight and neonatal head and mid-upper-arm circumferences. This was a landmark study, which gave important data regarding micronutrient and nutritional status of the pregnant females and its relation to the neonatal outcome. Usually the circumstances that lead to undernutrition are frequently associated with multiple micronutrient deficiencies as well. Hence there is a necessity for multiple micronutrient supplementations with either pharmaceutical preparations or micronutrient-dense foods.

So far, the available data on the efficacy of single- or multiple-micronutrient supplementation are inconclusive about pregnancy outcomes except for folate and iodine, which are critical at periconception, and iron and folate supplementation in tropical areas where dimorphic and megaloblastic anemia exist. Data is even scantier for their effect on infant mental development and cognitive function. Hence more data is needed on the other micronutrients before their use can be considered as a routine measure at the population level.

BREASTFEEDING AND MENTAL DEVELOPMENT

Breastfeeding is the ideal nutrition for infants upto the age of 6 months and it provides all the necessary nutritional components essential for optimal cognitive development. Since the cognitive development of an infant is a complex process influenced by multiple genetic and environmental factors that interact with one another, therefore adjustment for various covariates is necessary to assess the effect of exclusive breast-feeding on cognitive development. It is not possible to perform randomized controlled trials in this area, so a number of observational cohort and case-control studies have been performed.

Ever since the first report of its benefit on cognitive development was published in 1929,[27] there have been a number of studies that have addressed this issue. A meta-analysis of 20 studies[28] comparing the mean difference in cognitive function between breast-fed and formula-fed groups showed that an unadjusted benefit of 5.32 (95% CI: 4.51, 6.14) points in cognitive function was observed for breast-fed compared with formula-fed children. After adjustment for covariates, the increment in cognitive function was 3.16 (95% CI: 2.35, 3.98) points. This adjusted difference was significant and homogeneous. Low birth weight infants showed larger differences (5.18 points; 95% CI: 3.59, 6.77) than did normal birth weight infants (2.66 points; 95% CI: 2.15, 3.17) suggesting that premature infants derive more benefits in cognitive development from breast milk than do full-term infants. It also concluded that the cognitive developmental benefits of breast-feeding increased with the duration of breastfeeding. In addition, there is an increased maturation of the sleep-wake cycle in terms of less indeterminate sleep and more quiet (NREM) sleep observed in human milk-fed infants in comparison to formula fed ones, and their Bayley scale at 18 months also demonstrated better developmental indices.

EFFECT ON BEHAVIOR

Most cross-sectional studies have found significant associations between height-for-age and children's cognitive development. A small number of studies have been undertaken assessing the behaviour of mildly to moderately underweight infants or school-aged children who were also stunted to some degree. The results were fairly consistent, with unsupplemented young children being quieter, reserved, withdrawn, and timid, and having greater difficulty making up their minds and also had a fear of novel situations.[29] When they were older, the children spent less time on task in the classroom, and cried and slept more than the supplemented children. Underweight children tended to be more anxious, less imaginative in their problem-solving approaches, and less environmentally involved than children of normal weight.[30]

Stunting has also been associated with poor fine motor skills in children,[31-32] and poor neurosensory integration in children.[33] Cognitive function is more likely to be detrimentally affected by short-term hunger in stunted children than in non-stunted children.[34] Preliminary data from Jamaica also suggest that stunted children have higher levels of stress hormones (cortisol) and higher heart rates, implying that they may be less able to cope with environmental stressors and may have heightened arousal of the hypothalamic-pituitary-adrenal or autonomic nervous systems.[35]

A supplementation study aimed specifically at stunted children was conducted among stunted Jamaican children 9 to 24 months of age who had poor development and received nutritional supplementation for two years, with or without psychosocial stimulation.[36] The results showed that supplementation and stimulation produced independent benefits to the children's mental and motor development. The benefits from a combination of supplementation and stimulation were additive, and only the children receiving both treatments caught upto the non-stunted control group in developmental levels. The implications of these findings are that at least part of the deficit in the development of stunted children is due to poor nutrition. However, both stimulation and supplementation are necessary to improve the development of stunted children to culturally appropriate levels.

The precise mechanism linking stunting to poor mental development is unknown. It is possible that the mechanism varies according to which nutrients are deficient, or that several hypothesized mechanisms could act separately or together. One hypothesis is that undernutrition causes poor motor development and subsequent low activity levels. It also causes apathy and lack of interest in the environment. The children thus explore their environment less and fail to acquire skills at the normal speed.[37] These behaviours have been described in children with deficiencies of iron,[38] zinc,[39-40] and energy.[41] The caretakers may in turn be less stimulating towards an apathetic child, which may exacerbate the effects on development.[42] Another possible mechanism is that the children's small size could lead adults to treat them like younger children and not provide age-appropriate stimulation.

ROLE OF SPECIFIC NUTRIENTS

Several animal and human studies have assessed the role of specific nutrients in overall neurodevelopment and they highlight the importance of obtaining balanced nutrition in early life. In the initial few months of life, breast milk provides ideal nutrition, provided the nutritional intake and health of the mother is adequate. During the weaning and subsequent stages, nutritional deprivation may set in and cause long-term neuromorbidity, if corrective measures are not instituted promptly. We now examine the role of specific nutrients in contributing towards mental development and cognitive functioning and present the existing scientific evidence that highlights their role.

ROLE OF LIPIDS

The role of long-chain polyunsaturated fatty acids in neurodevelopment is an important field of ongoing research. The parent essential fatty acids (EFAs) like Linoleic Acid (LA 18: 2 w6) and a Linolenic Acid (LNA 18:3 w3) are the precursors of w6 and w3 fatty acids, which undergo further metabolism. Docosahexaenoic Acid (DHA, 22:6 w3) is a product of omega 3 FA metabolisms, whereas Arachidonic Acid (AA, 20:4 w6) and Docosapentaenoic Acid (DPA 22:5 w6) are end products of w6 metabolisms, respectively. These lipids are essential membrane components and form a number of bioactive compounds.[43]

The dry weight of the human brain is predominantly made up of lipids, with 22% of cerebral cortex, and 24% of white matter being made up of phospholipids. The fatty acid composition of membrane structural lipids affects a number of membrane properties like thickness, fluidity or interaction with proteins.

During development, there are important changes in neural membrane physical properties and excitability. Long Chain PUFAs regulate cell growth and differentiation by modulating gene expression, which occurs at the transcriptional level and is mediated by transcription factors that bind *cis*-regulatory elements of target genes.[44] The effect of DHA on functional maturation of the retina is mediated by its effect on photoreceptor differentiation.[45] The transport of opsin and rhodopsin to the apical process via post-golgi membranes is coupled to DHA transport. DHA supply also modifies the phospholipid molecular species present in neural tissues, thus possibly affecting overall function. Membrane fatty acid composition affects the ability of photons to transform Rhodopsin to the active state. Therefore, the corresponding physiologic phenomenon is the increase in retinal light sensitivity associated with DHA supply in the diet, and by affecting light transduction early in life, DHA may have long-lasting effects on the function and organisation of the visual cortex. Hence early dietary essential fatty acid supply may affect visual and brain maturation and this has been corroborated in a number of clinical studies using electrophysiologic findings.

A meta-analysis of studies evaluating the effect of long chain PUFAs on visual acuity maturation of term infants demonstrated a positive effect for assessments conducted during the first 4 months of life. Subsequent evaluation at 6 months showed equivocal results but at 12 months results were consistently positive. The analysis concludes that there is a significant overall advantage in LCPUFA supplemented infants in terms of visual acuity maturation.[46]

Very Low Birth Weight (VLBW) babies are especially vulnerable to EFA deficiency because of the almost complete absence of adipose tissue at birth, the physiologic immaturity of the fatty acid elongation/desaturation pathways, and their inadequate intake of EFAs due to formula feeding. A number of clinical studies in this subgroup of VLBW babies have shown the favourable effects of LNA or LNA plus DHA supplementation on plasma and tissue lipid composition, retinal electrophysiologic function, maturation of visual cortex and other measures of infant growth and development.[47] Carlson's and Werkman's RCT[48] did show better visual acuity at 4 months age in preterm infants supplemented with PUFAs but after this age, control infants "caught up" in visual function measures with supplemented ones, even though their test group showed more rapid visual processing at 6-12 months of age. Similar results have been reported in other studies where delayed responses become normal by 1 year of age. Should we therefore dismiss this phenomenon as transitory and of limited significance or assume that the authors failed to detect significant change at later ages because the tools applied were not sensitive enough? Therefore unless sensitive outcome measures are used and sufficient follow-up is provided, it is impossible to negate the possible long-term consequences on neurodevelopment.

That also raises questions regarding the significance of PUFA supplementation of full-term formula fed infants and for this, a number of studies have shown benefits in these term babies as well. The breast-fed group were found to have higher plasma and RBC phospholipid DHA concentrations throughout first year of life and their Stereo Acuity, as measured by Operant Preferential Looking Techniques, was more mature as compared to the formula fed group.[49] Jorgensen *et al* found better visual acuity at 4 months in breastfed infants as compared to formula fed infants, which correlated with their high DHA levels in RBC-phosphatidylcholine.[50] A number of trials providing DHA supplementation in preterm formula fed infants showed significant differences in VEPs as compared to formula fed controls.

The principal source of PUFA for infants is human milk and its content depends on the mother's diet during pregnancy and lactation. Human milk contains 0.3 to 0.4% DHA, with levels varying between populations and individuals due to dietary intake differences. Hence, human milk remains the best and the only time-proven source of fats and EFAs in the infant diet.

EFFECT OF PROTEIN INTAKE ON NEUROTRANSMITTER FORMATION

L-tryptophan (L-Trp) is an essential amino acid and is a precursor for synthesis of Serotonin (5-HT). It's the free fraction of L-Trp that crosses the blood-brain barrier to enter serotonergic neurons to activate the synthesis of 5-HT, whereas the albumin bound fraction cannot. Studies in rats malnourished during gestation or lactation showed that there is accelerated synthesis of brain 5-HT. The changes may be seen in fetal period itself, with increased brain L-Trp and Trp Hydroxylase levels suggesting activation of serotonergic system during the period of nutritional stress. Serotonin has important role in morphogenesis and neurogenesis is involved a number of neurologic and psychopathologic states. However, the overall functional consequences of these changes related to malnutrition are not fully understood yet.[51]

Similarly tyrosine is the precursor of monoamine neurotransmitters like Dopamine (DA) and Norepinephrine (NE). Catecholamine synthesis rates in the brain parallel the tyrosine changes produced by diet and one possible function of these dietary neurochemical relationships may be to provide a signal to the brain (in the form of modified neurotransmitter synthesis and release) regarding the animal's success in acquiring adequate protein in the diet. Such information may be employed by appetite circuits in the brain to direct protein-seeking behaviour. Since these findings are from animal studies, therefore their implications are not fully understood yet.[52]

ROLE OF IRON

Iron is an important cofactor for several intracellular enzymes and its deficiency has been shown to cause cognitive and learning impairment in infants and young children. According to the National Family Health Survey (NFHS-2) data, 74% of the children between the ages of 6 to 35 months in our country are anemic.[53] In a study of children from 6-36 months in an urban slum in Delhi, 64% of the children were found to be anemic, of which 44% were in the moderate to severe category.[54] The effects of iron deficiency on the developing brain are well documented and the deficits may permanent.

During the first 6 months of life, iron stores are adequate in most healthy term babies; and as the baby grows, it is mobilized for hemoglobin synthesis, and production of myoglobin and several enzymes. Thus half of the iron stores are mobilized and most term babies do not become iron deficient before 6 months of age.[55] But after 4-6 months of age, iron stores are no longer sufficient to meet the requirements of growth and subsequent dietary patterns influence the development of anemia in infancy. Approximately 20-40% of infants fed only non iron-fortified formula or whole cow's milk and 15-25% of breast-fed infants are at risk for iron deficiency by ages 9-12 months.[56-57] The iron content of human milk is the highest in transitional milk and then declines progressively during lactation to about 0.3 mg/L by 5 months of age.[58] The overall bioavailability of iron from breast milk is about 50% but it is not enough to sustain the body's requirements beyond 6 months of age. Hence, subsequent dietary changes and complementary feeding practices determine the iron status; but after the age of 2 years, the prevalence of anemia tends to fall as children begin to consume a more varied diet.

In preterm or low birth-weight babies,[59] or babies born to anemic mothers,[60] the iron stores are already low to begin with and iron deficiency may manifest in them within the first 3 to 6 months of life. The Committee on Nutrition of the American Academy of Pediatrics recommends that full term infants be provided with iron 1 mg/kg/d, starting at not later than four months of age and continuing until three years of age.[61] For low birth weight infants, the requirement is 2 mg/kg/d, to a maximum of 15 mg/d, starting at not later than two months of age. Higher doses have been suggested for in the lowest birth weight categories.[62] Infants with birth weights between 1,000 and 1,500 g should receive 3 mg/kg/d and infants with birth weight less than 1,000 g should receive 4 mg/kg/d. For these infants iron supplementation at higher doses should continue throughout the first year of life.

The International Nutritional Anemia Consultative Group (INACG), based on a iron dose of 2 mg kg body weight for prevention of anemia, have recommended a uniform dose of 12.5 mg in 6-24 mo old children.[63] This is based on assumption[64] of 5 percent iron absorption, which is a very conservative estimate of absorption. National Nutritional Anemia Control Program (NNACP) in India has recommended 20 mg of iron per day for children below the age of 5 years.[65] Based on 5% iron absorption this dose would provide 1 mg of absorbed iron. National Consultation on Control of Nutritional Anemia has recommended this dose in liquid form to be targeted to 6-24 mo old children.[66] If the average body weight of 6-24mo old children is taken as 10 kg, the prophylactic dose of 20 mg turns out to be 2 mg/kg/day. However, for treatment of iron deficiency anemia, a dose of 3 mg/kg of elemental iron is recommended.

Iron has an important role in the overall development and functioning of the brain. It has an important role to play in myelination and its deficiency is known to affect the dopaminergic system. The neurochemical basis of this effect is related to down-regulation of striatal dopamine D2 receptors[67] and increased striatal and ventral tegmental endogenous opiate peptides (dynorphin B and enkephalins). In addition, there is degeneration of C1 and C2 areas of hippocampus.[68] If these changes occur during a critical state of brain development and neural differentiation, iron supplementation may not necessarily correct the cognitive impairment and the changes may be permanent.

Several longitudinal studies have consistently shown that children anemic in infancy continue to have poorer cognition, school achievement, and more behavior problems into middle childhood. However, there are a number of confounding factors that prevent causal inferences from being made and these include: poor socio-economic status, lack of stimulation at home (especially maternal warmth), poor maternal education and low IQ, single parent families, maternal depression, low birth weight (<2.5kg), early weaning, recurrent parasitic infections, malnutrition and elevated blood lead levels.

In anemic children <2 years old, short-term trials of iron treatment do not benefit development and most longer trials lacked randomized placebo groups and failed to produce benefits (Table 17.3[69-73]). Similarly, the few preventive trials have had design problems or produced no or questionable benefits only. For children >2-year-old, even though the evidence from RCT is reasonably convincing but it is not conclusive. Hence, more RCTs of iron treatment are warranted especially in younger children, with larger study size and longer follow-ups.

Section 5

Table 17.3. Trials of iron treatment given to anemic children under two years of age for at least two months[69-73]

Study	*Sample*	*Treatment*	*Test*	*Results*
Aukett *et al.* (1986) UK	n = 97 IDA 17-19 mo Random assignment to treatment or placebo	Fe and vitamin C for 2 mo; placebo was vitamin C	Denver Test	No significant treatment effect on Denver scores; significantly more treated children achieved normal rate of development
Lozoff *et al* (1987) Costa Rica	1. 12-24 mo, n = 52 IDA, n = 35 non-IDA Random assignment to treatment or placebo 2. Children from group 1 after the 1-wk Bayley Test; all IDA group treated, non-IDA group given placebo	Oral or intramuscular Fe for 1 wk	Oral Fe for 12 wk	Bayley Test. Initially anaemic group had lower MDI and PDI scores; no treatment effect after 7 days IDA children who had complete Fe status recovery after 3 mo, not significantly different from nonanaemic MDI & PDI at 15 mo; anaemic group with partial recovery still had significantly lower scores
Walter *et al.* (1989) Chile	1. n = 196, 3 mo stratified by BF, randomly assigned to treatment or placebo; no baseline measures 2. n = 39 IDA, n = 30 not IDA, from pooled group at 12 mo randomly assigned to treatment or placebo 3. All children from group 2 given Fe treatment	1. Fe-fortified food from 3 to 12 mo; tested at 12 mo 2. Oral Fe for 10 days 3. Oral Fe for 3 mo	Bayley Test	1. Groups pooled, anaemic children had lower MDI and PDI at 12 mo 2. No treatment effect on MDI or PDI 3. No difference in change in MDI or PDI between anaemic and control groups
Idjradinata & Pollitt (1993) Indonesia	12-18 mo 50 anaemic (IDA) 29 non-anaemic Fe-deficient 47 Fe-sufficient Each randomly assigned to treatment or placebo	4 mo Fe treatment	Bayley Test	Initially IDA significantly lower MDI and PDI than other 2 groups, IDA significantly improved and caught upto the other 2 groups
Lozoff *et al.* (1996) Costa Rica	12-23 mo n=32 IDA n = 54 non-IDA All IDA treated and non-anaemic randomly assigned to treatment or placebo	6 mo Fe treatment	Bayley Test	IDA significantly lower MDI on enrolment and showed no improvement, PDI lower (non-significant) and remained so throughout

Abbreviations: BF, breastfeeding; IDA, iron-deficiency anaemia; MDI, mental development index of the Bayley Test; NS, not significant; PDI, psychomotor development index of the Bayley Test.

ROLE OF IODINE

Iodine deficiency is the most common preventable cause of mental subnormality[74] and is a major public health issue. The goals set by UNICEF and WHO to achieve universal salt iodization have reduced the overall prevalence but people living in areas with low-salt iodine content (especially the Himalayas) continue to be at risk. A meta-analysis of 18 studies of iodine deficient individuals versus controls showed an average IQ-difference of 13.5 points between the two groups.[75]

Iodine is an essential nutrient involved in thyroid hormone biosynthetic pathway. Oral administration of iodized oil to pregnant women pre-conception or during the first trimester has been shown to increase placental weight, reduce rates of prematurity, stillbirths, and abortions, and eliminate abnormal hormone levels in newborns.[76-77] Several studies have also investigated the effects of iodized oil given to women before and during pregnancy on their children's mental development (Table 17.4)[78-87] but the study design had many problems, including non-blinded treatment and inadequate matching. Therefore, it is not possible to draw firm conclusions about the effects of supplementation on mental development from these data. The data from childhood supplementation studies are less clear than those from maternal supplementation studies, probably because there are only a few studies and only one had a randomized design with pre- and post-treatment measures.

Several randomized trials have been conducted to examine the impact of iodine supplementation on the cognitive performance of children in iodine-deficient areas (Table 17.5).[88-96] However, results have not been consistent. When iodine deficiency occurs *in utero*, it leads to fetal hypothyroidism and irreversible neurological and cognitive deficits manifested as cretinism. Neurological cretinism includes mental retardation, primitive reflexes, visual problems, facial deformities, stunted growth and diplegia.[97] Hence in children to mothers living in iodine deficient areas, the effects of postnatal iodine deficiency may be difficult to separate from the effects of possible intrauterine deficiency.

At present, roughly 50% of households in our country consume iodized salt[2] and there is still a long way to go before the goal of universal consumption of iodized salt is achieved. The UNICEF has set a goal for sustainable elimination of iodine deficiency disorders by 2005. Although iodized salt is the most desirable option, other possible forms of fortification do exist. According to WHO,[98] iodized oil should be used in situations in which the prevalence of iodine-deficiency disorders is moderate or severe, cretinism and neonatal hypothyroidism are present, or universal salt iodization programmes would not reach women of reproductive age in one to two years. Although it is certain that women of reproductive age should be given iodine at all costs, it is not yet clear if schoolchildren should also be given priority. Single oral doses of Lipiodol, 240 mg for 6 months or 480 mg for 12 months, have been shown to prevent the worst iodine-deficiency disorders, such as hypothyroidism and cretinism, and doses much higher than 400 mg are usually not recommended.[99-102]

ROLE OF ZINC

Zinc deficiency is associated with complications of pregnancy and birth out comes[103] impaired immune function,[104] and increased duration and severity of diarrhea in children.[105] It also causes growth retardation, and several studies have shown that zinc supplementation can produce a significant growth response in height and weight-for-height.[106-108] It is common where diets contain little meat and high levels of phytate or fiber, which reduce zinc bioavailability. In addition, there is competitive interaction with copper and iron and cow's milk also reduces its bioavailability whereas breast milk does not affect its absorption.

Requirements for zinc are increased during periods of rapid growth, such as infancy and pregnancy, and in addition, increased loss in the stool occurs in diarrhea. Zinc is involved in RNA and DNA synthesis and is important for cellular growth, differentiation and metabolism. Studies have used indirect measures of zinc status and only a very small percentage is present in plasma, majority being localised in muscle, bone and liver, where it has a slow turnover.[109] The consequences of zinc deficiency in humans are assessed by randomised trials of zinc supplementation in susceptible populations. In addition to the demonstrated beneficial effects of Zinc supplementation on growth, diarrhea and pneumonia related morbidity and mortality in children; there are also studies that assess its effects on their cognitive functioning, including activity and attention.

There is concern that zinc deficiency may detrimentally affect children's mental development and behaviour. Of the six zinc supplementation trials (Table 17.6)[110-113] conducted to examine its effects on development and activity in preschool children, three trials showed greater activity with zinc supplementation. Of the three trials in school age children, one study found no impact whereas two studies showed benefits in neuropsychological processes, especially reasoning. These studies have yielded inconsistent results possibly because of differences in the preexisting zinc status of the study subjects; the content and bioavailability of zinc in the local diets; and the incidence of common infections that can affect an individual's zinc status. Moreover, methodologic aspects of these studies, such as variations in the dose, chemical form, and method

Table 17.4: Iodine intervention studies with mothers[78-87]

Source	*Sample*	*Intervention*	*Outcome measures*	*Results*
Ramirez *et al.* (1969) Ecuador	Two I-deficient villages: pregnant women in 1 treated not in the other. Group I: children of mothers treated during mo 4-7 of pregnancy Group II: children of mothers treated before conception Controls: children of untreated mothers	Mothers treated with iodized oil (regular doses to maintain urinary excretion of 50 μg/g creatinine until 4-5 yr after 1st injection). Iodized salt available in area for 1 yr before treatment	Stanford-Binet	Difference between group II and controls ($p < .002$) No differences between group I and controls
Ramirez *et al.* (1972) Ecuador	Group I: children of mothers who received I before 6th mo of pregnancy Group II: children of untreated mothers	Same as above	Gesell	Higher % of children < 4 yr old in village receiving iodized oil performed in normal range of IQ scores than children in control village
Pretell *et al.* (1972) Peru	n = 456 newborns 56% iodized group 44% placebo, I- deficient	Mothers received dose of I during pregnancy and another dose 3 yr later	Stanford-Binet Brunet-Lezine Physical examination Urinary I	No significant differences, but scores higher in iodized group
Thilly *et al.* (1980) Zaire	Double-blind randomized trial in area of severe I deficiency All children assessed at 4-25 mo n = 115 treated at average 28th wk of pregnancy n = 104 placebo	500 mg iodized oil, or I-free vitamins 1 treatment	Brunet-Lezine scale (DQ) Thyroid function	In children whose mothers were treated: higher DQ(115> 104**), lower infant mortality rate*, higher maternal I concentration**
Cao *et al.* (1994) China	All children 2 yr n = 120 infants whose mothers were treated during 1st or 2nd trimester n = 752 whose mothers were treated in 3rd trimester	400 mg iodinated oil Treated again at 6 mo or annual reevaluations	Bayley Scales (DQ) Anthropometry	In children whose mothers were treated earlier: higher DQ (90 > 75***), decreased prevalence of moderate or severe neurological abnormalities (2% v. 9%**), decreased prevalence of microcephaly (11% v. 27%**)
Pharoah *et al.* (1971) Papua New Guinea	Families in 16 villages randomly assigned to treatment or placebo 498 births to treated mothers 534 births to untreated mothers	Same as above	Incidence of cretinism, maternal T3 and T4 levels	Higher number of cretins born to unsupplemented mothers
Connolly and Pharoah (1979) Papua New Guinea	Children from 5 of above villages births to treated mothers 11% 79 births to untreated mothers	Same as above	Same as above and manual dexterity (bead threading, pegboard)	Better values in treated group for pegboard*, bead threading**
Pharoah *et al.* (1981) Papua New Guinea	Same 5 villages Children aged 6-11yr of women who had thyroid function measured n = 37 or 35 for some tests	Same as above	Same as above	Significant correlations between motor ability of child and maternal T4 level
Pharoah *et al.* (1984) Papua New Guinea	Same 5 villages n = 20 children aged 10-12 yr whose mothers had thyroid function measured in pregnancy	Same as above	Same as above and Pacific Design Construction Test	Significant correlations between both intellectual and motor ability of child and maternal T4 level
Connolly *et al.* (1989) Papua New Guinea	Same 5 villages n = 44 children aged 14-16 yr whose mothers had thyroid function measured during pregnancy	Same as above	Motor performance, cards orting	Significant correlations between all mental and motor scores and maternal T4 level

*p < .05, **p < .01, ***p < .001. Abbreviations: DQ, developmental quotient; IQ, intelligence quotient.

Section 5

Table 17.5: Observational studies of children from iodine-deficient areas[88-96]

Source	*Study type and sample*	*Outcome measures*	*Results*
Azizi *et al.* (1995) Iran	n = 271,6-16 yr, similar SES, education levels, school teachers, exposed to many of same influences (radio, TV, toys) 95 from A: 93% visible goitre, 39% low T4,70% high TSH 103 from B: 66% visible goitre, 7% high TSH 73 from C: 22% visible goitre, normal thyroid function	Raven's IQ Bender-Gestalt ENT evaluation Endocrine evaluation	Ravens IQ: C > B* > A**(116>96>89) More errors when taking Bender-Gestalt Test in A & B than C** Hearing threshold lower in I-deficient group**
Tiwari *et al.* (1996) India	*n* = 200, boys 9-15 yr, case-control design 100 children from 10 severely I-deficient villages: goitre > 60%, cretinism 3.4%; cretins excluded from study 100 children from 4 mildly I-deficient control villages: goitre < 10%, no cretinism Matched for SES, formal education level, age	Human maze learning Verbal learning rate Pictorial learning Achievement motivation scale	Children from I-deficient villages: lower scores in human maze learning**; slower verbal learning in serial learning** (not in free recall); worse performance in pictorial learning**; less motivation**; interaction between I deficiency and age
Azizi *et al.* (1993) Iran	n = 105,6-15 yr, children from 3 different villages 54 from Randan, area with hyperendemic goitre 20 from Zangoon, 2 mountainous regions with hyperendemic goitre 31 from Tehran, high goitre, normal thyroid function	Bender-Gestalt Test Hearing Thyroid function (T3, T4, etc.)	Thyroid function and somatic growth are normal Difference in IQ*** Tehran > Zangoon > Randan (117 > 102 > 89) Many other differences in social background
Vermiglio *et al.* (1990) Italy	n = 1089, 6-12 yr, living in 2 areas 368 from A, endemic cretinism 351 from B, no endemic cretinism 370 from C, no goitre or cretinism	Bender-Gestalt Test Neurological examination	Bender-Gestalt Test results of A and Bv.C.*** (223 v.27 performing defectively or borderline) More neuromuscular and neurosensory abnormalities in A and B***
Fenzi *et al.* (1990) Italy	6-14 yr, living in 2 areas 384 from representative sampling of 1 area of moderate I deficiency, goitre prevalence of 52% 352 sex- and age-matched from control, I-sufficient area, with 5.6% goitre prevalence (some tests on subsample in class 3 and 5)	WISC-R Thyroid size Thyroid function Neuropsychological studies (in 50 children from each group) PM47	No overall difference in PM 47 WISC or In children from class 3: verbal IQ*(105 < 111); information* (9.5 < 12.1); vocabulary** (11.1 < 13.9); coding* (8.3 < 10.3) No differences in children from class 5
Boyages *et al.* (1989) China	*n* =270, 7-14 yr, from urban and rural areas 141 born during iodized-salt prophylaxis in I- deficient rural village 51 from I-sufficient rural village 78 from I-sufficient urban populations (2 cities) Rural villages matched for several variables Urban areas not matched for any variables	Griffiths Mental Development Scales Hiskey-Nebraska Test of Learning Aptitude	Mean IQ lower*** in children from I-deficient village, in spite of iodized salt prophylaxis Treated rural: 72.4 Untreated rural: 84.4 Urban control 1:108.6 Urban control 2: 106.3
Bleichrodt *et al.* (1987) Spain	*n* = 355, 0-12 yr, from 7 different villages 162 from I-deficient area, goitre rate 66%, endemic cretinism 13% 193 from non-I-deficient area, goitre rate 13%, endemic cretinism 4% Matched for SES, degree of isolation, health care, education quality	Mental development: Bayley McCarthy, Catell Motor development: Bayley, Oseretsky, Bender-Gestalt, fine motor	Lower scores of mental development in children from I-deficient areas for all age groups* More mentally retarded children in I-deficient group Infants: lower psychomotor score** Older group: lower manual dexterity and speed of reaction**
Bleichrodt *et al.* (1987) Indonesia	*n* = 245, 6-20 yr, from 2 villages 106 from I-deficient village, goitre rate 68%, endemic cretinism 4.5% 139 from non-I-deficient area, goitre 3%, no endemic cretinism Matched for SES, degree of isolation, size	Test Intelligensi Anak and Test Intelligent Koletip, Indonesia Raven's Matrices Mental development (fluency, block design, vocabulary)	Lower scores of mental development in children from I-deficient area in all age groups* Differences in motor development after age 2.5 yr (eye-hand coordination, reaction time, balance)
Mehta *et al.* (1987) India	*n* = 60,6-16 yr, from 2 villages Both villages severely I deficient Children selected randomly from school, all goitrous; compared IQs of these children with those of normal rural Indian school children	WISC IQ Bhatia's Test Bender-Gestalt Test Goitre graded Urine samples Anthropometry Nutritional status	49 test children with IQ < 89, 11 with IQ > 90 Children from test village scored worse** than normal school children on digit span, similarities, and Koh's Block Design
Querido *et al.* (1978) Indonesia	*n* = 245,6-20 yr 139 from village with 3% goitre rate 106 from village with 58% goitre rate Villages matched for employment, population, altitude	Motor development tests: pinboard, tapping, balance, reaction time, throwing balls, figure comparison	Treated children (6-8 yr) scored higher in pinboard**, tapping* Treated children (9-12 yr) scored higher in all tests** Treated adolescents (13-20 yr) scored higher in reaction time, tapping, figure comparison

*p < .05, **p < .01, ***p < .001.

Abbreviations: ENT, ear, nose and throat; IQ, intelligence quotient; SES, socio-economic status; WISC, Weschler Intelligence Scale for Children.

Table 17.6: Studies of the effect of zinc treatment on children's behavioral and cognitive functions[110-113]

Source	*Sample size and study design*	*Treatment*	*Outcome*	*Results*
Penland *et al.* (1997) China	*n* = 372, 6-9 yr Double-blind RCT; 3 groups	A. 20 mg Zn daily B. 20 mg Zn daily plus micro-nutrients C. Micro-nutrients only 10 wk duration	Growth: knee height Neuropsychological functions: visual motor tracking, continuous performance, visual perception, short-term visual memory, concept formation, abstract reasoning, linger tapping	Knee height: B > C > A Neuropsychological findings: significant treatment effect after A or B compared with C for continuous performance, visual perception, visual memory, tracking, concept formation, finger tapping
Bentley (1997) Guatemala	*n* = 108 6-9 mo Double-blind RCT	10 mg Zn or placebo 7 mo duration	Behaviour observed at baseline and 3 and 7 mo later	No difference at baseline or 3 mo 7 mo: supplemented group sat and played more, cried less Major milestones not different
Sazawal *et al.* (1996) India	*n* = 93 children 12-23 mo Double-blind RCT	10 mg elemental Zn given daily for 6 mo to treatment group	Behaviour observation or 2 confsecutive days, 5 h/day	Significant increase with treatment in high-movement activities Significant treatment effect on children's activity rating score and on energy expenditure score
Cavan *et al.* (1993) Guatemala	*n* = 162, ~81.5 mo Double-blind RCT	Before study all were given multivitamin and mineral supplement without Zn Treatment: 10 mg Zn daily or placebo 25 wk duration	Anthropometry Bio-chemistry functional assessments Taste acuity, cell-mediated immunity, cognition (letter sequences, oral directions, design reproduction)	Significant treatment effect for mid-arm circumference and triceps skinfold only, not significant for height and weight No significant treatment effect for functional physiological and cognitive measurements
Friel *et al.* (1993) Canada	*n* = 52 VLBW infants, mean gestational age 29 wk RCT	Supplemented 6 mo: 11 mg/L Zn, 0.9 mg/L Cu Unsupplemented: 6.7 mg/L Zn, 0.6 mg/L Cu Assessed at 3, 6, 9, 12 mo	Biochemistry: blood and hair samples Anthropometry Cognition: Griffiths developmental assessment	Significant difference in growth velocities and Griffiths motor subscale between supplemented and unsupplemented group No significant difference in Griffiths global score between supplemented and unsupplemented group
Gibson *et al.* (1989) Canada	60 boys aged 5-7 yr Double-blind RCT	10 mg Zn daily, or placebo 12 mo duration	Anthropometry: height, weight, weight-for-height dietary assessment Biochemistry Cognition: 4 sub-tests of Detroit Tests of Learning Aptitude (sentence imitation, word sequence, oral directions, design reproduction) Hair Zn	No overall treatment effect on anthropometry biochemistry, or cognition Growth response seen among children who had impaired taste acuity and hair Zn <1.68 μmol/g at initial assessment

of administration of zinc and duration of supplementation, may have influenced their results. Finally, in some cases, the sample sizes may have been inadequate to detect potentially important differences in growth with statistical confidence. Hence, the evidence linking zinc deficiency to children's cognitive and motor functioning suggests a relationship among the most vulnerable children but lacks a clear consensus, highlighting the need for additional research into the timing of zinc deficiency and the co-occurrence with other micronutrient deficiencies.

ROLE OF VITAMIN B_{12}

Because animal products are the only source of vitamin B_{12}, infants breastfed by mothers with low intakes of these products, and also children who do not consume them, are at risk for vitamin B_{12} deficiency. Most of the research linking vitamin B_{12} deficiency to cognitive functioning has been conducted in the elderly, where it has been associated with dementia and neurobehavioral deficits.[114] There are two observational studies in children; the first one showed that infants of macrobiotic mothers had poorer motor and language development as compared to that of infants of omnivore mothers.[115] At 12 years of age, these children had higher methylmalonic acid levels and scored lower than the omnivores on standardized assessments, including the Raven's progressive matrices, Digit Span and Block Design, even though their current diet contained almost their recommended daily intake of vitamin B_{12}.[116]

The second study was conducted among Guatemalan school-age children with vitamin B_{12} deficiency. It showed that these children had slower reaction time on neuropsychological tests of perception, memory and reasoning, along with academic problems including lower academic performance, lower teacher ratings, more attention problems

Section 5

and more delinquent behavior.[117, 118] These observational studies provide evidence that vitamin B_{12} deficiency is associated with poorer cognitive performance, but intervention trials are needed for confirmation.

ROLE OF VITAMIN E

Vitamin E, an antioxidant regulates brain prostaglandin, leukotriene synthesis, controls nucleic acid synthesis and gene statement. The neuropathological lesions associated with vitamin E deficiency are characterized by axonal degeneration in the posterior columns and a selective loss of large caliber myelinated sensory axons in the spinal cord and peripheral nerves. Neurological signs including posterior column, spinocerebellar, retinal, peripheral nerve deficits and problems with fine motor coordination are being increasingly recognized in vitamin E deficiency states. Kalra *et al.*[122] reported that malnourished children (PEM grade II-III) had significant neurological deficits akin to those observed with low vitamin E levels. The subjects revealed significantly low a-tocopherol levels.[119] In a supplementation study on the same cohort with oral aqueous vitamin E, serum a-tocopherol levels normalized and many of the observed neurological signs in PEM subjects reversed. This raises issue of routine vitamin E supplementation in Vitamin D deficiency may result malnutrition, especially in developing countries.[120]

OTHER VITAMINS

Rickets and the associated hypocalcemia may cause tetany and seizures. Thiamin deficiency (beriberi) causes three types of neurological manifestations namely, peripheral neuropathy, Wernicke's encephalopathy and Korsakoff syndrome. The neuropathy is a mixed polyneuropathy with dominant sensory features, affecting the distal parts of the limbs. The histology shows non-inflammatory degeneration of myelin sheaths.

Wernicke's encephalopathy presents with vomiting, nystagmus, ophthalmoplegia, fever and progressive mental deterioration resulting in a global confusional state that may progress to coma and death. Korsakoff syndrome consists of retrograde amnesia, impaired ability to learn and confabulation. Patients who die in the acute stages of Wernicke-Korsakoff disease show symmetrical necrotic lesions in the paraventricular regions of the thalamus and hypothalamus, mammillary bodies, periaqueductal region of the midbrain, floor of the 4th ventricle and anterior-superior folia of the cerebellum.

Niacin deficiency causes Pellagra and diarrhea, dermatitis and dementia (3Ds) are the triad of manifestations associated with pellagra. Fatigue, insomnia and apathy precede the development of the encephalopathy, which is characterized by confusion, disorientation, hallucination, loss of memory and, eventually, frank organic psychosis. The mental changes are considered to be associated with diminished conversion of tryptophan to serotonin. The pathological changes are noticeable in the large Betz cells of the motor cortex.

NUTRITIONAL RECOVERY SYNDROME

The nutritional recovery syndrome is observed in kwashiorkor. Neurologic manifestations include tremor, truncal ataxia and upward gazing of the eyes.

Its pathogenesis is not well understood. The demands of renewed rapid brain growth may be exposing an underlying and unknown deficiency or, an imbalance in the production of such components as glutamic acid decarboxylase or g-aminobutyric acid, which has an inhibitory effect on nerve cells. The abnormality may accrue from a temporary fault in myelination during recovery due to an imbalanced metabolism of the essential fatty acids.[121]

According to an alternative hypothesis, it has an endocrinal origin.[113,114] That in PEM the function of the pituitary and its target glands is set at a lower ebb is widely recognized. This response of the pituitary to the state of poor dietary intake appears to be an adaptive mechanism that permits survival of the patient by reducing body activity and metabolic rate, and by retarding growth. During nutritional rehabilitation, the greater utilization of the hormone by the body stimulates the piuitary to produce its trophic hormones. This results in a response by the target glands. Thus, it appears that the nutritional recovery syndrome is caused by an increase in estrogen level and by a variety of trophic hormones produced by the recovering pituitary gland.[116,117,123]

SUMMARY AND CONCLUSIONS

Mental development and cognitive functions are complex phenomena that involve interplay of several factors, which affect the overall outcome and quality of life. Nutrition in prenatal as well as postnatal life contributes in a big way towards timely and appropriate maturation of brain function. A greater understanding of the effects and mechanisms of specific nutrients in neurodevelopment will help in devising appropriate interventions for achieving optimal mental development for all children, and could possibly help in reducing the long-term morbidity of malnutrition.

REFERENCES

1. UNICEF website. State of World's Children 2005. Available from URL: www.unicef.org. Accessed 13 March 2005.
2. Bellamy C. Childhood under threat. In: *The State of the World's Children 2005* . New York: UNICEF 2004.
3. Lecours AR, Mandujano M, Romero G. Ontogeny of brain and cognition: Relevance to nutrition research. *Nutr Rev* 2001;59:S7-S12.
4. Lucas A. Programming by early nutrition in man. In: *The Childhood Environment and Adult Disease* (CIBA Foundation Symposium). Chichester: Wiley, 1991: 38-55.

Section 5

5. Uauy, R.; Mena, P.; Peirano, P.: Mechanisms for nutrient effects on brain development and cognition. In: Fernstrom JD. Uauy R, Arroyo, P (eds): *Nutrition and Brain* (Nestle Nutrition Workshop Series) Vivey: Karger 2001:41-72.
6. Winick M. Nutrition and cellular growth of the brain. In: Winick M (ed): *Malnutrition and Brain Development*. New York: Oxford University Press 1976: 89-94.
7. Udani PM. Protein Energy Malnutrition (PEM), brain and various facets of child development. *Indian J Pediatr* 1992;59:165-186.
8. Levitsky, D.A, Strupp BJ. Malnutrition and the brain: Changing concepts, changing concerns. *J Nutrition* 1995; 125:2212S-2220S.
9. Chopra JS, Sharma A. Protein-energy malnutrition and the nervous system. *J Neurol Sci* 1992; 110: 8-20.
10. Agarwal, KN, Agarwal DK, Kumar A, Upadhyay, SK. Sequelae of early undernutrition on reaction time of rural children at 11-14 years. *Indian J Med Res* 1998;107:98-102.
11. Chavez A, Martinez C. Neurological maturation and performance on mental tests. In: *Growing Up in a Developing Community*. Mexico: Institute of Nutrition of Central America and Panama (INCAP) 1982.
12. Shaffer D, O'Connor P.A, Shafer, SQ, Prupis S. Neurological "soft signs": Their origins and significance for behavior. In: Rutter M (ed) *Developmental Neuropsychiatry*. New York: Guford 1983;144-163.
13. Galler JR, Ramsey G, Solimano G, Kucharski T, Harrison R. The influence of early malnutrition on subsequent behavioral development IV. Soft neurological signs. *Pediatric Res* 1984; 18: 816-821.
14. Agarwal KN, Agarwal DK, Upadhyay SK. Impact of chronic undernutrition on higher mental functions in Indian boys aged 10-12 years. *Acta Paediatr* 1995; 84: 1357-1361.
15. Grantham-McGregor S. A review of studies of the effect of severe malnutrition on mental development. *J Nutr* 1995; 125: 2233S-2238S.
16. Hesse H, Rivera MF, de Diaz I, Guirk GJ. Central somatosensory conduction time in severely growth-stunted children. *Am J Clin Nutr* 1998; 67: 93-96.
17. Durmaz S, Karagol U, Deda G, Onal MZ. Brainstem auditory and visual evoked potentials in children with protein-energy malnutrition. *Pediatr Int* 1999; 41: 615-619.
18. Gunston, GD, Burkimsher D, Malan H, Sive AD. Reversible cerebral shrinkage in Kwashiorkor: An MRI study. *Arch Dis Child* 1992; 67:1030-1032.
19. Fall CHD, Yajnik CS, Rao YS, Davies AA, Brown N, Farrant HJW. Micronutrients and fetal growth. *J Nutr* 2003;133:1747S–1756S.
20. Ashworth A. Effects of intrauterine growth retardation on mortality and morbidity in infants and young children. *Eur J Clin Nutr* 1998;52:S34-S42.
21. Barker DJP. *Mothers, Babies and Health in Later Life*. London: Churchill Livingstone. London 1998.
22. Hamadani JD, Fuchs GJ, Osendarp SJM, Huda SN, Grantham-McGregor SM. Zinc supplementation during pregnancy and effects on mental development and behaviour of infants: A follow-up study. *Lancet* 2002;360:290-294.
23. Yajnik CS, Fall CHD, Coyaji KJ, Hirve SS, Rao S, Barker DJP, Joglekar C, Kellingray SD. Neonatal anthropometry; the thin-fat Indian baby. The Pune Maternal Nutrition Study. Int J *Obstetr* 2003;27:173-180.
24. Rao S, Yajnik C S, Kanade A, Fall C H D, Margetts B M, Jackson A, *et al*. Intake of micronutrient-rich foods in rural Indian mothers is associated with the size of their babies at birth. Pune Maternal Nutrition Study. *J Nutr* 2001;131:1217-1224.
25. Fall CHD., Yajnik CS, Rao S, Coyaji KJ, Shier RP. The effects of maternal body composition before birth on fetal growth: The Pune Maternal Nutrition and Fetal Growth Study. In: O'Brien, PMS, Wheeler T, Barker DJP (eds): *Fetal Programming*. London: Royal College of Obstetricians and Gynecologists Press 1999:231-245.
26. Kinare AS, Natekar A S, Chinchwadkar M C, Yajnik CS, Coyaji KJ, Fall CHD, Howe DT. Low mid-pregnancy placental volume in rural Indian women: A cause for low birthweight? (The Pune Maternal Nutrition and Fetal Growth Study). *Am J Obstet. Gynecol* 2000;182:443-448.
27. Hoefer C, Hardy MC. Later development of breastfed and artificially fed infants. *J Am Med Assoc* 1929; 92:615-620.
28. Anderson JW, Johnstone BM, Remley DT. Breast-feeding and cognitive development: A meta-analysis. *Am J Clin Nutr* 1999;70:525-535.
29. Chavez A, Martinez C. Consequences of insufficient nutrition on child character and behavior. In: Levitsky DA (ed): Malnutrition, Environment, and Behavior: New Perspectives. New York: Cornell University Press 1979:238-255.
30. Barrett DE, Radke-Yarrow M. Effects of nutritional supplementation on children's responses to novel, frustrating and competitive situations. *Am J Clin Nutr* 1985;42:102-120.
31. Meeks-Gardner JM, Grantham-McGregor SM. Physical activity, undernutrition and child development. *Proc Nutr Soc* 1994;53:241-248.
32. Grantham-McGregor SM, Walker SP, Chang SM, Powell CA. Effects of early childhood supplementation with and without stimulation on later development in stunted Jamaican children. *Am J Clin Nutr* 1997;66:247-253.
33. Cravioto J, DeLicardie E, Birch H. Nutrition, growth and neurointegrative development: an experimental and ecologic study. *Pediatrics* 1966;38:319-372.
34. Meeks-Gardner JM, Grantham-McGregor SM. Physical activity, undernutrition and child development. Proc Nutr Soc 1994;53:241-8. 143. Fernald LC, Grantham-McGregor SM. Effects of early childhood under-nutrition on stress response. *Trans R Soc Trop Med Hyg* 1997;91:500.
35. Grantham McGregor SM, Powell CA, Walker SP, Himes JH. Nutritional supplementation, psychosocial stimulation, and mental development of stunted children: The Jamaican Study. *Lancet* 1991:338:1-5.
36. Levitsky DA. Malnutrition and hunger to learn. In: Levitsky DA (ed): *Malnutrition,Environment and Behavior*. New York: Cornell University Press 1979:161-79.
37. Lozoff B, Wolf AW, Urrutia JJ, Viteri FE. Abnormal behavior and low developmental test scores in iron-deficient anemic infants. *J Dev Behav Pediatr* 1985:6:69-75.
38. Sazawal S, Bentley M, Black RE, Dhingra P, George S, Bhan MK. Effect of zinc supplementation on observed activity in low socio economic Indian preschool children. *Pediatrics* 1996:98:1132-1137.
39. Bentley ME, Caulfield LE, Ram M, Santizo MC, Hurtado E, Rivera JA, Ruel MT, Brown KH. Zinc supplementation affects the activity patterns of rural Guatemalan infants. *J Nutr* 1997:127:1333-1338.

Section 5

40. Torun B, Viteri FE. Energy requirements of pre-school children and the effects of varying energy intakes on protein metabolism. In: Torun B, Young VR, Rand WM, eds. Protein-energy requirements of developing countries: Evaluation of new data. Tokyo: United Nations University, 1981:229-241.
41. Viteri FE, Torun B. Nutrition, physical activity and growth. In: Ritzen M, Aperia A, Hall K, Larson A, Zetterberg A, Zetterström R, eds. The biology of normal human growth. New York: Raven Press, 1981:265-273.
42. Chavez A, Martinez C. Growing up in a developing community. Guatemala City: Institute of Nutrition of Central America and Panama, 1982.
43. Uauy R, Mena P. Lipids and Neurodevelopment. *Nutr Rev* 2001;59:S34-S48.
44. Clark CD, Jump DB. Dietary polyunsaturated fatty acid regulation of gene transcription. *Ann Rev Nutr* 1994;14:83-98.
45. Rodriguez de Turco E, Deretic D *et al.* Post Golgi vesicles co-transport docosahexaenoyl phospholipids and rhodopsin during frog photoreceptor membrane biogenesis. *J Biol Chem* 1997;272:10494-10497.
46. SanGiovanni JP, Berkey C, Dwyver JT, Colditz GA. Dietary essential fatty acids, long chain polyunsaturated fatty acids, and visual resolution acuity in healthy full term infants: A systematic review. *Early Hum Dev* 2000;57:165-188.
47. Uauy R, Birch DG, Birch EE, *et al.* effect of dietary omega 3 fatty acids on retinal function of very low birth weight neonates. *Pediatr Res* 1990;28:485-492.
48. Carlson SE, Werkman SH, Peeples JM, Wilson WM III. Visual acuity development in healthy preterm infants: Effect of marine oil supplementation. Am *J Clin Nutr* 1998; 58: 35-42.
49. Birch D, Birch E, Hoffman D, *et al.* Breast-feeding and optimal visual development. *J Pediatr Ophthalmol Strabismus* 1993;30: 33-38.
50. Jorgensen MH, Hernell O, Lund P, *et al.* visual acuity and erythrocyte Docosahexaenoic acid status in breast-fed ad formula-fed term infants during the first four months of life. *Lipids* 1996;31:99-105.
51. Hernández-Rodriguez J, Manjarrez-Gutiérrez G. Macro-nutrients and Neurotransmitter Formation During Brain Development. *Nutr Rev* 2001;59:S49-S59.
52. Fernstrom JD, Fernstrom MH. Monoamines and protein intake: Are control mechanisms designed to monitor a threshold intake or a set-point? *Nutr Rev* 2001;59:S60-S68.
53. Report. *National Family Health Survey-2 1998-1999.* Mumbai: International Institute of Population Sciences 2000.
54. Kapur D, Agarwal KN, Sharma S, Kela K, Kaur I. Iron status of children aged 9-36 months in an urban slum integrate child development services project I Delhi. *Indian Pediatr* 2002;39:136-144.
55. Simes MA, Salmenpera L, Perheentupa J. Exclusive breast-feeding for 9 months: Risk of iron deficiency. *J Pediatr* 1984;104:196-199.
56. Dallman PR, Siimes MA, Stekel A. Iron deficiency in infancy and childhood. *Am J Clin Nutr* 1980;33:86-118.
57. Pizarro F, Yip R, Dallman PR, Olivares M, Hertrampf E, Walter T. Iron status with different infant feeding regimens: Relevance to screening and prevention of iron deficiency. *J Pediatr* 1991;118:687-692.
58. Siimes MA, Vuori E, Kuitunen P: Breast milk iron: A declining concentration during the course of lactation. *Acta Paediatr Scand* 1979;68:29-31.
59. Siimes MA. Iron nutrition in low birthweight infants. In: Stekel A (ed): *Iron Nutrition in Infancy and Childhood.* New York: Raven Press, 1984:85-91.
60. Blot I, Diallo D, Tchemia G, Iron deficiency in pregnancy: Effects on the newborn. Current Opinions Hematol 1999;6(2):65.
61. Committee on Nutrition. Iron supplementation for infants. *Pediatrics* 1976; 58: 765-768.
62. Dallmen PR. Progress in the prevention of iron deficiency anemia in infants. *Acta Pediatr Scand Suppl* 1990;365:28-37.
63. Stoltzfus R, Dreyfuss M. *Guidelines for the Use of Iron Supplements to Prevent and Treat Iron Deficiency Anemia.* INACG/WHO/UNICEF Report 1998.
64. FAO/WHO. *Report of a Joint FAO/WHO Expert Consultation: Requirements of Vitamin A, Iron, Folate, and Vitamin B_{12}.* FAO Food and Nutrition Series No.23,1988.
65. National Nutritional Anemia Control Program. Policy on Control of Nutritional Anemia. New Delhi: Ministry of Health and Family Welfare, Government of India 1991:1-8.
66. Report. *National Consultation on Control of Nutritional Anemia in India.* New Delhi: Ministry of Health and Family Welfare. Government of India 1998.
67. Youdim MBH, Yehuda S. The neurochemical basis of cognitive deficits induced by brain iron deficiency: Involvement of dopamine-opiate system. *Cell Mol Biol* 2000;46:491- 500.
68. Shoham S, Youdim MBH. Iron involvement in neuronal damage and microgliosis in models of neurodegenerative diseases. *Cell Mol Biol* 2000; 46:743-760.
69. Idjradinata P, Pollitt E. Reversal of developmental delays in iron-deficient anemic infants treated with iron. *Lancet* 1993,341:1-4.
70. Lozoff B, Brittenham GM, Wolf AW. Iron deficiency anemia and iron therapy: Effects on infant developmental test performance. *Pediatrics* 1987,79:981-995.
71. Lozoff B, Wolf AW, Jimenez E. Iron-deficiency anemia and infant development: Effects of extended oral iron therapy. *J Pediatr 1996*;129:382-389.
72. Walter T, de Andraca I, Chadud P, Perales CG. Iron deficiency anemia: Adverse effects on infant psychomotor development. *Pediatrics* 1989;84:7-17.
73. Aukett M, Parks Y, Scott P, Wharton B. Treatment with iron increases weight gain and psychomotor development. *Arch Dis Child* 1986;61:849-857.
74. Stanbury JB. *The Damaged Brain of Iodine Defciency.* New York: Cognizant Communication 1994.
75. Bleichrodt N, Resing, W. Measuring intelligence and learning potential in iodine-deficient and noniodine deficient populations. In: Stanbury JB (ed) *The Damaged Brain of Iodine Deficiency.* New York: Cognizant Communication 1994 :27-36.
76. Chaouki ML, Benmiloud M. Prevention of iodine deficiency disorders by oral administration of lipiodol during pregnancy. *Eur J Endocrinol* 1994;130:547-551.
77. Pedersen KM, Laurberg P, Iversen E, Knudsen PR, Gregersen HE, Rasmussen OS, Karsen KR, Eriksen GM, Johannsesn PL. Amelioration of some pregnancy-associated variations in thyroid function by iodine supplementation. *J Clin Endocrinol Metab* 1993;77:1078-1083.
78. Ramirez I, Fierro-Benitez R, Estrella E, Jaramillo C, Diaz C, Urresta J. Iodized oil in the prevention of endemic goiter and associated defects in the Andean region of Ecuador II. Effects

Section 5

on neuromotor development and somatic growth before two years. In: Stanbury JB (ed):*Endemic Goiter*. Washington: Pan American Health Organization 1969:341-359.

79. Ramirez I, Fierro-Benitez R, Estrella E, Jaramillo C, Diaz C, Urresta J. The results of prophylaxis of endemic cretinism with iodized oil in rural Andean Ecuador I. In: Stanbury JB, Kroc RL (eds): *Human Development and the Thyroid gland. Relation to Endemic Cretinism*. New York: Plenum Press, 1972:223-237.
80. Pretell EA, Torres T, Zenteno V, Cornejo M. Prophylaxis of endemic goiter with iodized oil in rural Peru. *Adv Exp Med Biol* 1972:30:249-265.
81. Thilly CH, Lagasse R, Roger G, Bourdoux P, Ermans AM. Impaired fetal and postnatal development and high perinatal death-rate in a severe iodine deficient area. In: Stockigt JR, Nagataki S (eds): *Thyroid Research VIII*. Oxford: Pergamon 1980:20-23.
82. Cao X-Y, Jiang X-M, Dou Z-H, Murdon AR, Zhang M-L, O'Donnell K, Tai M, Amette K, DeLong N, Delong GR. Timing of vulnerability of the brain to iodine deficiency in endemic cretinism. *N Engl J Med* 1994;331:1739-1744.
83. Pharoah POD, Buttfield IH, Hetzel BS. Neurological damage to the fetus resulting from severe iodine deficiency during pregnancy. *Lancet* 1971;1:308-310.
84. Connolly KJ, Pharaoh POD, Hetzel BS. Petal iodine deficiency and motor performance during childhood. *Lancet* 1979,2:1149-1151.
85. Pharoah POD, Connolly KJ, Hetzel BS, Ekins RP. Maternal thyroid function and motor competence in the child. *Dev Med Child Neurol* 1981;23:76-82.
86. Pharoah POD, Connolly KJ, Ekins RP, Harding AG. Maternal thyroid hormone levels in pregnancy and the subsequent cognitive and motor performance of the children. *Clin Endocrinol* 1984:21:265-270.
87. Connolly KJ, Pharoah POD. Iodine deficiency, maternal thyroxine levels in pregnancy and developmental disorders in the children. In: Delong GR, Robbins J, Condliffe PG (eds): *Iodine and the Brain*. New York: Plenum, 1989:317-331.
88. Azizi F, Kalani H, Kimiagar M, Ghazi A, Sarshar A, Nafarabadi M, Rahbar N, Noohi S, Mohajer M, Yassai M. Physical, neuromotor and intellectual impairment in non-cretinous schoolchildren with iodine deficiency. *Int J Vitam Nutr Res* 1995;65:199-205.
89. Tiwari BD, Godbole MM, Chattopadhyay N, Mandal A, Mithal A. Learning disabilities and poor motivation to achieve due to prolonged iodine deficiency. *Am J Clin Nutr* 1996;63:782-826.
90. Azizi F, Nafarabadi M, Ghazi A, Kimiagar M, Noohi S, Rahbar N, Bahrami A, Kalantari S. Impairment of neuromotor and cognitive development in iodine-deficient schoolchildren with normal physical growth. *Acta Endocrinol* 1993;129:501-504.
91. Vermiglio F, Sidoti M, Finocchario MD, Battiato S, Lo Presti VP, Benvenga S, Trimarchi F. Defective neuromotor and cognitive ability in iodine-deficient schoolchildren of an endemic goiter region in Sicily. *J Clin Endocrinol Metab* 1990;70:379-384.
92. Fenzi GF, Giusti LF, Aghini-Lombardi F, Marcocci C, Santini F, Bargagna S, Brizzolara D, Ferretti G, Falciglia G, Monteleone M, Marcheschi M, Pinchera A. Neuropsychological assessment in school children from an area of moderate iodine deficiency. *J Endocrinol Invest* 1990;13:427-431.
93. Boyages SC, Collins JK, Maberly GF, Jupp JJ, Morris J, Eastman CJ. Iodine deficiency impairs intellectual and neuromotor development in apparently-normal persons. *Med J Aust* 1989;150:676-682.
94. Bleichrodt N, Garcia I, Rubio C, Morreale de Escobar G, Ecobar del Rey F. Developmental disorders associated with severe iodine deficiency. In: Hetzel B, Dunn J, Stanbury J (eds): *The Prevention and Control of Iodine Deficiency Disorders*. Amsterdam: Elsevier 1987:65-84.
95. Mehta M, Pandav CS, Kochupillai N. Intellectual assessment of school children from severely iodine deficient villages. *Indian Pediatr* 1987;24:467-473.
96. Querido A, Bleichrodt N, Djokomoeljanto R. Thyroid hormones and human mental development. *Prog Brain Res* 1978;48:337-344.
97. Halpern J. The neuromotor deficit in endemic cretinism and its implications for the pathogenesis of the disorder. In: Stanbury JB (ed) *The Damaged Brain of Iodine Deficiency*. 15-24. New York: Cognizant Communication 1994.
98. World Health Organization. Safe use of iodized oil to prevent iodine deficiency in pregnant women. *Bull WHO* 1996:74:1-3.
99. Elnagar B, Eltom M, Karlsson FA, Ermans AM, Gebre-Medhin M, Bourdoux PP. The effects of different doses of oral iodized oil on goiter size, urinary iodine, and thyroid related hormones. *J Clin Endocrinol Metab* 1996:80:891-897.
100. Benmiloud M, Chaouki ML, Gutekunst R, Teichert H-M, Wood WG, Dunn JT. Oral iodized oil for correcting iodine deficiency: Optimal dosing and outcome indicator selection. *J Clin Endocrinol Metab* 1994:79:20-24.
101. Ermans AM. Prevention of iodine deficiency disorders by oral iodized oil. *Eur J Endocrinol* 1994:130:545-546.
102. Dunn JT, Thilly CH, Pretell EA. Iodized oil and other alternatives to iodized salt for the prophylaxis of endemic goiter and cretinism. In: Dunn JT, Pretell EA, Daza CH, Viteri FE (eds): *Towards the Eradication of Endemic Goiter, Cretinism and Iodine Deficiency*.Washington: Pan American Health Organization 1986:170-181.
103. Goldenberg RL, Tamura T, Neggers Y, Copper RL, Johnston KE, DuBard MB, Hauth JC. The effect of zinc supplementation on pregnancy outcome. *JAMA* 1995; 274:463-468.
104. Castillo Duran C, Heresi G, Fisberg M, Uauy R. Controlled trial of zinc supplementation during recovery from malnutrition: Effects on growth and immune function. *Am I Clin Nutr* 1987;45:602-608.
105. Walravens PA, Krebs N, Hambidge KM. Linear growth of low income preschool children receiving a zinc supplement. *Am J Clin Nutr* 1983;38:195-201.
106. Walravens PA, Hambidge KM, Koepfer DM. Zinc supplementation in infants with a nutritional pattern of failure to thrive: A double-blind, controlled study. *Pediatrics* 1989; 83:532-538.
107. Ninh NX, Thissen JP, Collette L, Gerard G, Khoi HH, Ketelslegers JM. Zinc supplementation increases growth and circulating insulin-like growth factor I (IGF-I) in growth-retarded Vietnamese children. *Am J Clin Nutr* 1996;63:514-519.
108. Jackson MJ. Physiology of zinc: General aspects. In: Mills CF (ed): *Zinc in Human Biology*. London: Springer-Verlag 1989:1-14.
109. Penland JG, Sandstead HH, Alcock NW, Dayal HH, Chen XC, Li JS, Zhao F, Yang JJ. A preliminary report: Effects of zinc and micronutrient repletion on growth and neuropsychological

function of urban Chinese children. *J Am Coll Nutr* 1997;16:268-272.

110. Bentley ME, Caulfield LE, Ram M, Santizo MC, Hurtado E, Rivera JA, Ruel MT, Brown KH. Zinc supplementation affects the activity patterns of rural Guatemalan infants. *I Nutr* 1997;127:1333-1338.
111. Cavan KR, Gibson RS, Graziosa CF, Isalgue AM, Ruz M, Solomons NW. Growth and body composition of periurban Guatemalan children in relation to zinc status: A longitudinal zinc intervention trial. *Am J Clin Nutr* 1993:57:344-352.
112. Friel JK, Andrews WL, Matthew JD, Long DR, Cornel AM, Cox M, McKim E, Zerbe GO. Zinc supplementation in very-low birthweight infants. *J Pediatr Gastroenterol Nutr* 1993:17:97-104.
113. Gibson RS, Smit Vanderkooy PD, MacDonald AC, Goldman A, Ryan BA, Berry M. A growth-limiting, mild zinc deficiency syndrome in some Southern Ontario boys with low height percentiles. *Am J Clin Nutr* 1989;49: 1266-1273.
114. Rosenberg IH, Miller JW. Nutritional factors in physical and cognitive functions of elderly people. *Am J Clin Nutr* 1992; 55: 1237S–1243S.
115. Schneede J, Dagnelie PC, Van Staveren WA, Vollset SE, Refsum H, Ueland PM. Methylmalonic acid and homocysteine in plasma as indicators of functional cobalamin deficiency in infants on macrobiotic diets. *Pediatr Res* 1994; 36: 194-201.
116. Gupte S. Nutritional recovery syndrome. *N Engl J Med* 1974; 501.
117. Gupte S, Gomez EM. Pediatric Nutrition and nutrition deficiency states. In: Gupte S (ed): *The Short Textbook of Pediatrics,* 11th edn. New Delhi: Jaypee 2009: 129-153.
118. Louwman MW, Van Dusseldorp M., Van de Vijver F J, Thomas CM, Schneede J, Ueland PM, Refsum H, Van Staveren WA. Signs of impaired cognitive function in adolescents with marginal cobalamin status. Am. *J Clin Nutr* 2000; 72: 762-769.
119. Allen LH, Penland J G, Boy E., DeBaessa Y, Rogers LM. Cognitive and neuromotor performance of Guatemalan schoolers with deficient, marginal and normal plasma B-12. *FASEB* J 1999; 13: A544.
120. Penland, J., Allen LH., Boy E., DeBaessa Y, Rogers LM. Adaptive functioning, behavior problems and school performanceof Guatemalan children with deficient, marginal and normal plasma vitamin B_{12}. *FASEB* J 2000; 14: A561.
121. Kalra V, Grover J, Ahuja GK, Rathi S, Khurana DS. Vitamin E deficiency and associated neurological deficits in children with protein-energy malnutrition. *J Trop Pediatr* 1998; 44: 291-295.
122. Kalra V, Grover JK, Ahuja GK, Rathi S, Gulati S, Kalra N. Vitamin E administration and reversal of neurological deficits in protein-energy malnutrition. *J Trop Pediatr* 2001; 47: 39-45.
123. Alleyne GAO, Hay RW, Picou DI, Stanfield JP, Whitehead RG. The pathology of protein-energy malnutrition. In: *Protein-Energy Malnutrition*. New Delhi: Jaypee 1989.

Suraj Gupte • CA Gopalan

18 Prevention and Control of Malnutrition

INTRODUCTION

According to the World Health Organization (WHO),[1] malnutrition, especially in infancy and childhood, is a "global problem", having adverse effects on the survival, health performance and progress of population groups. The adverse effects are of the highest order in the developing countries.

Despite several advances on the nutritional front, including remarkable hike in cereal production, child malnutrition continues to be rampant. India is included amongst countries where child nutrition is worse than expected by GNP per capita by the World Bank. Right now, India has 75-80 million strong force of under-5 malnourished children, the situation in Rajasthan, Bihar, Orissa and UP being the worst.[2]

Fighting such a vital problem of tremendous dimension in the Third World, including India, is, therefore of paramount importance. Much more important than the treatment of individual cases suffering from overt nutritional deficiencies or preventing the occurrence of malnutrition in the individuals is prevention of malnutrition at a large scale. This can eventually be accomplished through improvement in the socio-economic status and coordinated as also well-planned efforts in the field of agriculture, education, social services and public health.

Preventive action should be at the following levels:

- Family level.
- Community level.
- National level; and
- World level.

ACTION AT FAMILY LEVEL

The most significant in the preventive measures at family level is what is called "nutrition education". Nutrition education consists of targeting several areas.

Good Antenatal Care With Emphasis on Nutrition

All attempts should be made so that mother's own nutrition remains upto the mark and she does not develop malnutrition and anemia. This of much help in reducing the incidence of intrauterine growth retardation and low birthweight infants—the predecessors of malnourished children in very many instances.

Breastfeeding

Encouragement to the mothers to breastfeed the infants for as long as they can. Even if the mother is not in a position to breastfeed the infant for some reason, it is of advantage to express her milk and feed it to him. Of course, she must take good diet and adequate amounts of fluids to maintain her lactation. In case of prolonged breastfeeding, it is to be confirmed that the lactation performance of the mother is adequate. Else, adequate supplementation of feeding becomes imperative.

Down with the Bottle

The practice of shifting to artificial feeding in the form of bottle feeding with diluted cow milk or tinned milk should be discouraged, particularly in the poor in whose families it is virtually impossible to prevent occurrence of contamination of the bottle and the formula.

Complementary Feeding

After the age of 6 months, the infant should start receiving complementary foods, in addition to breastfeeding. These should be combination of cereals, protein-rich foods (say legumes) and fruits such as mashed banana. The combination helps to make up deficiency of limiting aminoacids. Rather than juices and soups, it is advisable to bank on energy dense and thick consistency food items. Supplementing with high biological value protein-rich foods, say egg, meat, and fish improves the net dietary protein value.

Improvement in Knowledge, Attitudes and Practices Concerning Nutrition

There is considerable evidence that education of the family members as also the health providers regarding correct

KAPs on maternal and infant and young child feeding contributes considerably to containment of malnutrition and improving nutrition.

Dietary Care During Illness

The families need to know and practice good nutrition during illness of the child. The old belief and practice of semistarvation as and when the child suffers from diarrhea (any illness, in fact) does grave damage to the nutritional status of the child.

Nutrition of the Girl Child

Usual neglect of the female child in India is well known. Such a child often grows as a "weakling" and may become an undernourished mother who gives birth to low birthweight infants. The cycle continues. Social and nutrition education is capable of changing this unfortunate state of affairs.

Down with Teenage Marriage and Pregnancy

Teenage brides may well be biologically capable of conceiving but they certainly are not suited for pressure of pregnancy and rearing children, much the less well nourished children.

Spacing of Pregnancies

Reasonable gap between two pregnancies allows mothers to prepare well for the next pregnancy and to provide good care and nutrition to children.

Immunization

Timely immunization plays a pivotal role in safeguarding from vaccine-preventable diseases and, thereby, prevent malnutrition.

ACTION AT COMMUNITY LEVEL

Nutrition Education

Here again nutritional education is of vital importance. Its delivery may be either through mass media such as radio, television, posters, documentary, films, etc. or imparting knowledge to the mothers at group meetings or at the doorstep of the family by the health auxiliary.

Nutritional Surveillance and Growth Monitoring

Surveys to detect cases of mild to moderate malnutrition, using preferably age-independent criteria, should be conducted. Such children may be kept under surveillance and, if required, given nutritional supplements.

Supplementary Nutrition Programs

The supplementary feeding programs in India include:

- Applied nutrition program.
- Midday meal program for school children.
- Nutritional program.
- Vitamin A prophylaxis program.
- Anemia prophylaxis program.
- Integrated child development services (ICDS).

The principal beneficiaries of such programs are the nutritionally vulnerable preschoolers, school-going children and pregnant and lactating mothers. Ample evidence is now available to support the contention that adequate supplementation through the feeding programs results in improvement of nutritional status of the target population, provided that operational efficiency is ensured.

ACTION NATIONAL LEVEL

Overview

There is a near consensus that prevention of malnutrition in children needs comprehensive and systemic analysis and planning at national level. Schemes and projects aimed at prevention of malnutrition must be result oriented, both short-term and long-term. Effective steps for arresting Government attention should include data concerning the long-term effects of malnutrition, failure of malnourished children to attain full potential in intellectual ability, the way malnutrition reduces the work output, high cost of treatment and rehabilitation, etc.[3] Health personnel need to provide guidelines for the government to focus on the priority groups that need focused action.

Nutrition education is a powerful tool for improving nutritional status of children. The content of nutrition education should be flexible, varying from situation to situation. The areas for nutrition education include mothers with weaning child who is at risk of PEM and breastfeeding itself. The recommendations of the 27th World Health Assembly in 1974 for reversing the trend of declining breastfeeding must be followed in letter and spirit.

According to Ghosh,[2] the association of maternal eduction with child survival and growth and development is consistent and strong. Educated women are likely to have reasonable knowledge of child rearing and child nutrition and are flexible in changing erratic beliefs and practices. This contributes to better nutrition of the child.

In addition to nutrition education, non-nutritional interventions are important for prevention of malnutrition. The leading ones are those addressed to prevention of infection and infestation, say immunization, malaria control, spacing of children to provide the mother ample time to care for each child properly, nutrition of the girl child, avoidance of early marriage and avoidance of teenage pregnancy.

All in all, the preventive action at the national level consists of measures to:

- *Improve food production.*
- *Control price-rise.*
- *Make available cheap supplementary foods.*

- *Fortify and enrich foods.*
- *Prevent adulteration.*
- *Irradiate certain foods such as wheat, potato and onion.*
- *Nutrition education.*
- *Nutritional-related health activities.*
- *Socio-economic development.*
- *Containment of population explosion are of paramount importance.*

India's National Nutrition Policy and National Plan of Action

In India, we have a well-conceived National Nutrition Policy since 1993 (Table 18.1) and a National Plan of Action (Table 18.2).[4, 5] The aims and objectives of NNP are:

1. To identify vulnerable groups requiring immediate action.
2. To identify key areas for action in the field of food production, supply, information, nutrition education, rural development, health care, monitoring and surveillance.

Table 18.1: Noteworthy components of India's National Nutrition Policy

- Fortification of essential foods.
- Control of micronutrient deficiencies.
- Improvement of dietary pattern through production and demonstration.
- Land reforms.
- Popularization of low-cost nutritious food.
- Public distribution system.
- Prevention of food adulteration.
- Health and family welfare.
- Nutrition surveillance.
- Communication and community participation.

Table 18.2: Some Noteworthy features of India's National Plan of Action

- Reduction in moderate and severe malnutrition among preschool children by one-half.
- Reduction in chronic undernutrition and stunted growth in children.
- Reduction in incidence of low birthweight (LBW) infants to less than 10%.
- Elimination of vitamin A deficiency (VAD)-related blindness.
- Reduction in iron deficiency anemia (IDA) in pregnant woman to less than 25%.
- Universal iodization of salt and to reduce iodine-deficiency disorders (IDD) to less than 10%.
- Empowerment of all women to breastfeed their children exclusively for 6 months and to continue breastfeeding with complementary foods well into the second year.
- Production of sufficient foodgrains.
- Improving household food security through poverty alleviation programs.
- Promoting appropriate diets and healthy lifestyles.

India's National Nutrition Programs

The programs mentioned under "Action at Community Level" revolve around supplementary nutrition are indeed our national nutritional programs as well. It is now believed that in order that a supplementary nutrition program indeed delivers good it should also incorporate:

- Nutrition education.
- Immunization to control infection.
- Improvement in health as such and quality of life of the population (QOL).

In keeping with the contention of the Joint FAO/WHO Expert Committee on Nutrition,[6] that food and nutrition planning has got to be an integral part of the overall socio-economic development, over and above the nutrition intervention programs, India has also undertaken the following actions at national level to improve the nutritional status:

1. Rural development.
2. Increase in agriculture production.
3. Stabilization of population through birth spacing and small family norm.
4. Nutrition-related health activities.

ACTION AT WORLD LEVEL

Efforts to intensify various international food programs like those of WHO, FAO, UNICEF, CARE, World Bank, and UNDP to fight the ghost of PEM are gaining popularity globally. Enhanced international cooperation not just to mitigate the effects of natural disasters such as famines, floods and earthquakes but also to solving the problem of malnutrition on ongoing basis is the need of the hour. International cooperation forms the crux of the action at world level, especially when it comes to acute disasters/ emergencies caused by floods, earthquakes, typhoons, etc.

REFERENCES

1. World Health Organization. *Nutrition and Malnutrition*. Geneva: WHO 1984.
2. Ghosh S: Current nutrition scenario. In: Gupte S, Gupte SB (eds): *Recent Advances in Pediatrics (Special Vol. 1 Nutrition, Growth and Development)*. New Delhi: Jaypee 1997; 1-7.
3. Alleyne GAO, Hay RW, Picou DI, Stanfield JP, Whitehead RG. *Protein-energy Malnutrition. London*/Edward Arnold 1989.
4. Gupte S, Gomez EM. Nutrition and nutritional deficiency states. In: Gupte S (ed). *The Short Textbook of Pediatrics,* 10th edn. New Delhi: Jaypee 2004.
5. Government of India. *National Nutrition Policy*. New Delhi: Department of Women and Child Development, Ministry of Human Resource Development 1983.
6. Joint FAO/WHO Expert Committee on Nutrition. *Report of the Joint FAO/WHO. Expert Committee on Nutrition*. Geneva: WHO 1976.

Priyali Shah (Pathak) • Umesh Kapil

19 Vitamin A Deficiency (VAD) Disorders

INTRODUCTION

Vitamin A is an essential nutrient needed in small amounts for the normal functioning of the visual system, growth and development, maintenance of the epithelial cellular integrity, immune function and reproduction. Function of vitamin A in the visual system and cell differentiation is well defined. More recently, its involvement in the embryonic development has also been reported.[1] In addition, vitamin A is needed for various bodily functions such as growth, erythropoiesis, and maintaining the immune system.

Vitamin A is essential in the body for the integrity of the epithelial tissue and this function is pronounced in the respiratory and gastrointestinal tract. In the absence of vitamin A, the integrity of the specific epithelium in these structures is lost since it is replaced by non-functional keratinized tissue, leading to various types of infections in these two physiological systems. Diarrhea, bronchitis and several types of acute respiratory infections have been proved to have roots in vitamin A deficiency. Recent studies have very clearly demonstrated the possible therapeutic role of vitamin A in diarrhea in children through repair of intestinal epithelium and their functional improvement.[2]

Also, vitamin A appears to increase the absorption of non-heme iron by preventing the inhibitory effects of phytates and polyphenols on iron absorption.[2] These findings have special significance for India where grains rich in phytates form the bulk of the daily diet and the prevalence of iron deficiency anemia is alarming.

Vitamin A deficiency (VAD) results when body stores are depleted to the extent that physiological functions are impaired, even though clinical eye signs may not be evident. The depletion of the body stores of vitamin A occurs when the dietary content of vitamin A is too less to replace the amounts used by the tissues or reduced by breastfeeding. The implications of such VAD, however, vary by the group at risk. In preschool children, VAD can lead to increased risk of mortality and morbidity and to blindness; in pregnant and lactating women, it can lead to night blindness and appears to have implications for maternal morbidity and mortality.[3]

> Vitamin A deficiency (VAD) is the single most important cause of childhood blindness in developing countries. It also contributes significantly, even at sub -clinical levels, to morbidity and mortality from common childhood infections. VAD is the result of two primary factors: persistent inadequate dietary intake of vitamin A that is frequently exacerbated by other dietary circumstances; and a high frequency of infections. An estimated 2.8 million pre-school age children are at risk of blindness from VAD, and the health and survival of 251 million others are seriously compromised.

ETIOLOGY OF VITAMIN A DEFICIENCY

Inadequacy of Dietary Intake

Inadequate dietary intake of vitamin A or its precursor (β–carotene) is the most important contributory factor leading to VAD. Maternal malnutrition is high in India, particularly in low income group families, leading to low dietary intakes of nutrients. Pregnant and lactating women in the rural areas consume quantitatively the same diets as those of non-pregnant non-lactating women. They do not make any extra dietary provision to satisfy the additional dietary needs. As a result the offspring is born with poor liver stores of vitamin A. Though during infancy, the mother's milk protects the child from VAD, the intake of vitamin A by the children either during the weaning period or at later age is inadequate and provides only 25-30 percent of the recommended intakes. Consequently, the hepatic stores of vitamin A in children are depleted gradually leading to VAD.

Illiteracy and Ignorance

Due to female illiteracy and consequent ignorance, supplementation of children with vitamin A rich foods is delayed and certain rich sources of β– carotene (provitamin A) like green leafy vegetables and papaya are avoided with the belief that these are harmful to the health of the children.

Poverty

Low purchasing power of the communities and their consequent inability to meet the nutrient requirements even after spending 80-90 percent of their income on food is another important factor leading to VAD. Animal foods like eggs, milk, and liver provide preformed vitamin A. But these are expensive, and the poor families cannot afford these and consequently depend on plant foods that provide only provitamin A.

Infections

Infections like measles, diarrhea, respiratory tract infections, and worm infestations interfere with the absorption of vitamin A. During acute infections, due to impaired appetite, food intake is reduced. Serum levels of vitamin A are also significantly reduced during acute infections. As a result, the nutritional status of these marginally nourished children worsens leading to clinical forms of malnutrition. Measles, not only interferes in the absorption of vitamin A, it also reduces the immunity, increasing the susceptibility of any child to infections. Thus, any such infection can aggravate VAD.

MAGNITUDE OF VITAMIN A DEFICIENCY IN INDIA (MALNUTRITION IN SOUTH ASIA)

Vitamin A deficiency remains widespread in many countries of South and South-East Asia and contributes to a considerable proportion of preventable blindness, although there have been encouraging declines in overt xerophthalmia over the last decade in India.[4, 5]

Preschool Children and Infants

Nutrition surveys in the late 1960s and early 1970s carried out in different parts of India showed that about 5-15 percent of children and clinical signs of VAD. In 1974, a countrywide survey conducted by the Indian Council of Medical Research had shown that about 7 percent of pre-school children had clinical signs of VAD. It was estimated in India that there were more than one million cases of blindness arising from VAD.

Although prevalence of xerophthalmia has decreased significantly over the past 15 years, there remains clinical and biochemical evidence of VAD. Table 19.1 indicates the gradual reduction of VAD prevalence over the past years as revealed through various surveys. An estimated 5-7 percent pre-school children suffer from xerophthalmia which causes al least 60000 children to go blind each year. Prevalence rates of VAD vary greatly among states. Statewise data presented in India Nutrition Profile (1998) indicate that 7 states of India namely, Orissa, Mizoram, Maharashtra, Karnataka, Tamil Nadu, Andhra Pradesh, and Madhya Pradesh still have a prevalence rate of much over 0.5 percent for Bitot's spot which is the cut-off point suggested by WHO for considering it as a public health problem (Table 19.2). Another four states namely, Arunachal Pradesh, Assam, Nagaland and Dadra Nagar Haveli following closely have the VAD prevalence level of 0.30 percent and above.[6]

Table 19.1: Reported prevalence of vitamin A deficiency in India

Source	*Prevalence (%)*	*Criteria*
ICMR (1971-4)*	2.0	Nutritional Blindness
NNMB (1975-79)****	2.0	Bitot's Spots
WHO (1988-1990)****	0.7	Bitot's Spots
India National Survey 1989*	0.04	Total Blindness
WHO 1995**	1.4	Bitot's Spots
UNICEF, 1997**	0.7	Bitot's Spots
India Nutrition Profile***	0.21	Bitot's Spots
	0.11	Corneal Xerosis
	0.05	Keratomalacia
	0.05	Corneal Opacity

* Textbook of Human Nutrition, Oxford & IBH Publishing Co., New Delhi, 1996.
** WHO-MDIS, 1995 and UNICEF Field Office Report, 1995.
*** India Nutrition Profile, DWCD, Ministry of Human Resource Development, 1998.
**** National Nutrition Monitoring Bureau, 1991.

School Children and Adolescents

The early vitamin A surveys demonstrated an increased prevalence of VAD with increasing age. A survey conducted in pre-school children showed that the prevalence of Bitot's Spots increased from 0.9 percent in 1 year old to 7.3 percent in 5-year-old children. The prevalence was even higher among school age children.[4,7,8]

Women of Reproductive Age Group

Night blindness during pregnancy and lactation has been reported since the 1960s but the magnitude of the problem in India has not been established. Studies conducted in India have reported prevalence of night blindness amongst pregnant women as 2.9, 4.8, 6.0, 15.9 and 38.9 percent.[9-13] The recent National Family Health Survey–2 conducted in India reported 13% prevalence of night blindness amongst pregnant women.[14] A multicentric study conducted in 16 districts of India reported a prevalence of night blindness amongst pregnant women in the range of 0.59–19.62[15] (14 pm-vita-srf-pap). Earlier data from population based studies conducted in rural areas of South and Southeast Asia indicate maternal night blindness prevalence rates of 10 to 20 percent in pregnant women.[16]

HEALTH CONSEQUENCES OF VITAMIN A DEFICIENCY

Health consequences of VAD can be ocular and /or nonocular and at clinical and subclinical levels depending

Table 19.2: Statewise prevalence of vitamin A deficiency

State/UT	*Bitot's Spots*		*Corneal Xerosis*		*Keratomalacia*		*Corneal Opreats*	
	Male	*Female*	*Male*	*Female*	*Male*	*Female*	*Male*	*Female*
Haryana	0.26	0.23	NA	NA	NA	NA	NA	NA
Himachal Pradesh	0	0.12	NA	NA	NA	NA	NA	NA
Punjab	0.08	0	NA	NA	NA	NA	NA	NA
Rajasthan	0.24	0.21	0.17	0.14	0.12	0.07	0.02	0.02
Chandigarh	0	0	0	0	0	0	0	0
Delhi	0.04	0.05	0	0.04	0.02	0.05	0.01	0
Bihar	0.18	0.11	0.1	0.06	0.04	0.07	0.06	0.05
Sikkim	0.16	0.22	0.99	0.66	NA	0.02	0.09	0.05
Arunachal Pradesh	0.35	0.33	0.34	0.38	0.02	0.28	0.26	0.23
Assam	0.20	0.3	NA	NA	NA	NA	NA	NA
Manipur	0.14	0.14	0.1	0.05	0.02	0.01	0.08	0.16
Meghalaya	0.26	0.1	0.1	0.03	0.11	0.08	0.09	0.11
Mizoram	2.6	3.33	1.13	1.14	0.33	0.24	0.76	0.63
Nagaland	0.33	0.37	0.57	0.03	NA	NA	0.10	0.03
Tripura	0.02	0.02	0.12	0.12	0.07	NA	NA	0.05
Dadra Nagar Haveli	0.43	0.32	NA	NA	1.11	0.11	NA	NA
Daman Diu	NA	NA	NA	NA	NA	NA	NA	0.1
Goa	NA	NA	0.13	0.06	NA	NA	NA	NA
Gujarat	0.2	NA	NA	NA	NA	NA	NA	NA
Maharashtra	0.72	NA	NA	NA	NA	NA	NA	NA
Kerala	0.25	NA	NA	NA	NA	NA	NA	NA
Karnataka	0.77	NA	NA	NA	NA	NA	NA	NA
Tamil Nadu	3.11	NA	NA	NA	NA	NA	NA	NA
Andhra Pradesh	0.79	NA	NA	NA	NA	NA	NA	NA
Madhya Pradesh	2.62	NA	NA	NA	NA	NA	NA	NA
Orissa	0.86	NA	NA	NA	NA	NA	NA	NA
WHO Cut-off	> 0.5%	> 0.01 %	> 0.01 %	> 1.0 %				

Source: National Nutrition Profile (1998), Department of Women and Child Development, Ministry of Human Resources Development, Goa, 1998.

NA: Data Not Available.

on the severity of VAD. Common clinical signs of VAD are night blindness and xeropthalmia, the latter covers all the eye signs including changes in cornea and retina. Based on the severity of VAD, the stages of xeropthalmia have been defined by WHO as night blindness (XN), conjunctival xerosis (X1A), Bitot's Spot (X1B), corneal xerosis (X2), corneal ulceration/keratomalacia (X3) and corneal scar (XS).[3, 17]

Night Blindness (XN)

Vitamin A plays an essential part in the mechanism of vision in dim light. It is a useful screening tool and correlates closely with other evidence of VAD. It can be elicited in the case of young children by the detailed questioning of the parents/guardians. The children cannot usually see in dim light, either at dusk or dawn. Observant mothers can easily notice the inability of their children to see the plate of food kept in front of them, or children frequently stumbling in dim light. The value of night blindness will depend on the care with which the questions are asked and upon the degree to which the phenomenon of night blindness is recognized by the community. In India, there is a specific term for night blindness in different languages (e.g. "*Rataundhi*").[16,18]

The role of retinol (preformed vitamin A) in vision in dim light is based upon the formation of rhodopsin (visual purple) of which retinoaldehyde is an essential component. The visual purple gets bleached in presence of light and stimulates the rods of retina. This process in highly dependent upon adequate availability of retinol and, therefore, the first symptom of VAD is night blindness, also known as *nyctalopia*.[16,18]

Conjunctival Xerosis (X1A)

It manifests as dry patches of non-wettable conjunctiva. When the eye is exposed for about 30 seconds and when the child ceases to cry, the tears appear to emerge like sand-bank at receding tide. It may be associated with various degrees of thickening, wrinkling and pigmentation (muddy coloring) of the conjunctiva. Conjunctival xerosis is subject to investigators bias, making it absolutely essential for standardization of all the investigators in its correct diagnosis.[3]

Bitot's Spot (X1B)

These are more an extension of the xerotic process. These are raised muddy and dry triangular grayish or glistening white patches formed of desquamated thickened conjunctival epithelium. They are firmly adherent to the underlying conjunctiva. These spots consist of epithelial debris, fatty globules and often masses of xerosis bacilli. These are generally bilateral on the temporal sides of cornea[3] (Fig. 19.1).

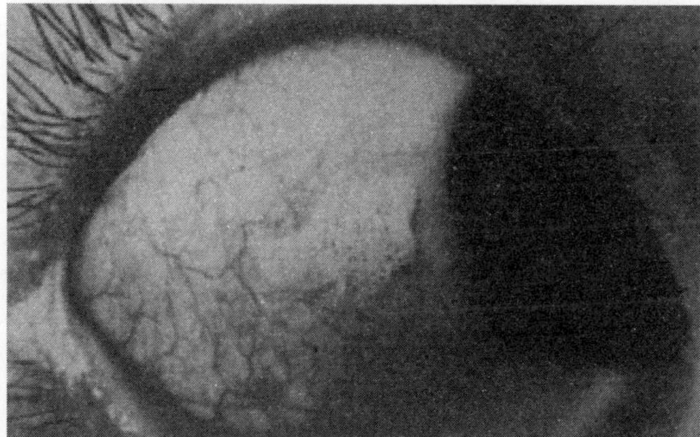

Fig. 19.1: VAD. Note the Bitot's spot (X1B) on temporal side of right cornea (See for colour figure Plate 1)

Corneal Xerosis (X2)

This is diagnosed by the presence of haziness or dryness of cornea on clinical examination. Generally, the changes start at the lower portion of the eye. The cornea takes ground-glass appearance.[3]

Corneal Ulceration/Keratomalacia (X3)

Subsequently, corneal ulceration may occur. These are characteristically circular and sharply demarcated. If properly managed, these corneal changes usually heal leaving useful vision. Only children, in whom stroma is deeply affected, develop blindness. Keratomalacia represents rapidly progressive necrosis and death of tissue affecting the full thickness of the cornea. This for the child is the point of no return and may end up in extrusion of intraocular contents or complete atrophy of the eye.

Corneal Scar (XS)

These are white opaque patches on the cornea as a result to healing of corneal ulcer. Vision may be seriously affected, depending on the size of the scar.

In addition to these eye signs, it is reported, though controversial, that VAD increased morbidities (like diarrhea and respiratory infections in children) and mortality. Children having VAD are 2-3 times more prone to infections than children with adequate vitamin A status. It is known that diarrhea and respiratory tract infections account for 50 percent of all deaths in 1-4 years children in India.

On the other hand, measles has been shown to "starve" the child of vitamin A making the child vulnerable to illnesses such as diarrhea and respiratory tract infections.

RECOMMENDED DIETARY ALLOWANCES OF VITAMIN A

Preformed vitamin A (retinol) is not produced in the body and has, therefore, to be ingested like all other vitamins. It can either be ingested through foods which contain preformed vitamin A (retinol) which are found in the animal kingdom or as its precursor pro-vitamin A, the carotenoids, which are found in the vegetable kingdom. After ingestion of the precursor carotenoids, these are converted in the body to retinol. However, carotenoids are not as effective as retinol, if one considers these on weight for weight basis. In technical terms, 1 μg of retinol is equivalent to 1 IU of vitamin A, while 6 μg of carotenoids has 1IU of vitamin A activity.

Vitamin A is present in fish liver oil and foods of animal origin such as liver, eggs, butter milk and fatty fish. All plant foods contain carotenoids. Rich sources of vitamin A are Halibut liver oil, cod liver oil, Shark liver oil, Shark liver oil (Indian Pharmacopoeia), Liver (sheep, goat, ox, or pig). Good sources of vitamin A are butter, ghee, egg (hen) whole, egg yolk, milk powder (full cream) and cheese (fatty type). Fair sources of vitamin A are milk (cow/buffalo; whole), human milk, and fatty fish. Some sources of carotene are green-leafy vegetables (amaranth leaves, cabbage, coriander leaves, curry leaves, drumstick leaves, fenugreek leaves, radish leaves, mint, spinach) carrot, yellow pumpkin, jack fruit, ripe mango, orange, and ripe tomato.

The vitamin A requirements for the different age groups recommended by the FAO/WHO Expert Group on vitamin requirements and ICMR Expert Groups are given in Table 19.3.

THE NATIONAL PROPHYLAXIS PROGRAM FOR PREVENTION OF BLINDNESS DUE TO VITAMIN A DEFICIENCY

The National Prophylaxis Program for Prevention of Blindness due to VAD aims at protecting children 6 months–5 years at risk from VAD. The prophylaxis program comprises a long-term and short-term strategy. While the short-term intervention focuses on administration of mega doses of vitamin A on periodic basis, dietary improvement is the long-term ultimate solution to the problem of VAD. This program is implemented through the Primary Health Centers and its sub-centers.

Prevention of Vitamin A Deficiency

Promoting Consumption of Vitamin A-rich Foods

- Regular dietary intake of vitamin A-rich foods by pregnant and lactating women and by children under 5 years of age must be promoted.

Table 19.3: Recommended dietary intakes of vitamin A or carotene (μg/day)

Age	*ICMR Expert Group*		*FAO/WHO Expert Group*	
	Vitamin A Retinol (μg)	*Carotene (μg)**	*Vitamin A Retinol (μg)*	*Carotene (μg)***
Upto 1 year	350	1400	300	1800
1 – 3 years	400	1600	250	1500
4 – 6 years	400	1600	300	1800
7 – 9 years	600	2400	400	2400
10 – 12 years	600	2400	575	3450
13 – 15 years	600	2400	725	4350
Adolescents	600	2400	750	4500
Adults (M/F)	600	2400	750	4500
During pregnancy	600	2400	750	4500
During lactation	950	3800	1200	7200

Source: Gopalan C, Ramashastri BV. Nutritive Value of Indian Foods, NIN, ICMR, Hyderabad 2001;p 156.
Swaminathan M. Vitamins. In: Advanced Textbook on Food and Nutrition. Vol. I, 1993;p 250

* Vitamin A equivalent calculated on the assumption that 4 μg carotene in the diet will have the same biological activity as 1 μg vitamin A retinol.

** Vitamin A equivalent calculated on the assumption that 6 μg carotene in the diet will have the same biological activity as 1 μg vitamin A retinol.

Section 6

- The women attending antenatal clinics and immunization sessions as well as mothers and children enrolled in the ICDS Program must be made aware of the importance of preventing VAD.[19-22]
- Breastfeeding, including feeding of colostrums, must be encouraged.
- Feeding of locally available β carotene (precursor of vitamin A) rich foods such as green-leafy vegetables and yellow and orange vegetables and fruits like pumpkin, carrots, papaya, mango, oranges, etc. along with cereal and pulse to a weaning child must be promoted widely. In addition, whenever economically feasible, consumption of milk, cheese, paneer, dahi (yoghurt), ghee, eggs, liver, etc. must be promoted.
- For increasing availability of vitamin A-rich food, growing of vitamin A-rich foods in home gardens and consumption of these must be promoted.

Administration of Massive Dose of Vitamin A

Unlike most other micronutrients, vitamin A is stored in the body for prolonged periods. Hence, periodic administration of massive dose ensures adequate vitamin A nutriture.

- Administration of massive dose of vitamin A to preschool children at periodic intervals is a simple, effective and most direct intervention strategy. This is a short-term strategy.
- Under the massive dose program, every infant 6-11 months and children 1-5 years is to be administered vitamin A every 6 months. Priority is to be given for coverage of children 6 months-3 years since the highest prevalence of clinical signs of VAD is reported in this age group. The recommended schedule is as follows:

6-11 months	one dose of 100, 000 IU
1-5 years	200, 000 IU / 6 months

- A child must receive a total of 9 oral doses of vitamin A by its fifth birthday.
- The contact with an infant during administration of measles vaccine between the age of 9-12 months is considered a practical time for administration of the vitamin A supplement–100, 000 IU for infants.

TREATMENT OF VITAMIN A DEFICIENT CHILDREN

- All children with clinical signs of VAD must be treated as early as possible.
- Treatment schedule is to administer 200, 000 IU of vitamin A immediately after diagnosis. This must be followed by another dose of 200, 000 IU 1-4 weeks later.
- Infants and young children suffering from diarrhea, measles or acute respiratory tract infections must be monitored closely and encouraged to consume vitamin A-rich food. In case, early signs of VAD are observed, the above treatment schedule must be followed.

Concentrated Vitamin A Solution–Important Guidelines

- Vitamin A concentrate is available at primary health centers and sub-health centers in the form of flavored syrup at a concentration of 100,000 IU/ml or 100,000 IU/capsule.
- Vitamin A syrup should be administered using the 2 ml spoon/dispenser provided with each bottle of vitamin A solution. A marked level full 2 ml spoon of vitamin A contains 200,000 IU vitamin A.
- Vitamin A solution must be kept away from direct sunlight. It should be stored in a cold dark room. Vitamin A solution kept at room temperature is stable for a minimum of one year.
- Vitamin A solution bottle once opened must be utilized within 6-8 weeks.

- Regular consumption of dark green leafy vegetables or yellow fruits and vegetables prevents vitamin A deficiency (Fig. 19.2).
- Breastfeeding protects against vitamin A deficiency. Colostrum is rich in vitamin A.
- Oral Prophylactic dose of vitamin A (Fig. 19.3):
  - One dose of 100, 000 IU to infants 6-11 months.
  - Six monthly dose of 200, 000 IU to children 1-5 years.
- Treatment of vitamin A deficient cases:
  - Single oral dose of 200, 000 IU of vitamin A immediately at diagnosis.
  - Follow-up dose of 200, 000 IU of vitamin A one-four weeks later.

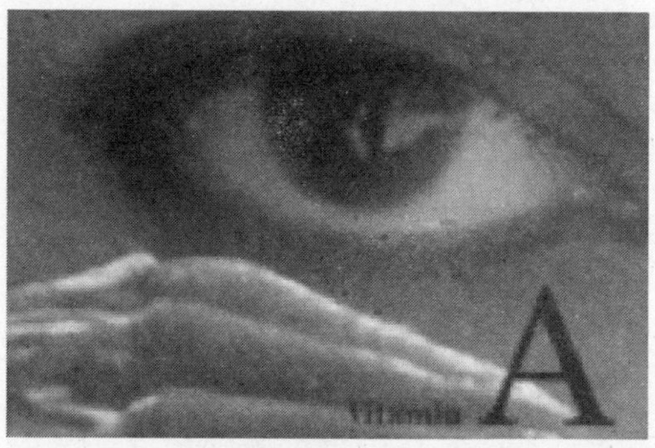

Fig. 19.2: Carrots are good source of vitamin A and, therefore, vision-friendly (See for colour figure Plate 1)

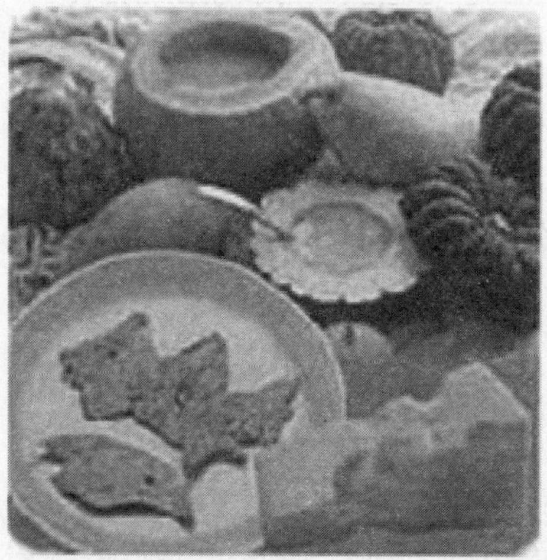

Fig. 19.3: Fruits and vegetables are a good source of vitamin A (See for colour figure Plate 1)

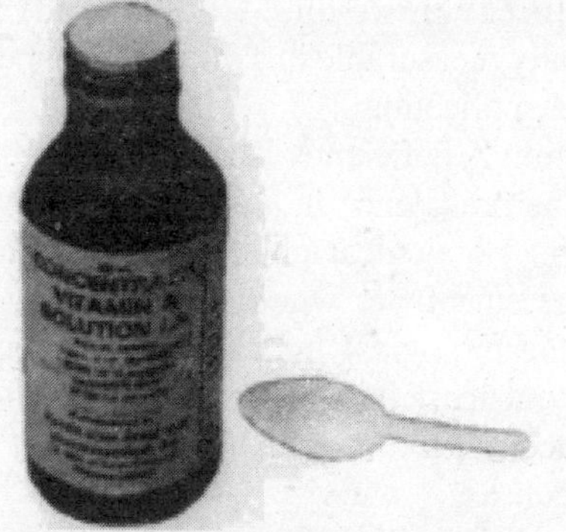

Fig. 19.4: Vitamin A for prophylatic and therapeutic use

ASSESSMENT OF VITAMIN A DEFICIENCY

Assessment of VAD requires indicators that are operationally simple, cost-effective and reliable. To define VAD status, clinical and sub-clinical indicators are utilized. The most sensitive group used for detection of VAD in preschool children aged 6-71 months.

Clinical and subclinical indicators of vitamin A status cut-off levels that define deficiency and minimum prevalence levels that define VAD as a public health problem are presented in Table 19.4.

Indicators for Vitamin A Deficiency

Night Blindness

The prevalence of individuals with a history of night blindness (or local names for this condition) can serve as a useful indicator of VAD. Specialists can make quantitative measurements of dark adaptation, but these measurements can be difficult to standardize under field conditions. Also, the low prevalence of positive findings limits the use of night blindness in populations with mild to moderate levels of vitamin A deficiency.

Xerophthalmia

Eye signs such as conjunctival xerosis and Bitot's spots can indicate the existence of VAD. However, these signs are somewhat variable and subjective. Health workers must be carefully trained for accurate diagnosis. Additionally, the low prevalence of these findings means that very large samples are required to establish the disorder with any certainty, especially if only mild or moderate levels of deficiency are present. For these reasons the quantitative assessment of xerophthalmia is not likely to be a practical measure in populations with mild or moderate deficiency.

Conjunctival Impression Cytology

In this technique filter paper is applied to the conjunctiva to remove epithelial cells, which are then classified histologically as positive or negative.[23] The method is simple and minimally invasive and may provide an indication of the likelihood of deficiency for surveillance purposes. However, the results indicate only the positive findings and do not provide a continuous scale of deficiency. Moreover, interpreting the samples requires careful training and standardization. For these reasons conjunctival impression cytology falls short of providing a reliable, quantitative index of vitamin A status.

Serum Retinol

Measurement of retinol has been widely used to determine vitamin A status at the population level. The proportion of individuals with low retinol levels reflects the risk of deficiency. However, retinol does not reflect liver stores of vitamin A and may be affected by other factors such as infection and protein-energy malnutrition. Also, the method may not be practical under field conditions because of the need for venous blood samples, careful storage and transport of specimens, and sophisticated laboratory analysis. Retinol can be measured in a microsample of serum. The use of a filter paper and the Dried Blood Spot (DBS) method has been developed and used in India, Liberia, Mexico and Nepal,

Table 19.4: Indicators of vitamin A deficiency

Indicator	*Individual Level*		*Population Level (%) (to be defined as a public health problem)*		
	Moderate	Severe	Mild	Moderate	Severe
Eye signs: Night blindness (XN) (children 24-71 months)	(present- y/n)	(present- y/n)	>0 to <1	≥ 1 to <5	≥ 5
Conjunctival xerosis (X1A) (children 6-71 months)	(present- y/n)	(present- y/n)	—	—	—
Bitot's Spots (X1B) (children 6-71 months)	(present- y/n)	(present- y/n)	—	0.5% (n ≥ 3058)	—
X2, X3A, X3b (children 6-71 months)	(present- y/n)	(present- y/n)	—	0.01% (n ≥ 153,650)	—
Corneal Scars (XS) (children 6-71 months)	(present- y/n)	(present- y/n)	—	0.05% (n ≥ 30,718)	—
Blood signs: Serum Retinol (children 6-71 months)	<0.7 umol/l	<0.35 umol/l	>0 to <10 (<0.7 umol/l)	≥ 10 to <20 (<0.7 umol/l)	≥ 20 (<0.7 umol/l)
Other signs: Breast milk retinol (children 6-71 months)	< 1.05 umol/l (< 8μg/g milk fat)	—	<10	≥ 10 to <25	≥ 25
RDR (children 6-71 months)	< 20%	—	<20	≥ 20 to <30	≥ 30
MRDR (children 6-71 months)	Ratio > 0.06	—	<20	≥ 20 to <30	≥ 30
CIC/ICT (children 6-71 mo)	abnormal	abnormal	<20	≥ 20 to <40	≥ 40

Sources: Blood signs from Prevention of Micronutrient Deficiencies Ch4: Prevention of Vitamin A Deficiency Table 4-2 by Barbara Underwood, 1998.

Section 6

with the advantage that only a finger-prick by sterile lancet is required.

Breastmilk Vitamin A Concentration

This is a unique indicator of vitamin A status because it provides information about the vitamin A status of both the mother and the breast-fed infant. The mother's secretion of vitamin A into the milk is directly related to her vitamin A status, at least when her vitamin A status is inadequate. All infants are born with low stores of vitamin A, thus the concentration of vitamin A in the breastmilk also serves as an indicator of an infant's likely vitamin A status.

Relative Dose Response (RDR)

Dose response tests, based on measuring retinol response to an administered dose of vitamin A, measure vitamin A status more accurately. These tests have the significant advantage of reflecting liver stores of vitamin A; however, their acceptability is limited by the requirement that two blood samples be drawn. The modified relative dose response (MRDR) test requires only a single venous sample, but it is complex for field application and its use as an indicator in continuing ongoing surveillance may be limited.

Retinol-binding Protein

The potential for retinol-binding protein to indicate vitamin A status is being explored. This test is highly correlated with serum retinol because it is the carrier protein for retinol in the circulation. When used as an indicator it has many of the limitations of serum retinol, including depression in response to infections and the lack of the ability to reflect liver stores. However, it has the advantage of being potentially measurable in a dried blood spot sample suitable for field application.

Vitamin A deficiency is a public health problem when:

a. The prevalence in a population of at least two of the above biological indicators of vitamin A status is below the cut off, or when,
b. One biological indicator of deficiency is supported by at least four of demographic and ecological risk factors (two of which are nutrition and diet related) such as:
   - IMR > 75/1000 live births; under 5-year MR > 100/1000 live births.
   - Full immunization coverage or, particularly measles immunization coverage in < 50 percent of children at 12-23 months of age.
   - Less than 50 percent prevalence of breast-feeding in 6-month-old infants.
   - Median dietary intake < 50 percent of recommended safe level of intake along 75 percent of children 1-6 years of age.
   - Two-week period prevalence of diarrhea > 20 percent.
   - Measles case fertility rate > 1 percent.

Table 19.5: Relative ranking of indicators on a population base

Indicators	*Risk Assessment*	*Targeting Programs*	*Evaluating Effectiveness*
Night Blindness	+++	+++	+++
Breast Milk Retinol (lactating mothers and breastfed infants)	++	+++	++
Serum Retinol	++	+	++
RDR/MRDR	+++	+++	+++
CIC/ICT	+	—	—

- No normal schooling for > 50 percent of women 15-44 years of age.
- Less than 50 percent households with safe water source.

Biological indicators are the most specific and useful indicators for determining VAD risk assessment, targeting programs and evaluating their effectiveness. Table 19.5 depicts a relative ranking of the usefulness of indicators of VAD.

REFERENCES

1. Sommer A. *Vitamin A Deficiency and its Consequences: A Field Guide to their Detection and Control*, 3rd edn. Geneva: World Health Organization 1995.
2. Gopalan C, Venkatachalam K. *Nutrition Atlas of India*. New Delhi: Indian Council of Medical Research 1971.
3. World Health Organization. Indicators for assessing vitamin A deficiency and their Application in Monitoring and Evaluating Intervention Programs. Geneva: World Health Organization 1996 WHO/NUT/96.10.
4. United Nations Children's Fund. *Malnutrition in South-East Asia: A Regional Profile*. Kathmandu: UNICEF 1996.
5. Indian Council of Medical Research. *Blindness*. Annual Report, New Delhi: ICMR 1974.
6. Government of India. *India Nutrition Profile*. New Delhi: Department of Women and Child Welfare, Ministry of Human Resource Development 1998.
7. Rao NP, Singh D, Swaminathan MC. Nutritional status of pre-school children of rural communities near Hyderabad city. *Indian J Med Res* 1969, 57: 2132-2246.
8. Khamgaonkar MB, Ramkrishnan S, Ghuliani KK, Murthy GV, Nayar S, Vidwans P. Vitamin A intake and vitamin A deficiency in rural children. *Indian Pediatr* 1990;28:443 -446.
9. Radhika MS, Bhaskaram P, Balakrishna N, Ramalakshmi BA, Devi S, Kumar BS. Effects of vitamin A deficiency during pregnancy on maternal and child health. *Br J Obstet Gynecol*. 2002; 109: 689-693.
10. Kapil U, Pathak P, Tandon M, Singh C, Pradhan R, Dwivedi SN. Micronutrient deficiency disorders amongst pregnant women in three urban slum communities of Delhi. *Indian Pediatr*1999; 36: 983-989.
11. Biswas AB, Mitra NK, Chakraborty I, *et al.* Evaluation of vitamin A status during pregnancy. *J Indian Med Assoc* 2000; 98:525.
12. Pathak P, Singh P, Kapil U, Raghuvanshi RS. Prevalence of iron, vitamin A, and iodine deficiencies amongst adolescent pregnant mothers. *Indian J Pediatr* 2003;70:299-301.
13. Dixit DT. Night-blindness in third trimester of pregnancy. *Indian J Med Res* 1966;54:791-795.
14. Anonymous. *National Family Health Survey–India (NFHS-II) 1998-99*. Mumbai: International Institute of Population Sciences 2000.
15. Toteja GS, Singh P, Dhillon BS, Saxena BN. Vitamin A deficiency disorders in 16 districts of India. *Indian J Pediatr*. 2002;69:603-605.
16. International Vitamin A Consultative Group (IVACG). *IVACG Statement. Maternal Night Blindness: Extent and Associated Risk Factors*. Washington: IVACG 1997.
17. Trowbridge FL. Surveillance of micronutrient deficiency. *Food and Nutr Bull* 1994; 15: 290-293.
18. International Vitamin A Consultative Group (IVACG). *IVACG Statement. Maternal Night Blindness: A New Indicator for Vitamin A Deficiency*. Washinton: IVACG 2002.
19. World Health Organization. *Using Immunization Contacts as the Gateway to Eliminating Vitamin A Deficiency. A Policy Document*. Geneva: World Health Organization 1995.
20. Gopalan C, Ramashastri BV. *Nutritive Value of Indian Foods*, Hyderabad: NIN/ ICMR 2001.
21. World Health Organization. *Vitamin A Supplements: A Guide to their Use in the Treatment and Prevention of Vitamin A Deficiency and Xerophthalmia*, 2nd edn. Geneva: World Health Organization 1995.
22. Government of India. *Policy on Management of Vitamin A Deficiency*. New Delhi: Ministry of Health and Family Welfare 1991.
23. Stoltzfus RJ, Miller KW, Hakimi M, Rasmussen KM. Conjunctival impression cytology as an indicator of vitamin A status in lactating Indonesian women. *Am J Clin Nutr*. 1993; 58:167-173.

Section 6

Pankaj Abrol

20 Vitamin B Complex Deficiencies

INTRODUCTION

Vitamin B complex consists of various factors or vitamins having different composition and function. These are important constituents of enzyme system and act as coenzymes in many vital reactions occurring in our body. Some of these vitamins are synthesized in our body by the microbial flora. As diets deficient in one B complex factor are deficient in other B complex factors also, it is more practical to treat the patient deficient in one B complex factor with all B complex factors.[1]

Vitamin B complex includes following compounds: thiamine (B_1), riboflavin (B_2), niacin (B_3), pyridoxine (B_6), folic acid and cyanocobalamin (B_{12}). Pantothenic acid (B_5), choline and inositol are also included in B complex group, but at present specific clinical syndromes are not well defined in children due to their deficiencies.[2] Vitamins of B complex are water-soluble and are not stored in human body. Therefore, toxicity is generally not observed. Most of vitamins of this group are heat stable, except B_1 which is heat labile.[3]

THIAMINE (B_1)

Thiamine is water-soluble and heat labile vitamin. It is usually available in tissues as thiamine pyrophosphate (TTP). It is also known as carboxylase. It is required for acetylcholine synthesis and thus has a role in nerve conduction. It acts as a coenzyme in transketolation and in decarboxylation of a-ketoacids. It has a role in carbohydrate and protein metabolism. In thiamine deficiency utilization of pyruvic acid is decreased, increasing tissue and blood levels of pyruvic acid and lactic acid.[3]

Milk (breast milk or cow's milk), whole grain cereals, dried yeast, pulses, oilseeds, eggs and fruits are the dietary sources of thiamine. Meat and green vegetables are relatively poor sources of thiamine. An enzyme factor destructive to thiamine is present in some varieties of fish. If a lactating mother is deficient in thiamine, her infant may develop beriberi. Thiamine deficiency may occur in a child because of lack of dietary intake, lack of absorption in prolonged diarrhea, excess use as in hyperthyroidism, surgery, stress and fever; or impaired use in liver disease.

Recommended dietary intake

0.4 mg/1000 kcal/day.

Deficiency State

Pathology

In fatal cases, the lesions are mainly located in heart, peripheral nerves, subcutaneous tissue and serous cavities. Fatty degeneration of myocardium and dilated heart are usual findings. Serous effusions, edema over the legs and venous congestion may be present. Degeneration of myelin and axon cylinders with Wallerian degeneration is seen in peripheral nerves. Nerves of lower extremities are first to get involved. Intra-cranial hemorrhage following vascular dilatation may be seen.

Clinical Features

Thiamine deficiency leads to beriberi. It is more common in communities whose staple food is polished rice. Early symptoms include fatigue, irritability, depression, poor memory, sleep disturbance, chest pain, anorexia, constipation and abdominal pain. The disease mainly affects the heart, peripheral nerves, subcutaneous tissues and serous cavities. The signs of progression include peripheral neuritis, paresthesias of toes and feet, areflexia, loss of vibration sense, tender legs with cramps, congestive heart failure and psychic disturbances. Ptosis of eyelids along with hoarseness/aphonia due to paralysis of laryngeal nerve may occur. Muscle atrophy may be followed by ataxias. Later signs of increased intracranial pressure, meningismus or coma may occur. Nervous system involvement is termed dry beriberi. It occurs usually in older children and when poor caloric intake and relative physical inactivity is present.

In Wernick's encephalopathy, there is vomiting, ophthalmoplegia, ataxia, horizontal nystagmus and altered sensorium due to thiamine deficiency. It occurs infrequently in malnourished children. Encephalopathy has occurred in children on total parenteral nutrition. Other causes include infection, malignancy and gastrointestinal disorders including malabsorption. In Korsakoff psychosis there is retrograde amnesia, inability to learn and confabulation. The combination of these two is called Wernicke-Korsakoff syndrome.

Wet beriberi usually presents with palpitation, tachycardia, dyspnea and edema. It is the consequence of high caloric intake and high level of activity in the absence of adequate thiamine required for carbohydrate metabolism. In chronic wet beriberi there are various stages. In the first stage there is peripheral vasodilation leading to high cardiac output failure. This leads to salt and water retention due to renin-angiotensin mediated aldosterone secretion in kidneys. In response to loss of volume, kidney responds by conserving salt. This leads to fluid overload and edema of the dependent extremities. Trying to maintain the cardiac output to end organs, the heart gets fatigued and undergoes myocardial ischemic injury presenting as chest pain. A more rapid form of wet beriberi is termed acute fulminant cardiovascular beriberi or **Shoshin beriberi.**[4] In this the predominant injury is to heart muscle. Instead of edema, the patient may present with cyanosis of hands and feet, tachycardia, distended neck veins, restlessness and anxiety. The response to thiamine therapy is fairly quick. If untreated death ensues rapidly.

Infantile beriberi is seen in breastfed infants of mothers with inadequate thiamine intake. It occurs in 2nd or 3rd month of life.[1]

Diagnosis

Deficiency can be diagnosed by demonstrating decreased levels of RBC transketolase and high blood or urinary glyoxylate values. Therapeutic response to thiamine remains the best test for thiamine deficiency.

Prevention

Infantile beriberi can be prevented by the maternal diet rich in thiamine. Older children require thiamine rich diet. Thiamine requirement increases with carbohydrate rich diet.

Treatment

When a breastfed infant gets beriberi, both mother and the baby should be treated with thiamine. The daily therapeutic dose for the adults is 50 mg and for the children is 10 mg. Oral administration is effective except when the child has gastrointestinal disturbances. It is given by parenteral (intramuscular or intravenous) route when cardiac failure is there.[5] There is dramatic improvement initially followed by complete cure over some weeks. Damage to heart is irreversible. Other B complex factors should also be given, as their deficiencies are usually associated.

RIBOFLAVIN (VITAMIN B_2)

Isolated riboflavin deficiency is rare. Usually it is associated with deficiency of other B complex factors. It is a yellow fluorescent water-soluble substance stable to heat and acids but rapidly destroyed by light and alkalis. It is involved in many oxidative enzyme systems in energy metabolisms, synthesis of glycogen and erythropoiesis. Riboflavin is required for synthesis of coenzymes flavin mononucleotide and flavin adenine dinucleotide (FAD). These nucleotides play important role in electron transport. Riboflavin is required for growth, tissue respiration and light adaptation.[6]

Sources

Liver, kidney, brewer's yeast, meat, eggs, milk, cheese and green leafy vegetables. Cow's milk contains five times riboflavin as much as in human milk.

Recommended Dietary Allowance

0.6 mg/1000 kcal consumed.

Deficiency State

Deficiency is usually caused by inadequate dietary intake or decreased absorption in chronic diarrhea, biliary atresia, hepatitis, post-operative states; or in those getting drugs like probenecid, phenothiazine and oral contraceptives.[6]

Clinical Features

In riboflavin deficiency a child can have cheilosis (angular stomatitis), glossitis, keratitis, conjunctivitis, photophobia, lacrimation and marked corneal neovascularization. Cheilosis begins at the angle of mouth. It may be followed by superficial linear scars on healing. Grayish white exuberant lesions may result from super infection by Candida albicans. In glossitis tongue is smooth with loss of papillary structures. It may appear sore, magenta or red. Cutaneous lesions may affect the nasolabial folds, alae nasi, ears, eyelids, scrotum and labia majora. These may become red, scaly and greasy. Seborrheic dermatitis may also be seen. Peripheral neuropathy with hyperaesthesia and altered temperature and pain sensation may appear. These patients may have normocytic, normochromoic anemia with bone marrow hypoplasia.

Diagnosis

Diagnosis is established by urinary riboflavin excretion of < 30 mg/24 hours. A level of erythrocyte glutathionine reductase activity reflects the stores of riboflavin.

Prevention

It can be prevented by taking diet rich in riboflavin. The diet should contain milk, eggs, leafy vegetables, liver and lean meat.

Treatment

Treatment consists of oral administration of 3-10 mg of riboflavin/day. Intramuscular riboflavin in the doses of 2-5 mg can be given three times a day if there is no response to oral therapy. The child should also get a balanced diet and other B complex factors for associated deficiencies.

NIACIN DEFICIENCY (PELLAGRA)

Niacin (nicotinic acid), also called vitamin B_3, is an important component of NAD and NADPH enzymes required for glycolysis and electron transfer. Nicotinic acid plays a crucial role in cellular respiration. It is required for DNA synthesis and repair.[7] It is found in foods like yeast, liver, red meat, fish, lean pork, poultry, whole grain cereals, legumes etc. As dietary tryptophan can only partially substitute for niacin other sources of niacin are necessary. Milk and eggs contain little niacin but are rich in tryptophan. Niacin deficiency is common in people whose staple diet is maize or sorghum (jowar).[3] These cereals are rich in leucine but are deficient in tryptophan. Leucine itself is known to inhibit endogenous biosynthesis of niacin.[3] Niacin can be synthesized in the body from tryptophan—an essential amino acid. Only small losses occur while cooking.

Deficiency State

Deficiency of niacin is called pellagra (*pellis*: skin; *agra*: rough). Pellagra can be either primary or secondary.

Primary pellagra results when the diet is extremely deficient in niacin-rich foods. *Secondary pellagra* occurs when the diet contains adequate niacin but there is a disease interfering with its absorption and/or processing. The various causes are chronic diarrhea, cirrhosis of liver, alcoholism, prolonged use of isoniazid, malignant carcinoid tumor and Hartnup disease.

Pathology

In pellagra there is edema and degeneration of superficial collagen of the dermis layer of skin. Engorgement of papillary vessels and perivascular lymphocytic infiltration is also observed. The epidermis is hyperkeratotic and later on progresses to atrophy. Comparable changes are seen in the tongue, buccal mucous membrane and vagina. Colonic walls may be thickened and inflamed with a pseudo-membrane. Mucosa may get atrophied. There may be associated secondary infection and ulceration. In central nervous system patchy demyelinization and degeneration of ganglion cells; and demyelination of posterior and lateral columns may occur.

Recommended Dietary Allowance

6.6 mg /1000 kcal consumed. It may range from 5 mg in an infant to 20 mg in adults.

Clinical Features

Initial symptoms are vague. Weakness, anorexia, lassitude, numbness, dizziness may present as prodromal symptoms. Prolonged deficiency may present as the classical triad of dermatitis, diarrhea and dementia. The characteristic cutaneous manifestations presenting as erythematous rash may be precipitated by some irritant or intense sunlight. These appear on exposed parts first— hands (*pellagrous gloves*), foot and legs (*pellagrous boot*) and neck (*casal necklace*). These are sharply demarcated lesions and their distribution may change frequently. Sometimes vesicles and bullae may appear. It may get infected or may disappear after desquamation. Sometimes pigmentation remains.

Sometimes gastrointestinal manifestations precede cutaneous lesions. These may present as diarrhea, glossitis and vomiting. The entire tongue may become red, swollen and ulcerated. Bloody diarrhea may occur.

Initial mental changes appear as insomnia, fatigue and apathy. These may lead to memory loss, confusion, depression and hallucinations. Prolonged deficiency of niacin, if untreated can result in death.

Classical symptoms are sometimes not seen in infants and children. Alternate constipation and diarrhea may appear. Moderate anemia and evidence of deficiency of other B complex vitamins may be seen.

Diagnosis

Usually made from clinical picture of glossitis, symmetric dermatitis, diarrhea and mental changes. Rapid therapeutic response to niacin is an important confirmatory test. No chemical tests are available for definitive diagnosis of pellagra.

Prevention

A well balanced diet consisting of meat, vegetables, eggs, milk and milk products is the best way of prevention of pellagra. Breast-fed babies of mothers having pellagra require niacin supplementation.

Treatment

Pellagrous child should get a well-balanced diet along with 50-300 mg/24 hr of niacin. Severe cases and those with intestinal malabsorption should get 100 mg of niacin by intravenous route. After getting large doses of niacin the patient gets sense of warmth, flushing and burning in skin (not with niacinamide). Large dose of niacin is hepatotoxic and can cause cholestatic jaundice. Avoid sun exposure in acute cases.

Emollients can be applied to skin for soothing effect. The child should also get other vitamins, particularly B complex. Iron may be required to treat accompanying hypochromic anemia.

PYRIDOXINE (VITAMIN B_6) DEFICIENCY

Vitamin B_6 includes a number of pyridine derivatives—pyridoxal, pyridoxine and pyridoxamine. These are converted to pyridoxal-5-phosphate or pyridoxamine-5-phosphate and these coenzymes play an important role in amino acid metabolism, e.g. transamination, decarboxylation and desulpharation.[8] It helps in formation of serotonin, and also in the metabolism of glycogen and fatty acids. It is also required for breakdown of kynurenine; therefore its deficiency leads to appearance of xantherunic acid in urine. Pyridoxine is required for proper functioning of the nervous system. Its deficiency leads to seizures and demyelination of peripheral nerves leading to peripheral neuropathy. Pyridoxine is necessary for normal brain metabolism.[1]

Sources

Pyridoxine is widely distributed in foods—liver, meat, yeast, fish, legumes and cereals. Adequate amount is present in both human and cow's milk. Prologed heating required for processing of milk destroys it.

Recommended Daily Allowance

0.5–1.0 mg/day.

Deficiency State

Etiology

Use of processed milk/foods and malabsorption disorders like celiac disease can cause pyridoxine deficiency. Isoniazid used in tuberculosis is pyridoxine antagonist. Requirement is also increased in pregnancy and with use of drugs like penicillamine, hydralazine and oral contraceptives.[9]

There are some vitamin B_6 dependent syndromes like pyridoxine dependent convulsions, pyridoxine responsive anemia, xanthurenic aciduria, homocystinuria and cystathioninuria. These patients respond to high dose of pyridoxine.

Clinical Features

Deficiency symptoms are less commonly seen in children, compared to adults. Various presentations can be there. Infants fed on pyridoxine deficient formula for 1-6 months may have irritability and generalized seizures. Convulsions due to pyridoxine dependency can occur several hours after birth to as long as 6 months of age. Myoclonic seizures and hypsarrythmic pattern in electroencephalogram (EEG) are observed. Many cases give the history of several doses of pyridoxine in pregnant mother for the control of emesis.

Children with pyridoxine deficiency have microcytic and hypochromic anemia. Serum iron concentration and saturated iron binding protein are increased. Hemosiderin deposits in liver and bone marrow are also increased. There is non-utilization of iron for hemoglobin synthesis. Pyridoxine deficiency can cause pyridoxine responsive sideroblastic anemia in young children.

Treatment of tuberculosis with isoniazid (INH) may cause peripheral neuropathy. This may respond to supplementation with pyridoxine or reduction of dose of INH. This side effect is less common in children.

Pyridoxine deficiency may also cause dermatitis. There may be seborrhea around eyes, nose and oral cavity. Cheilosis and glossitis may also be associated. These patients may have lymphopenia, decreased antibody formation and recurrent infections. Some children have failure to thrive, hyperirritability and hyperaccusis.

Xanthurenic aciduria can appear after loading with tryptophan. Cyst athioninuria can also appear. Both of these respond to high dose of pyridoxine.

Diagnosis

1. After administration of 100 mg / kg of tryptophan, large amount of xanthurenic acid is excreted in patients of pyridoxine deficiency. None is excreted in a normal individual. The test may also be normal in pyridoxine deficiency.
2. Diagnosis is suspected in a convulsing infant when more common causes like hypocalcemia, hypoglycemia and sepsis are excluded. Pyridoxine deficiency is suspected when convulsions respond to a dose of 100 mg of injectable pyridoxine. Older children may show response to 100 mg of Intramuscular pyridoxine while EEG is being recorded. In such situations tryptophan loading test is indicated.
3. In pyridoxine deficiency erythrocyte glutamic pyruvic transaminase is reduced.

Prevention

Balanced diet containing adequate amounts of pyridoxine is the best way to prevent deficiency. Babies of mothers having large doses of pyridoxine during pregnancy are at increased risk to develop pyridoxine dependence. A child receiving pyridoxine antagonist like isoniazid should be observed closely for signs of pyridoxine deficiency. In case these signs appear, the child should either be supplemented with pyridoxine or the dose of antagonist drug reduced.

Treatment

In pyridoxine responsive seizures, possibly due to deficiency, 100 mg pyridoxine should be given by intramuscular route. This should be followed by adequate daily dietary intake. In patients having dependence, 2-10 mg intramuscularly or 10-100 mg orally may be required daily for 4-6 weeks.

VITAMIN B_{12} DEFICIENCY

Vitamin B_{12} is also called cyanocobalamin due to presence of a cyano group and a cobalt atom. Another name is extrinsic factor of Castle.[3] The cyano group may be replaced by nitrate or hydroxyl group to give nitrosocobalamin or hydroxycobalamin, both of which are hemopoietically active forms of the vitamin. Vitamin B_{12} is converted to the coenzymes such as methyl-cobalamin and 5-deoxy-adenosyl-cobalamin which are required for various metabolic reactions. This vitamin also plays an important role in nucleic acid metabolism and protein synthesis.[10]

Vitamin B_{12} is derived from cobalamin in food, which is from animal sources and is produced by microorganisms. Humans do not synthesize vitamin B_{12}. It is found in many foods–all animal sources. Deficiency is rare, can occur in extreme dietary restriction or in absolute vegetarians (vegans)—those who do not use even animal milk products.[11] Plants do not synthesize vitamin B_{12}. In the acidic media of stomach cobalamins are released and combine with R proteins and intrinsic factor (IF). This complex passes through duodenum. The pancreatic enzymes break down R proteins. Intrinsic factor-cobalamin complex gets absorbed in the distal ileum. Some amount of vitamin B_{12} is also absorbed directly through diffusion across the intestinal and buccal mucosa. In blood it is mainly bound to transcobalamins (TC) mainly TC II and partly to TC I, and TC III.[1]

Sources

Primary source of vitamin B_{12} is intestinal microbial flora. Besides liver, kidney, egg, fish, and milk are good sources.

Recommended Daily Allowance

Children 0.2-1.0 mg.

Deficiency State

The causes of vitamin B_{12} deficiency are:

1. Inadequate dietary intake.
2. Breastfed infants of vitamin B_{12} deficient vegetarian mothers.
3. Following administration of certain drugs—neomycin, para amino salicylic acid, colchicine.
4. Malabsorption due to blind loop syndrome, tropical sprue, Crohn's disease, intestinal tuberculosis.
5. Surgery/resection of part of stomach and/or terminal ileum.
6. Lack of secretion of Intrinsic Factor (IF)—Juvenile pernicious anemia.
7. Consumption/inhibition of B_{12}-IF complex.
8. Abnormality of receptor sites in terminal ileum.
9. Deficiency of transcobalamin II (TC II).

Vitamin B_{12} is excreted in urine as well in feces. Deficiency impairs DNA synthesis and repair. There is defective myelin formation. Erythropoiesis is megaloblastic and arrested in later stages in bone marrow. Peripheral blood shows macrocytic and normochromic anemia. Life span of red cells is reduced. Demyelination of large nerve fibres of spinal cord, and fibres in lateral and posterior columns occurs.

Clinical Features

The symptoms of juvenile pernicious anemia appear at 9 months – 11 years. Anemia due to deficiency of vitamin B_{12} occurs between 4-7 months of age. The symptoms usually occur when *in utero* stores of vitamin B_{12} are exhausted. Early signs are tingling and numbness in fingers and toes. There is weakness, irritability, anorexia and listlessness. The tongue is smooth, red and painful. There is anemia, which becomes severe with the passage of time. Neurological manifestations are ataxia, paresthesias, hyporeflexia, clonus, positive babinski and coma. The advanced stage is called "subacute combined degeneration of the cord".

Vitamin B_{12} has been implicated in the etiology of infantile tremore syndrome.[10]

Diagnosis

Macrocytic anemia with macro-ovalocytosis is seen in peripheral blood. Large and hypersegmented polymorphs (polycytes) are also seen in the blood film. Advanced cases can have anemia, neutropenia and thrombocytopenia mimicking aplastic anemia. Bone marrow shows megaloblastic erythropoiesis. Serum vitamin B_{12} levels are less than 100 pg / ml, though serum LDH is markedly raised. Levels of folic acid and iron may be normal or elevated. Serum bilirubin may be raised to 2-3 mg/dl. Methyl malonic aciduria is a reliable and sensitive index of vitamin B_{12} deficiency. In contrast to adult pernicious anemia, serum antibodies directed against parietal cells of stomach or intrinsic factor are not detected in children. Gastric acidity also may be reduced initially but returns to normal once vitamin B_{12} therapy is started. Gastric histology is also normal in children.

Schilling test is used to assess the absorption of vitamin B_{12}. When a normal person is given vitamin B_{12} into which radioactive ^{57}Co is incorporated, it combines with intrinsic factor (IF) in stomach. The complex is absorbed in terminal ileum and then the absorbed vitamin gets bound to TC II. Little or none is excreted in urine. Now if a large dose (1 mg) of non-radioactive vitamin B_{12} is injected parenterally after 2 hours, 10-30 % of radioactive vitamin B_{12} is excreted in urine in 24 hours. Children having pernicious anemia usually excrete 2 % or less. To find out whether absence of IF is the reason for non-absorption of vitamin B_{12}, 30 mg of IF is given with second dose of the radioactive vitamin, normal amount is excreted in urine. In case, malabsorption of the vitamin is due to absence of ileal receptor sites or some other cause, no improvement occurs with IF.

Treatment

There is prompt hematological response with reticulocytosis to parenteral administration of 1 mg of vitamin B_{12}. It occurs in 2-4 days. As the physiological requirement is only 1-5 mg of the vitamin, response can occur with such small doses and this can be very well used as therapeutic test. When there is neurological involvement, 1 mg should be injected by intramuscular route daily for at least 2 weeks. This should be followed by monthly intramuscular administration of 1 mg of vitamin B_{12} for maintenance throughout life.[12] Oral therapy is not preferred due to uncertain absorption.

FOLIC ACID

Folic acid and related compounds with folic acid activity are given the generic name folacin. The word folacin is derived from the word folium meaning leaf. Folic acid is essential for the maturation of red blood cells. After absorption it is reduced to its coenzyme form tetrahydrofolic acid (THFA). This reaction requires NADPH. Some infections and certain drugs increase the requirement of folic acid resulting in its deficiency. These conditions also compound dietary deficiency. Drugs like phenytoin and mysoline cause folic acid deficiency. Methotrexate is also antifolinic. Patients with hemolytic anemia and compensatory erythropoiesis also require supplementation with folic acid. Indian way of cooking destroys folic acid. Goat's milk is deficient in folic acid. Cow's milk and human milk provide adequate amounts of folic acid, provided that the mothers themselves are well nourished. Folate requirements are markedly increased during pregnancy, so as to meet the fetal needs. Folic acid should be supplemented in the dose of at least 400 mg/24 hr from the beginning of pregnancy, in order to prevent neural tube defects and meet the growth needs.

DNA of cells can be damaged through attacks by free radicals. Folic acid is required in addition to protect DNA and ensure its replication. Folic acid deficiency is implicated in Alzheimer disease, depression, dementia, hearing loss, cleft lip/palate and neural tube defects.[13]

Sources

Green-leafy vegetables such as spinach, cabbage and broccoli. Besides yeast, liver, kidney and eggs are also good sources.

Recommended Daily Allowance

100 mg/24 hours. It increases in pregnancy and lactation to 350 mg / 24 hours.

Deficiency State

Deficiency of folic acid in a patient can be isolated or present along with deficiency of other vitamins like vitamin B_{12}, minerals like iron and proteins. DNA synthesis is impaired resulting in defective cell division. All rapidly dividing cells like bone marrow and intestinal mucosa are affected. Hence the deficiency leads to megaloblastic anemia and diarrhea.

Clinical Features

Very low birthweight (VLBW) infants may have anemia. Therefore, routine supplementation in VLBW infants with folic acid is advised. Megaloblastic anemia as such appears earlier than iron deficiency anemia. The usual age of presentation in infancy is 4-7 months, whereas iron deficiency anemia (IDA) in full term babies with adequate weight occurs usually after 9 months of age. The children are pale, irritable and may have chronic diarrhea with growth failure. The children look sicker compared to the degree of anemia. There is increased pigmentation of back of hands, fingers and toes. Some infants have tremors and developmental retrogression. The patient may bleed because of thrombocytopenia. The patient may also have associated malnutrition as kwashiorkor or marasmus. In contrast to megaloblastic anemia due to vitamin B_{12} deficiency, which is more common in infants, megaloblastic anemia due to folic acid deficiency is more often after first year of life.

Laboratory Findings

The anemia is macrocytic (MCV>100 fl) with normochromic morphology. Variations in red cell size and shape are not uncommon. Reticulocyte count is low and nucleated red cells with megaloblastic morphology are seen. Anemia specially if prolonged may be associated with neutropenia and thrombocytopenia. Large hypersegmented polymorphs with counts more than 5% of total neutrophils having 5 or more lobes may be seen. Bone marrow is cellular with erythroid hyperplasia. Megaloblastic changes are prominent, although some normal erythroid precursors may also be seen. Giant metamyelocytes with cytoplasmic vacuolization may be seen. Nuclei of megakaryocytes may also be seen. Normal serum folic acid level is 5-20 ng/ml. It may be reduced to 3 ng/ml. RBC folate is a better index, which is reduced. Normal RBC folate level is 150-600 ng/ml. Serum lactic dehydrogenase (LDH) level is markedly elevated. Levels of vitamin B_{12} and iron may be normal or elevated.

Treatment

Folic acid is used in the dose of 1-5 mg/24 hours by oral or parenteral route. In doubtful cases, 50-100 mg/24 hr. of folate may be used for a week for diagnostic test. In folic acid deficiency, folic acid should be continued for 3-4 weeks. Folic acid should be avoided in patients of suspected vitamin B_{12} deficiency or pernicious anemia as there is every possibility for neurological symptoms to deteriorate.

BIOTIN DEFICIENCY

Biotin deficiency is rare as it can be synthesized by intestinal flora.

Dietary Sources

Whole cereals, liver, kidney, yeast, legumes and peanuts. It is also synthesized by intestinal flora.

Daily Requirements

Infants–50 mg/day; child–100 mg/day; adolescent–150-200 mg/day.

Deficiency State

Etiology

1. Consumption of raw-egg white can however produce biotin deficiency symptoms by inhibiting absorption of biotin. Raw-egg white contains a glycoprotein avidin, which acts antagonist to biotin and forms avidin-biotin complex. On cooking the egg white, avidin gets inactivated and cannot bind biotin.[3]
2. Children receiving parenteral nutrition for prolonged periods at risk to develop biotin deficiency.
   Babies of mothers having biotin deficiency can also suffer from biotin deficiency.

Clinical Features

Macuolo-squamous and brawny dermatitis, orofacial lesions, anorexia, lassitude, hypotonia, muscle pain, somnolence, hallucinations and hyperesthesias. These children may have anemia and decreased immunity. Genetic defects with biotin deficiency include Rett's syndrome and carboxylase defects.

Prevention and Treatment

Parenteral solutions when administered for long periods must include biotin. Therapeutic dose is 10 mg.

PANTOTHENIC ACID (VITAMIN B_5)

It is present in coenzyme A and acyl carrier protein. It acts as H ion donor and receptor in the metabolism of cholesterol, fatty acids, lipids and sterols. It is required for synthesis of cholesterol in our body. It is essential for infantile growth. It participates in fatty acid and acetylcholine synthesis. Deficiency affects both nervous system and digestive system.[14]

Dietary Source

Yeast, liver, eggs, potatoes, whole cereals and legumes.

Daily Requirements

1.5-5 mg for infants, 5-10 mg for school children.

Deficiency State

Clinical Features

Headache, fatigue, weakness, vomiting, impaired motor activity, muscle cramps, disturbed sleep, depression and gastrointestinal disturbances. It is useful in burning feet syndrome, healing of ulcers and bedsores. It is useful in variety of other conditions like alcoholism, allergies, hair loss, graying of hair, autism, heart diseases, celiac disease, seborrhea, muscular dystrophy, multiple sclerosis and obesity.

Treatment

The principal form of supplementary pantothenic acid is calcium D-panthotenate. Usual therapeutic doses range from 10-50 mg/day.

CHOLINE

Choline is an essential constituent of phospholipids. It is involved in mobilization and transport of fats and cholesterol. It is a lipotropic factor.[3] In its absence neutral fats and cholesterol accumulate in liver. Hemorrhagic necrosis of kidney and accumulation of free radicals in liver, heart and kidney also results. Immunity may be depressed. Choline gets acetylated in the body to get converted to acetylcholine –a chemical mediator of synaptic transmission.

INOSITOL

Inositol is believed to play an important role in health at cellular level. It is found in fair concentration in lens of human eye and heart. It plays important role in the health of cell membrane especially of specialized cells in brain, bone marrow, eyes and intestine. It is said to promote healthy hair, hair growth and helps in controlling estrogen levels in blood. It also reduces blood cholesterol levels. Deficient patients may have eczema, hair loss, constipation, abnormalities of eyes and raised blood cholesterol. Not much is known about this factor at this time.

Sources of inositol include wheat germ, brewer's yeast, bananas, liver, brown rice, nuts and vegetables. Coffee destroys inositol.

REFERENCES

1. Curran JS, Lewis AB. Vitamin deficiencies and excesses. In: Behrman RE, Kliegman RM, Jenson HB (eds): *Nelson Textbook of Pediatrics*, 16th edn. Philadelphia: Saunders 2000: 176-184.
2. Berger H, Gracey M. Water soluble vitamins. *Clinical Nutrition of the Young Child*. Vol 2. New York: Nestec Vevey / Raven Press 1994: 518-534.
3. Lal H. Vitamins. In: Lal H (ed) *A Textbook of Biochemistry*. New Delhi: CBS 2004: 75-99.
4. Shivalkar B, Engelmann I, Carp L. Shoshin syndrome: Two case reports representing opposite ends of the same disease spectrum. *Acta Cardiol* 1998; 53: 195-199.
5. Beers MH, Berkow R, Rogin RM. *The Merck Manual.* 17th edn. New Jersey: Merck and Co 1999:45-46.

6. Rivlin RS. Hormones, drugs and riboflavin. *Nutr Rev* 1979;37:241.
7. Swendseid ME, Jacob RA. Niacin. In: Shils ME, Olson JA, Shike M (eds) *Modern Nutrition in Health and Disease,* 8th edn. Philadelphia: Lea and Febiger, Year: 376-382.
8. Frye RE, Jabbour SA. Pyridoxine deficiency. Citkowitz E, Talavera F, Cooper M, Griffing GT (eds): *E-Medicine.* Last updated on December 12, 2002.
9. Bender DA. Vitamin B_6 requirements and recommendation. *Eur J Clin Nutr* 1989;43:289-309.
10. 10. Gupte S. Infantile tremor syndrome. In: Gupte S (ed) *Textbook of Pediatric Emergencies,* 2nd edn. New Delhi: Peepee 2008:142-148.
11. Rauma AL, Torronen R, Hanninen O, Mykannen H. Vitamin B_{12} status of long-term adherents of a strict uncooked vegan diet is compromised. *J Nutr* 1995;125:2511-2515.
12. Berlin R, Berlin H, Brante G, Pilbrant A. Vitamin B_{12} body stores during oral and parenteral treatment of pernicious anemia. *Acta Med Scand* 1978;204:81-84.
13. Hans RL. Folic acid. International Health News http://www.yourhealthbase.com. Downloaded on March 18, 2005.
14. Plesofsky-Vig N. Pantothenic acid. In: Shils ME, Olson JA, Shike M, Ross AC (eds) *Modern Nutrition in Health and Disease.* 9th edn. Baltimore: Williams and Wilkins 1999: 423-432.

Harmesh Singh Bains • Sanjeev Gupta • Shivani Kansal

21 Scurvy

INTRODUCTION

Ascorbic acid (vitamin C) deficiency results in scurvy. Historically scurvy is an ancient disease. Francis Glisson reported the earliest case of infantile scurvy in 1650 after observing it among infants with rickets.[1] The increased incidence of infantile scurvy was attributed to the consumption of heated milk and proprietary foods deficient in vitamin C.[1,2]

PATHOPHYSIOLOGY

Ascorbic acid plays an important role in oxidation of tyrosine and phenylalanine, in formation of hydroxy proline, in preventing depolarization of collagen and maintaining integrity of ground substance and in hemopoiesis. Deficiency of Vitamin C results in tendency to hemorrhage, defective tooth dentin and loosening of teeth and defective formation of osteoid.[3]

ETIOPATHOGENESIS

Scurvy may occur in following conditions:[4]

1. Primary protein-energy malnutrition (PEM) though during periods of gross retardation of growth overt scurvy is not seen.
2. Secondary PEM as in malabsorption.
3. Infants not on breast feed.
4. Breast fed infants born to mother with vitamin C deficiency.
5. Infections which lead to increased requirement of vitamin C.
6. Food faddism.
7. Child neglect.

CLINICAL FEATURES

Scurvy can occur at any age but presents usually in infants between the age of 6 months to 2 years. It is unusual in newborn.[3, 5]

Infantile Scurvy

Initial symptoms are nonspecific and include the following:

- Gross irritability.
- Excessive crying.
- Tenderness to touch.
- Tachypnea.
- Digestive disturbances.
- Diarrhea.
- Poor weight gain.
- Low-grade feverde.

Peudoparalysis: The infant adopts the so-called frog position with hips and knees semiflexed and externally rotated feet. The posture of lower limbs gives an impression as though these are paralysed. In some cases subperiosteal hemorrhage can be felt at the end of femur which may contribute to pain, thus preventing movements of legs further; the affected child looks apprehensive.

Subperiosteal hemorrhage: The lower end of femur and tibia are the most frequently involved sites.

Petechial hemorrhage: These can occur into the skin and mucus membrane.

Spongy gums: Hemorrhage into the gums may result in spongy swollen, bluish purple gums especially about the erupted teeth.

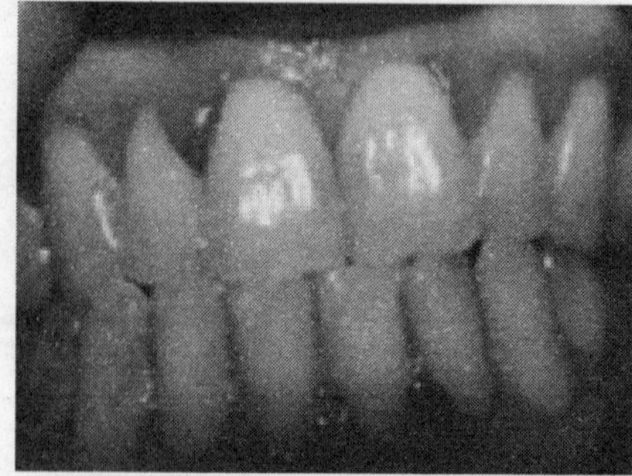

Fig. 21.1: Spongy gums in scurvy (See for colour figure Plate 1)

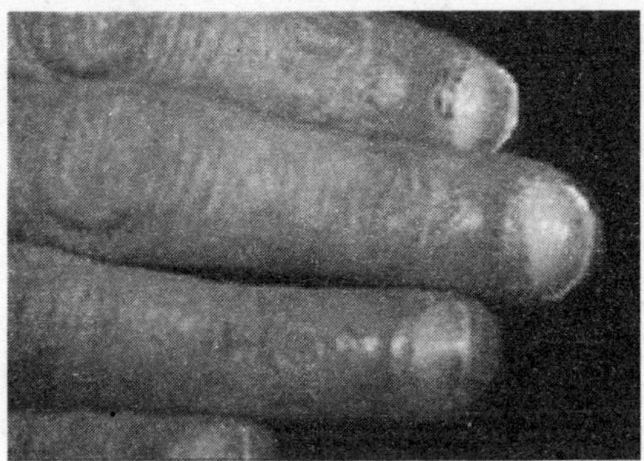

Fig. 21.2: Periungual hemorrhage in scurvy (See for colour figure Plate 1)

Internal hemorrhage into the internal organ may cause hematuria, malena, and subdural swelling.

Proptosis of eyeball can occur secondary to orbital hemorrhage.

Scorbutic rosary at the costochondral junction result from posterior displacement of sternum. It is tender, sharp and angular.

Depressed sternum can also occur in scurvy.

Anemia: Mild to moderate anemia is present due to inability to utilize iron or impaired folic acid metabolism.

Childhood scurvy present as:

- Swollen joints.
- Follicular hyperkeratosis with development of minute hemorrhage at roots of hair follicles.
- Petechial hemorrhage.
- Purpuric swelling into the skin.
- Bleeding into gums may occur.
- Subperiosteal hemorrhage–Rarely.
- Poor wound healing.

Hyperkeratosis, corkscrew hair, and sicca syndrome are typically observed in adult scurvy but rarely occurs in infantile scurvy.[4]

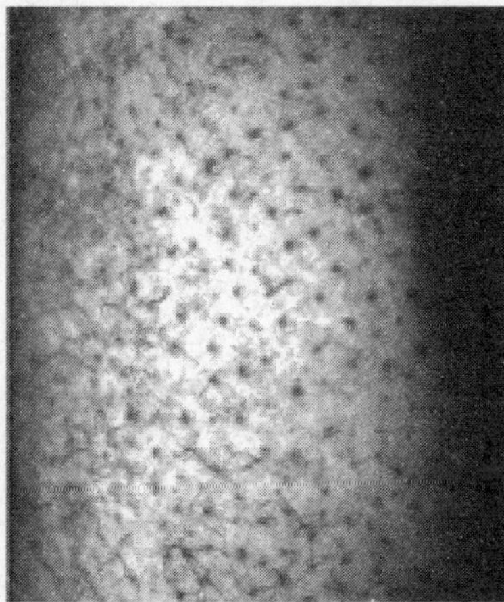

Fig. 21.3: Corkscrew skin in scurvy (See for colour figure Plate 1)

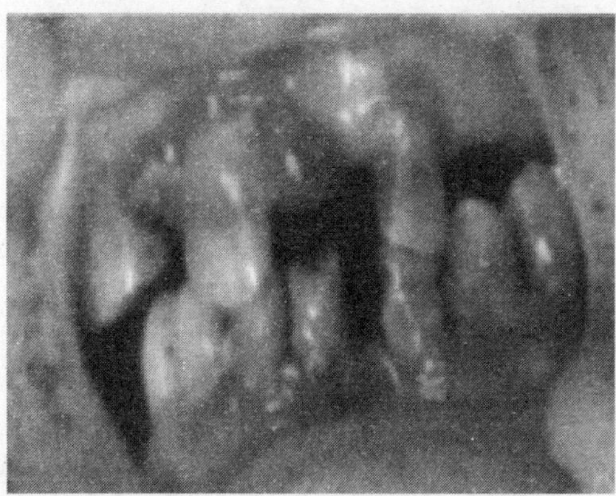

Fig. 21.4: Severe scurvy (See for colour figure Plate 1)

COMPLICATIONS

- Scurvy, if untreated, can be fatal and has been associated with sudden death.
- Loss of function at the site of the hemorrhage and anemia are typical sequelae in scurvy.

DIAGNOSIS

Biochemical

1. Ascorbic acid level in serum/wbc/buffy coat in scurvy is less than 0.1mg/dl. Normal value is 25-40 mg/dl.[3, 8, 9]
2. Urinary excretion of ascorbic acid < 80% of test dose within 3-5 hours after loading dose. Normal value is > 80% of test dose.[3,8]
3. Fasting serum vitamin C level of > 0.6 mg/dl excludes scurvy.[3]

X-ray Changes

Diagnosis of scurvy is based on radiological appearance mainly seen at lower end of femur and upper end of tibia and fibula.[9,10]

White line of Fraenkel: A dense irregular line at the metaphysic represents the zone of well calcified cartilage. White line is also seen in healed rickets, lead poisoning, acute leukemia and congenital syphilis.

Trummerfeld zone: Proximal and parallel to line of Franenkel occurs an area of destruction or rarefaction.

Wimburger sign or Signet ring sign: Epiphyseal centers of ossification are surrounded by a white ring.

Corner sign: Margin of metaphysic project laterally which leads to formation of a spur called Pelkan spur.

Subperiosteal hemorrhage: It results in periosteal elevation and effected bone look like a dumbbell.

Pencil thin cortex: The cortex is thinned because of generalized osteoporosis and trabeculae have ground glass appearance.

Table 21.1: Differential diagnosis of scurvy

- Pseudoparalysis of scurvy needs to be differentiated from that in the following conditions:
  - **Syphilis**: Usually occurs at an earlier age than scurvy and is accompanied by other signs of syphilis.[3,6,7]
  - **Suppurative arthritis/Osteomyelitis:** Acute skeletal infection, bacterial in etiology, characterized by erythema and edema of skin, soft tissue overlying site of infection.
  - **Trauma:** History of trauma is usually present.
  - **Myositis:** Viral in etiology and myalgia is a common complaint.
- In **poliomyelitis**: The paralysis is truly flaccid.
- Bleeding into the skin and mucus membrane needs to be differentiated from **bleeding diathesis** of purpura and leukemia.
- In **Menkes disease** (due to copper deficiency) radiological changes simulate scurvy but clinically characterized by distinctive facies, chubby rosy cheeks, kinky colorless hairs, hypotonia and myoclonic seizures.
- **Child abuse**: The bony pathology associated with scurvy could potentially be confused with physical abuse of a child. A good history and response to treatment establishes the diagnosis and clears confusion. Nevertheless, in the developed world, vitamin C deficiency in children may be associated with neglect as a form of child abuse, even in the absence of overt sign of physical trauma.

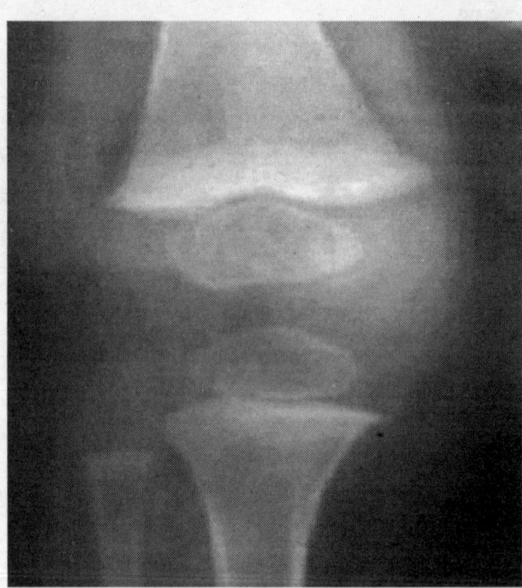

Fig. 21.5: X-ray knee joint in scurvy

TREATMENT

Vitamin C

Dose: Loading dose of 500 mg is followed by dose of 100-200 mg daily for several weeks.[3,10,11]

Route: Oral administration of vitamin C is good enough.[3]
Clinical response occurs in 24-48 hours.[3,10,11]
Radiological changes takes 1-2 weeks.[3]

Contraindication

- G-6-PD deficiency—large doses may precipitate hemolysis.
- Conditions aggravated by acid loading (gout, renal tubular acidosis, paroxysmal nocturnal hemoglobinuria).

Drug Interactions

- Large doses of vitamin C interfere with the absorption and metabolism of vitamin B_{12}.
- Decreases effect of warfarin and fluphenazine.
- Increases aspirin level.[12]

Side-effects

- Large doses can cause renal stones and diarrhea.
- Long-term high intake has been associated with metabolic tolerance/ resistance and the expression, either clinically or biochemically of vitamin C deficiency.[12]

MORTALITY/MORBIDITY

- Sudden death due to cardiac failure is reported in infants and adults.
- Predominant morbidity is due to hemorrhage into various tissues. Subperiosteal hemorrhage in the tibia and femur cause excruciating pain.

PREVENTION

- Encouragement of breastfeeding.
- Not to boil fruit juices.
- Supplement of vitamin C in infants on artificial feed.
- Diet adequate in vitamin C can prevent the development of scurvy. The dietary requirement of vitamin C sufficient to prevent deficiency vary with the age of the individual. The following are the Food and Nutrition Board of the National Academy of Sciences, National Councils minimum recommended dietary allowances of vitamin C.[13-15]
- Infant 30-40 mg.
- Children and adult: 45-60 mg.
- Pregnant women: 70 mg.
- Lactating mother: 90-95 mg.
- Food sources rich in vitamin C include the following:[14,15] Citrus fruits, Berries, Broccoli, Cauliflower, Cabbage, Spinach, Potatoes.

PROGNOSIS

- Typically, scurvy carries an excellent prognosis if diagnosed and treated appropriately.

REFERENCES

1. Wilson LG. The clinical definition of scurvy and the discovery of Vitamin C. *J Hist Med* 1975; 30: 40-60.
2. Carpenter KJ. *The History of Scurvy and Vitamin C.* New York: Cambridge University Press 1986: 1-288.
3. Gupte S, Gomez EM. Pediatric Nutrition and nutritional deficiency states. In: Gupte S (ed): *The Short Textbook of Pediatrics*, 10th edn, New Delhi: Jaypee 2004;125-166.
4. Greene HL. Disorders of the water soluble vitamin B complex and vitamin C. In: *Textbook of Pediatric Nutrition*, 2nd edn. New York: Raven Press 1993: 86-88.

5. Akikusa JD, Garrick D, Nash MC. Scurvy: Forgotten but not gone. *J Pediatr Child Health* 2003;39:75-77.
6. Woodruff CW. Ascorbic acid—Scurvy. *Prog Food Nutr Sci* 1975;1:493-506.
7. Park EA, Guilod HG, Jackson D. The recognition of scurvy with special reference to the early X-ray changes. *Arch Dis Child* 1965;4:82-89.
8. Hess AF. Scurvy: Past and Present. Philadelphia: JB Lippincott 1920.
9. Sauberlich HE. Human requirements. Vitamin C status: Methods and findings. *Ann NY Acad Sci* 1975; 258: 438-450.
10. McDonald, McDonalol A. Scruvy: Not yet out 1 Br. Nutr Surv. 1999;7:204-29.
11. Berger H, Gracey M. Water soluble vitamins. In*: Clinical Nutrition of Young Child,* Vol 2. New York: Nestec Vevey / Raven Press 1994: 518-534.
12. Jacob RA. Three eras of vitamin C discovery. *Subcell Biochem* 1996;25:1-16.
13. ICMR. *Nutrient Requirements and Recommended Dietary Allowances for Indians*. A Report of the Expert Group of Indian Council of Medical Research 1990.
14. Shils ME, Olson JA, Shike M, *et al. Modern Nutrition in Health and Disease*, 9th edn. Baltimore: Williams and Wilkins 1999:305-483.
15. Bowman BA, Russel RM. *Present Knowledge in Nutrition*, 8th edn. Washington, DC: ILSI Press 2001:127-270.

Harmesh Singh Bains • Sanjeev Gupta • Shivani Kansal

22 Rickets

INTRODUCTION

Vitamin D is also known as the "sunshine vitamin" due to the fact that humans can manufacture the vitamin internally from the action of sunlight on the skin.[1,2] Rickets is a disease of growing children in which the bones become softened and deformed due to failure of normal mineralization of bones and epiphyseal cartilage due to vitamin D deficiency. Rickets and osteomalacia are manifestations of the same pathologic process in childhood and adulthood, respectively. Precisely, rickets is a disease of childhood, while osteomalacia is of adult life.

ETIOPATHOLOGIC CONSIDERATIONS

Though most often, the term, *rickets,* refers to deficiency rickets (usually vitamin D), a large number of additional conditions such as malabsorption, renaltubular defects and such factors as prolonged treatment with anticonvulsant agents may contribute to its etiology (Table 22.1).

Table 22.1: Etiological classification of rickets

Deficiency rickets
- Vitamin D deficiency
- Calcium deficiency
- Phosphorus deficiency
- Chelators in diet

Absorptive rickets
- Gastric abnormalities
- Hepatobiliary disease
- Enteric absorptive defects
- Chronic pancreatic insufficiencies

Renal tubular rickets
- Proximal tubular lesion
- Distal tubular lesion

Renal osteodystrophy

Unusal causes of rickets
- Fibrous dysplasia
- Neurofibromatosis
- Soft tissue and bone neoplasms
- Anticonvulsants
- Hypophosphatasia

CLINICAL MANIFESTATIONS

Rickets is a disease of growing bones, usually manifesting in the latter half of first year or in second year. It is uncommon in infants under 3 months of age. Preterm infants have higher incidence of rickets compared to full term infants. Clinical picture of rickets depends upon the following factors:
- Age of child.
- Severity of disease.
- Cause of deficiency state.

The earliest manifestations are quite vague and nonspecific. These include irritability, restlessness, and profuse sweating over the head (more so during sleep).

In infants and young chidren, the child is listless, apathetic, irritable and has hypotonia and flabby muscle. Abdomen gets protruded due to hypotonia of abdomen muscle. There is delay in developmental milestones specially dentition and motor mile stones.

In florid rickets, the child is unable to walk, stand or even sit without support.

Skin

Pallor, at times profound anemia is seen in rickets.

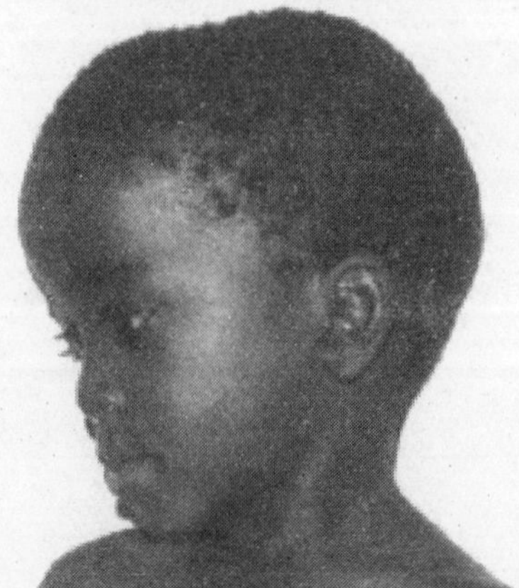

Fig. 22.1: Bossing of skull (See for colour figure Plate 2)

Ligaments

Laxity of ligaments is common.

Skull

- Asymmetrical contours.
- Craniotabes—It is one of the earliest signs of rickets and is due to thinning of the outer table of the skull. In this condition, on pressing occipital or posterior part of parietal bone a ping-pong ball-like sensation can be felt.
- Widening of sutures.
- Patent and wide anterior and posterior fontanels.
- Macrocephaly with flattening of vertex (caput quadratum or box head).
- Bossing of skull (frontal and parietal bones).

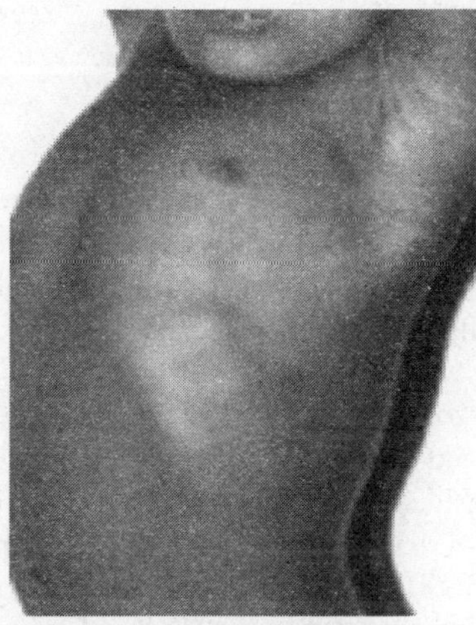

Fig. 22.2: Rachitic rosary (See for colour figure Plate 2)

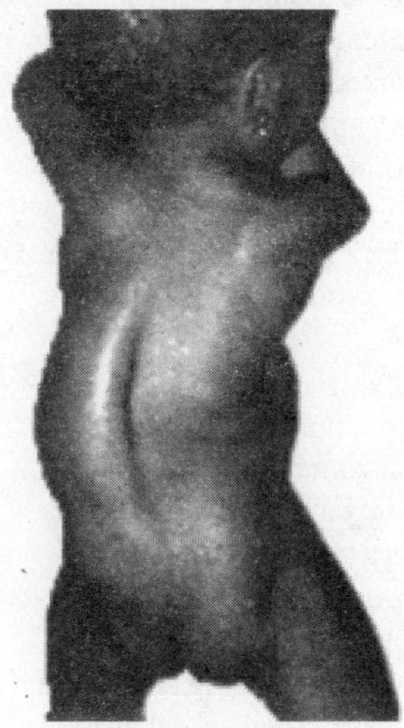

Fig. 22.3: Scoliosis in rickets (See for colour figure Plate 2)

Thorax

- Rachitic rosary-palpable enlargement of costochondral junction (smooth, rounded, nontender).
- Pigeon chest.
- Pectus excavatum (rare).
- Harrison groove or sulcus—a depression along the insertion of diaphragm into the ribs is seen along the lower border of chest.

Abdomen

- Rachitic pot-belly: Abdomen becomes protuberant because of marked hypotonia of abdominal wall muscles.

Spine

- Rachitic cat back.
- Waddling gait.
- Lumbar lordosis.
- Rarely scoliosis.

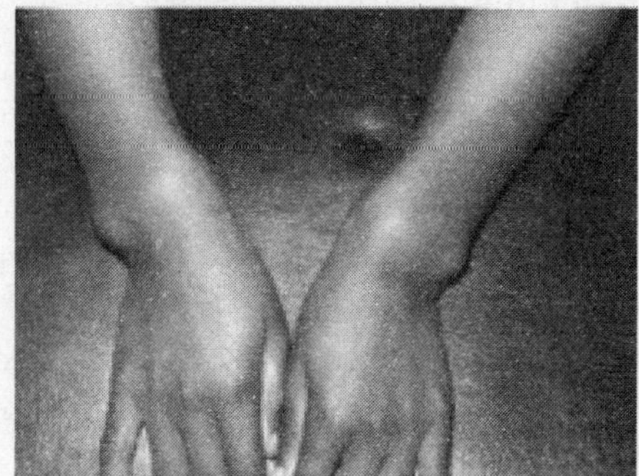

Fig. 22.4: Widening of wrist joints (See for colour figure Plate 2)

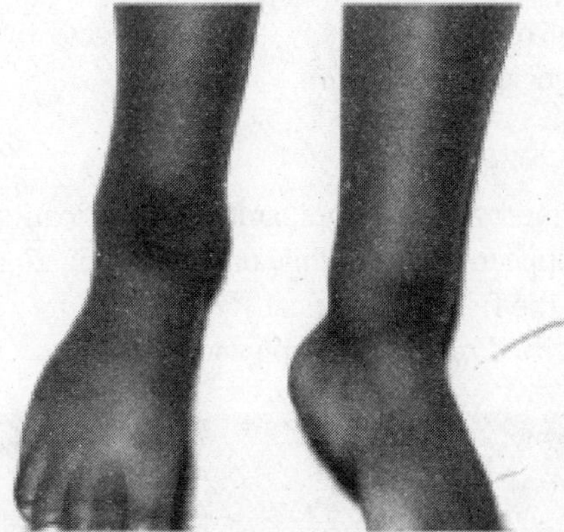

Fig. 22.5: Widening of ankle joints (See for colour figure Plate 2)

Extremities

- Bow legs—due to bending of softened shafts of the femur, tibia and fibula.
- Coxa vera.
- Knock knee.

- Widening of wrist knee and ankle joint.
- Greenstick fracture.

Deformities of spine, pelvis and legs result in rachitic dwarfism.

DIAGNOSIS

Biochemical Abnormalities

- Low or normal serum calcium.
- Serum phosphorus level almost always less than 4 mg/dl.
- Raised alkaline phosphatase levels.
- Elevated urinary cyclic AMP level.
- Low serum 1,25 dihydroxy calciferol level-sensitive index of rickets.
- Nonspecific finding include aminoaciduria, a low bone citrate level, impaired renal acidification, phosphaturia and rarely glucosuria.

Radiological Findings

Active Rickets Ray wrist is the best site for early diagnosis as characterstic changes occur early in ulna and radius. Following features are evident:

- Widening of distal end of radius and ulna.
- Cupping (saucer like depression) and fraying (blurring of margins of metaphysis) of distal ends.
- Splaying (flaring of the metaphysic on either side).
- Increased distance between distal ends of forearm bones and metacarpal bones.
- Decreased bone densities of shaft with prominent trabecular pattern.
- Green stick fracture.
- Periosteal reaction (lifting)—due to excess of osteoid lying under the periosteum.

Healed Rickets

- Well defined zones of preparatory calcification—This result in appearance of a white line of calcification, which hailed as the first radiological sign of healing.
- Well calcified rachitic metaphysic.

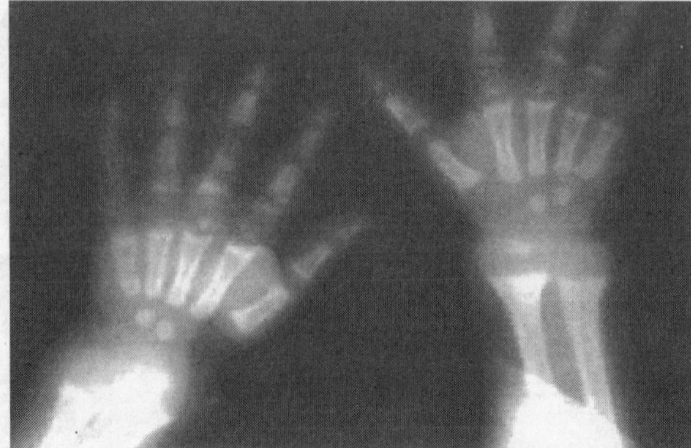

Fig. 22.6: X-ray wrist showing active rickets

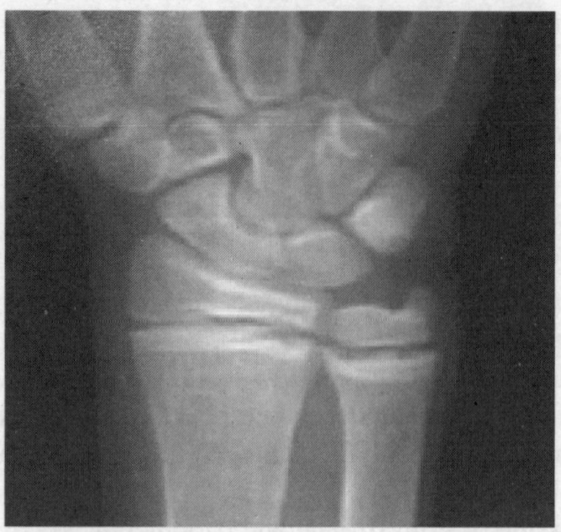

Fig. 22.7: Healed rickets

MANAGEMENT[3-8]

Vitamin D

- **Dose**—Vitamin D is given in a singe dose of 1500 μg (600,000 IU).
- **Route of administration:** Orally or intramuscularly.

Healing is rapid, if there is no sign of healing line on skiagram within 3-4 weeks of therapy, same dose can be repeated.

Refractory rickets: If there is no response within 3-4 weeks of second dose, then diagnosis of refractory rickets should be considered and investigation should be initiated. After healing of rickets, normal daily requirement of vitamin D (10 μg or 400 IU) should be continued. Serum alkaline phosphatase and phosphorus tend to return to normal within 5 days. Deformities of bone may occasionally need surgical correction e.g. osteotomy.

- **Contraindications**
  - Documented hypersensitivity.
  - Hypercalcemia.
  - Malabsorption syndrome.
  - Decreased renal function.
- **Side-effects:** High doses of vitamin D result in
  - Anorexia, vomiting.
  - Hypotonia.
  - Irritability.
  - Polydipsia, polyuria.
  - Hypercalcemia, hypercalciuria.
  - Metastatic calcification on X-ray.
- **Drug Interactions**
  - Cholesyramine and colestipol decreases absorption of calcitriol.
  - Magnesium containing antacids and thiazide diuretics can increase effect of calcitriol.

COMPLICATIONS OF RICKETS

- Short stature, pelvic deformation, and abnormal gait are potential serious outcome of severe rickets.

Section 6

PREVENTION

Rickets can be prevented by:

- Exposure to sunlight.
- Oral administration of 400 IU of vitamin D daily.
- Breast fed infants whose mothers are vitamin D deficient, dark skinned infants.
- Infants born during the winter months in temperate climate should receive vitamin D supplementation.
- Health education of parents against overclothing the infants and young children and proper housing should be given.
- Child should be encouraged to play outdoors for longer period.

VARIANTS OF RICKETS

1. Renal Rickets

- Deficiency in the tubular reabsorption of phosphate—phosphate rickets or late rickets. Manifestation appear in later age and usually resistant to dose of Vitamin D.
- Cystinosis (Fanconi syndrome) characterized by multiple renal tubular defect that is glycosuria, aminoaciduria, tubular acidosis, phosphaturia and uricosuria.This condition needs heavy dose of Vitamin D (50000-3 lakh IU/d) for healing.

2. Pseudodeficiency Rickets (Vitamin D Dependent Rickets)

- **Type I:** autosomal recessive disorder, due to deficiency of 25 hydroxy D3-1 alfahydroxylase deficiency resulting in low level of 1,25 dihydroxy D3.There is hypocalcemia, hypophosphatemia and high PTH level. Treatment: Vitamin D 20000 – 1 million IU/d or Calcitriol 0.5- 2 μg/d.
- **Type II:** Due to marked reduction of binding of 1,25 dihydroxy D3 to its receptors and defective nuclear translocation. Other features include alopecia and short stature.Treatment: Calcitriol 15-30 μg/d.

3. Celiac Rickets: Rickets associated with any major malabsorption state.

4. Primary Hypophosphatemia (X-linked Vitamin D Resistant Rickets)

Mode of inheritance is X-linked and it is most common non-nutritional form of rickets.

Defect occurs in the proximal tubular reabsorption of phosphate and in conversion of 25 hydroxy D3 to 1,25 dihydroxy D3. The activity of the Na- dependent phosphate transporter in the renal PCT is reduced, resulting in excessive urinary phosphate excretion.

Clinical features:The children with familial hypophosphatemia present with bowing of legs, waddling gait, coxa vara, genu varus, genu valgum and short stature. Rachitic rosary and Harrison sulcus are not evident. Pulp deformities and a lesion known as intra globular dentin are characteristic tooth abnormalities. Enamel defect are rare.

Laboratory finding:

- Low or normal serum calcium.
- Reduced serum phosphate.
- Elevated alkaline phosphatase.
- Normal PTH.
- Increased urinary phosphate excretion.
- Absent aminoaciduria, bicarbonaturia and kaliuria.

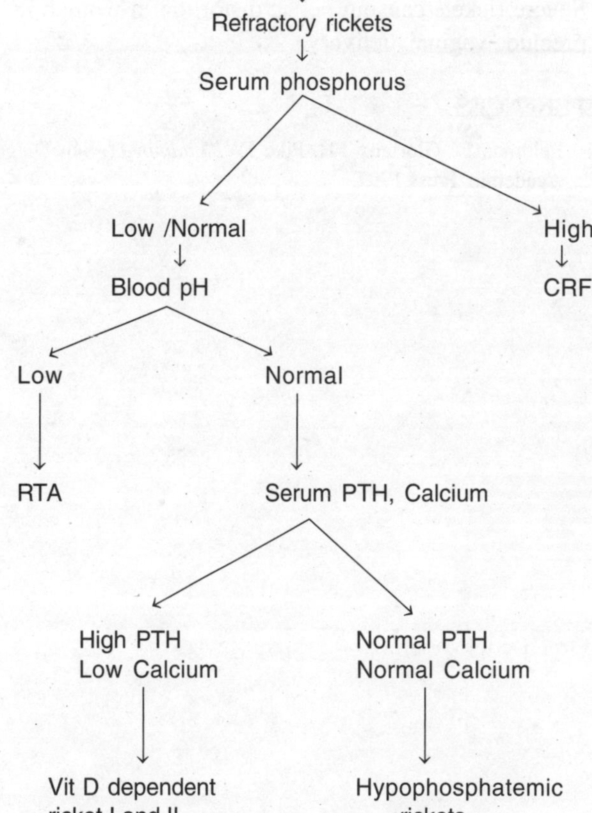

Fig. 22.8: Approach to vitamin D resistant rickets

Treatment

- Oral phosphate supplements
  - Young children—0.5-1 g/day at least 5 times a day.
  - Older children—1-4 g/day.

  Main side-effect is diarrhea.
- Vitamin D:

  It is administered to complete bone healing and prevention of secondary hyperparathyroidism.
  - Dihydrotachysterol—0.02 mg/kg/d; or
  - Calcitriol–50-60 ng/kg/d.

5. Hepatic Rickets

It occurs in children with hepatic disorders especially hepatic. Biliary atresia, neonatal hepatitis and following damage induced by TPN. It is due to decreased vitamin

D absorption because of failure of bile salt secretion.

Treatment

- Vitamin D2-4000-10000 IU/d; or
- Calcitriol–0.2 μg/kg/d along with oral calcium.

6. Oncogenous Rickets

Associated with tumors of mesenchymal origin, due to deficiency of phosphorus. It resolves with removal of tumor.

MORTALITY/MORBIDITY

1. Skeletal deformity and short stature may occur.
2. Severe rickets causing pelvic distortion in women may preclude vaginal delivery.

REFERENCES

1. Feldman D, Glorieux FH, Pike JW. *Vitamin D*. San Diego: Academic Press 1997.
2. Harrison HE, Harrison HC. *Disorders of Calcium and Phosphorus Metabolism in Childhood and Adolescence*. Philadelphia: WB Saunders 1979.
3. Shah BR, Finberg L. Single Day therapy for nutritional vitamin D deficiency rickets: A preferred method. *J Pediatr* 1994;125:487-490.
4. Zmora E, Gorodischer R, Bar-Ziu J. Multiple nutritional deficiencies in infants from a strict vegetarian community. *Am J Dis Child* 1979;133:141.
5. Indian Council of Medical Research. *Nutrient Requirements and Recommended Dietary Allowances For Indians: A Report of the Expert Group of Indian Council of Medical Research*. New Delhi: ICMR 1990.
6. Argo EA, Heubi Je. Fat soluble vitamin deficiency in infants and children. *Current Opin Pediatr* 1993;5:562.
7. Shils ME, Olson JA, Shike M, *et al. Modern Nutrition in Health and Disease*, 9th edn. Baltimore: Williams and Wilkins 1999:305-483.
8. Bowman BA, Russel RM. *Present Knowledge in Nutrition*, 8th edn. Washington: ILSI Press 2001:27-270.

KE Elizabeth

23 Micronutrient Deficiency Disorders (MDDs)

INTRODUCTION

The fascinating sementic, *micronutrient,* has gained popularity in the recent past. The term refers to substances that are needed in small quantities by the body, say vitamins and minerals that are in 'milligrams per day' requirement (usually < 10 micrograms / day), in contrast to the major nutrients which are required in 'grams per day'.[1] They form less than 0.01% of the body weight of a child.[2]

Three of them have been signed out in the World Summit for Children 1990, namely vitamin A, iron and iodine.[3] These are already in limelight, have relevance on a public health scale and have national /global prophylaxis programs associated with them. For example, the vitamin A prophylaxis program for children, the anemia prophylaxis programme for children and mothers and the universal iodization of salt. Recently folic acid, which has gained momentum as periconceptional folic acid, has been found to reduce the incidence of neural tube defects. Micronutrients include vitamins (both water soluble and lipid soluble) and trace elements.

Microminerals or trace elements include iron, cobalt, chromium, copper, iodine, manganese, selenium nickel, fluorine, vanadium, zinc and molybdenum. Currently, some experts have opined that the definition of essential micronutrients be broadened to include some carotenoids and flavonoids, as well as various human metabolites, such as coenzyme Q10, carnitine, and alpha-lipoic acid, which are also dietary constituents.[4]

MICRONUTRIENT MALNUTRITION

Micronutrient malnutrition compromises both survival and quality of survival. According to National Nutrition Monitoring Bureau of India, over 50% of apparently healthy looking children have subclinical or biochemical deficiencies of vitamin A, vitamins B_2, B_6, folate and vitamin C. Over two-third of children have clinical evidences of iron deficiency while deficiency of trace minerals like iodine and zinc is quite common in certain populations. Iron deficiency contributes to 20% of maternal deaths and lowers IQ points in children by 9 points.[5]

Children have food preferences and they are quite reluctant to take green leafy vegetables and fruits, thereby compromising their intake of micronutrients from dietary sources. The full genetic potential of the child for physical growth and mental development may be compromised due to subclinical deficiencies of micronutrients which are commonly referred to as "hidden hunger".

IMPORTANCE OF MICRONUTRIENTS IN HUMAN HEALTH

Micronutrients are cofactors of enzymes, gene activators and scavengers of free radicals. These are considered as "magic bullets" by many clinicians and patients as well. Those items that promote brain growth and function are also referred to as "smart nutrients".[6] Some of micronutrients are powerful antioxidants and they have also found to be important in stress, mood changes, depression and dementia.[7] Micronutrients are required for the integrity and optimal functioning of immune system. Children with subclinical deficiency of micronutrients are more vulnerable to develop frequent and more severe common day-to-day infections, triggering a vicious cycle of undernutrition and recurrent infections.

NEURONAL GROWTH AND DEVELOPMENT OF COGNITION IN CHILDREN AND PREVENTION OF NEUROLOGICAL DISEASE

Undernutrition and deficiencies of iodine, iron, and folate are all important for the development of the brain and the emergent cognitive functions. There is some evidence to suggest that zinc, vitamin B_{12}, and omega-3 polyunsaturated fatty acids may also be important. The term, *supernutrients*, is used to refer to four nutrients which are essential for brain development and function. These include vitamin A, iron, folic acid and omega 3 fatty acids.[8]

Among the B complex factors B_1, B_2, B_3, B_6, B_{11} and B_{12} are essential for the synthesis of various neurotransmitters.[9] Thiamine (B_1) is essential for the functioning of the brain and peripheral nerves. B_1 deficiency decreases the ability to utilize glucose. Deficiency is also associated with insomnia, memory loss, decreased visual acuity, Wernickes encepahalopathy, Korsakoff's psychosis and absent knee jerk. Riboflavin (B_2) deficiency is associated with neuromotor incoordination, personality changes and impaired performance in psychomotor tests. Niacin (B_3) deficiency leads to pellagra with dementia and impaired cognition. Pyridoxine (B_6) is essential for the synthesis of GABA, the inhibitory neurotransmitter and its deficiency may cause convulsions and peripheral neuropathy. Folic acid deficiency is associated with neural tube defects. It is also associated with chronic diarrhea, attention deficit hyperactivity disorder, stroke and autism. Folic acid and choline are also responsible for myelin synthesis. Cobalamine (B_{12}) deficiency is associated with sub acute combined degeneration of the cord.

Vitamin C deficiency is associated with reduced IQ score, altered behavior and increased incidence of stroke. Vitamin E is a potent antioxidant. Its deficiency is associated with transient ischemic attacks (TIAs), stroke, oxygen toxicity and Alzheimer's disease.[10]

Among the minerals, iodine, iron and copper and zinc have been found to have effects on brain and cognition. These are addressed in some detail later in this very chapter as well.

Section 7

MICRONUTRIENTS AND PREVENTION OF CANCER

Adverse dietary factors account for approximately 30% of all cancers. Over consumption of energy is undoubtedly one of the major risk factors, but dietary composition is also very important. In particular, a low consumption of fruits and vegetables appears to double the risk of carcinomas of the lung and alimentary tract. Epidemiological studies suggest that high plasma levels of selenium, carotenoids and ascorbic acid are protective against cancer. However, intervention studies with antioxidant nutrients have given mixed results, and it has not been established that the benefits of a high intake of fruits and vegetables are invariably related to the prevention of oxidative DNA damage. Folic acid supplementation appears to protect against colo-rectal neoplasia, probably by preventing mutations associated with the repair of uracil mis-incorporation. However, there are indications from animal studies that exposure to high levels of folic acid at certain stages of development may lead to epigenetic effects that are, as yet, poorly understood.

All in all, there seems little doubt that micronutrients contribute to the protective effects of plant foods against cancers of the lung and alimentary tract. Nevertheless, it has not been established that these benefits can be achieved using supplements.[11]

MICRONUTRIENTS IN MAINTAINING THE GENOMIC STABILITY

The focus on diet as a key factor in determining genomic stability is more important than previously imagined because we now know that it has an impact on all relevant pathways i.e. exposure to dietary carcinogens, activation/detoxification of carcinogens, DNA repair, DNA synthesis and apoptosis. This is because all of these critical pathways are dependent not only on enzymes but also on the provision of substrate and co-factors some of which are only available at the right concentration when dietary intake of key minerals and vitamins is adequate. Effectively this means that dietary deficiency in key micronutrients required for DNA maintenance may produce similar effects as inherited genetic disorders that impair activity of enzymes required for genomic stability and may damage DNA to similar extents as significant exposure to known carcinogens such as ionizing radiation.[12, 13]

Table 23.1: Micronutrients in genomic stability and deficiency consequences

Micronutrient/s	*Role in genomic stability*	*Consequence of deficiency*
Carotenoids, Vitamin C, Vitamin E	Prevention of oxidation to DNA and lipid oxidation.	Increased base-line level of DNA strand breaks, chromosome breaks and oxidative DNA lesions and lipid peroxide adducts on DNA.
Folate and Vitamin B_{12}	Maintenance methylation of DNA; synthesis of dTMP from dUMP and efficient recycling of folate.	Uracil misincorporation in DNA, increased chromosome breaks and DNA hypomethylation.
Niacin	Required as substrate for poly (ADP-ribose) polymerase (PARP) which is involved in cleavage and rejoining of DNA and telomere length maintenance.	Increased level of unrepaired nicks in DNA, increased chromosome breaks and sensitivity to mutagens.
Zinc	Required as a co-factor for Cu/Zn superoxide dismutase, endonuclease IV, function of p53, Fapy glycosylase and in Zn finger proteins such as PARP.	Increased DNA oxidation, DNA breaks and elevated chromosome damage rate.

INTERACTION OF MICRONUTRIENTS WITH CARDIOVASCULAR SYSTEM

Micronutrients have a host of obvious and subtle interactions with the cardiovascular system.

Iron deficiency anemia can lead to cardiac decompensation (usually with a hemoglobin level < 5 g/dl). Excess iron as seen in hemochromatosis can lead to a dilated cardiomyopathy.

Copper deficiency usually seen in milk-fed premature babies, babies recovering from PEM and LBW babies can result in ECG changes and arrhythmias.

Magnesium deficiency, usually seen in premature babies (80% transferred in the third trimester from the mother), causes ECG changes, say low amplitude QRS, prolonged PR, T wave inversion in precordial leads and occasionally supra-ventricular arrhythmia.

Endomyocardial fibrosis is hypothesized to be due to Magnesium-cerium interaction at the cellular level (the geochemical theory states that in the presence of magnesium deficiency, increased dietary cerium enters and replaces the magnesium in the mitochondria leading to myocyte injury). Excess magnesium can cause heart block. Cobalt in excess can cause dilated cardiomyopathy.

Selenium is an integral portion of glutathione peroxidase and is linked to vitamin E. Its deficiency leads to dilated cardiomyopathy common in certain parts of China endemic DCM (Keshan's disease).

Carnitine is a cofactor in the transfer of long chain fatty acids into mitochondria for energy production and deficiency can cause depletion of intracellular fatty acids. Carnitine deficiency syndrome includes both a systemic and myopathic variety. Both can produce DCM (with a endocardial fibroelastosis picture on muscle biopsy).[14]

Thiamine deficiency of the wet beri beri type typically presents in an infant 1-4 months of age with progressive right heart failure. Shoshin beri beri presents with severe CCF and shock, and can be a cause of sudden cardiac death in infancy.

ANTIOXIDANTS

Antioxidants are agents both endogenous and exogenous which reduce oxidative stress in the tissues. Vegetables, fruits and tea contain micronutrients and antioxidants. The usual antioxidants are vitamin C, vitamin E and beta carotenes.

Vitamin E may reduce CVD risk factors by preventing the oxidation of unsaturated lipids in LDL and preventing events leading to atheromatous plaque formation.

Vitamin C in addition to antioxidant properties has been linked to the maintcnancc of normal BP.

Carotenoids are a group of over 500 yellow, orange and orange-red fat soluble pigments present in vegetables and fruits. That imparts color to them. Beta carotene is most popular among them and is the provitamin A compound. The less understood, lycopene, is now found to be much more abundant in human blood and tissues and a more potent antioxidant than beta carotene. It is rich in red tomatoes, water melon, guava, papaya and pink grapes. It is twice as effective as beta carotene in limiting cell membrane tissue damage by free radicals. Lycopene is said to be protective against CVD.

However, routine administration of antioxidants is not warranted and is not recommended by the American Heart Association (AHA).[15,16] Evidence from animal experiments and human observational studies suggests that some dietary micronutrients may protect against the development of type 1 diabetes. The most promising data so far have been obtained for a beneficial role of vitamin D. Beneficial effects of vitamin E (or other antioxidants) in diabetes development remain hypothetical.[17]

MICRONUTRIENT DEFICIENCY DISORDERS

Iron Deficiency Anemia (IDA)

It is the most common micronutrient deficiency across the globe affecting all ages and all socioeconomic status. Up to 30-60% of pregnant mothers and children have varying grades of anemia.[18] All India level data available from National Family Health Survey (NFHS-2) (1998-99) for children in the age group 6 months to 35 months indicated an overall prevalence of anemia of 74.3%. The prevalence of anemia was generally the highest in the northern and eastern regions and the lowest in the southern region. The anemia level was the highest among children in the age group 12-23 months (77.7%) as compared to children in the age group 6-11 months (71.7%) and 24-35 months (72%). An analysis of community based work published from 1950 to mid 2002 indicated a high prevalence of anemia among infants (80%) and in 1 to 2 year-old children (78%). The prevalence was 74% among 2-3 years old children. The mean hemoglobin level was low (9.0 g/dL) in both infants and children aged upto three years of age, increasing to only 10.0 g/dL by the age of 6 years.[19]

The grading of anemia as per the WHO criteria is given in Table 23.2.[20]

Table 23.2: Hemoglobin levels (g %) indicative of anemia

Subject	*Non anemic*	*Anemic*	*Mild anemic*	*Moderate anemic*	*Severe anemic*
Pregnant women	≥ 11	< 11	> 10-10.9	7-10	< 7
Women	≥ 12	< 12	> 10-11.9	7-10	< 7
Men	≥ 13.5	< 13.5	> 10-13.4	7-10	< 7
New born	≥ 14.5	—	—	—	—
2 mo	≥ 9	—	—	—	—
6 mo-6 yrs	≥ 11	< 11	> 10-10.9	7-10	< 7
>6 yrs	≥ 12	< 12	> 10-11.9	7-10	< 7
Adolescent girls	≥ 12	< 12	> 10-11.9	7-10	< 7
Adolescent boys	≥ 13	< 13	> 10-12.9	7-10	< 7

Anemia during pregnancy and childhood increases the risk of LBW, maternal morbidity and mortality and also child morbidity and mortality. Apart from increasing morbidity and mortality, iron deficiency anemia (IDA) decreases physical stamina, learning ability, concentration and work efficiency. It leads to headache, lack of concentration, impaired auditory and visual evoked potentials.[21, 22]

Cytochrome oxidase in mitochondria is an iron-dependent enzyme and oligodendrocytes require iron for the synthesis of myelin.[23] IDA during the critical period of brain growth may lead to irreversible changes in the brain by decreasing dopaminergic receptors and increasing opiate receptors. This has an adverse effect on learning ability. Iron is also important in maintaining the levels of serotonin and GABA (Fig. 23.1).

In treating anemia, daily iron is required till the anemia gets corrected and the stores get replenished, which may take up to 100 days.[24] But in prophylaxis, weekly iron has revolutionized the situation.[25] The intestinal cells are shed and renewed in 4-5 days. The iron that is taken into the mucosal cell is released into the body only as per the need and the rest gets shed with the mucosal cells. The scope of weekly iron is thus conclusive theoretically. UNICEF has also supported weekly iron in anemia prophylaxis.[26] It is an effective strategy to give weekly iron to adolescent girls, and also boys, to prevent anemia. It is expected to reduce the future prevalence of anemia during pregnancy and improve pregnancy outcome.

The economic consequences of IDA include cognitive delays in children, lower productivity among adults, low birth weight, increased morbidity and mortality among children and mothers. Iron also can correct menstrual irregularities, headache, minor learning problems, lack of concentrations etc. This weekly iron program is in full swing in some states of India like Tamil Nadu and is implemented as a directly observed swallow pill on Saturdays. Saturdays are now being earmarked for adolescent care and counselling clinics.

The habit of drinking fruit juice especially lime juice will enhance iron absorption from a good meal where as coffee and tea will hinder iron absorption. Cooking in iron pots may improve iron bioavailability. The greens, grams and grains (3 Gs) are rich in iron, but the bioavailability is very low compared to heme iron. The newer iron preparations are GI friendly but it is their bioavailability that is questionable. Iron polymaltose complex is ferric iron. The conventional ferrous iron is better absorbed than the ferric iron. Recently carbonyl iron is replacing iron polymaltose in the market. The addition of folic acid with iron is found to improve the outcome.

There are some suggestions that iron supplementation may result in increased risk of infectious morbidity. In a malnourished child with diarrhea and vomiting, iron is often poorly tolerated and may aggravate the GI problem. As long as carrier proteins are not available, unbound iron in the gut may facilitate proliferation of *E coli.* In a well-nourished and stable patient, this risk is less. So iron supplements are advised only after stabilizing the patient and preferably after giving deworming.

Vitamin A Deficiency (VAD)

Vitamin A deficiency is now declining and florid vitamin A deficiency (VAD) leading to blindness is rare. Still, it is prevalent in some backward pockets of the community and among some pregnant mothers who often complain of night blindness. The overall prevalence of VAD in India is upto 6%; in some backward pockets it is upto 12%.[18] Vitamin A Prophylaxis Program was started in 1977 and was integrated with Immunization Program in 1992. It is warranted if the prevalence of VAD is above 0.5%.[27]

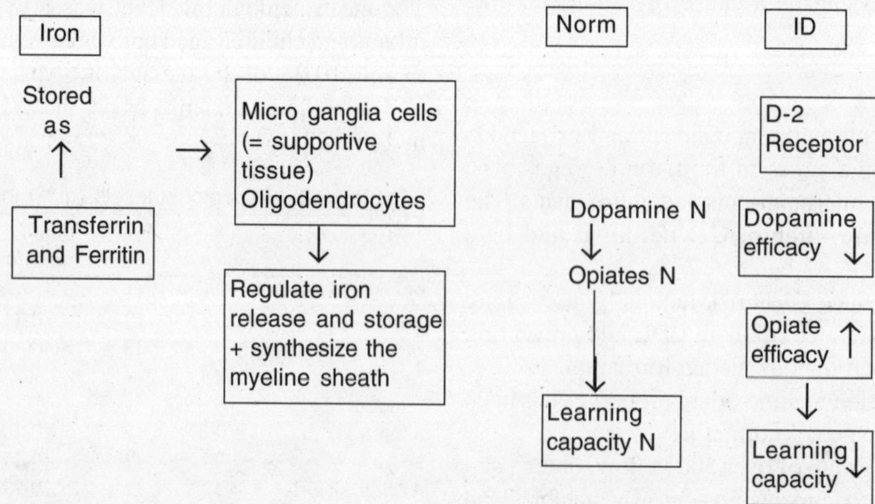

Fig. 23.1: Interaction between iron deficiency anemia (IDA) and learning capacity

Section 7

The indicators for vitamin A deficiency are given in Table 23.3.

Table 23.3. Indicators of clinical and functional vitamin A deficiency that signifies a public health problem

Indicator	*Minimum Prevalence*
Night blindness(24-71 months)	> 1%
Bitot's Spot (6-71 months)	> 0.5%
Corneal scars/ulcer (6-71 months)	> 0.05%
Keratomalacia (6-71 months)	> 0.01%

(*Ref:* WHO. Indicators for assessing vitamin A deficiency and their application in monitoring and evaluating intervention programmes. WHO/NUT/1996.10)

For treatment of VAD, the WHO/UNICEF/IVACG Task force 1998 recommends Vitamin A concentrate 1 lakh units < 1yr and 2 lakh units >1 yr of age × 2 doses on 2 consecutive days and repeat doses at 6 months interval. In severe PEM, apart from the initial 2 doses, monthly doses are recommended till recovery. In GI upset, severe deficiency and impending blindness, injectable Vitamin A (Aquasol A) may be given. But it should be followed up with vitamin A concentrate to ensure storage. Water soluble injections do not serve this function of storage.

Hypervitaminosis A and the side-effects of vitamin A also require mention in this context.[28] The important ones are its teratogenic effect, hyperostosis of tibia, benign intracranial hypertension (BIH), and the so-called *Gulf syndrome*. The Gulf syndrome refers to hypervitaminosis A and D due to excessive intake of the attractive Vitamin A and D fish oil pearls that are brought from Middle-East countries.

Vitamin A maintains the integrity of the skin and the mucus membrane and reduces bacterial binding to the mucosa and protects the surface tracts like GIT and respiratory tract and is also shown to decrease morbidity and mortality due to ADD and ARI. This is highly effective in post-measles cases. Hence one dose of vitamin A is recommended in all measles cases.

IODINE DEFICIENCY DISORDERS (IDDS)

Iodine is a critical vitamin in early nervous system growth. Intrauterine deficiency can cause mental retardation.[29] Goiter, growth retardation and mental sub- normality occur in iodine deficient areas. Iodine deficiency disorder (IDD) is now identified as a major public health problem all over India, including the coastal districts. The prevalence is reported to be around 16% among preadolescent children.[18] Endemic goiter is due to overt deficiency, simple colloid goiter is thought to be due to subclinical deficiency, which is rampant even in coastal districts of Kerala, where it was thought to be not a problem. If the prevalence of goiter is >5%, endemic goiter is suspected and the urinary iodine will be low in these deficient subjects. A reagent treated testing strip or dipstick is being designed to do spot analysis of urine.[3] When urinary iodine is not low in such goitrous areas, goitrogens should be suspected as the cause of goiter. Other causes are cobalt deficiency, selenium deficiency and certain infections like Yersinia.

WHO criteria for assessing severity of IDD based on urinary iodine are given in Table 23.4.

Table 23.4: Epidemiological criteria for assessing severity of IDD based on median urinary iodine levels

Median Value (g/L)	*Severity of IDD*
<20	Severe IDD
20-49	Moderate IDD
50-99	Mild IDD
≥100	No deficiency

Universal Salt Iodization (USI) Program was started in 1984. Upto 30-50 ppm potassium iodate is fortified at the manufacturing level to ensure at least 15 ppm to the beneficiary. Excess iodine can lead to iodism, dermatitis, goiter and rarely thyrotoxicosis. USI Program has had major setbacks due to the disparity in price and quality among the various products available in the market. It is high time that the Government ensures the right quality of iodized salt at the right price. Double fortified salt with iodine and iron is another breakthrough in the research field. This is being tried out in Andhra Pradesh. Benefits of such research should reach the community.

Folic Acid/Folate (Vitamin B_{11})

It is important in cell maturation, especially RBC maturation. Deficiency leads to megaloblastic anemia and concurrent iron and folic acid deficiency leads to dimorphic anemia. Folic acid and B_{12} deficiency may also produce periungual and knuckle pigmentation. The pteroyl polyglutamate available in some vegetables and leaves are less bioavailable than pteroyl monoglutamate (folic acid). It is now known that it is the most critical vitamin during the first 4 weeks of gestation that regulate neurulation and neural tube closure.[30] Deficiency may also lead to nutritional anemia, premature birth and low birthweight. Addition of folic acid to iron in pregnancy has led to significant positive impact. In India the multicentric randomized clinical control ICMR study has shown a reduction of recurrence of open NTD by about 60 per cent with folate supplementation of 4 mg as compared to the placebo group.[31] The dose recommended is 400 mcg/day. It seems to be an ideal wedding gift to a couple who are thinking of the family way. It should also be given to mothers who already had a similar problem in a previous pregnancy. It is also found to be beneficial in megaloblastic anemia following anticonvulsant therapy. Some cases of sub-acute combined degeneration, homocystinuria and stroke syndromes also benefit from folate supplementation.

Other B Complex Factors

Vitamin B_1 (Thiamine) deficiency causes beriberi, which could be dry or wet type. Wet type is usually cardiac and the dry type is neurologic. Infant with beriberi present by one to four months with progressive right heart failure with cardiomegaly; pulmonary artery hypertension (PAH), murmurs and ECG showing low voltage QRS, prolonged QT interval and inverted T waves. The CNS manifestations are peripheral neuropathy, Wernicke's encephalopathy (cerebral beriberi) and Korsakoff Syndrome. Thiamine responsive inborn errors of metabolism include thiamine responsive megaloblastic anemia, which is due to decreased cellular transport of thiamine; thiamine responsive lactic acidosis, which is due to low activity of the pyruvate dehydrogenase complex; thiamine responsive branched–chain ketoaciduria, which is due to low activity of a branched chain α-keto acid dehydrogenase; and a subset of subjects with Leigh's encephalopathy due to abnormality of E1 alpha subunit of pyruvate dehydrogenase.

Vitamin B_2 (riboflavin) deficiency is the most common deficiency in South India, where polished rice is the staple diet. Stomatitis, glossitis and neovascularisation of the cornea are the common manifestations.

Vitamin B_3 (niacin and niacinamide) results in pellagra and is associated with diarrhea, dermatitis and dementia. The neurologic symptoms consist of both an encephalopathy and peripheral neuropathy. Early nonspecific symptoms consist of insomnia, fatigue, anxiety, nervousness, irritability, and depression.

Vitamin B_5 (pantothenic acid) deficiency is associated with burning feet syndrome. The Greek word '*pantos*' means everywhere and it is present in animal and plant sources. It is important in handling stress, in memory and concentration. It leads to conversion of choline to acetylcholine.

Vitamin B_6 (pyridoxine) deficiency and dependency states include peripheral neuropathy, B_6 responsive anemia, B6 dependent convulsions and homocystinuria. B_6 excess also may cause sensory neuropathy.

Vitamin B_{12} (cyanocobalamin) deficiency causes pernicious anemia with spinal cord degeneration. B_{12} and folic acid may benefit some patients with homocystinuria because methyl tetrahydro folate is a substrate and methyl cobalamin is a cofactor in remethylation of homocyseine to methionine.

Biotin deficiency produces hyperesthesia, hallucination and dermatitis. It is synthesized by the microbes in lower GIT.

Inositol supports the cells and nervous system along with other B complex vitamins. Deficiency may lead to high blood cholesterol, constipation, eczema and hair loss. Biotin, choline and niacin have good relaxing effect and niacin is called 'Nature's valium'. Inositol supplementation has been proposed for folate resistant neural tube defects.[32]

Pyrroloquinoline quinone (PQQ) is the first new vitamin to be discovered since 1948, when vitamin B_{12} was found. PQQ was discovered in 1979 from a bacterium, and afterward it was reported to be present in common foods PQQ, which must be supplied by the diet, acts as a cofactor in enzyme-catalyzed reduction-oxidation (redox) reactions, much as nicotinamides and flavins. As a mammalian redox cofactor necessary for the degradation of the amino acid lysine, PQQ qualifies as a member of the B vitamin family. Researchers noted decreased conception and fertility in PQQ-deficient mice, and the babies born to PQQ-deprived mothers grew at slower rates than offspring from mice given supplemental PQQ.

Vitamin C (Ascorbic Acid)

Vitamin C deficiency leads to scurvy, delayed wound healing and so on. It was one of the early prototypes of a deficiency disorder that can be effectively treated by dietary intervention. It converts proline to hydroxy proline which is a constituent of collagen.

Bioflavanoids are water-soluble compounds that help in absorption of vitamin C. Vitamin C is also a powerful antioxidant by virtue of its reducing function.

Vitamin K

Vitamin K deficiency is the cause of hemorrhagic disease of the newborn. It is synthesized by the intestinal flora and deficiency may occur in prolonged use of antibiotics and GI upsets. It participates in oxidative phosphorylation and coagulation.

Vitamin E

Vitamin E is called the "Shady lady of nutrition" as many of its magic properties are still in shade. In 1997, the American Heart Association hailed the discovery of vitamin E as one of the top 10 discoveries of the century.

The vitamin E family is large, consisting of at least 8 closely similar structural forms or isomers that are grouped into two clans–the tocopherols and the tocotrienols. The former have more biological activity as measured by conventional means, but the latter have more antioxidant potency in biological systems. Tocotrienols help in reduction of blood cholesterol, regression of carotid artery plaques in stroke, inhibition and spread of breast cancer and strengthening the bones.

Hemolytic anemia of prematurity is shown to respond to vitamin E. By virtue of its antioxidant properties, it has been proposed that vitamin A supplementation may be beneficial in preterm babies to prevent retinopathy of prematurity (ROP), bronchopulmonary dysplasia and other oxygen toxicity states. However, a recent meta-analysis showed that vitamin E supplementation in preterm infants reduced the risk of intracranial hemorrhage but increased the risk of sepsis. In very low birthweight infants it increased the risk of sepsis, and reduced the risk of severe retinopathy and blindness among those examined. Hence, current evidence does not support the routine use of vitamin E supplementation by intravenous route at high doses, or aiming at serum tocopherol levels greater than 3.5 mg/dl.[33]

Vitamin D

It is essential for bone growth and calcium absorption. It is synthesised in the body from 7-dehydrocholesterol with the help of U-V light. It is hydroxylated to 1-25- di hydroxy chole calciferol in the liver and kidney respectively. Vitamin D deficiency leads to rickets in growing children and osteomalacia in adults. LBW babies especially preterm have rapid catch up growth and there is a chance to develop rickets in the rapidly growing bone as the demand may not match the supply. They are generally overprotected and kept indoors. Lack of exposure to sunlight also may add to the problem. Changes may be visible as early as 2-3 months. If there is associated zinc deficiency, serum alkaline phosphatase may not be raised as in a case of rickets.

Other Microminerals (Trace Elements)

Zinc is a cofactor in various enzymes and in protein and nucleic acid synthesis. Overt zinc deficiency states like acrodermatitis enteropathica are rare. Zinc supplementation trials have shown a role in immunity, growth and prevention of infections. In those with PEM and especially stunting, zinc supplementation has shown improvement in nutritional status especially height gain.[34, 35] This is warranted in those with rapid catch up growth and eroded body stores. Meta-analysis of various studies has shown reduction in diarrhea and pneumonia by about 15-20%, especially in those with PEM.[36] It is helpful in those with PEM, stunting, persistent diarrhea, preterm etc.[34-37] But, there is no need to prescribe it to promote growth and development in normal children. Excess zinc can lead to reduced copper and iron absorption. This property is made use when zinc sulphate is prescribed in Wilson's disease. S. alkaline phosphatase (SAP) is a zinc dependent enzyme, which can easily be measured. Low levels of S. thymulin and SAP are markers of zinc deficiency.

Copper is rightly called the "iron twin". It is involved in cross-linkage of connective tissue, hemopoiesis, neurotransmission, lipid metabolism, iron absorption and oxidative enzymes. Copper deficiency produces refractory hypochromic anemia, neutropenia, hypopigmented hair, osteoporosis, subperiosteal hematoma and soft tissue calcification. The source are cereals, pulses, nuts, fish etc. Excess of copper is associated with Indian childhood cirrhosis (ICC). Inherited copper deficiency in males is encountered in Menke's disease and inherited copper toxicosis in Wilson's disease.

Cobalt is part of vitamin B_{12} and is required for iodine utilization. It increases iron absorption. Its deficiency causes anemia and goiter and excess can cause dilated cardiomyopathy, which is indistinguishable from primary dilated cardiomyopathy. Its excess may also cause goiter.

Selenium is an integral part of glutathione peroxidase, is linked to vitamin E and is an important antioxidant cofactor. Its deficiency leads to dilated cardiomyopathy which used to be common in certain geographical parts of China ("Endemic DCM/ Keshan disease"). It was first described in 1979 and may occur in young children and women. It is a preventable cardiomyopathy, but once DCM sets in, total reversal to normality is not possible even with selenium supplementation. Four forms of Keshan's disease are recognized: an acute variety with shock, a subacute variety with both hypotension and CHF, a chronic variety with CHF and the fourth one, presenting as asymptomatic cardiomegaly. It is virtually indistinguishable from various presentations of primary DCM. Deficiency may also cause liver necrosis, arthritis and myopathy. Its excess may cause dental caries, alopecia and garlic odour in breath.

Chromium deficiency is associated with poor glucose tolerance and neuropathy. It facilitates insulin action. Its excess can lead to dermatitis and renal failure.

Manganese is an enzyme cofactor in superoxide dismutase, oxidative phosphorylation and bone mineralization. Deficiency may produce growth retardation, weight loss, red hair and hypocholesterolemia. Excess may cause cholestasis, encephalopathy, basal ganglia disorder, goiter and cardiomyopathy.

Fluorine is a component of bone and teeth. Upto 1 ppm in drinking water is desirable. Deficiency leads to caries tooth and excess to fluorosis.

Molybdenum is important in uric acid metabolism. Deficiency may lead to tachycardia, irritability, central scotoma and upper GIT cancers. Excess may unmask gout and cause bony defects like genu valgum.

Nickel is a component of urease and nickel plasmin. Excess may produce dermatitis, liver necrosis and lung cancer.

Vanadium deficiency is associated with nutritional oedema.

Silicon is important in cross linkage of collagen and deficiency may produce defective bone growth. Excess may cause fibrosis lung.

Arsenic is important in skin and nail formation.

ROLE OF MATERNAL MICRONUTRIENT SUPPLEMENTATION IN ALTERING PERINATAL OUTCOME

Maternal micronutrient deficiency has been related to adverse fetal effects. It is believed that micronutrient supplementation during pregnancy may improve fetal and neonatal outcome. Despite biological plausibility, the evidence base for individual micronutrient benefit on neonatal morbidity, mortality, growth and development is patchy and often contradictory, except for the role of folic acid in prevention of neural tube defects.[38]

Iron supplementation during pregnancy improves the hematological parameters in the mother. Limited data from developed countries suggest a benefit in terms of fetal or neonatal survival but a Cochrane review could not draw any valid conclusion about beneficial effect of routine iron supplementation in pregnancy.[39,40]

Severe zinc deficiency is associated with fetal loss and neonatal death in experimental animal models. However, marginal zinc deficiency does not seem to be having a significant effect on fetal or neonatal survival. Observational studies on zinc status and pregnancy outcome are confusing mainly because of the lack of a valid indicator of zinc nutriture. The results of the supplementation trials of zinc also do not suggest a beneficial effect on fetal or neonatal survival in the short term. However, preliminary data suggests that antenatal zinc supplements may cause reduction in later diarrheal and infectious morbidity in infants.[41]

Vitamin A deficiency is associated with reduced fetal survival in animal models. This correlation has not been proved in humans.

The effect of other vitamins like thiamin, riboflavin, pyridoxine, cobalamin, ascorbic acid, cholecalciferol or tocopherol on neonatal survival has not been evaluated.[38]

MICRONUTRIENT SUPPLEMENTATION IN THE NEWBORN

Studies have demonstrated micronutrient deficient states in our setting and benefits of supplementation of micronutrients among newborns and children with malnutrition, diarrhea, pneumonia etc. However, as per the current level of knowledge, we do not have a "rule of thumb" to suggest specific micronutrient supplementation. Term babies who are thriving well on exclusive breast-feeding do not need any supplements. Among the LBW babies, there appears to be a differential rational among preterm vs term IUGR babies. Preterms are definite to benefit from supplements as most of the micronutrient transfer occurs in the third trimester. Cord blood levels of micronutrients are reported to show a preferential concentration compared to maternal serum.

A study is ongoing in the Department of Pediatrics, SAT Hospital, Thiruvananthapuram, India, on cord blood micronutrient levels among LBW *vs* normal weight and preterm *vs* term small for gestational age (SGA). The preliminary data has shown that micronutrient levels were the lowest in preterm followed by term SGA babies. In both groups, the levels were lower than term normal babies. This study highlights the importance of judicious supplementation of micronutrients in preterm and term SGA babies, irrespective of maternal nutritional status. Exclusively breastfed babies in the first semester of life do not have significant micronutrient deficiencies, but meeting the demands during and after initiation of complementary feeding is an area of concern.

MICRONUTRIENT DEFICIENCY DURING COMPLEMENTARY FEEDING

Complementary feeding or weaning is now identified as the "weakest link in child nutrition". By 5-6 months of age, when complementary feeding is initiated, breast milk supply reaches the maximum and plateaus off subsequently. Birth weight doubles by 5 months and by that time; the calcium and iron stores get depleted. In our part, where complementary feeding is mostly on to vegetarian items and cow's milk, there is a risk of developing deficiency of calcium, iron, zinc, vitamin A, folic acid, vitamin C, vitamin B_{12} and so on. Nonavailability of heme iron and intake of cow's milk increases iron deficiency. Nonheme iron is only 5% bioavailable as against 35% from heme iron. Reduced bioavailability of calcium due to increased phosphate in cow's milk may add to calcium deficiency. Lack of green, yellow, orange, red (GYOR) vegetables and fruits in the diet leads to MDDs especially vitamin A deficiency (VAD) and lack of citrus fruits lead to vitamin C deficiency. Lack of nonvegetarian items pose the risk of vitamin B_{12} and zinc deficiency.

IMPORTANT INTERACTIONS BETWEEN MICRONUTRIENTS AND THE IMPLICATIONS FOR PREVENTIVE AND THERAPEUTIC PRESCRIPTIONS

The interactions among the various micronutrients are well-known and have important implications. As for example; zinc depletes copper and competes with iron absorption, high phosphorus hinders calcium absorption and may be severe enough to cause hypocalcemic tetany in artificially fed babies, in spite of high content of calcium in cow's milk. There are some useful interactions also, as for example vitamin A and C enhances iron absorption.

INTERACTIONS BETWEEN MICRONUTRIENTS AND DEVELOPMENTAL BIOLOGY

Human development proceeds as a series of complex interdependent, yet distinct and precisely integrated, biological program. Following fertilization, developmental programs are initiated by selective reading of the genetic code leading to the generation of the various cell types, organs and organ systems that constitute mammals. These programs are dependent on the expression of the maternal and fetal genomes and regulated by maternally derived supply of nutrients. In fact, most developmental programmes, including organogenesis, limb formation, and central nervous system (CNS) maturation, requires specific nutrients for their initiation and progression. Nutrients serve as informational molecules that interact with the genome and trigger or facilitate developmental programmes. Micronutrients act as gene activators.

Mammalian development is dependent critically upon the function of the maternal and foetal genomes and the availability of maternally or placentally synthesized small molecules including hormones, cytokines and growth factors. Mammalian development proceeds as a precisely orchestrated temporal program that requires coordinated changes in foetal and maternal gene expression as well as a complete and regulated maternally derived nutrient supply as in the Figure 23.2.

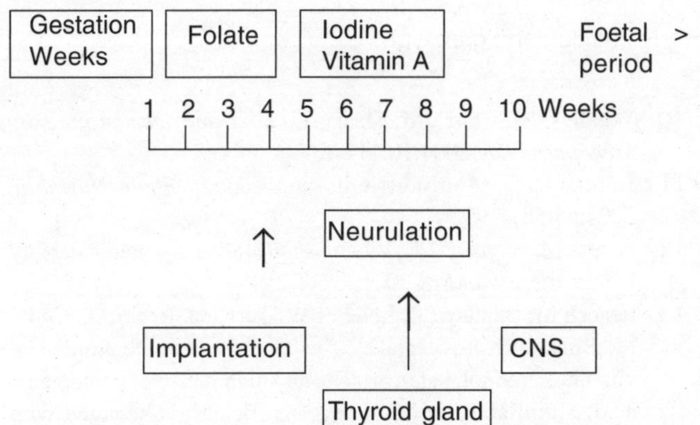

Fig. 23.2: Role of nutrients at a critical time of developmental process—"critical window"

During more advanced stages of fetal development, nutrient deficiencies can impair the progression of morphogenic processes resulting in developmental impairments of varying severity. In many cases, deficiency or excess of particular nutrients at a critical time will impair specific genetically programmed developmental processes. Therefore, the risk of these impairments is associated with specific developmental period or "critical window". Nuclear receptors, otherwise known as ligand activated transcription factors, represent a common mechanism where by individual nutrients specifically can target and influence maternal and fetal gene expression and thereby determine cell lineage in the fetus. With the genetic code now solved, nutrition is the safest and most effective means to modify genome structure and function.

METABOLIC PROGRAMMING

Metabolic programming refers to the process by which an event operating at a critical or sensitive period results in a long-term change in the structure or function of the organism.

Early nutrition affects not only brain development, growth and body composition but also metabolic programming. This influences the occurrence of diet related adult chronic diseases, immunity, coping up with stress, capacity for physical work, cognitive and educational performance.

In the past decade, data from numerous epidemiological studies have indicated strong inverse associations between birthweight and risk of coronary heart disease, hypertension, type 2-diabetes, and other diseases in adulthood. The "Barker hypothesis" thus postulates that a number of organ structures and functions undergo programming during embryonic and fetal life.[42] This developmental programming determines the set points of physiological and metabolic responses in adult life. Alterations of nutrient availability during gestation may lead to developmental adaptations *via* hormonal maneuvers by the embryo and fetus that readjust these set points. These adaptive measures have short-term benefits to the embryo and fetus, so that the newborn will be better prepared for the adverse environment (e.g., undernutrition). However, adequate nutritional support during postnatal life that enables catch-up growth may create metabolic conflicts that predispose the adult to aberrant physiological functions and, ultimately, increased risk of disease. Metabolic programming has been found to continue even into extrauterine life. Early malnutrition in extrauterine life independent of birthweight has an adverse effect on insulin sensitivity, glucose tolerance, and lipid profile in young men.[43]

The role of a variety of micronutrients in the regulation of fetal growth and their potential as programming stimuli has yet to be explored in detail. However, there is already some evidence of their potential importance. The discovery of a variety of polymorphisms for homocysteine metabolism has revealed an association between increased homocysteine levels and not only coronary heart disease but also a variety of complications in pregnancy, including intrauterine growth restriction and pre-eclampsia. Folate supplementation in pregnancy is commonly recommended because it reduces the incidence of birth defects. It appears that at least part of this effect is via effects on homocysteine levels. One role of folate is its involvement in donation of methyl groups in the placenta when serine is converted to glycine with the generation of single carbon methyl groups. These methyl groups in turn can be used for the generation of nucleotides and phospholipids, essential for cell division and cell membranes. Thus folate availability may be critical in fetal and placental growth as well as adult disease risk.

CURRENT RECOMMENDATIONS FOR MICRONUTRIENT NUTRITURE

The methods for micronutrient nutriture are medical supplementation, food fortification and dietary diversification and increased consumption. The former two are expensive and

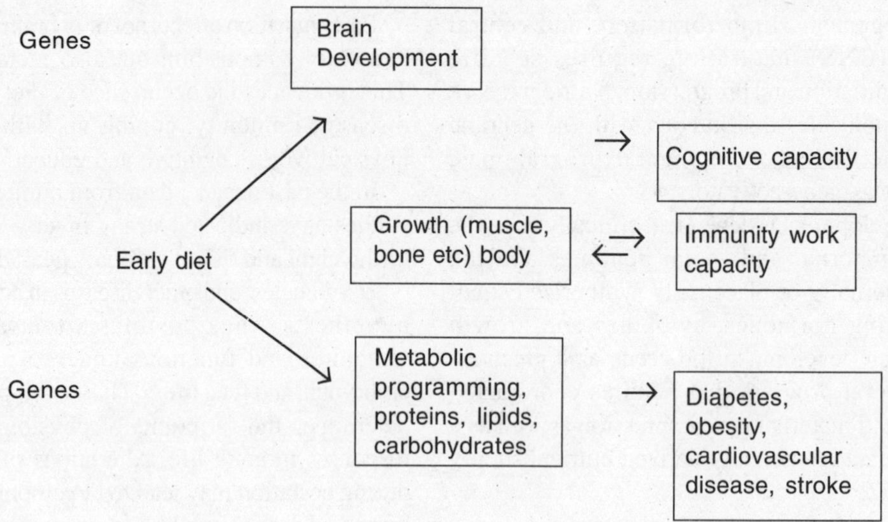

Fig. 23.3: Interaction between early nutrition and genotype

not available to poor and weaker sections of the community. There may also be side-effects and drug interactions. So, the best way to improve micronutrient nutriture and to prevent micronutrient deficiency disorder (MDDs) is food diversification and healthy eating practices. The 'rainbow revolution' should be intensified to improve supply and consumption of micronutrients. Nutrition action plan should be designed and implemented to achieve this goal. Micronutrient fortification strategies like double fortification of salt with iodine and iron also should reach the needy community. Biological products like spirulina, which is a treasure source of micronutrients, should be tapped instead of pills for each micronutrient which may act as 'double edged sword' due to toxicity and drug interaction.

Section 7

REFERENCES

1. Burtis CA, Asherwood ER. *Teitz Textbook of Clinical Chemistry*, 2nd edn. Philadelphia: Saunders 1994:1275-1353.
2. McLaren DS, Burman D. *Textbook of Pediatric Nutrition*, 2nd edn. NewYork: Churchill Livingstone 1982:143-191.
3. UNICEF. *The State of the World's Children*. 1998 New York: UNICEF 1998.
4. Challem JJ.Toward a new definition of essential nutrients: Is it now time for a third 'vitamin' paradigm? *Med Hypotheses*. 1999;52:417-422.
5. Singh M Role of micronutrients for physical growth and mental development. *Indian J Pediatr* 2004;71:59-62.
6. Elizabeth KE. Smart nutrients and brain development. *Indian J Pract Pediatr* 2003; 5:149-154.
7. Glatthaar I. Micronutrients and Stress. *S A J Clin Nutrition* 1998:89 :16-22.
8. Bryan J, Osendarp S, Hughes D, Calvaresi E, Baghurst K, van Klinken JW. Nutrients for cognitive development in school-aged children. *Nutr Rev* 2004;62:295-306.
9. Elizabeth KE. Micronutrients. In: *Nutrition and Child Development*, 3rd edn. Hyderabad: Paras 2005:93-132.
10. Whalley LJ, Starr JM, Deary IJ. *Diet and Dementia. J Br Menopause Soc* 2004;10:113-117.
11. Johnson IT. Micronutrients and cancer. *Proc Nutr Soc* 2004;63:587-595.
12. Fenech M, Ferguson LR. Vitamins/minerals and genomic stability in humans. *Mutat Res* 2001;475(1-2):1-6.
13. Fenech M, Baghurst P, Luderer W, Turner J, Record S, Ceppi M, Bonassi S. Low intake of calcium, folate, nicotinic acid, vitamin E, retinol, beta-carotene and high intake of pantothenic acid, biotin and riboflavin are significantly associated with increased genome instability—results from a dietary intake and micronucleus index survey in South Australia. *Carcinogenesis* 2005;26:991-999.
14. Zulfikar A. *Micronutrients and the CVS: Update on Pediatric Nutrition and Healthy Living*. Thiruvananthapuram: Department of Pediatrics SAT Hospital 2003.
15. Shah D, Garg K and Chowdhary P. Oxidants and antioxidants in pediatric nutrition and disease. Nutrisearch 2001,8:2-8.
16. Berger MM Can oxidative damage be treated nutritionally? *Clin Nutr* 2005 ;24:172-183.
17. Hypponen E. Micronutrients and the risk of type 1 diabetes: Vitamin D, vitamin E, and nicotinamide. *Nutr Rev* 2004;62:340-347.
18. Toteja GS, Singh P, Dhillon BS, Saxena BN. *Micronutrient Deficiency Disorders in 16. Districts of India*. New Delhi: ICMR 2001.
19. Kapil U. Editorial: *Indian Pediatr* 2003; 40:293-295.
20. World Health Organization. *Nutritional Anemia*. Geneva: World Health Organization, 1968.
21. Agarwal KN. Iron and brain: Neurotransmitter receptors and magnetic resonance spectrometry. *Br J Nutr* 2001; 85 Suppl 2:S 147-150.
22. Harahap H, Jahari AB, Husaini MA, Saco-Pollitt C, Pollitt E. Effects of an energy and micronutrient supplement on iron deficiency anaemia, physical activity and motor and mental development in undernourished children in Indonesia. *Eur J Clin Nutr* 2000; 54 Suppl 2: S114-S119.

23. Connor JR, Menzies SL. Relationship of iron to oligodendrocytes and myelination. *Glia* 1996;17:83-93.
24. Dubey AP. Iron deficiency anemia. *Nutrisearch* 2002; 9:1-3.
25. Kapur D. *Iron Supplementation: A strategy for Prevention and Control of Anemia. Technical Consultation for Strategies for Prevention and Control of Iron Deficiency Anemia.* New Delhi: Human Nutrition Unit, AIIMS 2002.
26. Seshadri S. Nutritional anemia in South Asia. In: Gillespie S (eds): *Malnutrition in South Asia.* Kathmandu: UNICEF/ ROSA 1997;75-125.
27. WHO. *Indicators for Assessing Vitamin A Deficiency and their Application in Monitoring and Evaluating Intervention Programs.* Geneva:WHO 1996.
28. Gopalan C. The vitamin A fiasco. *Nutrisearch* 2001;8:1-2.
29. Bernal J. Iodine and brain development. *Biofactors* 1999;10:271-276.
30. Butterworth CE, Bendich A. Folic acid and the prevention of birth defects. *Ann Rev Nutr* 1996;16:73-97.
31. ICMR. Central Technical Co-ordinating Unit, ICMRCentral Technical Coordinating Unit, ICMR. Multicentric study of efficacy of periconceptional folic acid containing vitamin supplementation in prevention of open neural tube defects from India. *Indian J Med Res* 2000;112:206-211.
32. Greene ND, Copp AJ. Inositol prevents folate-resistant neural tube defects in the mouse. *Nat Med* 1997;3:60-66.
33. Brion LP, Bell EF, Raghuveer TS. Vitamin E supplementation for prevention of morbidity and mortality in preterm infants. *Cochrane Database Syst Rev*.2003;4:CD003665.
34. Elizabeth KE, Sreedevi P, Narayanan NS. Outcome of nutritional rehabilitation with and without zinc supplementation. *Indian Pediatr* 2000;37:650-655.
35. Sachdev HPS. Zinc deficiency. *Nutrisearch* 2001;8:1-6.
36. Bhutta ZA, Black RE, Brown KH, Gardner JM, Gore S, Hidayat A, *et al.* Prevention of diarrhea and pneumonia by zinc supplementation in children in developing countries: Pooled analysis of randomized controlled trials. *J Pediatr* 1999;135:689-697.
37. Elizabeth KE. Status of micronutrients in malnutrition before and after rehabilitation. *Indian Pediatr* 2000;37:912-913.
38. Dheeraj H, Sachdev H PS. Maternal micronutrients and fetal outcome: Symposium on micronutrient deficiency disorders. *Indian J Pediatr* 2004;71:985-990.
39. Mahomed K. Iron supplementation in pregnancy (Cochrane Review). The Cochrane Library, Issue 3, 2003;CD000117. Oxford: Update Software.
40. Preziosi P, Prual A, Galan P, Daouda H, Boureima H, Hercberg S. Effect of iron supplementation on the iron status of pregnant women: Consequences for newborns. *Am J Clin Nutr* 1997; 66: 1178-1182.
41. Shah D, Sachdev HPS. Effect of gestational zinc deficiency on pregnancy outcomes: Summary of observation studies and zinc supplementation trials. *Br J Nutr* 2001;85(Suppl 2):S101-S108.
42. Lau C, Rogers JM Embryonic and fetal programming of physiological disorders in adulthood. *Birth Defects Res C Embryo Today* 2004;72:300-312.
43. Smith A, Anderson EA. Early malnutrition and its consequences. *Nutr Update* 2004;7: 314-319.

Praveen C Sobti • Shivani Kansal

24 Iron Deficiency Anemia

INTRODUCTION

Iron is one of the most important nutrients required throughout life by an individual. Whereas the strength of iron and steel industry determines the economic status of a country, the iron content of the human body makes a significant difference between health and disease for individuals.

ROLE IN HUMAN BODY

Iron in the human body is present as:

Essential Iron

Heme iron
Cytochromes
Iron requiring enzymes.

Storage Iron

Ferritin
Hemosiderin.

Essential Iron (Functional Iron)

It is the iron involved in the normal metabolism of human body and is divided into 3 groups

Heme Iron

Heme proteins—hemoglobin, myoglobin, catalases, peroxidases

Hemoglobin and myoglobin are the most abundant essential iron compounds in the human body. These consist of an iron–porphyrin prosthetic group attached to the protein globin.

Catalase is a heme containing enzyme found in blood, bone marrow, mucus membranes, bones and kidney. It comprises four heme groups. It destroys hydrogen peroxide formed in the tissues.

Peroxidases are found in milk, erythrocytes, leucocytes and lens fibres. It contains protoheme as the prosthetic group and weighs 44,100 for example-glutathione peroxidase reacts with reduced glutathione and catalyses the destruction of hydrogen peroxide.

$$H_2O_2 + 2\,GSH \xrightarrow[\text{(se-containing)}]{\text{Glythione peroxidase}} H_2O + \underset{\text{(Oxidised glutathione)}}{G\text{-}S\text{-}S\text{-}S}$$

Cytochromes

These are pigment containing molecules having ferrous ions as a component.

Iron Requiring Enzymes

a. Iron requiring enzymes which use riboflavin as coenzyme.
   For example—xanthine oxidase, cytochrome c-reductase, acyl coA dehydrogenase, NADH reductase.
b. Enzymes which require iron as co-factor such as succinate dehydrogenase, aconitase, ribonucleotide reductase.
c. Ferrous ion (Fe^{2T}) are also required for the conversion of superoxide radical to free hydroxyl radical. This is called Haber's reaction.

Storage Iron: Discussed Subsequently

Thus, it is evident that iron has wide and varied functions in the human body, therefore the deficiency of this micronutrient is associated with great morbidity.[1]

SOURCES OF IRON

Exogenous

Animal sources: Meat, Fish, Liver, Spleen, shellfish. Provide 2-6 mg/100 g. of iron. Milk especially cow's milk has a low iron content. Human breast milk provides 0.7 mg/l of iron.

Vegetable sources: Cereals provide 2-8 mg/100 g. Legumes, molasses, nuts, amaranth leaves and dates are other rich sources of iron.

Considerable amount of iron may be added to the diet by cooking in iron utensils.

Endogenous

Iron can also be utilized from ferritin of reticuloendothelial system, intestinal epithelial cells and also from old and effect RBCs.

Table 24.1: Sources of iron

Exogenous sources	*Endogenous sources*
Meat, fish, liver, shell fish, milk Cereals, legumes, molasses, nuts, dates	Ferritin, intestinal epithelial cells, RBCs

FATE OF INGESTED IRON

Ingested iron is of two types–Hem iron and non-hem iron. Hem iron is that which is derived from meat and other animal sources while non hem iron is the one that is derived from vegetable sources. The absorption of non-hem iron is significantly influenced by the presence of other substances in diet as phytates, phosphates and ascorbic acid while that of hem iron is independent of the presence of these substances.[1]

Iron is absorbed only in the ionic state and that too primarily in the ferrous form. Ferric ions are soluble at low pH but tend to polymerize and become unavailable for absorption as the pH in the duodenum rises.[1] Ferrous ions do not undergo such marked polymerization and moreover they are more soluble at any given pH as compared to ferric irons—hence have a higher bio-availability.[2] Hem iron released from the food in the stomach enters the intestinal epithelial cells unchanged. Polymerization of hem is prevented by the presence of other protein degradation products in the lumen of duodenum and jejunum. These also help to maintain its availability to the mucosal cells.[2]

The absorption of non-hem iron is limited by phytates and phosphates through the formation of insoluble complexes. This can however be overcome by an increased level of either iron or calcium in the diet. Ascorbic acid increases iron absorption by reducing ferric ions to ferrous ions and also by forming soluble iron ascorbate chelates. Fructose also forms iron chelates which remain soluble at an alkaline pH.

In patients with pica, clay eating causes the formation of insoluble complexes as also injection of tetracyclines with iron salts. Tannin in tea is also an inhibitor of iron absorption.[2]

Absorption of iron is most efficient in the duodenum and proximal jejunum. Non-hem iron attaches to surface glycoprotein receptors on the brush border of the mucosal cells.[1]

The mechanism determining the amount of iron to be transported to the plasma is located in the epithelial cells. These are exquisitely sensitive to the iron requirements of the body even in healthy and non-anemic subjects. When iron stores are decreased in the body or when there is severe iron deficiency, the iron absorption from intestinal lumen is increased. In states of iron overload this is however, decreased.[2]

The absorbed iron is rapidly transported across the cell into the portal circulation for distribution to the iron stores. The remaining iron in the mucosal cells binds with apoferritin to form ferritin. The ferritin containing cells are subsequently exfoliated at the end of their lifespan of 2-3 days and the iron excreted in the feces.[1]

Though the absorption of hem iron is not influenced by the simultaneous administration of phytates, desferrioxamine, EDTA or ascorbic acid but it is less rapid as compared to non-hem iron. It has been observed in experimental models that when hemoglobin and ferrous iron are administered simultaneously then hem iron absorption is decreased. This lag may result from the evidence of a hem splitting mechanism in the epithelial cells possibly involving xanthine oxidase and hem oxygenase found in a number of tissues.[2]

IRON STORES

Iron stores at the time of birth depend upon the blood volume and hemoglobin concentration. The blood volume depends upon the weight and the time in which the cord is clamped. Delay in cord clamping for 3 minutes results in a 58% increase in red cell volume.[3]

The absolute amount of iron has been found to vary from 50 mg in infants weighing 1 kg to 372 mg in infants weighing more than 4 kg. Most of the iron stores are built in the third trimester of pregnancy. Pre-term infants are therefore born with low iron stores. The iron stores are of the greatest importance as has been demonstrated by studies of Smith *et al.*[3] They showed that, at 1 year, 70 percent of hemoglobin iron and, at 2 years, 40 percent of hemoglobin iron is of maternal origin.[3]

With the growth of the baby the iron stores also increase. Each kilogram gain in weight involves an increase of 35 to 45 mg of body iron. During the first year especially the second half of first year 200 mg of iron needs to be absorbed to maintain the storage iron in the average infant. From the age of 2 years to puberty, the growth rate is approx at the rate of 2.5 kg/yr leading to an iron requirement of 100 mg/yr or 0.3 mg/day. At puberty there is an increase of 30 kg weight over 7 years in boys and a little less in girls. Thus the iron requirement increases to 170 mg/yr or 0.5 mg/day. In girls an additional 0.6 mg/day is required to compensate the menstrual loss.

Forms of Storage Iron

- Ferritin.
- Hemosiderin.

In a normal individual iron stores are equally divided between the reticuloendothelial cells (spleen, liver and bone marrow), hepatic parenchymal cells skeletal muscles and bone marrow.

Ferritin predominates in the hepatocytes while hemosiderin is the major form in the reticuloendochelial cells. In states of iron overload hemosiderin increases to a greater extent than ferritin. Iron represents 23 per cent of the dry weight of the ferritin molecule and about 25-40 per cent of dry weight of hemosiderin molecule. It is believed that as the ferritin molecule ages, there is a partial denaturation of apoferritin and a corresponding increase in the iron content, with hemosiderin being gradually formed.

ETIOLOGY OF IRON DEFICIENCY ANEMIA (IDA)

Iron deficiency is the most common cause of anemia in the tropics. It has been estimated that more than 50 per cent of children of all ages and 92 per cent of children below the age of two years suffer from iron deficiency anemia. There is an even higher incidence if estimated from serum iron.[4]

Causes of iron deficiency are:

- Lack of dietary intake.
- Increased demands of a growing body.
- Increased losses.

Lack of Dietary Intake

Human breast milk efficiently caters to the iron needs of a growing term neonate and infant till 4-6 months of life. Thereafter the depletion of maternal iron stores coupled with increasing requirements of a growing body account for increased iron demands. This demand, if not fulfilled through on adequate diet rich in iron, leads to iron deficiency anemia. Too much reliance on milk (any form) and inadequate solid diet accounts for most cases of iron deficiency anemia in the first 2 years of life.

IDA between 2 to 14 years is linked to dietary patterns. Most children are fussy eaters. Over reliance on junk food and less consumption of fresh fruits and vegetables is largely responsible for a high incidence of anemia. Strictly vegetarian diet may also lead to low iron stores especially if the non-hem iron is being consumed with foods containing large amounts of phytates and phosphates as in wheat, rice and tannins of tea.

Increased Demands

The first 14 years of life are those of rapid growth and development. Thus, there is a concomitant increase in the requirement of dietary iron. This, if not taken care of, leads to IDA. Failure to meet these demands could be due to ignorance in the parents regarding the needs of the growing child, poverty leading to inadequate diet, frequent infections or a combination of these.

Increase Losses

Hookworm infection is a widely prevalent infection in children. Children in most Indian villages are seen playing bare which provides an easy passage to the hookworm larvae. Chronic infestation leads to acute blood loss which over a long period of time becomes significant enough to cause iron deficiency.

Bilharzial polyposis is also a cause of acute blood loss although not so common in India.

Intestinal malabsorption leading to poor absorption of iron can also lead to iron deficiency. The establishment of an iron deficiency state may further lead to the loss of a significant amount of iron from the gastrointestinal tract owing to villous atrophy and cause or aggravate intestinal malabsorption leading to a further depletion of iron. This cycle may progress to such a state of morbidity that it cannot be easily interrupted by replacement of nutrients alone. The damaging effects of iron deficiency on the gastrointestinal treat may be mediated through decreased activity of the various iron containing enzymes such as aconitase succinic dehydrogenase, cytochrome and cytochrome oxidase.

Sequence of Changes in Iron Deficiency Anemia

Whenever the condition of iron deficiency arises the body stores of iron start getting mobilized. The stores in the bone marrow followed by hemosiderin in the liver are the first to get depleted. Following this there is a decrease in the serum ferritin level to less than 10 ng/ml. This is accompanied with an increase in total iron binding capacity and in free erythrocyte porphyrin levels. This subsequently manifests as microcytic hypochromic anemia.[5]

Decreased supply iron
↓
Depletion of body stores
Bone marrow iron
Hemosiderin in liver
↓
↓ Serum ferritin
↓ Transferrin saturation
↓
↑ TIBC (total iron binding capacity)
↑ FEP (free erythrocyte porphyrin)
↓
MCHC anemia
(Microcytic hypochromic anemia)

Fig. 35.1: Sequence of events in development of IDA

CLINICAL FEATURES

IDA has a wide spectrum of clinical features from being absolutely asymptomatic to florid symptoms and signs, including cognitive deficits. In mild to moderate deficiency (Hb 8-10 g/dl), most patients have few symptoms owing to compensatory mechanisms like—2,3-DPG and shift of oxygen dissociation curve to right.[6]

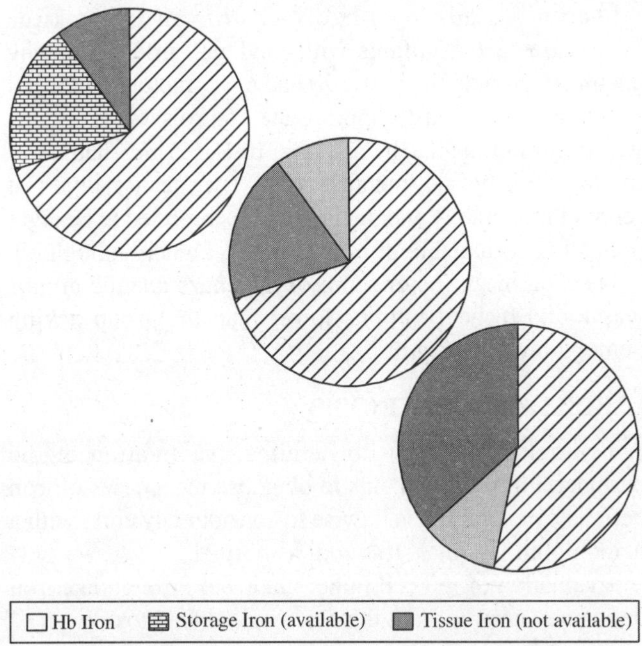

Fig. 24.2: Stages in development of iron deficiency anemia[1]

Normal Values

World Health Organization Scientific Group[4] (1968) has defined anemia according to age groups as per Table 24.2.

Table 24.2: Anemia cutoff point in terms of hemoglobin value as per WHO[4]

	Hb (g/dl) (less than)
Children aged 6 months–6 years	11
Children aged 6 years–14 years	12
Adult males	13
Adult non-pregnant females	12
Adult pregnant females	11

Pallor is the most common symptom; the others being easy fatiguability and failure to thrive.

Koilonychia and platynychia (flattening of nails) is common in the tropics and when present is almost diagnostic of iron deficiency. Evaluation of nail changes in 845 subjects in a village survey showed that in 100 subjects with hemoglobin less than 10 g/dL, 8 had koilonychia while another 17 had definite flattening of the nails. 10 subjects of the remaining 745 whose hemoglobin was more than 10 g/100 ml had koilonychia while another 41 had flattening of the nails making a total incidence of 9 per cent.[4] Koilonychia, in its severest form is characterized by the flattening and even concavity of the nail plate instead of the normal convexity. The distal part of the nail becomes thin and brittle. It is most common in patients with a long duration of anemia but it has also been observed in patients who are sideropenic but not anemic.[7] This should be distinguished from congenital koilonychia especially in young children. Congenital koilonychia is characterized by equal severity of koilonychia in finger and toe nails and presents shortly after birth.

Glossitis, a painful red tongue with flattening and atrophy of the lingual papillae, is also observed in iron deficiency anemia. Histologically, moderate atrophy is seen as loss of filiform papillae and decreased number of prickle cells while a severely affected tongue is characterized by a marked thinning of the epithelium and absence of papillae in the substantia propria.

It cannot be distinguished either histologically or clinically from glossitis due to pernicious anemia.

Angular stomatitis, cracking and fissuring at the angle of the mouth, has also been reported, but is less specific than koilonychias in IDA.

Riboflavin and pyridoxine deficiency can both produce oral lesions similar to those seen in IDA. Jacobs and Cavill[7] in a study of 25 patients having these features however showed that all had a normal red cell total riboflavin content. A reduction of red cell pyridoxine activity was also observed in these patients but a consistent improvement in oral symptoms was not observed after supplementation with these vitamins alone. Black pigmentation of the tongue often accompanies glossitis and disappears with iron supplementation.[4]

Some workers have described a painless parotid swelling also as a feature of iron deficiency anemia but it is now believed to be a part of a multiple nutritional deficiency state.

IDA may cause in young or middle aged adults, especially females, the so-called Patterson Kelly syndrome or Plummer Vinson syndrome. It is secondary to obstruction caused by a web of tissue passing back from the cricoid. It rapidly responds to treatment with iron supplements although without a significant radiological improvement.

Chronic iron deficiency may also be accompanied with all degrees of gastric mucosal change from superficial gastritis to complete gastric atrophy. The spleen becomes palpable in 10 per cent patients with IDA.

Breath holding attacks and pica have both been described in iron deficiency anemia but a cause and effect relationship has not been established as yet in either case.

IRON AND INFECTION (NUTRITIONAL IMMUNITY)

Most living organisms have developed efficient mechanisms for the transport and storage of iron as it has an important role in redox reactions and oxygen transport. In human beings, transferrin and lactoferrin are the major transport proteins and ferritin is the important proteins and ferritin is the important non-functional storage form. At the time of an infectious insult to the human body, various inflammatory mediators are released, one of which is interleukin-1

(IL-1). This IL-1 enhances the production of acute phase reactant proteins like fibrinogen, ferritin, cerruloplasmin, haptoglobin and amyloid-A protein. Increased ferritin synthesis blocks release of iron causing a reduction in circulating iron levels. This 'hypoferremia' is one of the most constant features of infection and has been suggested by some to be an important defense mechanism. The term 'nutritional immunity' was coined by Kochan [9] in 1973 to describe this mechanism of iron deprivation as an immunity against growth of invading organisms. Studies on microbial cultures have shown that while iron supplements enhance the growth of some microbial like *E. coli* and *Vibrio cholrae*, iron deprivation may also enhance the virulence of some organisms like *Corynebacterium diphtheria*, *Clostridium tetani* and *Shigella.* Hence, the use of iron supplements in management of diphtheria in the early 19th century.

Both iron deficiency and iron overload have been found to have adverse effect on the human immune system. Iron deficient neutrophils have been found to have a reduced bactericidal activity due to respiratory burst suppression, while lymphocytes have been seen to have reduced proliferative response to mitogens despite maintaining a normal activation and effector function. Antibody mediated immunity in iron deficient individuals appears normal. Neutrophils of patients with transfusional overload on the other hand have been found to have severe impairment of phagocytosis and myeloperoxidase activity inversely correlated with serum ferritin concentrations. This could be reversed with desferrioxamine treatment.[8]

Section 7

IRON DEFICIENCY AND COGNITION

One of the most devastating long-term consequences of iron deficiency is on behavior and cognition.[10]

Iron deficiency is most prevalent in children in the age range of 6-24 months. which is also the age of brain growth spurt. Several studies done all over the world over the last decade have demonstrated this relationship. Dr. Walter *et al.* performed a study in association with a field trial in the city of Santiago. Infants from a community clinic in the city of Santiago were included in the study at 3 months of age and followed till 12 months of age. Anthropometeric, nutritional, morbidity and socioeconomic data were collected. Full hematological assessment of blood samples obtained by venepuncture was performed at the ages of 9 months and 12 months. At 12 months of age the first Bayley Scale for Infant Development was applied 7-10 days after the first clinic visit. Iron sulphate or a placebo was then given for 10 days and then the second Bayley Scale for Infant Development was applied. All infants were given iron sulphate drops for an additional 3 months after which the third Bayley scale for infant development was applied. It became clear after this study that a decrease in hemoglobin leading to overt anemia was necessary to affect mental and psychomotor development scores.

Another study by Lozoff *et al.*[12] in Costa Rica demonstrated that infants with moderate iron deficiency anemia (Hemoglobin < 10 g/dl) had lower motor and mental scores as compared to appropriate controls while infants with only mild anemia (hemoglobin 10.1-10.5 g/dl) had lower motor scores but not mental scores. The mean mental test score of moderately anemic infants was reported to be eight points lower than that of infants with a higher hemoglobin value. The mean motor score of the entire anemic groups was found to be 10 points lower than the group having hemoglobin > 10.5 g/dl.[11]

LABORATORY DIAGNOSIS

A hemoglobin level with detailed examination of the peripheral blood film helps to diagnose most cases of iron deficiency anemia. It is unwise to consider any child with a hemoglobin less than 10.5 g/dl as normal.

Evaluation of red cell indices helps to differentiate iron deficiency anemia from thalassemia and lead toxicity.

Table 24.3: Differential diagnosis of iron deficiency anemia[1]

Disease	*Ferritin*	*S. Iron*	*TIBC*	*Saturation*
Iron deficiency anemia	Decreased	Decreased	Increased	Decreased
Anemia of chronic disease	Normal/ increased	Decreased	Normal/ decreased	Decreased
Thalassemia	Normal	Normal	Normal	Normal
Sideroblastic anemia	Normal/ increased	Normal/ increased	Normal	Normal/ increased

Peripheral Blood Film

It can be particularly useful while evaluating a case of anemia. The best place to search for properly spread erythrocytes is several millimetres inside the feathered edge of the smear.[13] The characteristic changes in the blood film are time related and a function of the severity of the anemia. The morphological changes of hypochromia and microcytosis do not appear until the hemoglobin is less than 12 g/dl. The red cell count may be near normal but the cells have anisocytosis and poikilocytosis besides being hypochromic. The degree of hypochromia varies from a slight increase in central pallor to an extremely large area of central pallor surrounded by a small rim of hemoglobin. A large number of cells will be microcytic while a small number may be macrocytic and polychromatic. Reticulocyte count may also be increased from 2 to 5 per cent especially after hemorrhage. Target cells and pencil cells are not uncommon.[1] Target cells are caused by alterations in erythrocyte surface area which in dried smears results in an outward bulge of excess membrane into the region of central pallor, creating the characteristics target appearance.[13]

Red Cell Indices in Iron Deficiency Anemia

Hb	↓
Hct	↓
MCH	↓
MCHC	↓
MCV	↓
RBC Count	↓
RDW	↑

Biochemical Findings

- **Serum iron:** It is decreased to values less than 300 μg/dl.
- **Total iron binding capacity:** It is increased, occasionally to levels more than 350 mg/dl.
- Transferrin saturation is often less than 15 per cent.
- Serum ferritin is less than 12 μg/dl in uncomplicated cases. A level in the normal range, however, does not rule out iron deficiency. In patients having chronic infection or malignancy, serum ferritin less than 50 μg/ml may be associated with iron deficiency.[1]

Free Erythrocyte Protoporphyrin

If iron is not available in sufficient quantity protoporphyrin is not converted into heme. So free erythrocyte protoporphyrin level is increased to values between 100-600 mg/dl (normal 20-40 mg/dl). This helps to diagnose iron deficiency before the development of overt hypochromic anemia.[1] Ratio of free erythrocyte protoporphyrin to hemoglobin also helps in diagnosis. Values more than 2.8 indicate iron deficiency. In thalassemia minor, free erythrocyte protoporphyrin is not increased.

Bone Marrow

Marrow examination is seldom necessary for diagnosis. There is erythroid hyperplasia with an increase in the mature forms. Polychromatic normloblasts are the predominant cells however these may be smaller than normal. Erythropoiesis is thus described as being micronormoblastic. Granulopoietic cells and megakaryocytes are normal in numbers and morphology. Potassium ferrocyanide staining (Prussian Blue reaction) of the trephine biopsy indicates a diminished reticuloendothelial iron and sideroblasts.[1] This test is especially helpful in differentiating true iron deficiency from iron deficient erythropoiesis from inflammatory anemias where stainable reticuloendothelial iron is adequate and also from other hypochromic anemias and sideroblastic states not due to iron deficiency.

Unutilized stainable marrow iron may however be found in true iron deficiency anemia when a large dose of iron dextran has been injected.[14]

Other Tests

- Radioactive iron absorption is increased early in states of iron depletion and is a sensitive index of iron deficiency but is not of generally appreciable usefulness.[14]
- Examination of feces for occult blood.
- Urine routine to rule out hematuria.
- Stool routine for worm infestation.
- Fecal fat estimation, stool pH for malabsorption.

Table 24.4: Various parameters in different stages of iron deficiency

	Depleted iron without anemia	*Iron deficiency*	*Iron deficiency anemia*
↓ S. ferritin	—	—	→
↓ Trasnsferrin saturation		—	→
↑ Erythrocyte protoporphyrin			
↓ Hemoglobin —	→		
↓ MCH			
↓ MCV			→
Microcytic hypochaomic PBF			→

TREATMENT

The aim is to identify the underlying cause, remove it and correct the present deficiency.

Treat Underlying Cause

- Worm infestation—deworm the patient.
- Stool for occult blood positive, rule out cow's milk protein intolerance.
- Dietary counselling and supplementation if poor intake—Discussed subsequently.

Iron Therapy

The only indication of iron therapy is the presence of a demonstrable iron deficiency state. Prophylactic iron therapy is indicated in prematurely born neonates, twins and small for gestation age neonates.[14]

Oral Therapy

Various iron preparations are commercially available. Ferrous salts are better absorbed than ferric. The various preparations differ in their content of elemental iron. Consumption of iron preparation with meals decreases the absorption but also the incidence of adverse effects. The absorption of iron is increased in deficiency states and it starts decreasing as the deficiency state improves.

Some of the commercially available salts of iron are listed in Table 24.5.

Dose

3-6 mg/kg/day elemental iron start with lower dose first and then gradually build it upto avoid unpleasant

Table 24.5: Salient details of commercially available iron salts

Salt	*Elemental iron*	*Commercial name*
Iron hydroxide polymaltose	50 mg/5 ml	Syp Ferich
Iron hydroxide polymaltose	50 mg/5 ml	Syp Ferose
Iron hydroxide polymaltose	50 mg/5 ml	Syp Ferrium
Iron hydroxide polymaltose	50 mg/5 ml	Syp Iris
Ferrous fumarate	33 mg/5 ml	Vitcofol
Ferrous calcium citrate	25 mg/5 ml	Racicap
Ferrous ammonium citrate	60 mg/5 ml	Ferrochelate
Ferrous gluconate	15 mg/5 ml	RB tone
Ferrous sulphate	80 mg/5ml	Tonoferon
Ferrous sulphate	55 mg/5ml	Fesovit
Drops		
Iron hydroxide polymaltose	50 mg/ml	Feritin
Iron hydroxide polymaltose	50 mg/ml	Ferich
Iron hydroxide polymaltose	50 mg/ml	Ferrium
Ferric ammonium citrate	20 mg/ml	Ferrochelate

gastrointestinal side-effects. Phytates, and tannins in food decrease absorption.

With this hemoglobin rises at the rate of 0.15 g/dl/day.

Duration

It is continued till 6-8 months after normal hemoglobin levels are reached.[5]

Table 24.6: Response to iron therapy[15]

12-24 hrs	Replacement of intracellular iron subjective improvement as decreased irritability and improvement in appetite
36-48 hrs	Initial bone marrow responses erythroid hyperplasia
48-72 hrs	Increased reticulocytes peak in 5 to 7 days
4-30 days	Increase in hemoglobin
1-3 months	Repletion of stores

Section 7

Adverse Effects

Iron salts are astringent, hence may produce unpleasant gastrointestinal side-effects as gastritis, heart burn, nausea, diarrhoea and constipation. These may become a cause of poor compliance in some patients. These are avoided by starting iron supplements at a lower dose, administration of the drug with meals and also by starting with a preparation having lower elemental iron. No significant difference in the incidence of adverse affects has been observed between the various iron salts.

Failure of Oral Therapy

- **Poor compliance:** Unacceptably high side-effects leading to poor compliance. Psychological factors as a cause of poor compliance are less frequent in children.
- **Malabsorption:** Chronic or persistent diarrhoea can lead to malabsorption.
- Continuing blood loss either as occult blood loss due to hookworm infestation or cow's milk protein intolerance can lead to failure of therapy.

Parenteral Iron Therapy

Indications

- Genuine intolerance of oral preparations or inability on part of the patient to understand and follow the instructions properly.
- Malabsorption syndromes chronic or persistent diarrhoea a primary gut disorder affecting iron absorption e.g. ulcerative colitis.
- Continued bleeding with which oral iron cannot keep pace e.g. hereditary haemorrhagic telangiectasia, menorrhagia in adolescent girls.
- Patient is unable to maintain iron balance on treatment e.g. hemodialysis.
- Patient is donating large amounts of blood for auto transfusion programmes.

Preparations and Administration[1]

1. Iron-dextran complex (Imferon) IM/IV is available as 50 mg per ml of solution.
2. Iron sorbitol–citric acid complex is also available under the trade name Jectofer.

Iron-Dextran Complex

It is combination of ferric hydroxide with dextran. After an intravenous injection it is cleared in a half life period of 2 to 3 days. It requires two to three weeks for complete clearance from the circulation. Initially there is a rapid delivery of iron from the reticuloendothelial cells to transferrin but it quickly decreases accompanied with a parallel increased in serum iron. The serum iron returns to normal or even deficient levels in two weeks. The rise in serum iron is reflected by a stimulated erythropoiesis in the bone marrow which may initially increase to 6 to 7 times the normal but falls to twice normal by the fifth or seventh week.[14]

Iron dextran administered by the i.m. route is taken up by the lymphatics. Twenty five per cent of the injected dose can be detected at the infection site after three weeks.

Dose: It is calculated based on the amount needed to correct hemoglobin and also replenish the stores.[1]

Iron to be injected in miligrams is

$$\text{Wt (kg)} \times (14.5 - \text{Hb. Conc.}) \times 80/100 \times 3.4 \times 1.5$$

$$\downarrow$$

$$\text{wt. (kg)C (Hb deficit) C 4.1}$$

1 g of hemoglobin contains 3.4 mg of iron. If hemoglobin deficit is 'x' then the amount of iron required to raise the hemoglobin to the desired amount is 3.4x. Blood volume is 80 per cent of body weight is 80/100 wt.

Hence to raise the hemoglobin to normal level in the whole body, amount of iron required is

3.4 × 80/100 wt.

Where '×' is hemoglobin deficit. Half of the amount calculated from this formula is given extra to replenish the stores.

Method of Administration

After testing the drug for hypersenstivity 2 ml of the iron dextran complex is injected. Intravenously undiluted at the rate of 1 ml/min.

Total Dose Infusion (TGI)

Entire calculated dose is given as an infusion after dilution in saline or 5% dextrose. 5 ml of iron dextran complex is diluted in 100 ml of the diluent (NS/Dextrose). Initial flow rate is set at 20 drops per minute for five minutes. Thereafter if no side-effects are observed the drop rate is increased to 40-60 drops per minute. Temperature, pulse rate and blood pressure are recorded every half hour initially and every one hour subsequently.

Adverse Effects

Local pain at injection site, discoloration of skin and tender regional lymphadenopathy lasting a few weeks. A faster rate of administration than recommended can cause pain at the injection site, flushing and metallic taste. This improves by slowing the rate of infusion.

Systemic

Immediate Hypotension, malaise, urticaria, nausea and anaphylactoid reactions. Delayed lymphadenopathy, myalgia, fever and arthralgia.

Most reactions are mild and transient except for the anaphylactoid reaction which may be life threatening.

Intramuscular Route

It is given as a deep intramuscular injection in the upper and outer quadrant of the buttock. The skin should be displaced laterally and a Z-track should be followed to prevent staining of skin; 0.5 ml dose should be given first to check for hypersensitivity; after one hour the full dose may be given.

Iron Sorbitol Citric Acid Complex (Jectofer)

This is given only as an intramuscular injection. It is an inhomogenous injection comprising molecules weighing between 3000 to 4000 units. The small molecular size enables rapid diffusion from the injection site. It can also be excreted in saliva. Nearly 40 percent of the dose may be lost in the first 24 hours–due to urinary excretion.

Blood Transfusion

This is indicated only in severe iron deficiency anemia with severe morbidity.

In chronic anemia the rate of transfusion should be low around 8-10 drops per minute, and may be given in smaller aliquots of 10 ml/kg.

In cases of congestive cardiac failure or impending failure, partial exchange should be done.[5]

PREVENTION OF IDA

It is a widely acknowledged fact that IDA is one of the most widely prevalent nutritional disorders. More than forty per cent children in developing countries suffer from this malady in various forms. Children in the age group of 6 to 24 months are most vulnerable to the effects of iron deficiency anemia as this is also the age of maximum brain growth. It has been demonstrated unequivocally by numerous studies that nutritional deficiency in this period of life can cause serious cognitive, behavioral and motor disability.[10] Thus it would not be irrelevant to talk of prophylaxis of iron deficiency anemia with iron supplements.

Iron stores accumulated at the time of birth are all utilized by the age of six months. Breast milk iron though having a high co-efficient of absorption cannot fulfil the needs of a growing infant beyond six months. Weaning foods in most developing countries are usually cereal or root based and hence low in available iron. This accentuates the risk of iron deficiency anemia.

Beyond twelve months of age the child increasingly partakes the family food, the diversification of diet increases. So, the risk of iron deficiency anemia is marginally less. Providing iron supplements between six and twelve months would ensure protection for the first twelve months of life and if the supplements are continued till fifteen months of life enough iron stores would accumulate to ensure protection for two years of life.

Fortification of Food with Iron

One of the methods of preventing iron deficiency anemia is to fortify routine foodstuffs with iron salts such that they take care of eighty to ninety per cent of the iron needs of the child. For successful fortification the foodstuff chosen must be routinely consumed by all the members of the community for example salt, sugar and bread. Fortification should not produce any undesirable alteration in the colour, taste, storability, cost and texture of the food. Ferrous sulphate is the most commonly used fortificant. Bakery products and wheat flour have been fortified to varying levels with iron for several decades now in several countries. This accounts for nearly forty per cent of the dietary intake in Sweeden, twenty per cent in the United States of America and ten per cent in the United Kingdom. The iron added is in two forms viz ferrous sulphate and elemental iron. Ferrous sulphate is satisfactory as a fortificant to bread and bakery products but produces organoleptic problems in stored wheat flour. Elemental iron is used for fortification in the United States while ferric pyrophosphate and ferric orthophosphate are used in Europe.

Among developing countries, several African and South American countries require that iron be added to the flour but there are several logistic problems in this. These include lack of a central processing unit for most vehicles and a predominantly cereal based diet of most populations. Three strategies have been tried to overcome these problems. The first involves the use of a stable form of iron like iron orthophosphate together with an enhancer of iron absorption like ascorbic acid. Salt tolerates this combination moderately well but better results have been obtained from a combination of iron orthophosphate and sodium hydrogen sulphate. The colour, taste, storage properties and bioavailability were all reported to be good moreover it proved efficacious in a multicenter clinical trial.

The second strategy is to use an iron salt for fortification which is not affected by the presence of inhibitors in the diet. Sodium iron EDTA complex is one such salt which has a bioavailability 1.05 to 2.8 times that of ferrous sulphate when consumed between meals. It has been used as a fortificant in fish sauce, sugar and masala in three separate studies all of which demonstrated an improvement in iron nutrition. There has been some concern about the safety of EDTA but the Food and Drug Administration has concluded that it is a safe drug on the basis of long-term studies in rodents. The third strategy involves the use of bovine hemoglobin to overcome the problem of dietary inhibitors. Hemoglobin iron is well absorbed because it is not released from the porphyrin ring prior to uptake by mucosal cells and is therefore not affected by dietary inhibitors which reduce the absorption of non heme iron. While concerns regarding sterility of hemoglobin during collection and storage could lead to problems in gaining approval, its potential as a fortificant merits further investigation.

Problems in Fortification

The food to be fortified must be widely and regularly consumed by the community, and there should be a central processing policy of that food item. In India common salt is already being fortified with iodine. Addition of iron phosphate and acid sodium phosphate to iron fortified salt is not compatible. It can however be fortified with sodium iron EDTA, the only disadvantage being yellow discoloration of salt which may not be acceptable to traditional Indian households. Another problem with widespread use of iron fortified food items in India is the high prevalance of beta thalassemia. This condition is as such associated with a high iron absorption rate which is eight to ten times the normal, the consumption of iron fortified foodstuffs would aggravate the iron overload in these children.

Iron Supplements

The UNICEF/WHO Joint Committee on Health Policy 1995 endorsed a strategy for reduction of iron deficiency anemia. The strategy called for implementing a preventive iron supplement program for all infants and young children in regions where the prevelance of iron deficiency anemia is 30 per cent or more. Epidemiologic data show that in virtually all developing countries, more than forty per cent of infants and young children have iron deficiency anemia. The administration of an aqueous solution of ferrous sulphate or a ferric complex such as iron polymaltose could prove to be one of the most practical iron supplements for children between 6 and 24 months of age. A single, safe dose that is effective for all children under two years of age and that can be easily dispensed with by illiterate mothers is required.

Therapeutic dose in iron deficiency anemia is 4-6 mg/kg/day of elemental iron. In a prophylactic program, 1-2 mg/kg/day would be appropriate. A daily 12.5 mg dose of an oral supplement would meet eighty to ninety per cent of the recommended daily intake for a 12-month-old and an 18-month-old, respectively.

The supplement can be given as drops or syrup. One teaspoonful of syrup would be 5 ml and one drop would be 0.05 ml. A more concentrated solution of iron administered as drops would prove most economical due to the high cost of packaging and transport. As the risk of iron deficiency anemia is greatest between 6 and 24 months of age it would be worthwhile to start iron supplements by 6 months of age and continue the same till at least 15 months of age.

REFERENCES

1. Harrison KE. Iron deficiency: Changing concepts and concerns. *Nutr Update* 2001;4:68-73.
2. Jacobs A. The mechanism of iron absorption. *Cl Hematology* 1973: 2; 323-337.
3. Burman D. Iron deficiency in infants and children.*Cl Hematology* 1973:2;257-268.
4. Cowan B, Bharucha C. Iron deficiency in the tropics. *Cl Hematology* 1973:2;353-363.
5. Chandra J, Gupte S. Pediatric Hematology. In: Gupte S (ed) *The Short Textbook of Pediatrics*, 10th edn. New Delhi: Jaypee 2004:455-486.
6. Shendurnikar N, Shukla O, Madan S. Nutritional anemias in infancy and childhood. In: Parthasarthy A, Menon PSN, Nair MKC (eds): *IAP Textbook of Pediatrics*, 2nd edn. New Delhi: Jaypee 2002:500-504.
7. Chisholm M. Tissue changes associated with iron deficiency. *Cl Hematology* 1973:2;303-321.

8. Hershko C. Iron and infection. In: *Nutritional Anemias* (Nestle Nutrition Workshop Series 30). Vevey: Nestle 1992:53-59.
9. Kochan I. The role of iron in bacterial infections with special consideration of host tubercle bacillus interaction. *Ccrr Top Microbial Immunol*1973:60;1-30.
10. Walter T. Early and long-term effect of iron deficiency anemia on child development. In:*Nutritional Anemias (Nestle Nutrition Workshop Series 30)*.Vevey: Nestle1992:81-92.
11. Walter T, de Andraca, Chadud P, et al. Adverse effect of iron deficiency anemia on infant psychomotor development. *Pediatrics* 1989:84;7-17.
12. Lozoff B, Brittenham GM, Wolf AW, *et al.* Iron deficiency anemia and iron therapy effects on infant development test performance. *Pediatrics* 1987:79;981-995.
13. Walters MC, Abelson HT. Interpretation of the complete blood count. *Pediatr Clin North Am* 1996: 43;599-621.
14. Dagg JH, Goldberg A. Detection and treatment of iron deficiency. *Cl Hematol* 1973:2;365-380.
15. Gladder B. Anemias of inadequate production. In: Behrman RE, Kleigman RM, Jenson HB (eds) *Nelson Textbook of Pediatrics,* 17th edn. Philadelphia: Saunders 2004:1606-1617.

Umesh Kapil • Preeti Singh

25 Iodine Deficiency and Its Health Consequences

INTRODUCTION

Endemic goiter in India is an age-old problem. There are references to it in ancient Hindu scriptures dating back to 2000 BC. Iodine is one of the essential elements required for normal human growth and development. Its daily per capita requirement is 150 micrograms. Iodine is also required for the synthesis of the thyroid hormones, thyroxine (T_4) and triiodothyronine (T_3). T_4 and T_3, which are iodinated molecules of the essential amino acid tyrosine, regulate cellular oxidation and, hence, affect calorigenesis, thermoregulation, and intermediary metabolism. These hormones are necessary for protein synthesis, and they promote nitrogen retention, glycogenolysis, intestinal absorption of glucose and galactose, lipolysis, and uptake of glucose by adipocytes.

Synthesis and secretion of T_4 and T_3 are under the control of the thyroid-stimulating hormone (TSH) which is secreted from the anterior lobe of the pituitary gland. TSH stimulates iodide transport from the blood into thyroid cells, oxidation of iodide to iodine, and iodine binding to tyrosine. Synthesis of thyroid hormones is regulated by the levels of circulating free T_4 and T_3 as a negative feedback mechanism.[1]

ETIOLOGY OF IODINE DEFICIENCY

Unlike nutrients such as iron, calcium or the vitamins, iodine does not occur naturally in specific foods. Rather, it is present in the soil and is ingested through foods grown on that soil. Iodine is present in the superficial layers of the soil and absorbed by crops grown on it. Glaciations, heavy snow and heavy rain leach away iodine from the soil. This problem is further accelerated by deforestation and soil erosion.[2,3] Consumption of crops and plants grown on iodine deficient soils leads to iodine deficiency in populations solely dependent on this vegetation for their iodine requirements.[3]

High incidence of IDD has been documented from population residing in Himalayas, Andes, and Alps.[4] Ocean water contains adequate amounts of iodine. Only people eating a specific species of sea fish and sea products like *'kelp'* are more likely to be iodine sufficient, but these are not accessible to everyone. Moreover, eating seafood does not ensure adequate dietary iodine sufficiency.

Iodine deficiency in population residing at sea coast have been documented from pockets of Azores, Bangkok, Manila, Goa, Bombay, Kerala, Andaman and Nicobar Islands. New areas, which were relatively free of this problem, are now being identified as iodine deficient possibly because of intensive agricultural technologies and multiple cropping.[2] Presence of certain substances which adversely influence the utilization of iodine in staple foods is also recognized as a major etiological factor for IDD. These factors are called "goitrogens". They are generally present as thioglucosides or glucosinolates; the glucan portion of which is responsible for its goitrogenicity. Other chemical substances such as thiocyanates, thio-oxazazolidone, flavanoids, disulphides, phenols, phthalates, biphenyls and lithium, found in environment are also included in goitrogens category. These goitrogens are known to interfere with iodine metabolism at various stages or levels. Some of these substances are found in abundance in certain tubers and vegetables like tapioca, cabbage and cauliflower. Even common food items like sorghum, finger millets, mustard and groundnuts are known to contain fair amount of goitrogens.

MAGNITUDE OF IDD IN INDIA

IDD constitute a major nutrition deficiency disorder in India. Out of 587 districts in the country, 282 districts have been surveyed for IDD and 241 districts have been found to be endemic i.e. Total goiter rate of 10% and more in the population.[5] These districts are present in all the states and union territories of country (Table 25.1).

IODINE AND HEALTH CONSEQUENCES

Iodine deficiency has been called the world's major cause of preventable mental retardation. The healthy human body contains 15-20 mg of iodine, of which about 70-80% is

Table 25.1: Prevalence of iodine deficiency disorders and status of national iodine deficiency disorders program in different states/UTs of India

State	*Total No of Districts*	*No of District Surveyed*	*No of District Endemic*	*Ban Notification Issued*	*IDD Cell*
Andhra Pradesh	23	10	9	Partial*	Yes
Arunachal Pradesh	10	10	10	Complete	Yes
Assam	23	18	18	Complete	Yes
Bihar	55	22	21	Complete	Yes
Goa	2	2	2	Complete	Yes
Gujarat	25	16	8	Complete	Yes
Haryana	19	9	8	Complete	Yes
Himachal Pradesh	12	10	10	Complete	No
Jammu and Kashmir	15	14	11	Complete	No
Karnataka	27	17	6	Complete	Yes
Kerala	20	14	11	No ban	Yes
Madhya Pradesh	61	16	16	Complete	Yes
Maharashtra	35	29	21	Partial*	Yes
Mizoram	8	4	4	Complete	Yes
Manipur	9	8	8	Complete	Yes
Meghalaya	7	2	2	Complete	Yes
Nagaland	8	7	7	Complete	Yes
Orissa	30	4	4	Complete	Yes
Punjab	17	3	3	Complete	Yes
Rajasthan	31	3	3	Complete	Yes
Sikkim	4	4	4	Complete	Yes
Tamil Nadu	29	12	12	Complete	Yes
Tripura	4	3	3	Complete	Yes
Uttar Pradesh	83	34	29	Complete	Yes
West Bengal	18	5	5	Complete	Yes
Andaman and Nicobar Islands	2	2	2	Complete	Yes
Chandigarh	1	1	1	Complete	Yes
Dadra and Nagar Haveli	1	1	1	Complete	Yes
Delhi	1	-	1	Complete	Yes
Daman and Diu	1	1	1	Complete	Yes
Lakshadweep	1	-	-	Complete	Yes
Pondicherry	4	-	-	Complete	Yes
Total No. of districts	*587*	*282*	*241*		

present in the thyroid gland. The thyroid gland which weighs only 15 to 20 g possesses a remarkable concentrating power for iodine. In a day, 60 mg of circulating iodine needs to be trapped by the thyroid for adequate supply of T_3 and T_4. To extract this amount of iodine from the circulation, the thyroid daily clears several hundred litres of plasma of its iodine. This work can increase further by several times in severely iodine deficient environments. To cope up with this increased workload the thyroid enlarges in size, under the influence of Thyroid Stimulating Hormone (TSH), secreted from the pituitary gland. This compensatory mechanism triggered by the hypothalamus to increased TSH secretion from the pituitary causes remarkable enlargement of the thyroid gland (goitre).[6,7] Iodine deficiency affects all the stages of human development: fetus, neonate, child and adult. If a pregnant woman is starved of iodine, the fetus does not get adequate iodine and hence cannot produce enough thyroxin. This leads to fetal growth retardation. Hypothyroid fetuses often perish in the womb, and many infants die within a week of birth. Hypothyroid children are intellectually subnormal and have impaired school performance due to lowered IQ points. They are often incapable of completing school. In areas with prevalence of mild to moderate iodine deficiency , the school children are, on an average, 10 points of IQ below those of children living in areas where there is no iodine deficiency.[8] Children may also suffer from physical impairment. The spectrum of disorders caused due to iodine deficiency is presented in Table 25.2. The relationship between iodine intake and IDD is depicted in Table 25.3.

A linear relationship exists between the iodine content of domestic animal milk and the prevalence of goitre. The level of iodine in animal milk in goitrous regions has been found to be lower (20.6 mcg/L) than in non-goitrous regions (83.5 ug/L).[9]

i. *Maternal Thyroid Deficiency and Low IQ in the Offspring : Recent data.*

Table 25.2: The spectrum of iodine deficiency disorders

Stage in Life	*Health Effects*
Fetus	Abortions Stillbirths Congenital Anomalies Increased Perinatal Mortality Increased Infant Mortality Neurological Cretinism: • Mental deficiency • Deaf-mutism • Spastic diplegia • Squint Myxedematous cretinism: • Mental deficiency • Dwarfism
Psychomotor Defects	
Neonate	Neonatal goiter Neonatal hypothyroidism
Child and Adolescent	Goiter Juvenile hypothyroidism Impaired mental function Retarded physical development Adult Goiter with complications Hypothyroidism Impaired mental function

Table 25.3: Relationship between iodine intake and IDD

Nutritional Status	*Daily Iodine Intake (μg)*
Associated with cretinism	20 or less
Associated with goiter	20 - 50
Marginal	50 - 100
Normal	100 - 300
More than normal	300 and above

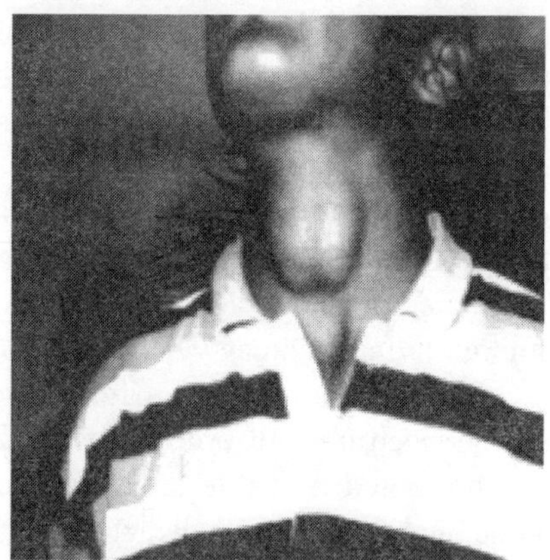

Fig. 25.1: An adolescent with Grade II goiter

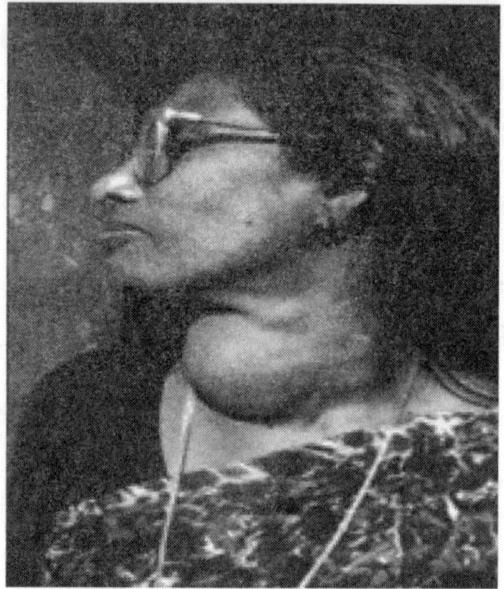

Fig. 25.2: A young lady with large goiter

It is known that thyroid deficiency in mothers during the second and third trimesters of pregnancy and the first month after delivery leads to development of mental retardation and other neurological deficits in the newborn. Whether thyroid hormones are needed by the foetus during the first trimester is less certain. If needed, they must be supplied by the mother, because the foetus does not secrete any until the fourteenth week of gestation.

A recent study was conducted in USA to determine whether inadequately treated or undetected thyroid deficiency during pregnancy is associated with lower IQ scores in the offspring even in the absence of congenital hypothyroidism. Serum samples of 25216 pregnant women were collected and were screened for their thyroid status. A total of 62 pregnant women with thyroid deficiency were selected based on the serum thyrotrophin and thyroxine levels. One hundred and twenty-four matched women with normal serum thyrotrophin and thyroxine values were taken as controls. When these children were 7-9 years old, their neuropsychomotor development was tested using 15 tests relating to intelligence, attention, language, reading ability, school performance and visual-motor performance. The performance of these children was lower in all the 15 tests. The study concluded that untreated hypothyroidism in mothers causes a reduction in the IQ of their children.[10]

ii. *Iodine and Brain Development*

In humans, the critical period for maximal brain growth and maturation comprises the last six months of gestation and the first year of life.[11] Iodine is required for the synthesis of thyroid hormones, which exert action through binding of triiodothyronine (T_3) to nuclear receptors. These nuclear receptors regulate the expression of specific sites in different brain regions following a precise developmental schedule.[12,13] Biochemical data indicates that thyroid hormones also have an effect on RNA polymerase II in assembling messenger RNA, influence t-RNA sulfurtransferase, which confers the release of polypeptide chains from ribosomes and play an important role in the timing, rate and quantity of brain cell proliferation.[11,14] Thus, the growth and differentiation of the Central Nervous System (CNS) is closely related to iodine and thyroid hormones and impairment of cerebral functions in the foetus is directly related to maternal thyroxinemia.[15]

Iodine deficiency during the foetal period leads to impairment of mitosis and differentiation of neural cells of the foetus. The insult involves impairment in the development of dendritic spines, their density and distribution along the apical shafts of deep pyramidal neurons of the most superficial layers of cerebral cortex.[16,17] This effect leads to a deficit in the general synaptology along apical shafts especially in the visual and auditory areas.[18] Iodine induced hypothyroidism during the foetal period also leads to a decrease in the proportion and density of radial glial cells fibres (one of the structures developing early in human pregnancy) of the hippocampal-formation of the brain.[19,20]

Extensive experimental studies have been done in rat to demonstrate effect of severe iodine deficiency on the brain of neonates. Postnatal morphogenesis of the nervous system in rats thyroidectomized at birth showed a decrease in axodendritic connections primarily in the neuropil, small size and abnormally densely packed perikarya and reduced number of axons and dendrites in the interperikaryonal space.[21] Similar studies on neonatal hypothyroid rats have shown:

- Alterations in shape and reduced brain weight.
- Decreased size and increased density of cortical neurons.
- Simplification of neuronal dendrites.
- Decreased numbers of cortical axons.
- Delayed disappearance of cerebral external granular layer.

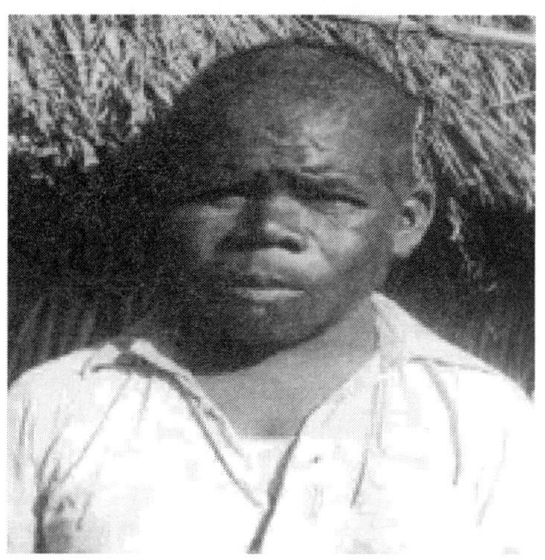

Fig. 25.3: An adult cretin

- Increased concentration of DNA with lowered RNA per unit DNA and.
- A reduction in myelin lipids with a lowered cerebral enzyme activities. These changes lead to a decreased rate of protein synthesis, reduced cell proliferation of the developing cerebrum and cerebellum, increased density of brain cells in cerebellum, delayed disappearance of external granular layer and reduced incorporation of ^{3}H leucine.[22,23]

iii. *Iodine deficiency and Intelligent Quotient*

A meta-analysis of 19 studies has demonstrated that, on an average, children living in iodine deficient areas have an intelligence quotient (IQ) 13.5 points lower than children living in iodine sufficient areas.[24] Similar results have been reported by other workers.[25]

iv. *Iodine and Cognitive Development*

It has been documented that unchecked iodine deficiency is likely to have widespread effects on cognitive performance and development due to the broad impact of hypothyroidism on neuronal development, structure, and function. The effect of iodine deficiency and hypothyroidism on cognitive development in children has been assessed in both cross sectional and randomized, controlled supplementation trials.

A meta-analysis of 18 studies completed by Bleichrodt and Born indicated a general loss of 13.5 IQ points, with an effect size of 0.90, in chronically iodine deficient populations compared with non-iodine-deficient groups.[24] Cross-sectional studies demonstrate that iodine deficiency has a negative effect on the cognitive performance of children, and that the symptoms of iodine deficiency can be alleviated by iodine supplementation. Some studies indicate that children with goiter perform significantly less well on tests of non-verbal reasoning ability[25-27] and other studies find no different between the groups on measures of general intelligence. Urinary iodine status has been found to be positively related to cognitive performance in a number of studies.[28,29]

RECOMMENDED DIETARY ALLOWANCES OF IODINE

Iodine requirements have been calculated based on:

a. Average daily loss of iodine in the urine which is 100-200 mcg/day; and
b. Balance studies to attain a positive balance which is 44-162 mcg/day.[30]

Based on scientific studies of iodine balance over a 24-hour period, a safe daily intake of iodine has been estimated to be between a minimum of 50 mcg and a maximum of 1000 mcg.[31] A generally accepted desirable adult intake is 100-300 mcg/day.

The average salt intake among adults is about 10 g/day, and at the current level of fortification of salt with 15 ppm of iodine at the consumer level, the iodised salt provides an additional amount of 150 mcg/day. Of which about 30% is lost during cooking. The remaining 105 mcg is ingested and from this about 70% is absorbed by the body. This means approximately only 73.5 mcg is absorbed per day from iodine fortified salt. The remaining requirement of iodine is met from the dietary sources. Thus, the total intake of iodine from iodised salt is much below the safe limit and therefore the iodised salt is unlikely to cause any harmful effects even in populations who are not iodine deficient. Also, it has been documented that at all intake levels, a proportionate amount of iodine is excreted in the urine, and hence minimum risk of toxicity.

NATIONAL IODINE DEFICIENCY DISORDERS CONTROL PROGRAM (NIDDCP)

Following the successful trial of iodized salt in the Kangra Valley, Himachal Pradesh, a National Iodine Deficiency Disorders Control Program (NIDDCP) was launched by the Government of India in 1962.[5] The objectives of the programme were: (i) Initial surveys to assess the magnitude of the iodine deficiency disorders (ii) Supply of iodised salt in place of common salt, and (iii) Resurveys to assess the impact of iodised salt after every 5 years.

Beneficiaries

All people residing in endemic and non-endemic areas for IDD. The population in known endemic area are given priority.

Activities and services provided under the NIDDCP:

The following activities are conducted under the NIDDCP:

i. Production and distribution of iodised salt.
ii. Notification for banning use of non-iodised salt.
iii. Establishment of goiter cell.

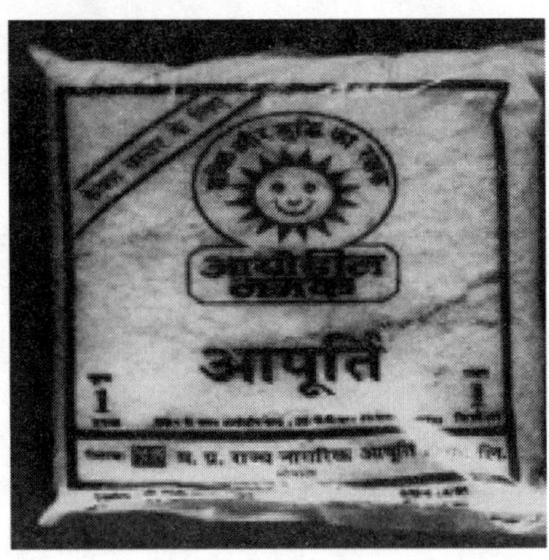

Fig. 25.4

iv. Information education and communication activities.
v. Intersectoral co-ordination.
vi. Laboratory support:
vii. Training under NIDDCP programs.
viii Evaluation.

Iodine content of Salt under NIDDCP at Beneficiary Level: Keeping in view of the mean daily intake of common salt of 10 g by the population in different parts of the country, it is mandatory under NIDDCP that a minimum of 15 ppm of iodine should be present in per gram of edible salt at the beneficiary level to ensure at least 150 µg of dietary intake of iodine per day through the salt.

Iodine Content of Salt under NIDDCP at Manufacturer Level: There is considerable loss of iodine during transportation and storage. Hence, under NIDDCP it is mandatory that a minimum of 30 ppm should be present in per gram of edible salt at the manufacturer's level.

The Impact of Salt Iodisation in India

Surveys have been conducted by the Central IDD Survey Team of Directorate General of Health Services, Government of India to monitor the progress of NIDDCP. The repeat surveys conducted under NIDDCP have shown a significant reduction in the total goiter prevalence after the supply of iodised salt.[32] A survey conducted in the National Capital Territory of Delhi in 1980 revealed a high prevalence of goiter (55.2%).[33] In 1989, the Universal Salt Iodisation programme was introduced in the state. A repeat survey conducted in 1996 revealed that the total goiter prevalence was reduced to 8.6%.[34] A more recent survey conducted in 2002 revealed a further reduction of TGR to 6.2% indicating the success of USI.[35]

Similarly, repeat surveys conducted by ICMR after a gap of 12 years in districts surveyed earlier revealed a significant reduction in total goiter prevalence in all the age groups (Table 25.4).[36] Studies conducted in selected districts of Uttar Pradesh have also revealed the lowering of incidence of neonatal hypothyoidism after introduction of iodised salt (Table 25.5).[37]

Table 25.4: ICMR repeat survey on IDD 1985-86 and 1997 total goiter rate

Age Gp.	*Dibrugarh*		*Viskhapattanam*		*Mandla*	
(in yrs)	85-86	98-99	85-86	98-99	85-86	98-99
<4	55.23	0.59	9.30	1.03	16.2	0.28
5-9	90.00	2.57	12.42	4.48	28.3	0.21
10-14	86.40	7.98	16.23	9.48	59.3	1.01
15-19	77.10	5.72	9.90	7.00	53.5	2.10
20-29	70.10	7.93	21.40	5.57	43.4	2.01
30-39	57.60	8.06	21.00	4.56	31.0	3.46
>40	32.30	5.14	13.80	2.47	25.6	3.70
Total	65.60	5.93	15.70	4.81	34.4	2.00
N	42347	6693	3350.8	7419	13088	8211

Table 25.5: Incidence of neonatal hypothyroidism in three endemic goiter districts of Uttar Pradesh, before and after successful salt iodization

Districts	*Incidence per 1000 birth*	
	Pre-iodation	*Post-iodation*
Deoria	133	16
Gonda	75	9
Gorakhpur	85	17

AIIMS collected a total of 21,546 urine samples through various research surveys from 116 districts during 1994 to 2001. Only 14.6% of the districts had median UIE levels less than 100 µg/l indicating iodine deficiency.

A multi-centric study conducted in 15 districts by Indian Council of Medical Research in which a total of 27,481 urine samples were collected. It was also found that only 3 districts had median UIE levels less than 100 µg/l (Table 25.6).[38]

Table 25.6: Median values (µg/l) of urinary iodine excretion levels for children (6 <12 years)[64]

Name of district	*No. of urine samples*	*Median value (µg/l)*
Northern Region		
Mandi	2001	150
Dehradun	1617	127
Lakhimpur Kheri	2003	90
Badaun	1978	118
Baramulla	2082	200
Bikaner	1824	118
Mainpuri	1050	90
Srinagar	1661	200
Eastern Region		
Bishnupur	2076	106
Gaya	1802	90
Patna	1671	109
Dibrugarh	2040	115
Nagaon	1836	115
Southern Region		
Mehboob Nagar	1748	150
Western Region		
Raigarh	2092	100
All Districts	**27,481**	

Lifting of Central Government Ban on Sale of Non Iodised Salt

The Government of India in 1998 implemented a central legislation banning sale of non-iodized salt for edible purposes in the entire country. However, in the year 2000, due to administrative and political compulsions, the GOI withdrew this central legislation.[39] Thereafter, the traders started procuring and selling of non-iodized salt for edible purposes. A decline in the production of iodised salt has been documented after the withdrawal of the central ban. The country's production of iodised salt has also decreased from 4.7 million tonnes (2001) to 3.6 million tonnes (2002).[40] In the year 2002, assessment of iodine content of salt in country conducted under the national Reproductive and Child Health Survey revealed that 63% of the families were consuming salt with iodine content less than 15 ppm.[41]

ASSESSMENT OF IDD

Sampling Procedure

Probability Proportionate to Size (PPS) cluster sampling methodology is recommended. Thirty clusters should be covered and should be selected as follows:

Firstly all population units/villages in the area to be surveyed is listed along with the population. Secondly, the cumulative frequency table is prepared and the total population in the survey area is calculated. Then by dividing total population with 30, the sampling interval is calculated. Subsequently the first cluster is selected at random and subsequent clusters are calculated by adding sampling interval. The number of subjects to be surveyed within each cluster depends on the following: (i) estimated prevalence of IDD, (ii) level of precision desired, (iii) variability of prevalence between clusters.

Selection of Target Groups for IDD Survey

The school age children (6-12 years) reflect the IDD status of the community, as they are vulnerable to deficiency and respond to the iodine supplementation intervention and hence have been recommended for the survey.

Indicators for Assessing IDD

The common indicators for assessment of IDD are:

i. Clinical indicators; and
ii. Biochemical indicators.

It is recommended that the assessment of iodine content of salt consumed by the subjects may also be included in the survey as data on this aspect provides the guideline for developing the immediate intervention measures for prevention of IDD.

Clinical Indicators

Thyroid size: The size of the thyroid gland changes inversely in response to alterations in iodine intake, with a lag of 6-12 months in children and young adults (i.e <30 years of age). The traditional method for determining thyroid size is inspection and palpation. It is recommended that if the proportion of children attending school is less than 50%, spot surveys should be done on two groups of children of the same age, i.e. those who attend school and those who do not, to ascertain if there is any significant difference between the two. If so, both groups should be studied separately, in all clusters, or an appropriate adjustment should be made in the rate found among school children.

The classification of goiter into various grades is depicted in Table 25.7. Table 25.8 gives the epidemiological criteria for establishing IDD severity based on goiter prevalence in school age children. It is recommended that a total Goiter rate (TGR, goiter grades 1 and 2) of 5% or more in primary school children (age range approximately 6 to 12 years) be used to signal the presence of a public health problem. The cut off of 5% allows some margin of inaccuracy of goiter assessment and for goiter that may occur in iodine replete population due to other causes such as goitrogens and autoimmune thyroid diseases. The previously recommended 10% cut off level has been revised downwards since it has been shown that goiter prevalence rates between 5% and 10% may be associated with a range of abnormalities, including inadequate urinary iodine excretion and/or sub normal levels of TSH among adults, children and neonates. The specificity and sensitivity of palpation are low in grades 0 and 1 due to a high inter-observer variation.

Table 25.7: Simplified classification of goiter

Grade 0 :	No palpable or visible goiter.
Grade 1 :	A mass in the neck that is consistent with an enlarged thyroid that is palpable but not visible (PNV) when the neck is in the normal position. It moves upward in the neck as the subject swallows. Nodular alteration(s) can occur even when the thyroid is not visibly enlarged.
Grade 2 :	A swelling in the neck that is visible (V) when the neck is in a normal position and is consistent with an enlarged thyroid when the neck is palpated

Table 25.8: Epidemiological criteria for assessing the severity of IDD based on the prevalence of goiter in school age children

Prevalence of Goiter	*Mild IDD*	*Moderate IDD*	*Severe IDD*
TGR	5.0-19.9%	20.0-29.9%	>30.0%

Biochemical Indicators

Urinary: Iodine Since most iodine that is absorbed is excreted, therefore the urinary iodine level is a good marker of a previous day's dietary iodine intake. However, since an individual's level of urinary iodine varies daily and even during a given day, data can be used only for making a population based estimate. Experience has shown that the

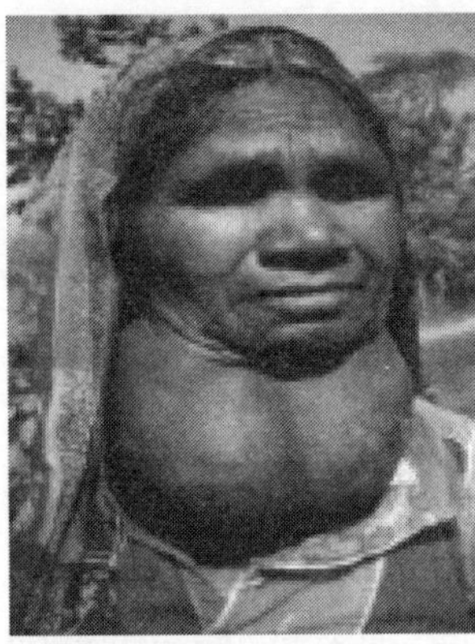

Fig. 25.5: A woman with multinodular goiter

iodine concentration in early morning urine specimens (child or adult) provides an adequate assessment of a population's iodine status; 24-hour samples are not necessary. Acceptability is very high and spot urine specimens are easy to obtain.

Small amount (0.5-1.0 ml) of urine is required. Specimens are collected in tubes, which are tightly sealed with screw tops they do not require refrigeration or the addition of a preservative. Iodine content remains stable throughout transport to the laboratory. The tightly sealed specimens can be refrigerated in the laboratory for several months before actual determinations are made. Should evaporation occur, iodine concentration will increase.

Since casual specimens are used, it is desirable to measure about 300 from a given population group to allow for varying degrees of subject hydration and other biological variations between individuals, as well as to obtain a reasonably small confidence interval. Smaller sample sizes are adequate to establish at the outset that iodine deficiency is the cause of the endemic goiter. The cut off points proposed for classifying iodine deficiency based on UIE levels into different degrees of public health significance are shown in Table 25.9. Frequency distribution curves are necessary for full interpretation, since urinary iodine values from populations are usually not normally distributed and therefore the median value should be used rather than the mean. The indicator of iodine deficiency "elimination" is a median value for iodine concentration of 100 ug/l (i.e. 50% of the samples should be above 100 ug/l, and not more than 20% of samples should be below 50 ug/l). As an IDD prevention Program progresses, Goiter rates become progressively less useful, and urinary iodine levels progressively more useful, as elimination criteria.

Table 25.9: Epidemiological criteria for assessing severity of IDD based on median urinary iodine levels

Median value	*Severity of IDD*
< 20	Severe IDD
20-49	Moderate IDD
50-99	Mild IDD
> 100	No deficiency

Assessment of IDD as a Public Health Problem

The common parameters used for assessment of IDD as a public health problem include goiter prevalence, median urinary excretion levels, TSH levels and median thyroglobin levels. The cut off levels of various parameters used to assess severity of IDD are depicted in Table 25.10. The criteria for achieving the elimination of IDD has been depicted in Table 25.11. A country can achieve IDD elimination by achieving all these parameters.

Section 7

Table 25.10: Criteria for a significant public health problem of IDD in a community

Indicator	*Target population*	*Severity of public health problem (prevalence)*		
		Mild	*Moderate*	*Severe*
Goitre grade > 0	SAC[a]	5.0-19.9 %	20.0-29.9 %	≥30.0 %
Thyroid volume > 97th centile by ultrasound[b]	SAC	5.0-19.9 %	20.0-29.9 %	≥30.0 %
Median urinary iodine level (mg/l)	SAC	50-99	20-49	<20
TSH > 5 mU/l whole blood	Neonates	30-19.9 %	20.0-39.9 %	≥40.0 %
Median Tg (ng/ml serum)[c]	C/A[d]	10.0-19.9	20.0-39.9	≥40.0

[a] **SAC = School-aged children.**
[d] C/A = Children and adults.
[b] Normative tyroid volume size values are available from WHO and ICCIDD in 1995.
[c] Different assays may have different normal ranges.

Table 25.11: Criteria for achieving elimination of IDD as a public health problem

	Indicator	*Goal*
1. Salt iodization	: Proportion of households consuming effectively iodized salt	>90%
2. Urinary iodine	: Proportion below 100 mg/l Proportion below 50 mg/l	<50% <20%
3. Thyroid size	: In school children 6-12 years of age: Proportion with enlarged thyroid by palpation ultrasound	 <5%
4. Neonatal TSH	: Proportion with levels >5mU/l whole blood	<3%

REFERENCES

1. American Medical Association. *Current Exposure to Iodine. Summary Report of a Workshop.* Newyork, Department of Foods and Nutrition. American Medical Association 1980.
2. Whitehead A. IDD: Issues and problems in developing world. Nutr Update 2002;5:126-135.
3. Hetzel BS. SOS for a billion—the nature and magnitude of iodine deficiency disorders. In: Hetzel BS, Pandav CV (eds*): SOS for a Billion: The Conquest of Iodine Deficiency Disorders.* 2nd edn. London: Oxford University Press, 1997: 1-29.
4. Anonymous. Iodine deficiency disorder (IDD). *ICCIDD Newsletter* 2001; 10:1-13.
5. Kapil U. Progress made in Elimination of IDD and possible impact of lifting ban on sale of non-Iodized salt. *J Acad Hosp Administr* 2000; 12: 33-41.
6. Ramji S. Iodine deficiency disorders: Epidemiology, clinical profile and diagnosis. In: Sachdev HPS, Choudhury P (eds) *Nutrition in Children: Developing Country Concerns.* New Delhi: BI Publications 1994: 245-249.
7. Stanbury JB. The iodine deficiency disorders: Introduction and general aspects. In: Hetzel BS, Dunn JT, Stanbury JB. *The Prevention and Control of Iodine Deficiency Disorders.* London: Elseiver Science Publishers 1987: 35-48.
8. World Health Organization. *Indicators for Assessing Iodine Deficiency Disorders and their Control through Salt Iodization.* Geneva: World Health Organisation 1994.
9. Government of India. *National Consultation on Benefits and Safety of Iodized Salt.* Jaipur: Salt Department, Government of India.
10. Haddow JE, Palomaki GE, Allan WC, *et al.* Maternal thyroid deficiency: Is it responsible for a low IQ in the offspring? *N Engl J Med* 1999; 341: 549-555.
11. Delong R. Neurological involvement in iodine deficiency disorders. In: Hetzel BS, Dunn JT, Stanbury JB (eds): *The Prevention and Control of Iodine Deficiency Disorders.* London: Elseiver 1987:49-64.
12. Bernal J, Nunez J. Thyroid hormone action and brain development. *Trends Endocrinol Metab* 2000; 133: 390-398.
13. Delange F. Endemic cretinism. In: Braveman LE and Utiger RD A (eds): *Fundamental and Clinical Text Thyroid.* Philadelphia: Lippincott; 1996:756-781.
14. Koibuchi N, Chin WW. Thyroid hormone action and brain development. *Trends Endocrinol Metab* 2000; 4:123-128.
15. Martinez-Galan JR, Pedraza P, Santacana M, Escobar del Ray F, Morreale de Escobar, Ruiz—Marcos A. *J Clin Invest* 1997; 99: 2701-2709.
16. Ruiz-Marcos A, Sanchez-Toscano FS, Salas J, Escobar del Rey F, Morreale de Esacobar G. Differential effects of hypothyroidism on the development of different areas and layers of the cerebral certex. In: Kochupillai N, Karmarkar MG, Ramalingaswami V (eds): *Iodine in Nutrition: Thyroxine and Brain Development.* New Delhi: Tata McGraw Hill 1986; 126-131.
17. Rakie P. Neurons in rhesus monkey visual cortex: Systematic relation between time of origin and eventual disposition. *Science* 1974; 183: 425.
18. Obregon MJ, Santisterban P, Rodriguez-Pena A, Pascual A, Carxegena P, Ruiz-Marcos A, Lamas L, Escobar del Rey F, Morreale de Escobar G. Cerebral hypothyroidism in rats with adult-onset iodine deficiency. *Endocrinology* 1984: 614-624.
19. Juan RMG, Pablo P, Maria S, Escobar del R, Morreale de Escobar, Antonio R. Early effects of iodine deficiency on radial glial cells of the hippocampus of the rat fetus. *J Clin Invest* 1997; 99: 2701-2709.
20. Ramie A, Rabie A. Effect of thyroid deficiency on the development of glia in the hippocampal formation of the rat: An immunocytochemical study. *Glia* 1988; 1: 337-345.
21. Earyrs JT. Endocrine influence on cerebral development. *Arch Biol* 1964; 75:529.
22. Bala´zs R, Brookbank BWL, Davidson S, Eayrs JT, Wilson DA. The effect of neonatal thyroidectomy on myelination in the rat brain. *Brain Res* 1969; 15:219.
23. Lie JQ, Wang X, Yan YQ, Wang KW, Qiw DK, Xin ZF, Wei J. The effect on foetal brain development in the rat of a severely iodine deficient diet derived from an endemic area-observation on the first generation. *Neuropathol-Appl-Neurobiol* 1986; 12: 261-276.
24. Bleichrodt N, Born MPH. A meta-analysis of research on iodine and its relationship to cognitive development. In: Stanbury JS (ed): The Damaged Brain of Iodine Deficiency: Cognitive, Behavioral, Servomotor and Educative Aspects. New York: Cognizant Communication Corporation 1994: 195-200.
25. Mehta M, Pandav CS, Kochupillai N. Intellectual assessment of school children from severely iodine deficient villages. *Indian Pediatr* 1987; 24: 467-473.
26. Haddow JE, Palomaki GE, Allan WC, Williams JR, Knight GJ, Ganhnon J, O' *et al.* Maternal thyroid deficiency during pregnancy and subsequent neuropsychological development of the child. *N Engl J Med* 1999; 341:549-555.
27. Azizi F, Kalani H, Kimiagar M, Ghazi A, Sarshar A, Nafarabadi M. Physical, neuromotor and intellectual impairment in non-cretinous school children with iodine deficiency. *Int J Vitam Nutr Res* 1995;65:199-205.
28. Pardede LV, Hardjowasito W, Gross R, *et al.* Urinary iodine secretion is the most appropriate outcome indicator for iodine deficiency at field conditions at district level. *J Nutr* 1998;128:1122-1126.
29. Van den Briel T, West CE, Bleichrodt N, van de Vijver FJ, Ategbo EA, Hautvast JG. Improved iodine status is associated with improved mental performance of school children in Benin. *Am J Clin Nutr* 2000;72:1179-1185.
30. Ranganathan S, Reddy V. Human Requirements of Iodine and safe Use of Iodized Salt. *Indian J Med Res* 1995; 102:227-232.
31. World Health Organization. *Evaluation of Certain Food Additives and Contaminants.* Thirtyseventh Report of Joint FAO/WHO Expert Committee on Food Additives. Geneva: WHO1997.
32. Salt Department. *Universal Salt Iodisation (USI)—India, Progress and Current Status.* New Delhi: Salt Department, Ministry of Industry, Government of India 1996.
33. Pandav CS, Pandav CS, Kochupillai N, Karmarkar MG, Ramachandran K, Gopinath PG, *et al.* Endemic goiter in Delhi. *Indian J Med Res* 1980;72:81-88.
34. Kapil U, Saxena N, Ramachandran S, Balamurugan A, Nayar D, Prakash S. Assessment of Iodine deficiency disorders using the 30 cluster approach in the National Capital Territory of Delhi. *Indian Pediatrics* 1996;33:1013-1017.
35. Kapil U, Sethi V, Goindi G, Pathak P, Singh P, 2003a. Tracking progress towards elimination of Iodine Deficiency Disorders in National Capital Territory of Delhi. *Indian J Pediatr* 2004; 71: 211-212.

36. Indian Council of Medical Research. *Repeat Survey on Prevalence of IDD in Selected Districts of India.* (Personal Communication with Indian Council of Medical Research Head quarters, New Delhi).
37. Kochupillai N. Neonatal hypothyroidism in India. *Mount Sinai J Med* 1992; 59: 111-115.
38. Indian Council of Medical Research. *Micronutrient Deficiency Disorders in 16 districts of India. Part 1 Report of an ICMR Task Force Study–District Nutrition Project.* New Delhi: Indian Council of Medical Research 2001.
39. Government lifts ban on noniodized salt. *Hindustan Times* 15th September, 2000.
40. Government of India. *Annual Report 2002-2003, Salt Department and Ministry of Commerce and Industry.* New Delhi: Government of India Press 2003.
41. Government of India. *Report of Reproductive and Child Health Project (Phase 1, Round 2, 2002).* Ministry of Health and Family Welfare and International Institute for Population Sciences, *Mumbai*. New Delhi: Government of India Press 2004.

B Vishnu Bhat • B Adhisivam

26 Zinc in Child Nutrition

INTRODUCTION

Zinc is the most ubiquitous of all trace elements involved in human metabolism. Zinc is the component of over 100 metalloenzymes with catalytic, regulatory or structural role. It has a fundamental role in cellular metabolism with profound effects on the immune system and the intestinal mucosa.

Micronutrient deficiency especially that of zinc is one of the causes for growth retardation and morbidity among children. Zinc deficiency is common in children from developing countries due to lack of intake of animal foods, high dietary phytate content, inadequate food intake and increased fecal losses during diarrhea. This deficiency occurs along with high rates of serious infectious diseases such as diarrhea, pneumonia, and malaria.[1]

Zinc deficiency is known to produce skin changes, persistent diarrhea, acrodermatitis enteropathica, defects in dark adaptation, delayed wound healing, thymic atrophy, altered immune function, candidial superinfection, abnormalities of taste sensation, neuropsychiatric disturbances like irritability and tremors and a syndrome of dwarfism, anemia, hepatosplenomegaly, dry skin, geophagia and hypogonadism.[2] Maternal zinc deficiency has been reported to result in low birthweight (LBW) babies.[3]

Improved dietary quality and intake, food fortification and cultivation of zinc-dense plants are some ways of mitigating zinc deficiency.

BIOLOGICAL FUNCTIONS OF ZINC

More than one hundred specific enzymes require zinc for their catalytic function. Zinc participates in all major biochemical pathways and plays multiple roles in the perpetuation of genetic material, including transcription of DNA, translation of RNA, and ultimately cell division. Research is beginning to clarify the molecular mechanisms underlying the action of zinc on the immune function.

It is clear that this trace element has a broad impact on key immunity mediators, such as enzymes, thymic peptides and cytokines, explaining the paramount importance of status of zinc on the regulation of lymphoid cell activation, proliferation and apoptosis. Zinc affects both non-specific and specific immune functions. In terms of non-specific immunity, it affects the integrity of epithelial barrier and function of neutrophils, monocytes and macrophages. With regard to specific immunity, both lymphopenia and declined lymphocyte function occur in zinc deficiency.

Ongoing and future studies regarding the immunological status of zinc deficiency 'at risk' groups could lead to public health interventions with nutritional doses of zinc supplements to prevent alteration of the immune system and improve resistance to infections.[4]

ZINC METABOLISM

Zinc is released from food as free ions during digestion. These liberated ions may then bind to endogenously secreted ligands before their transport into the enterocytes in the duodenum and jejunum. Specific transport proteins may facilitate the passage of zinc across the cell membrane into the portal circulation. With high intakes, zinc is also absorbed through a passive paracellular route.

The portal system carries absorbed zinc directly to the liver, and then released into systemic circulation for delivery to other tissues. About 70% of zinc in circulation is bound to albumin, and any condition that alters serum albumin concentration can have a secondary effect on serum zinc levels. Although serum zinc represents only 0.1% of the whole body zinc, the circulating zinc turns over rapidly to meet tissue needs. Loss of zinc through gastrointestinal tract accounts for approximately half of all zinc eliminated from the body. Considerable amount of zinc is secreted through the biliary and intestinal secretions, but most of it is reabsorbed and this process is an important point of regulation of zinc balance. Other routes of zinc excretion include the urine and surface losses (desquamated skin, hair, sweat).

HUMAN REQUIREMENTS

Since the mid-1990s, the World Health Organization (WHO), Food and Agriculture Organization (FAO), International Atomic Energy Association and the Food and Nutrition Board of the Institute of Medicine have convened expert committees to develop estimates of human zinc requirements and dietary intakes needed to satisfy these requirements (Table 26.1).[5]

Table 26.1: Estimated physiological requirements for absorbed zinc by age group and sex

	WHO	
Age	*Reference Weight (kg)*	*Requirement (mg/day)*
6-12 mo	9	0.84
1-3 yr	12	0.83
3-6 yr	17	0.97
6-10 yr	25	1.12
10-12 yr	35	1.40
12-15 yr	48	1.82
15-18 yr M	64	1.97
15-18 yr F	55	1.54
Pregnancy	—	2.27
Lactation	—	2.89

DIETARY SOURCES OF ZINC AND BIOAVAILABILITY

Zinc occurs in a wide variety of foods, but is found in highest concentrations in animal sources, particularly beef, pork, poultry and fish, and in lesser amounts in eggs and dairy products. Zinc content is relatively high in nuts, legumes and whole grain cereals and is lower in fruits and vegetables. The dietary components that have a substantial impact on the absorption of zinc are phytate and calcium (which inhibit zinc absorption) and protein which enhances zinc absorption. Phytate content is high in cereal grains, nuts and legumes. It is a strong chelator of minerals including zinc. Because phytate cannot be digested and absorbed, minerals bound to phytate also pass through the intestines unabsorbed. The inhibitory effect of calcium may result from the formation of insoluble calcium-zinc-phytate complexes in the intestinal tract. Both the total amount and the type of protein in the diet influence zinc absorption. Increasing protein intake results in a higher absorption of zinc. Animal protein such as meat and egg protein enhances absorption of zinc, while casein may have inhibitory effect.

CAUSES OF ZINC DEFICIENCY

The general causes of zinc deficiency include inadequate intake, increased requirements, malabsorption, increased losses and impaired utilization. Inadequate dietary zinc of absorbable form is the primary cause of zinc deficiency, in most situations. This may result from a combination of low dietary intake, heavy reliance on foods with low zinc content and/or with zinc that is poorly absorbable. Low intakes are further exacerbated by physiologic conditions associated with elevated zinc requirements, increasing the risk of zinc deficiency.

Malabsorption of zinc may occur in a number of situations. For example, acrodermatitis enteropathica is a rare genetic disorder that specifically affects zinc absorption. Malabsorption syndromes and inflammatory diseases of the bowel, resulting in poor absorption and loss of zinc, may lead to secondary zinc deficiency; particularly in the presence of marginal dietary intakes. Certain drugs such as phenytoin and tetracycline may reduce zinc absorption.[6] Several studies suggest that pharmacological doses of iron interfere with the absorption of zinc due to competitive interactions between these elements.[7] Utilization of zinc is impaired in the presence of infection, and decreased circulating levels of zinc reduce the availability of zinc to the tissues. Conditions that alter intestinal integrity not only reduce absorption, but also result in increased endogenous losses of zinc. For example, fecal excretion of zinc is increased during acute diarrhea, though it is not clear to what extent this represents unabsorbed zinc or zinc of endogenous origin. Not only does zinc deficiency increase the susceptibility to childhood diarrhea, but increased losses of endogenous zinc that occur during diarrhea may further deplete body zinc, setting up a vicious cycle.[8]

GROUPS AT HIGH RISK

1. **Infants and Children:** Young children are at greater risk of zinc deficiency because of the increased requirements during growth. Exclusively breast fed infants of mothers with adequate zinc levels can satisfy their zinc requirements for the first 5-6 months of life.[9] However, after this age, complementary foods containing absorbable zinc are required to meet the requirements. In many low-income countries, complementary feeding is delayed and cereal foods used for feeding have low content of total and absorbable zinc. These foods fail to meet the needs for zinc. Conversely, early introduction of such foods with high phytate may interfere with the absorption of zinc from breast milk.[10]

   Low birthweight infants have poor hepatic stores of zinc.[11] In those who are born prematurely, zinc status will be further compromised because most of the zinc is transferred during the last trimester of pregnancy. Moreover, preterm infants may have reduced absorption because of their immature gastrointestinal tract. These impairments result in increased zinc requirements during the neonatal period, although specific requirements for these infants have not been established.

   Zinc requirements of malnourished children are estimated to be between 2-4 mg/ kg body weight.[12] These requirements are much higher than those for healthy children (0.17 mg/kg at 1-3 years), presumably due to prior zinc depletion and problems of malabsorption due to changes in the intestinal tract.

2. **Adolescents:** The physiological requirements for zinc peak during adolescence at the time of the pubertal growth spurt, which generally occurs in girls between 10-15 years and in boys between 12-15 years. Even after the growth spurt has ceased, adolescents may require additional zinc to replenish tissue zinc pools depleted during puberty.
3. **Pregnant and lactating women:** Increased nutritional demands during pregnancy and lactation predispose women to develop zinc deficiency. These demands are greater during lactation, although physiological adjustments in zinc absorption help to meet the needs for lactation. Several studies have indicated that iron supplements reduce the absorption of zinc.[7]

ZINC AND DIARRHEAL DISEASES

The effects of zinc supplementation on prevention of diarrhea and the therapeutic benefits of zinc given during a diarrheal episode have been well evaluated. Majority of the studies were conducted in South East Asia, where zinc deficiency is common. Strong evidence exists that zinc supplements improve the prognosis of children being treated for diarrheal disease. A pooled analysis of randomised controlled trials of therapeutic zinc in children with diarrhea showed that children with acute diarrhea given zinc supplements had a 15% lower probability of continuing diarrhea on a given day compared with those in the control group; children with persistent diarrhea had a 24% lower probability of continuing diarrhea. In addition, children with persistent diarrhoea had a 42% lower rate of treatment failure or death if given zinc supplements.[14] Randomized controlled trials were conducted in children aged between 6 months and 3 years, using zinc doses ranging from 10 to 30 mg per day. Zinc supplemented children had 15% faster recovery with a 22% reduction in the odds of acute episodes lasting >7 days.[15] One study is of major interest as it measured impact on stool output, the most objective marker of severity and a useful proxy indicator for risk of dehydration, in hospitalized children with acute diarrhea and dehydration. In the zinc treated children, the total stool output was reduced by 31% than in the placebo group.[16] All studies showed that the effect of zinc did not vary significantly with age, or nutritional status assessed by anthropometry. The effects were not dependent upon the type of zinc salts: zinc sulfate, zinc acetate or zinc gluconate. There was little gain in efficacy when the commonly used 20 mg daily dose of elemental zinc was increased to 30-40 mg daily.[14, 15] The efficacy of 40 mg elemental zinc mixed with a litre of WHO ORS solution was compared with ORS without zinc and with zinc syrup administered separately from ORS.[17] While zinc-ORS was superior to ORS alone, it was less efficacious in reducing duration of the episode than zinc supplements given separately from the ORS solution. The data are currently too limited.

Therapeutic benefits of zinc administration during diarrhea are biologically plausible because of its effects on various components of the immune system and its direct gastrointestinal effects. Zinc is said to improve absorption of water and electrolytes by helping in early regeneration of intestinal mucosa, restoration of enteric enzymes and enhancing humoral and cellular immunity.[18]

ACRODERMATITIS ENTEROPATHICA

First described in 1942, the condition is now recognized as an inborn error of zinc metabolism that is inherited as an autosomal recessive disorder. Characteristic symptoms in infancy include periorificial and acral dermatitis (oral, anal, genital), diarrhea, behavioral and mental changes, neurological disturbances, and secondary bacterial and fungal infections. In older children, failure to thrive, anorexia, alopecia, nail dystrophy, and repeated infections are more common. Zinc deficiency may be due to inadequate intake, malabsorption, excessive loss, or a combination of these factors. If treated early, most of the symptoms are reversible and usually leave no sequelae.

History often reveals siblings or relatives with similar symptoms or death during infancy. Any history of diarrhea, anorexia, photophobia, behavioral changes (e.g., tearing, crying, and inability to be consoled), withdrawal from human contact, and pained expressions suggest AE as a possibility in the differential diagnosis. In general, patients are miserable and depressed. Infants are inconsolable and may withdraw from contact. Erythematous to vesiculo-bullous or pustular lesions leading to dry, scaly, or eczematoid lesions distributed around periorificial and acral areas of the body are characteristics of AE. The borders of affected areas are sharply demarcated and have an accentuation of craquel-like scale at the periphery. Paronychia may be present. Partial or total hair loss may be evident.

Table 26.2: Differential diagnosis for acrodermatitis enteropathica

- Biotin deficiency
- Atypical epidermolysis bulbosa
- Generalized and local candidiasis
- Atopic dermatitis
- Abnormality of essential fatty acid metabolism
- Seborrheic dermatitis
- Kwashiorkor
- Iatrogenic deficiency of branched chain amino acids (isoleucine) in restrictive diets for maple syrup urine disease or methylmalonic aciduria.

Other than acquired zinc deficiency, most of the differential diagnoses can be excluded easily. A successful zinc supplementation trial confirms the diagnosis. Plasma zinc concentrations are usually reduced (<50 mcg/dL). Collect specimens in plastic syringes or acid-washed Vacutainer tubes to prevent exogenous contamination that would lead to spuriously normal measurements. Reference range zinc concentrations have been reported in patients with AE. Hair, saliva, or urine zinc levels are rarely needed. Production of serum alkaline phosphatase depends on zinc. Therefore, a low level of alkaline phosphatase may support an AE diagnosis. Secondary infections may require cultures and additional therapy. Skin or intestinal mucosal biopsies are rarely needed. Intestinal mucosal biopsies show loss of villous architecture with increased cell infiltration in the lamina propria of patients with AE. The nuclei are enlarged with an open chromatin distribution. Complete normalization of the intestinal mucosa is observed in the mucosal biopsies after zinc sulphate treatment. Histopathology of cutaneous lesions discloses intracellular edema of epidermal keratinocytes. This finding is not pathognomonic and may be observed in other nutritional deficiency states.

Zinc gluconate or sulfate is administered orally at 1-3 mg/kg/d. Although the intravenous dose has not clearly been estimated, amounts of 300-1000 mcg/kg/d may be sufficient for rapid reversal of symptoms. Clinical response is observed within 5-10 days.

In AE, it is advisable to maintain zinc therapy throughout the patient's life span, although periods of remission have been reported. Exacerbation during pregnancy or the stress of disease may require an increase in therapy. In acquired zinc deficiency, treatment can be stopped after the precipitating cause has resolved. Warm compresses and petrolatum applied to areas of weeping or crusted dermatitis may enhance re-epithelialization when used concurrently with zinc replacement. Dietary advice should include oysters, crab, meat products, human milk, dried beans, and lentils.

Occasionally, high zinc supplementation may cause gastric upset. High zinc supplementation may also adversely affect copper metabolism. Untreated patients usually die within the first few years of life. They have severe growth retardation, dermatitis, alopecia, secondary bacterial and fungal infections, and neurological and behavioral changes. All of these conditions are reversible with therapy.

Therapy achieves a survival rate of 100%.

ROLE OF ZINC IN OTHER INFECTIONS

Case reports and observational studies provided initial evidence of a correlation between low plasma-zinc concentrations in children and a greater susceptibility to infections.[13]

i. **Respiratory Infections:** Fewer clinical trials have addressed the preventive benefits of zinc supplementation on lower respiratory tract infections than for diarrheal diseases. When results of 5 studies, of zinc supplementation in children aged between 4 and 36 months were pooled, the commutative reduction in episodes of pneumonia was 41%.[19,20] A large trial from India showed 26% reduction in clinical pneumonia diagnosed by two physicians using pre-defined criteria.[21] In Bangladesh, zinc supplementation resulted in 30% reduction in duration of severe pneumonia and significant shorter duration of individual markers of disease severity such as fast breathing, chest in drawing and hypoxia. There was a mean reduction of 25% in hospital stay, which is equivalent to one hospital day. In the other trial from Kolkata, zinc treatment significantly increased recovery rates from very ill status of severe acute lower respiratory tract infections by 2.6 times but these effects were only seen in boys.[22,23]

ii. **Malaria:** The information regarding the effect of zinc supplementation on malaria is limited. While supplementation with zinc showed no effect on various malarial indices in a community based cross-sectional surveillance it was found to reduce visits to health facilities for **Plasmodium falciparum** febrile episodes defined as fever with parasitemia in Papua New Guinea and Gambia.[24] Another trial in Burkina Faso found no effect of zinc supplementation on rates of fever in a community based surveillance of malaria.[25] The Zinc Against Plasmodium Study Group[26] evaluated the therapeutic effect of zinc given as an adjuvant to standard therapy during acute malaria in a large double-blind, randomized placebo-controlled clinical trial across 5 countries in Africa. Despite an improvement in mean serum zinc levels there was no effect on the median time to reduction of fever, parasitemia or a change in hemoglobin concentration in the initial 72 hours or during the four week follow-up.

EFFECT OF ZINC IN MORTALITY

A reduction in childhood mortality is anticipated because of the effects of zinc supplementation on reducing the incidence and severity of some of the most common childhood infectious diseases. A study conducted in Bangladesh[27] used a cluster-randomized design to evaluate the effect on mortality and morbidity of providing daily zinc for 14 days to children with diarrhea as part of the diarrhea treatment programme in the community. The children in the zinc cluster had a shorter duration and lower incidence of diarrhea than children in the control group. Lesser admission to hospital of children with diarrhea, and lower mortality due to non-injury deaths, notably diarrhea or pneumonia was reported in the zinc treated cluster. Preliminary evidence that routine zinc supplementation may have some effect on mortality in high risk group comes from a recent double blind randomized controlled trial in India which showed a 68% reduction in mortality in small for gestational age full term infants who were given 5 mg of zinc daily from 30 days to 284 days.[28]

ZINC AND PHYSICAL GROWTH

Studies from animal models and reports of severe zinc deficiency resulting in dwarfism and delayed sexual maturation in Iranian and Egyptian youths predominantly on a zinc depleted bread diet, suggested that zinc supplementation may have a significant role to play in improved child growth.[18] Zinc deficiency as early as during the intrauterine period may influence the dynamics of physical and intellectual development in humans. While the role of antepartum zinc deficiency and supplementation on immune function is being assessed, a few trials have also attempted to assess intrauterine well being in zinc supplemented mothers. A meta-analysis of 33 randomized intervention trials showed that zinc supplementation produced highly significant positive response in weight gain as well as linear growth.[29] Growth responses were greater in children with low initial weight-for-age or height-for-age Z scores. Thus, the beneficial effect of zinc on children's growth may be limited to populations with pre-existing growth failure.

ZINC AND THE NERVOUS SYSTEM

Zinc may act as a neurotransmitter and by influencing cell division, maturation, and growth early in fetal life it may determine later neurodevelopment and intellect. Although evidence from animal models, psychiatric patients and early studies from infants[30] suggests that zinc deficiency affects cognition, neuro-development, responses to stress and emotion, and motor activity, more trials will be needed to evaluate the critical period, risk groups and reversibility of the adverse effects of zinc deficiency on neurodevelopment.

MISCELLANEOUS EFFECTS OF ZINC

Large doses of zinc may reduce copper absorption from the gut and have been used in the treatment of Wilson's disease. Zinc has been found to be of benefit in the treatment of attention deficit hyperactivity disorder. Zinc lozenges are being used for treatment of common colds although the evidence presently at best is inconclusive.[1] The role of zinc in fertility and reproductive biology needs further research.

PREVENTION OF ZINC DEFICIENCY

WHO Task Force 2001, has recommended use of zinc in the treatment of diarrhea, given at a dose of 2 RDAs per day (10 to 20 mg per day) for 14 days. Zinc supplementation is also recommended as part of routine, standard case management in persistent diarrhea and in those with severe malnutrition. Further evidence is required for qualifying its use in treatment of other infective diseases like pneumonia and malaria.

There are several approaches to mitigate zinc deficiency. The most important would be to improve the dietary quality and intake of infants, children and women. Routine zinc supplementation in young children is a difficult task, given the past experience with iron supplementation. But supplementation of selected subgroups at highest risk of death (like low birthweight or the severely malnourished infants) may be possible. The other problem would be to combine zinc with other micronutrients as there may be significant interactions between them resulting in decreased bioavailability of the individual micronutrients. The effects of possible interactions in a combined formulation need to be assessed further on disease morbidity.

The other approach is of food fortification by encouraging cultivation of zinc dense plants or those that have a decreased concentration of zinc absorption inhibitors.

Finally, research in the field of zinc and health must be encouraged.[1]

ZINC TOXICITY

Individuals may be exposed to high intakes of zinc, either through supplemental zinc or by contact with environmental zinc. Overt toxicity symptoms, such as nausea, vomiting, epigastric pain, diarrhea and lethargy may occur with acute high intakes. Short-term exposure to high levels of contaminant zinc (>300 ppm) from improper storage of food or beverages in galvanized vessels has caused acute gastroenteritis.

Chronic overdosage of zinc, in the range of 100-300 mg zinc/day for adults may induce copper deficiency and alterations in the immune response.

SUMMARY

Zinc is an essential mineral and deficiency results in abnormal immune function and higher rates of infectious diseases. Randomized controlled trials of zinc supplementation have been conducted in children in developing countries to determine effects on infectious disease morbidity and mortality. Zinc-supplemented children have been found to have lower rates of diarrhea, pneumonia and malaria in comparison with children not given zinc. Zinc used as an adjunct to fluid and dietary management of acute and persistent diarrhea has been found to reduce diarrheal duration and severity. Preliminary evidence suggests that zinc supplementation in children in poor developing country settings may also reduce infant mortality. Preventive and therapeutic interventions should be implemented in developing countries where zinc deficiency is likely to be prevalent.

REFERENCES

1. Bhatnagar S, Natchu UM. Zinc in child health and disease. *Indian J Pediatr* 2004; 71:991-995.
2. Elizabeth KE, Sreedevi P, Narayanan SN. Outcome of nutritional rehabilitation with and without zinc supplementation. *Indian Pediatr* 2000;37:647-650.
3. Simmer K, Thompson RPH. Maternal zinc and intrauterine growth retardation. *Clin Sci* 1985; 68: 395-396.
4. Dardenne M. Zinc and immune function. *Eur J Clin Nutr* 2002;56 Suppl 3:S20-S23.
5. WHO, FAO, IAEA. *Trace Elements in Human Health and Nutrition*. WHO: Geneva 2002.
6. Aggett PJ, Harries JT. Current status of zinc in health and disease states. *Arch Dis Child* 1979; 54: 909-917.
7. O'Brien KO, Zavaleta N, Caulfield LE, Wen J, Abrams SA. Prenatal iron supplements impair zinc absorption in pregnant Peruvian women. *J Nutr* 2000;130;2251-2255.
8. Castillo-Duran C, Vial P, Uauy R. Trace mineral balance during acute diarrhea in infants. *J Pediatr* 1988; 113:452-457.
9. Krebs NF, Hambidge KM. Zinc requirements and zinc intakes of breast fed infants. *Am J Clin Nutr* 1998; 43: 288-292.
10. Bell JG, Keen CL, Lonnerdal B. Effect of infant cereals on zinc and copper absorption during weaning. *Am J Did Child* 1987;141:1128-1132.
11. Zlotkin SH, Cherian MG. Hepatic metallothionein as a source of zinc and cystine during the first year of life. *Pediatr Res* 1988;24:326-329.
12. Briend A, Golden MH. Treatment of severe child malnutrition in refugee camps. *Eur J Clin Nutr* 1993;47:750-754.
13. Bahl R, Bhandari N, Hambidge KM, Bhan MK. Plasma zinc as a predictor of diarrhea and respiratory morbidity in children in an urban slum setting. *Am J Clin Nutr* 1998; 68 (Suppl. 2): 414S- 417S.
14. Zinc Investigators Collaborative Group. Therapeutic effects of oral zinc in acute and persistent diarrhea in children in developing countries: Pooled analysis of randomised controlled trials. *Am J Clin Nutr* 2000; 72: 1516-1522.
15. Bhatnagar S, Bhandari N, Mouli UC, Bhan MK. Consensus statement of IAP National Task Force: Status report on management of acute diarrhea. *Indian Pediatr* 2004; 41: 335-348.
16. Bhatnagar S, Bahl R, Sharma PK, Kumar GK, Saxena SK, Bhan MK. Zinc treatment with oral rehydration therapy reduces stool output and duration of diarrhea in hospitalized children: A randomized controlled trial. *J Pediatr Gastroenterol Nutr* 2004; 38: 34-40.
17. Bahl R, Bhandari N, Saksena M, Strand T, Kumar G.T. Bhan MK *et al.* Efficacy of zinc fortified oral rehydration solution in 6-35 month-old children with acute diarrhea. *J Pediatr* 2002; 141: 677-682.
18. Hambidge M. Human zinc deficiency. *J Nutr* 2000; 130: 1344S-1349S.
19. Bhutta ZA, Black RE, Brown KH, Meeks-Gardner J, Gore S, Hidayat A, *et al.* Prevention of diarrhea and pneumonia by zinc supplementation in children in developing countries: Pooled analysis of randomized controlled trials. Zinc Investigators' Collaborative Group. *J Pediatr* 1999; 135: 689-697.
20. Black RE. Zinc deficiency, infectious disease and mortality in the developing world. *J Nutr* 2003; 133(5 Suppl 1):148S-149S.
21. Bhandari N, Bahl R, Teneja S, Strand T, Molbak K, Ulvik RJ *et al*. Routine zinc supplementation prevents pneumonia in children 6 months to 3 years of age: A randomized controlled trial in an urban slum. *BMJ* 2002; 324: 1358-1360.
22. Brooks WA, Yunus M, Santosham M, Wahed MA, Nahar K, Yeasmin S *et al.* Zinc for severe pneumonia in very young children: Double-blind placebo-controlled trial. *Lancet* 2004; 363: 1683-1688.
23. Mahalanobis D, Lahiri M, Paul D, Gupta S, Gupta A, Wahed MA *et al.* Randomized, double-blind, placebo-controlled clinical trial of the efficacy of treatment with zinc or vitamin A in infants and young children with severe acute lower respiratory infection. *Am J Clin Nutr* 2004; 79: 430-436.
24. Shankar AH, Genton B, Baisor M, Paino J, Tamja S, Adiguma T *et al.* The influence of zinc supplementation on morbidity due to plasmodium falciparum: A randomized trial in preschool children in Papua New Guinea. *Am J Trop Med Hyg* 2000; 62: 663-669.
25. VMuller O, Becher H, van Zweeden AB, Ye Y, Diallo DA, Konate AT *et al.* Effect of zinc supplementation on malaria and other causes of morbidity in West African children: Randomized double blind placebo controlled trial. *BMJ* 2001; 322: 1567-1573.
26. Zinc against Plasmodium Study Group. Effect of zinc on the treatment of Plasmodium falciparum malaria in children: A randomized controlled trial. *Am J Clin Nutr* 2002; 76:805-812.
27. Baqui AH, Black RE, El Arifeen S, Yunus M, Chakraborty J, Ahmed S, Vaughan JP. Effect of zinc supplementation started during diarrhoea on morbidity and mortality in Bangladeshi children: Community randomized trial. *BMJ* 2002; 325: 1059.
28. Sazawal S, Black RE, Menon VP, Dinghra P, Caulfield LE, Dhingra U et al. Zinc supplementation in infants born small for gestational age reduces mortality: A prospective, randomized, controlled trial. *Pediatrics* 2001; 108: 1280-1286.
29. Brown KH, Peerson JM, Rivera J, Allen LH. Effect of supplemental zinc on the growth and serum zinc concentrations of pre-pubertal children: A meta-analysis of randomized, controlled trials. *Am J Clin Nutr* 2002; 75: 1062-1071.
30. Bhatnagar S, Taneja S. Zinc and cognitive development. *Brit J Nutr* 2001;85: S139-S145.

Suraj Gupte • SK Gupta • Mohinder Pal • KR Sangra

27 Infantile Tremor Syndrome (ITS)

INTRODUCTION

That nutritional deficiencies, including those of micronutrients such as iron, vitamin B_{12}, thiamine, pyridoxine, zinc and magnesium, may be accompanied by varied neurologic manifestations sooner or later is well-known. What remains inadequately understood is the exact role and modus opertandi of various nutrients in their causation.

Etiologically poorly understood disorder, *infantile tremor syndrome (ITS)*, is such an example. It is characterized by coarse tremors, anemia, and regression of motor and mental milestones in subjects around one year of age.[1] Though once believed to be restricted to a few pockets in India, this clinical entity is beginning to receive attention globally following its discussion at international neurological and nutrition meets.

Dikshit[2] is credited for first reporting of ITS in 1957 from Hyderabad. Since most of his cases were malnourished and anemic and tremors were superimposed on the clinical manifestations, he gave this condition the new designation, "nutritional dystrophy and anemia". Subsequently, Pohowalla and associates[3] from Indore claimed to have seen similar cases in 1953. This group provided a more precise and clear description of the disorder and named it "infantile meningoencephalitic syndrome".

In the subsequent decades, the condition has been widely reported from across the country as also from other countries.

EPIDEMIOLOGY

Geographical Distribution

ITS is primarily reported from India though there are reports of its occurrence (or occurrence of identical cases) in rest of the developing world (Afghanistan, Pakistan, Nepal, Sri Lanka, Somalia, Nigeria, Southern Turkey, Iraq, Bangladesh, Myanmar) as also America and Italy. In India, cases have been reported from the length and breadth of the country. Nevertheless, Jammu and Kashmir, Delhi, Punjab, Chandigarh, Himachal Pradesh, Uttar Pradesh, Madhya Pradesh, Tamil Nadu, Andhra Pradesh, Tamil Nadu etc. are the areas from where a large chunk of cases are reported.[2-31]

Sementics employed for ITS by different workers are given in Table 27.1.

Table 27.1: Various sementics employed for infantile tremor syndrome in the literature

Author(s)	*Sementic(s) Employed for ITS*
Dikshit[2]	Nutritional dystrophy and anemia
Pohwalla *et al.*[3]	Infantile meningoencephalitic syndrome
Jadhav *et al.*[4]	Vitamin B_{12} deficiency in Indian infants
Kaul *et al.*[5]	Syndrome of tremor in infants
Schdeva *et al.*[6]	Syndrome of tremor, mental regression and anemia in infants
Deshpande and Ingle[13]	Tremor syndrome
Agarwal *et al.*[1,18,32]	Nutritional tremor syndrome
Srikantia and Reddy[7]	Megaloblastic anemia of infancy
Sharda and Bhandari[25]	Infantile neuro-motor-pallor-pigmentation syndrome Indian childhood tremor syndrome

Incidence

Until 1970s, ITS accounted for 1 to 2 percent of the pediatric admissions in some hospitals that had started recognizing this condition.[1] In 1971-74, it formed 1.9 percent of the admissions to the pediatric inpatient department of the Snowdon Hospital.[18] During 1975-77, it accounted for 1.1% of our pediatric admissions at the Goverment Children Hospital, Jammu.[22,24] Subsequently, the incidence showed considerable decline. In a pilot study conducted in mid 1990s, we found its incidence to be 0.2 percent in hospitalized infants and children.

In late 1990s and early 2000s, we have noticed a remarkable hike in the number of cases of ITS admitted with us. One time in mid-summer of 2000, we had as many as 15 cases in our wards. The sudden spurt in cases couldn't be convincingly accounted for by a reasonable explanation.

Age

Six months to 18 months age group, with a peak at 9 to 15 months, is the classical span for occurrence of ITS. As high as 80% cases are seen in this age profile. A few cases may be upto 24 months. Though it is unusual to see cases outside this age range, we vividly recall a 3-year-old and another 5-year-old with characteristic features of ITS.

Sex

Slight predominance of males is obvious in a large majority of the studies. But, not much need be read in this observation since male children get the priority when it comes to seeking medical advice and care.

Nutritional Background

A kinship of prolonged breastfeeding (usually without introduction of semisolids and solids) as such or with top feeds and a concomitant malnutrition is nearly a rule in most of the infants with ITS even though they appear plump and chubby. The latter observation seemingly had led many earlier workers to miss the *camouflaged* malnutrition in these infants.

Socio-economic Status

A vast majority of cases come from poor families, hailing from rural or periurban slum stock.

Birth Order

Most of the subjects are second, third or fourth born.

Seasonal Variation

Most of the ITS cases are encountered during the period February to June. During winter and rainy seasons, the incidence is minimal.

ETIOLOGY

Notwithstanding four decades of experience since its first recognition in 1957 in Hyderabad, a final word concerning the etiology of ITS remains to be said. It continues to be a theory-based disorder, the speculations ranging from nutritional deficiency to viral encephalitis and degenerative process. Yet, the massive weight of evidence strongly supports the "nutritional theory" (*vide infra*).

Nutritional Theory

Quite a few earlier documentations obliquely suggested that ITS appeared to be the result of megaloblastic anemia which responded to administration of vitamin B_{12} satisfactorily. This theory received support from the following observations:

- In the experience of protagonists of this theory, megaloblastic anemia was always present in ITS.
- Vitamin B_{12} levels were found to be always reduced in ITS by them.
- The administration of vitamin B_{12} to these cases caused regression of major manifestations of ITS.
- The syndrome resembled cases of megaloblastic anemia with neurologic manifestations observed in Italy and America.

In the subsequent years, experience has indicated that only a proportion of infants with ITS have megaloblastic anemia. In fact, in some studies, there has not been even a single infant with ITS showing megaloblastic anemia. Our experience which is now duly supported by many other workers has convincingly established that there are certainly ITS cases who demonstrate purely iron-deficiency anemia. Furthermore, even those suffering from megaloblastic anemia may well need folic acid alone or in conjunction with vitamin B_{12} for an adequate response. Yet, ITS infants without megaloblastic anemia may not need (in fact, usually they do not) vitamin B_{12} and folic acid in therapeutic doses and still show cure with correction of iron-deficiency anemia and improvement in the overall nutritional status.

Magnesium deficiency has been pointed out as a possible etiologic factor in ITS. Some workers have found significantly reduced magnesium in CSF of infants suffering from ITS. Low levels of serum magnesium too have been reported.[32] Such neurologic manifestations as tremors and rigidity of ITS could well be related to magnesium deficiency. This deficiency, however, fails to explain occurrence of hair changes, skin pigmentation, mental dullness, etc. which are important features of ITS.

Some workers have hypothesized that such micronutrients as selenium, copper and cadmium may well be deficient in ITS subjects and, thus, have an etiologic role. However, such a deficiency state has not so far been convincingly demonstrated in ITS.

Zinc deficiency appears to be an important etiologic factor in ITS. This hypothesis is now catching up attention of the contemporary workers. Zinc reduction in body tissues and fluids has been found by us and others. Table 27.2 shows hair zinc levels in ITS in relation to controls kwashiorkor and marasmus found by us in a recent investigation.[33,34] The levels in ITS were significantly lower than in normal controls (Table 27.2).[33,34] In view of the fact that zinc deficiency is known to cause such manifestations as growth retardation, mental dullness, tremors, skin changes, irritability, susceptibility to infections and emotional disturbances,[35] the role of zinc deficiency in causation of ITS seems to be quite probable. Our clinical observations have demonstrated gratifying response to zinc supplements along with overall nutritional rehabilitation in ITS, resulting in reduced morbidity and mortality in the last around 15 years or so.[28-31] We strongly suggest further well-controlled clinical trials in different centers in order to

Table 27.2: Hair zinc levels in ITS, kwashiorkor, marasmus, and normal controls as per study conducted in Government Medical College, Jammu, Jammu and Kashmir, India

Category of subjects	*No of subjects*	*Hair zinc level (mcg/g)*	*Significant(p) value*	*Comments*
Normal controls	50	162.53 ± 7.32		
ITS	85	125.32 ± 22.53	< 0.001	Highly significant
ITS with kwashiorkor	32	123.02 ± 17.16	< 0.001	Highly significant
Kwashiorkor	43	147.44 ± 9.45	< 0.01	Just significant
Prekwashiorkor	34	142.73 ± 10.42	< 0.01	Just significant
Marasmus	30	163.11 ± 10.56	> 0.005	Insignificant

Adopted from Gupte S, Sangra KR, Pal M, Gupta SK: Infantile tremor syndrome: Perspectives and projections. In: Gupte S (ed) *Recent Advances in Pediatrics (Special Vol 9: Neurology).* New Delhi: Jaypee 2001.

establish a cause and effect relationship between zinc deficiency and ITS.

Our recent work[36-38] shows that only infants with severe ITS reveal electroencephalographic (EEG) alterations in the form of high voltage sharp waves and spikes that are consistent with seizure activity. These EEG changes fail to revert soon after full cessation of the tremors. How long these take to disappear is yet to be studied by us through an extension of this particular study. Right now, we are of the opinion that this sort of EEG pattern is also quite indicative of nutritional factor(s) as its cause in ITS.

This raises a vital question: Why do some ITS infants show EEG changes while others do not?

In order to answer this question, it is important to understand that to produce electrophysiologic disturbances in the cortical neurons to the tune of being recorded as EEG changes, there has got to be some threshold level of stimulus or insult for these neurons. In case this threshold level is attained, the EEG records changes from the scalp surface as we observed in some of our cases of ITS (the severe ones, of course). Once the stimulus or insult restricts itself to the subthreshold level only, the EEG may not record changes as was the case with majority of our cases of ITS (pretremor state, mild to moderate severity cases). In other words, or perhaps, indirectly, one can speculate that greater the brain insult, severe the tremors during active tremor phase and, thereby, more the EEG abnormalities that are recorded. The recovery from this insult may be very gradual and even incomplete. Hence, persistence of EEG changes even after the tremors are fully controlled.

Viral Theory

According to this hypothesis, ITS may well be a sort of viral encephalitis. Acute onset of tremors, their occurrence after intravenous drip or blood transfusion in certain instances, seasonal variation and common accompaniment of respiratory infection are often cited in support of this hypothesis. However, no viral agent has so far been isolated from these subjects. The skin changes, hair changes and anemia too are difficult to ascribe to a viral agent. Moreover, absence of any consistent CSF change and course of the disease do not favor this hypothesis.

Degenerative Theory

The presence of cortical atrophy in brain biopsies and pneumoencephalographic studies and patchy fibrosis of muscle tissue and demyelination and swelling of the myelin sheath of nerves have suggested that ITS may well be a degenerative disorder. This view has not been substantiated.

Metabolic Theory

On the basis of the work carried out in Nagpur, it was postulated that a transient defect in tyrosine metabolism may be responsible for the hair changes in ITS and through involvement of the *substantia nigra* cause tremors and parkinsonian appearance with expressionless facies. This theory too has not received much support.

CLINICAL MANIFESTATIONS

Classically speaking, a typical case of ITS is an infant who is apparently plump in spite of presence of malnutrition. The striking plump look often camouflages the infant's signs of malnutrition. In fact, this factor contributed to erroneous observation by some workers[25] in the past that these infants are usually adequately nourished. Quite a proportion of the patients have clinically demonstrable edema over the pretibial region. In addition, they are characteristically listless, apathetic, and disinterested in the surroundings.

Scalp hair is characteristically sparse and light-colored (hypochromotrichia) as in kwashiorkor or prekwashiorkor.

Brownish dark pigmentation (reticular pigmentation) of skin is present, more so over the dorsal aspects of hands (especially over terminal phalanges close to the nailbeds), feet, knees, ankles, buttocks, axillae, lower abdomen and medial aspect of thighs. Table 27.3 gives the frequency of pigmentation observed by us and some other investigators.

Though some of the subjects have delayed developmental milestones, perhaps from early months, in a vast majority

Table 27.3: Frequency of pigmentary changes in ITS in different studies

Investigator(s)	*Distribution*	*Incidence (%)*
Gupte[28]	Dorsum of hands	100.0
	Dorsum of feet	75.5
	Thighs	60.3
	Generalized	12.5
Ramkumar and Pandove[21]	Dorsum of hands	53.6
	Dorsum of feet	50.5
	Thighs	56.8
	Generalized	7.3
Agarwal *et al.*[32]	Dorsum of hands	93.0
	Dorsum of feet	90.0
	Thighs	56.0
	Generalized	10.0

there is a regression of motor and mental milestones in the recent past. The infant has a dull expressionless (masklike) face with open mouth, drooling of saliva and listlessness. He fails to recognize mother and shows poor response to bright color objects.

The onset of tremors is usually preceded or accompanied by an acute stress in the form of an acute lower respiratory tract infection (LRTI), gastroenteritis, pertussis or measles (Table 27.4).

Table 27.4: Relative frequency of dominant precipitating/ aggravating factors in ITS in author's experience

Factor	*Frequency*
URTI	20%
LRTI	50%
AGE	20%
Infectious illnesses (measles, pertussis, chickenpox)	10%

Tremors, as a rule, have an acute onset. Initially, these are intermittent but become continuous in a few days. These are more prominent in distal parts of the limbs, head, face and tongue. Even trunk may be involved. A tremulous cry resembling the bleating of a lamb is quite characteristic. There is a tendency for the tremors to diminish or disappear during sleep. Tremors may be generalized or may involve one or more limbs, tongue, head, face in various combinations. The frequency of tremors varies between 60 and 140/minute. The site of origin of tremors appears to be cortical neurons.

Anemia is usually moderate. It may be of any morphologic type: microcytic-hypochromic, normocytic-normochromic, macrocytic/megaloblastic or dimorphic.

Hypotonia with flabbiness of the muscles, especially involving thighs, is common. In a small proportion of cases, there may be hypertonia. In some, muscle tone remains unaffected.

In addition to the associated protein-energy malnutrition, incidence of variable *nutritional deficiencies* is high (Table 27.5). In quite a significant proportion of cases, presence

Table 27.5: Relative incidence of concomitant infections/ nutritional deficiencies

Tuberculosis	20%
Intestinal parasitosis	30%
Skin infections	25%
PEM	100%
Anemia	100%
Vitamin deficiencies	75%

of pitting edema in pretibial area justifies the concomitant diagnosis of kwashiorkor. Interestingly, literature from other centers hardly makes mention about the concurrent occurrence of ITS and kwashiorkor (not even prekwashiorkor). This situation must not be confused with the so-called "Kahn's syndrome" which is characterized by coarse tremors, parkinsonian rigidity, bradykinesia and myoclonus. The most remarkable thing about this transient state is that it occurs 6 to several days after initiating nutritional rehabilitation in infants and children with advanced protein-energy malnutrition. The ITS, on the other hand, is a phenomenon that occurs before—rather much before— nutrition correction is instituted.

Incomplete forms of ITS, including the so-called "pretremor state" (all the cardinal features of the syndrome minus tremors), are too encountered. In our experience, left untreated, these infants are quite likely to develop tremors and, thereby, the full-blown ITS. We have made this observation time and again.[28-31]

According to contemporary thinking, it is advisable to identify ITS as a syndromal state comprising three phases, namely "pretremor", "tremor" and "posttremor" (Table 27.6).[1,27]

Table 27.6: Three phases of infantile tremor syndrome (ITS)

Pretremor (Prodromal) phase

Regression of motor and mental milestones as such or on top of "delay" right from the very early weeks or months of life, anemia, pigmentation, hair changes, plumpiness despite existence of malnutrition, expressionless facies with open mouth and drooling.

Tremor (Classical) phase

Appearance of parkinsonism-like coarse rhythmic tremors on top of the clinical features of pretremor phase. To begin, tremors are seen only on crying or feeding and involve fingers, face and tongue and are intermittent. Subsequently, these often become continuous and generalized.

Post-tremor (Recovery) phase

Regression of tremors and other features of the syndrome. Mental dullness continues for several months and, in a large proportion of cases, for quite a few years.

DIAGNOSIS

By and large, ITS is a clinical entity. A high index of suspicion and familiarity with the clinical profile of ITS constitute the cornerstone of its diagnosis. Invariably, the clinical picture is so striking that a clinician who has seen such a case earlier is able to recognize infants with ITS. No laboratory finding is, in any way, specific for this condition.

Investigations should, therefore, be limited to those directed at:

- Finding the extent and morphology of anemia through hemoglobin, peripheral blood film and bone marrow.
- Finding the nutritional status.
- Detecting coexisting infection/infestation through X-ray of the chest and multiple stool microscopy.

Occasionally, a lumbar puncture may become necessary to rule out a CNS infection. Else, there is absolutely no need to carry out LP as a routine in ITS (Table 27.7).

Electroencephalogram (EEG) may reveal changes in ITS with gross tremors. These are similar to those seen in seizure disorder and are in the form of high voltage sharp waves and spikes with a slow background activity of delta range.

Table 27.7: Investigations required in ITS

Usually recommended
- Hemoglobin
- Peripheral film/total and differential counts
- Serum proteins
- Bone marrow
- Chest X-ray
- Tuberculin (Mantoux) test/BCG diagnostic test
- Stool examination for ova and cysts

Occasionally recommended, especially when in doubt
- EEG
- CSF
- CT scan

MANAGEMENT

Anemia

The cornerstone of effective management of ITS is adequate treatment of accompanying anemia and nutritional deficiency states together with good nursing care. Zinc in therapeutic doses is very much in order. However, the earlier practice of giving high doses of vitamin B_{12} to every infant with ITS by some workers needs to be discouraged. The morphologic type of anemia should dictate the choice of hematinic(s) that are to be employed.

Some cases with severe anemia may need a blood transfusion.

Other Nutritional Deficiencies

It is usual to find direct or indirect evidence of associated nutritional deficiencies (say protein-energy, vitamin A and D, vitamin C and B-complex) which should be promptly treated for adequate response.

Tremors

Unless the tremors are mild, it is desirable to administer oral phenobarbital (3 to 5 mg/kg/day). The drug reduces the intensity of tremors and may even control these in due course. Furthermore, it protects the infant from endless exhaustion and provides much needed psychologic relief to the anxious parents. With its use, the period required for control of tremors too is likely to be reduced.

In case of poor response of tremors to phenobarbital (a situation which is quite infrequent in our experience, provided that we do not get impatient), alternative agents like chloropromazine, propranolol, carbamazepine, valproic acid, etc. (Table 27.8) may be employed.[1,30,39]

Their use should, however, be considered as "second line" tremor-control therapy.

Table 27.8 : Drugs used in controlling tremors in ITS

Drug	*Dose*
Usually	
Phenobarbital	3-5 mg/kg/day (O) in divided doses
In selected cases	
Chlorpromazine	2-3 mg/kg/day (O) in divided doses
Carbamazepine	10-20 mg/kg/day (O) in divided doses
Valproate	20-30 mg/kg/day (O) in divided doses
Propranolol	0.5–1.0 mg/kg/day (O) in divided doses

Associated Infections/Infestations

Over and above these measures, the infant must receive adequate treatment for associated infections, including URTI and LRTI, intestinal parasitosis, tuberculosis, etc. One of the vital factors contributing to poor control of tremors is inadequacy of treatment of coexisting infection(s). A noteworthy observation made by us and several other workers[27] is that response of ITS-associated pneumonia to conventional antibiotic therapy is often unsatisfactory, warranting institution of more energetic chemotherapy and other measures. These are the instances where the course of tremors may well be unduly prolonged, causing temptation to the attending physician to put the child on a stronger alternative agent for controlling the tremors.

Whereas onset of tremors is usually abrupt, their cessation is a slow process. To begin with, there is a gradual reduction in their amplitude and severity. Then, these become intermittent and finally stop. At times, these may persist in one extremity or more for a longer period than the rest of the body. Eventually, all cases become tremor-free in due course.

Prognosis and Course

The earlier impression that ITS is by and large a self-limiting condition does not appear to be entirely true in the light of recent experience. Though some of the cases with mild disease may show recovery with cessation of tremors without any medical intervention in 1 to 4 weeks time, severe illness usually needs correction of nutritional anemia and associated deficiencies together with phenobarbital and control of precipitating and or superimposed infection(s).

The cessation of tremors is, as a rule, slow. Pigmentary changes in skin and scalp hair take longer time to clear—usually around 3 months or so. Respiratory infections are not only common but take longer time to respond to adequate treatment.

Mental dullness and sluggishness last much longer. By now, we have a follow-up of several adequately treated cases spread over several years, including *some* who are in their 20s. Most of them continue to be relatively dull and physically retarded in relation to their peers from the same stock.

Electroencephalographic changes, encountered in advanced ITS, perhaps, take longer time to regress than the tremors. We are currently endeavoring to evaluate this aspect of ITS.[40]

No doubt, ITS *per se* is not a fatal disease. Nevertheless, fatalities as a result of a precipitating or superimposed illness such as bronchopneumonia, gastroenteritis, pertussis, measles, etc. are not infrequent.

Since, following treatment, ITS cases return to the same environment, the possibility of recurrence of tremors is always on the card. However, we have not as yet encountered any such occurrence amongst the cases we could follow-up.

With better understanding of its different aspects and improved care, the mortality rate has fallen over the years. This is borne out by our wide experience in relation to this movement disorder as summarized in Table 27.9.[41]

Table 27.9: Mortality in ITS observed in Government Children Hospital and SMGS Hospital, Government Medical College, Jammu, India

Representative period	*No. of cases*	*No. of deaths*	*Mortality (%)*
1975-1978	75	11	14.6
1985-1988	69	7	10.1
1995-1998	60	3	5.0
1998-2001	66	3	4.2
2001-2002	74	3	4.0
2002-2005[8]	72	3	4 %

[8]Data Courtesy Medical Superintendent and Record Section, SMGSs Hospital, Jammu, India.

Section 7

REFERENCES

1. Gupte S. Miscellaneous and unclassified issues. In: Gupte S (ed) *The Short Textbook of Pediatrics* 11th edn. New Delhi: Jaypee 2009;723-737.
2. Dikshit AK. Nutritional dystrophy and anemia. *Indian J Child Health* 1957;6:132-136.
3. Pohowalla JN, Koul KK, Bhandari NR, *et al.* Infantile meningo-encephalitic syndrome. *Indian J Pediatr* 1960;27:49-57.
4. Jadhav M, Webb JKB, Vaishnava S. Vitamin B_{12} deficiency in Indian infants: A clinical syndrome. *Lancet* 1962;2:903-906.
5. Kaul KK, Prasan N, Choudhary RM. Some clinical observations and impressions on a syndrome of tremors in infants from India. *J Pediatr* 1963;63:1158-1166.
6. Sachdev KK, Manchanda SS, Lal H. The syndrome of tremors, mental regression and anemia in infants and young children: A study of 102 cases. *Indian Pediatr* 1965;2:239-251.
7. Srikantia SG, Reddy V. Megaloblastic anemia of infancy and vitamin B_{12}. *Br J Hematol* 1976;13:949-953.
8. Bajpai PC, Misra PK, Tandon PN. Serum vitamin B_{12} in infantile tremor syndrome. *Indian J Med Res* 1968;56:1398-1405.
9. Bajpai PC, Misra PK, Tandon PN. Further observations on infantile tremor syndrome. *Indian J Pediatr* 1968;5:297-302.
10. Bajpai PC, Misra PK, Tandon PN, *et al.* Infantile tremor syndrome. *Indian Pediatr* 1969;6:249-253.
11. Garg BK, Srivastava JR. Infantile tremor syndrome. *Indian J Pediatr* 1969;36:213-228.
12. Mathur GP, Dayal RS, Prasad R, *et al.* Tremors, mental and physical retardation, light-colored hair and anemia in malnourished children. *Indian Pediatr* 1969;6:483-487.
13. Deshpandey TV, Ingle VN. Tremor syndrome in children. *Indian Pediatr* 1969;6:550-555.
14. Misra PK, Tandon PN, Bajpai PC. Infantile tremor syndrome. *Indian Pediatr* 1971;8:62-64.
15. Mahajan CM, Walia BNS, Dutta BN. Infantile tremor syndrome: Some aspects of serum biochemistry and liver histology. *Indian Pediatr* 1971;8:831-833.
16. Chhaparwal BC, Singh SD, Mehta S, *et al.* Magnesium levels in serum and in CSF in meningoencephalitic syndrome (tremor syndrome). *Indian J Pediatr* 1971;38:331-333.
17. Kaul KK. Syndrome of tremors in Indian infants. *J Indian Med Ass* 1972;59:473-477.
18. Gupte S, Pada V, Mullick DN. Infantile tremor syndrome in Chandigarh and Simla. *Indian Pract* 1973;26:45-49.
19. Agarwal SP, Katiyar GP. Infantile tremor syndrome. *Pediatr Clin India* 1972;7:203.
20. Sharma U, Saxena S. Infantile tremor syndrome. *Indian Med Gazette* 1974;14:140.
21. Ramkumar L, Pandove SP. Infantile tremor syndrome. *Indian J Pediatr* 1975;42:215-225.
22. Manchanda SS, Gupte S. Infantile tremor syndrome. In: Gupte S (Ed): *Newer Horizons in Tropical Pediatrics.* New Delhi: Jaypee 1977;297-301-307.
23. Gupta BD, Maheshwari RK, Miglani N. Infantile tremor syndrome. *Indian J Pediatr* 1978;45:221-228.
24. Gupte S, Pal M: Infantile tremor syndrome: Observations on north Indian children. *Indian Pract* 1979; 32:369-375.
25. Sharda B, Bhandari B. Infantile tremor syndrome. *Indian Pediatr* 1987;24:415-421.
26. Gupte S. Infantile tremor syndrome. *Indian Pediatr* 1987;24:1159.
27. Sharda B. Infantile tremor syndrome. In: Gupte S, Gupte SB (eds): *Recent Advances in Pediatrics, Vol.* 3. New Delhi. Jaypee 1993;155-164.
28. Gupte S. Infantile tremor syndrome: A growing Asian problem. *5th Intern Congr Child Neurol* Tokyo, 1990.
29. Gupte S. Perspectives in infantile tremor syndrome. *30th Nat Conf, Indian Acad Pediatr* Calcutta, 1992.
30. Gupte S. Infantile tremor syndrome: Newer insights. *Conjoint Meeting, Child Neurology Society/Intern Child Neurol Ass* San Francisco, 1994.

31. Gupte S, Pal M. Infantile tremor syndrome-1995. *9th World Congress of Pediatrics* London, 1995.
32. Agarwal R, Gupta BD, Agarwal DK, *et al.* A clinical study of nutritional tremor syndrome. *SDMJ* 1989;13:185-190.
33. Gupte S, Bhave R, Mary J. Hair zinc in infantile tremor syndrome. *Asian Med News* 1995;9:7.
34. Gupte S, Bhave R, Mary J, *et al.* Hair zinc in kwashiorkor, infantile tremor syndrome and other forms of malnutrition. *Asian Med News* 1997;11:15.
35. Gupte S. Zinc deficiency. *Am J Clin Nutr* 1976;29: 235.
36. Sangra KR, Gupte S, Pal M, Gupta SK. EEG changes in infantile tremor syndrome. *5th Intern Congs Trop Pediatr* Jaipur, 1999.
37. Gupte S, Pal M. Pediatric movement disorders (with special reference to ITS) in north India (Guest lecture). *6th Asian-Oceanian Congress of Neurology,* Singapore, 1999. Abstract No AOCN-V/39.
38. Gupte S. Infantile tremor syndrome (ITS). In: Gupte S (ed): *Recent Advances in Pediatrics (Special Vol. 6: Gastroenterology, Hepatology and Nutrition)* New Delhi. Jaypee 2000:509-517.
39. Kalra V, Marwaha RK. Propranolol in infantile tremor syndrome. *Indian J Pediatr* 1981;49:341-343.
40. Gupte S, Sangra KR, Pal M, Gupta SK. Infantile tremor syndrome: Perspectives and projections. In: Gupte S, Gupte SB (eds) *Recent Advances in Pediatrics (Special Vol 9: Neurology*) New Delhi. Jaypee 2001.
41. Gupte S. Guest lecture: Movement disorders with special reference to ITS. *Proceedings 6th International Symposium on Child Neurology*, Sydney 2003. Sydney: ISCN 2003. Abstract ISCN/N-3.

Section 7

Suraj Gupte

28 Acrodermatitis Enteropathica

INTRODUCTION

Also called *Brandt syndrome*, this uncommon genetic condition, was first described way back in 1942 by Danbolt and Closs. It is characterized by chronic diarrhea, skin lesions, alopecia and growth failure and is usually seen in 3 weeks to 18 months age group (often following shift from breast to cow milk or, occasionally, in neonates and infants on bottle feeding).[1-5] Zinc deficiency because of zinc malabsorption as a result of an inborn error of metabolism is responsible for the condition.

The classical form is a familial disorder with autosomal recessive inheritance. Recent studies show impairment of lymphatic function and free radical scavenging.

ETIOPATHOGENESIS

In the classical form, the fundamental defect is defective absorption of zinc, in all probability due to absence of a specific carrier protein. Such a malabsorption occurs in two situations:

1. At the time of weaning from breast to artificial feeding.
2. In a bottlefed infant, particularly a preterm baby, in first few weeks of life.

By and large, breast milk is supposed to be protective because of greater bioavailability of zinc in it than in bovine milk.

Since most of the zinc accretion in the fetus occurs in the last trimester, a deficiency in zinc stores may precipitate symptoms early in neonatal period in preterm babies. The condition may manifest in full-term babies later if the mother suffers from zinc deficiency with the production of low zinc level breast milk.

Recently, the focus for acrodermatitis enteropathica has been mapped to band 8q24.3.

In case of infants suffering from acrodermatitis enteropathica, the absence of a binding ligand appears to be contributing to zinc malabsorption.

CLINICAL FEATURES

Usually, manifesting after weaning, the condition is characterized by chronic diarrhea (sometimes with steatorrhea), a symmetrical rash or vesicobulbous, eczematous, dry, scaly or psoriasiform lesions, paronychia and dystrophy.

Notably, skin lesions are most marked over mucocutaneous junctions i.e. around body orifices (periorifacial) such as anus, genitalia, mouth and cheeks and extremities i.e. knees and elbows, hands and feet (acral).

Nail dystrophy may be encountered in some cases.

Hair loss, usually some alopecia, is often present, the leftover hair frequently demonstrating a characteristic redish tinge.

Ocular lesions include blephritis, conjunctivitis and photophobia.

Neurologic disturbances, irritability and behavioral changes may occur.

Superadded infections (both bacterial and fungal) may occur. Superimposed *Candida albicans* infection tends to modify the clinical picture.

Remaining accompaniments include stomatitis, glossitis, anorexia and delayed wound healing.

Left untreated, the child suffers from considerable failure to thrive and growth retardation.

Table 28.1 lists the clinical presentation in 32 children with this disorder seen by the author[3] over a span of three decades and William and William's series[7] comprising 110 cases.

DIFFERENTIAL DIAGNOSIS[1-5]

Differential diagnosis includes a similar syndrome manifesting as a result of:

- Long-term total parenteral nutrition (TPN) when unsupplemented with zinc.
- Chronic malabsorption.
- Advanced PEM.

Table 28.1: Salient features in 32 subjects with acrodermatitis enteropathica in an Indian series (32 cases) and an African series (110 cases)

Parameter	*Incidence*	
	African Series[6]	*Indian Series*[3]
Age	6 ± 2.1	9 ± 2.03
Skin lesions	90%	100%
Hair loss	82%	90%
Nail involvement	52%	50%
Chronic diarrhea	80%	100%
Failure to thrive	60%	75%
Anorexia	60%	90%
Irritability	66%	80%
Ocular lesions	50%	62%
Superadded infection	25%	40%
Mortality	5%	2%

- Breastfeeding by mothers who are zinc deficient.
- Immunodeficiency disease.
- Cystic fibrosis.
- Maple syrup urine disease.
- Organic aciduria.
- Essential fatty acid deficiency.
- Biotinidase deficiency.
- Methylmalonic acid deficiency.

DIAGNOSIS

Clinical judgement forms the cornerstone of diagnosis. The diagnosis must be considered in any infant presenting with chronic diarrhea, skin lesion around the body orifices, hair loss, and failure to thrive.

Investigations show reduction in serum zinc level (< 50 mcg/dl) and alkaline phosphatase level.

Endoscopic jejunal biopsy reveals paneth cell inclusions with parakeratosis and pallor of the upper epidermis.

MANAGEMENT

Response to zinc (as zinc sulfate or zinc gluconate) administration (1-2 mg/kg/day of elemental zinc) is dramatic, causing clearing of skin lesions and improvement in diarrheal state.

Now that medicinal zinc is readily available, use of diiodohydroxyquin which also yields gratifying result has become obsolete.[1] The risk of optic neuritis in children on diiodohydroxyquin weighed against its use.

Though most infants need zinc therapy just for a week or two, in some subjects, zinc administration needs to be continued indefinitely.[2]

PROGNOSIS

Timely treatment leads to excellent response though in a small proportion of cases prolonged therapy may be needed to safeguard from recurrences. Left untreated. It may end up with:

- Severe malnutrition.
- Superimposed infections.
- Death.

PREVENTION

The most important preventive measure is ensuring intake of high zinc-containing diet by the mother, especially during pregnancy and lactation,[7] say:

- Grains.
- Nuts.
- Cheese.
- Oysters.
- Meat.
- Egg.

REFERENCES

1. Gupte S, Anderson RA. Pediatric gastroenterology. In: Gupte S (ed): *The Short Textbook of Pediatrics*, 11th edn. New Delhi: Jaypee 2009;443-478.
2. Brown E. *Pediatric Dermatology*. London: Smith and Smith 2004.
3. Gupte S. Acrodermatitis enteropathica: Three decades' experience of a pediatrician. *Dermatol Chron* 2001;2:62-65.
4. Darmstadt GL, Schimdt CP, Wechsler DS, *et al*. Dermatitis as a presenting sign of cystic fibrosis. *Arch Dermatol* 1992;128:1358-1361.
5. Hansen RC, Lemon R, Revsin B. Cystic fibrosis manifesting with acrodermatitis enteropathica-like eruption. *Arch Dermatol* 1983;119:51-53.
6. Willian S, Willian C. Acrodermatis enteropathica: Observations on 100 cases. *S Afr J Dermatol Pract* 1979;7:231-236.
7. Murray MT. *The Healing Power of Foods*. Recklin: Prime 1993.

Suraj Gupte • Swati Ghosh • EM Gomez

29 Protein-Energy Malnutrition: Overview

INTRODUCTION

Nutritional deficiencies constitute a major public health problem in India and other countries of the Third World. The severe forms, *kwashiorkor* and *marasmus*, are the leading killers of our pediatric population. Whereas chronic malnutrition causes stunting in the long run, survivors of malnutrition in fetal life and infancy run the risk of cognitive dysfunction as well. Considerable morbidity (and, at times mortality) accompanies others such as nutritional anemias and vitamin deficiencies.

DEFINITION

The term, *protein-energy malnutrition*, refers to a class of clinical conditions that may result from varying degree of protein lack and energy (calorie) inadequacy. This nomenclature replaced the relatively older designation, i.e. protein-calorie malnutrition, on the recommendation of the World Health Organization (WHO) and Food and Agriculture Organization (FAO).[1-3]

This term has been adopted because it is now generally agreed that the major limiting factors in the diet of children, particularly in the countries of the Third World, are energy and proteins, usually more of the former. Deficiency of proteins is usually not primary and isolated. Almost always it appears to be due to poor intake of food (energy) as such. There is evidence that if child's energy is taken care of, it will be difficult for him to have significant protein deficiency. Else, if his energy consumption is poor, whatever proteins he takes are likely to be burnt to provide energy rather than to build the tissues.

Among the various factors that influence the clinical manifestations of protein-energy malnutrition (PEM) figure magnitude of deprivation, its duration, relative inadequacy of different principles of food and the accompanying infection or some other disease.

Broadly speaking, two major clinical syndromes, *kwashiorkor* and *nutritional marasmus*, are widely recognized. Kwashiorkor is said to result from gross deficiency of proteins though energy deficiency is also present. Nutritional marasmus, on the other hand, results from gross deficiency of energy though protein deficiency also accompanies. Thus, it is clear that there is deficiency of both, proteins and energy, in both the states. The predominance of the deficiency determines whether it is going to be kwashiorkor or nutritional marasmus.

Many malnourished children show overlap in the clinical picture, demonstrating features of both the deficiency states at a time. It is often quite appropriate to label them as *marasmic-kwashiorkor*.

But, the aforesaid severe form of PEM constitute only a tip of the widespread problem of malnutrition. A vast majority of the children suffering from mild to moderate forms of it remain hidden in the community for one or another reason. The two types of this subclinical malnutrition are: nutritional dwarfing and pre-kwashiorkor.

All these form of PEM, in actuality, constitute a continuous spectrum of the manifestations of malnutrition. Growth failure and poor tissue repair (due to protein lack) and energy shortage (due to calorie deficiency) are common to all the forms.

PREVALENCE AND MAGNITUDE

Around 25% (1 in every 4) of world's children suffer from significant PEM. Interestingly, a vast majority (70%) of them are in Asia and the remaining 30% in Africa, Caribbean and Africa.[4]

Just a word about the scenario in India! According to National Family Health Surveys (NFHS):

- Proportion of underweight children <3 years fell from 53% (1992-93) to 47% (1998-99).
- Proportion of several underweight children < 3 yeas fell from 20% (1992-93) to 18% (1998-99).
- Proportion of stunted children <3 years fell from 52% (1992-93) to 45% (1998-99).
- Proportion of severely stunted children <3 years fell from 29% to 23% (1998-99).

Evidently, though there has been some decline in prevalence of PEM in India over the past, the problem still continues to be of public health magnitude.[5,6] According to Ghosh,[7] "the intergenerational cycle of malnutrition is as widespread as before".

For, even now, around 60-75% of India's pediatric population is suffering from one or another nutritional deficiency. About 50-70% of the hospitalized children in our experience suffer from some degree or type of malnutrition. Around 25% of the pediatric beds are occupied by patients whose major problem is malnutrition or in whom malnutrition is indirectly responsible for hospitalization.

According to conservative estimates, gross malnutrition is said to kill around 5,00,000 of infants and children every year in India alone.

EVOLUTION

Dietetic Hypothesis

According to the widely-accepted *dietetic hypothesis*. Kwashiorkor is predominantly a protein deficiency and marasmus an energy deficiency. Of course, both proteins and energy, lack exist in both the syndromes. This hypothesis has a good deal of support from studies in the laboratory animals as well as work on human beings.

Gopalan's Adaptation Hypothesis

The noted nutritionist, Gopalan, has claimed that dietary background of children suffering from kwashiorkor and marasmus may well be the same. According to his postulation, the so-called *adaptation hypothesis*, marasmus is an extreme degree of adaptation to prolonged inadequacy of proteins and energy in the diet. Kwashiorkor is a stage of adaptation failure or dysadaptation which may follow two situations. First: Continued prolongation of the stress of malnutrition. Second: Sudden precipitation or aggravation by a fulminant infection such as measles, pertussis, bronchopneumonia or acute diarrheal episode.

Gopalan feels that whereas nutritional marasmus may be the result of extreme degree of adaptation and the kwashiorkor the result of dysadaptation, relatively mild effect of adaptation may be responsible for nutritional dwarfing. Since, according to Gopalan's hypothesis, kwashiorkor often follows occurrence of dysadaptation in a marasmic child, most of the cases are likely to show features of both, i.e., marasmic kwashiorkor.

Golden's Hypothesis of Free Radical Damage

According to Golden's *hypothesis of free radical damage*, kwashiorkor results from overproduction of free radicals (because of infection, toxins, iron, etc.) and breakdown of protective mechanism (provided by vitamin A and E, carotene, zinc, copper, selenium, manganese, etc.).

Free radical production is far more in kwashiorkor than in marasmus and can account for the full spectrum of clinical picture of kwashiorkor. For example, in kwashiorkor, free radical damage can explain development of:

- Edema (from damage to cell membrane and the resultant increase in permeability).
- Fatty liver.
- Dermatoses.

Hypothesis of Multiple Interactions and Sequelae

According to Jelliffe,[8] kwashiorkor is an intrinsically nutritional disorder with vulnerability to other factors, some identified and some unidentified. It is the cumulative result of a *mixture of interactions and sequelae* of dietary imbalances and/or deficiency, infections, parasitosis, emotional trauma from maternal deprivation due to abrupt weaning from breasts, toxins like aflatoxin or ochratoxin.

Aflatoxin Contamination

Recently, it has been postulated that *aflatoxin contamination* of food may well be an important factor in the causation of kwashiorkor.

PEM AND DISTURBANCES OF METABOLISM[9]

Many like to designate PEM as a "metabolic disorder". This is quite understandable if we recall that the disease is characterized by profound disturbances of water and electrolytes, minerals, protein, fat, carbohydrate and energy metabolism.

Water, Electrolytes and Minerals

Total body water: It has now become clear that total body water is increased in PEM, irrespective whether it is of kwashiorkor or marasmic type. Also, it has been convincingly demonstrated that a positive correlation exists between the magnitude of rise in body water and the extent of weight loss. Thus, lowest values are found in kwashiorkor and the highest in marasmus.

Whether the alteration is secondary to increased cellular mass which constitutes the active protoplasm of the body and reduction in the adipose tissue is not clearly understood.

A noteworthy point is that despite increased body water, a malnourished child is thirsty. This paradoxical observation is ascribed to the defective thirst mechanism in PEM.

Potassium

There is a definite reduction in the total body potassium by as much as 25%. All organs are depleted of potassium but the musculature suffers the most followed by the brain. There is evidence that potassium depletion is more marked in cases of PEM with diarrheal disease. In kwashiorkor, it is significant even in the absence of diarrhea. Whether potassium depleteion results from gastrointestinal losses through the gut or from defects in specific enzymes that have a role in carbohydrate metabolism, or both, is not clear. It is to be remembered that potassium deficiency may be existing despite absence of any clinical manifestations of dehydration and/or hypokalemia.

A very high frequency of pyelonephritis and acute renal failure is encountered in cases of severe malnutrition whose potassium depletion has not been attended to. Of course, the contributory role of concomitant dehydration and infection cannot be denied.

Sodium

Unlike potassium depletion, sodium is retained by the body. Sodium retention is primarily extracellular though muscle, skin, brain and viscera, too, are affected.

Intracellular sodium retention and potassium deficit may change the function of important enzymes in carbohydrate metabolism and oxidative phosphorylation.

Magnesium

Despite some confusion in the past, today it has been accepted that there is magnesium depletion in PEM. This deficiency may cause grave disturbances, including neurologic signs such as twitching, tremors and convulsions.

Phosphorus

Phosphorus metabolism in PEM has not yet been adequately investigated. The present consensus is that both forms of phosphorus—organic as well as inorganic—are decreased in the muscles of malnourished children. Adequate nutritional correction leads to increase in both the forms. The exact significance of this observation, particularly from a clinical angle, remains obscure.

Calcium

Calcium depletion is a common feature of PEM, more so when the assessment is based on blood levels. However, clinical evidence of tetany is infrequent.

Iron

Iron deficiency anemia is a common feature of PEM. It is, however, complicated by other deficiencies involving folic acid, vitamin B_{12} vitamin E and probably some other vitamins.

Copper

Low levels of copper in serum, hair and liver of subjects suffering from PEM have been documented. There may also be low levels of ceruloplasmin which plays the role of a "link" in copper and iron metabolism.

Chromium

Chromium deficiency has been blamed for the impaired glucose tolerance in malnourished children. There is evidence that it may contribute to poor growth of the child during the earlier stage of nutritional rehabilitation. Chromium therapy may accelerate growth in marasmic infants.

Zinc

Several investigations have suggested low serum as well as muscle and liver zinc values in PEM. Evidence collected from Middle-East has indicated that zinc deficiency may play an important role in the etiology of the *syndrome of growth retardation with short stature, hypogonadism, hepatosplenomegaly and anemia* in boys of those regions. The supplementation of zinc to such boys results in a dramatic improvement. Some time, within three weeks of initiating treatment, significant gain in weight and acceleration of sexual maturity are achieved.

Protein and Amino Acids

Total serum protein level is always reduced, principally due to hypoalbuminemia which is very remarkable in kwashiorkor. The level of beta-globulins is also reduced. Alpha and gamma-globulin level is variable in absolute terms; it is invariably high in relation to other serum protein fractions.

There is a remarkable reduction in the total body protein. Its turnover, unlike that of albumin, may be high rather than low.

Significant reduction in plasma amino acids occurs in kwashiorkor. Valine, leucine, isoleucine and tyrosine are the ones most affected. There is a rise in amino acid recycling in kwashiorkor. This mechanism, together with low urea synthesis, increased ammonia and urea nitrogen utilization for protein synthesis, contributes to increased nitrogen economy in protein deficiency.

Lipids

There is a reduction in fat absorption from the gut. Also, there is increase in fecal fat even when diet is free from fat. Free bile acids are increased whereas there is a decrease in the concentration of conjugated bile acids. The latter are supposed to be essential for dissolution of lipids in the lumen of the gut and their eventual absorption.

The transport of fat from liver to tissues as low density lipoproteins is considerably reduced though transport from gut to liver is not much altered.

Various factors that may contribute to the fatty liver of kwashiorkor are increased fat transport from tissues to liver, reduced synthesis of beta-lipoproteins, increased liver lipogenesis, and probably reduced level of essential fatty acids.

Carbohydrates and Energy

Hypoglycemia occurs frequently and may prove fatal in a proportion of cases. Glucose absorption is impaired due to deficiency of disaccharidase enzymes in the intestinal mucosa. Handling of intravenously administered glucose and galactose is abnormal. Circulating insulin levels are low. The levels fail to respond to stimulation with glucose or arginine.

Disaccharide intolerance is a common transient phenomenon. Hence, it is advisable to avoid large loads of lactose containing foodstuffs during early part of management of PEM.

Levels of growth hormone are high but of somatostatin low. Basal metabolic rate (BMR) is reduced. Thyroid function, too, is low.

PEM AND INFECTION

The interaction between infection and nutrition has been a subject of countless studies. Today it is widely recognized that there is a definite association between malnutrition and infection.

Malnutrition is the most common immunodeficiency in pediatric practice and breaks down the host resistance in by and large all segments. The most consistent abnormality detected in various studies has been the impairment in cell-mediated immunity (CMI). That explains why bacterial infections, which count on CMI for host's defence against them, are very severe in children suffering from PEM. Secondly, children with PEM are difficult to sensitize by repeated antigens. Thirdly, even the delayed hypersensitivity reactions that recall previous sensitization are also delayed.

There is evidence that iron deficiency anemia has an adverse effect on the cellular immune response.

The underlying mechanisms include lymphopenia, reduced number of T-lymphocytes in the peripheral blood, impaired response to mitogen and antigens, decreased lymphokine production and serum inhibition.

It has been demonstrated that levamisole improves the ability of lymphocytes to proliferate *in vitro* in response to phytomitogens and increases the number of rosetting T-lymphocytes. However, the effect on lymphocyte stimulation response is less than that achieved by nutritional supplementation both at 2 and 4-week intervals after initiation of therapy. When given together with nutritional rehabilitation, levamisole administration is associated with an increase in cell-mediated response *in vivo* and *in vitro*, the change being observed earlier than a significant gain in weight. The clinical significance of these observations is not yet clear.

Interrelationship between PEM and infection is summarized in Box 29.1.

Box 29.1: Interrelationship between PEM and infection

Causes of Malnutrition leading to Infection:
- Micronutrient deficiency: Iron, zinc, copper, selenium
- Vitamin deficiency: Vitamin A, C, E, B_6, folate
- Impaired cell-mediated immunity (CMI), phagocytic function and complement system
- Reduced cytokine production
- Reduced concentration of IgA, IgM and IgG

Causes of Infection leading to Malnutrition:
- Reduced intake of food, especially micronutrients
- Enhanced catabolic losses
- Reduced absorption of nutrients
- Metabolic inefficiency because of micronutrient deficiency

PEM AND FAMILY PLANNING

In developing countries, women (often malnourished) begin to produce children at a much younger age. They continue doing so quite frequently with poor spacing. Result: too many births. What is still more disturbing is that they continue doing so as long as they are not old enough.

This phenomenon leads to impaired nutritional status of both the mother and her babies, many of whom may be born after intrauterine growth retardation has already affected their bodies and perhaps brains. Such infants start life with a distinct disadvantage. They are also candidates for high morbidity and mortality.

Undoubtedly many of such deaths could be prevented. The biostatisticians call such deaths as excessive "reproductive wastage".

The question arises: why do women reproduce at such a high pace in developing world? The reason is simple. Unless parents can be assured that the children they have are going to survive into adulthood, they will be unwilling to consider limiting their reproductive activities. It has, therefore, been argued that nutrition and general health activities should be coordinated to provide major support for maintaining health and promoting survival of infants and children.

A strong plea is made for promoting the traditional breastfeeding with suckling done throughout the 24 hours each day. This practice is not only a safeguard against malnutrition but it also has an effect on ovulation and birth spacing.

PEM AND ENDOCRINAL STATUS

Cortisol: Contrary to earlier studies, now it has been convincingly shown that serum cortisol levels in gross PEM are high, suggesting hyperfunction of the adrenal cortex. Such factors as infection and hypoglycemia are said to contribute to this observation.

High cortisol levels mediate the following useful functions:

- Augmentation of lipolysis.
- Enhancement of muscle protein catabolism.
- Promotion of liver protein synthesis.

Somatomedins: Serum levels of insulin like growth factor (IGF-1and 2) are low due to one or more of the following factors:

- Low protein and/or energy supply in diet.
- Lack of essential amino acids.
- Low insulin/cortisol ratio.

Low somatomedins levels mediate the useful function of reducing energy and oxygen utilization by retarding growth.

Insulin: Impaired serum insulin levels are found in kwashiorkor and marasmic kwashiorkor but not in marasmus due to:

- High energy low protein ratio in diet.
- Low body potassium.
- Deficient insulinotropic factors and insulin transport by the damaged pancreas.

Growth hormone: Growth hormone levels are high in PEM, reflecting increased secretion rather than impaired clearance. The causative factors include:

- Low somatomedin levels.
- Hypoalbuminemia and low amino acid levels.
- Low serum tyrosine level.

The useful functions mediated by this observation include:

- Facilitation of the process of lipolysis.
- Boosting of glucogenesis.
- Decrease in catabolism of albumin.

Glucagon: Glucagon levels are high whereas insulin levels are low in PEM, leading to low insulin/glucagon ratio. The following useful functions may be mediated.

- Reduction in glucose uptake by muscles and adipose tissue, sparing heart and brain.
- Increased muscle protein catabolism.
- Increased lipolysis and fatty acid supply to peripheral tissues.

Thyroxine: Contrary to earlier observations, thyroid hormone production is either normal or high in kwashiorkor but normal or low in marasmus.

PEM AND DIARRHEA[2,3,10]

Diarrhea is a common accompaniment of the clinical picture of overt PEM. Its prevalence is 5 to 7 times more and its severity 3 to 4 times greater in malnourished children as compared to normal children. In the not-so-distant past, recurrent diarrhea in malnourished children was generally ascribed to superimposed infections and infestations. No doubt, malnourished patients are particularly susceptible to infection because of the impaired cellular immunity which is an important adverse sequel of malnutrition *per se*.

It was earlier suggested that, besides bacterial and parasitic contamination of the gut, gastrointestinal candidiasis may contribute to the common occurrence of diarrhea in malnutrition. The investigations from Indonesia and Australia lent support to this hypothesis.

Recently, it has been convincingly demonstrated that PEM may *per se* cause striking morphological as well as functional damage to the small intestinal mucosa, leading to malabsorption. Transitory secondary disaccharidase deficiency, causing lactose intolerance and osmotic diarrhea, has also been observed in significant proportion of the cases. The earlier reports suggesting existence of some monosaccharide malabsorption have now been substantiated. Moreover, it is to be noted that iron deficiency is a common occurrence in PEM. Since there is evidence that iron deficiency may itself contribute to an exudative enteropathy in childhood, the role of such anemia in etiology of diarrhea of malnutrition seems to be convincingly established.

A recent study has documented significant decline in histamine augmented maximum acid output as also presence of chronic gastritis and gastric mucosal atrophy in per oral gastric biopsies in marasmic children.

Finally, there is evidence that PEM may give rise to pancreatic atrophy and decreased enzyme secretion. Digestive disturbance and diarrhea may result.

Thus, it becomes obvious that diarrhea in malnutrition is of multifactorial etiology. An absolutely clear picture of the whole problem may emerge in the near future. The information as it stands today, however, does highlight some salient aspects which definitely have bearing on the line of management.

PEM AND CARDIAC FUNCTION

Gross malnutrition is known to considerably reduce the weight and the size of the heart. This is ascribed to atrophy of the cardiac muscle.

On the functional front, cardiac output is reduced in keeping with the severity of weight loss. There is prolongation of the systemic recirculation time, appearance time, bradycardia and reduced peripheral blood flow. Congestive cardiac failure may occur. ECG shows nonspecific changes. Radiology shows reduction in heart size. Not only does malnutrition *per se* affect cardiac function, but other factors such as accompanying severe anemia, reduced oxygen consumption and hypothyroid state too contribute to it.

PEM AND RENAL FUNCTION

PEM causes reversible impairment of renal function as manifested by:

- Reduction in glomerular filtration and renal plasma flow, especially when there is accompany gastroenteritis.
- Aminoaciduria, phosphaturia and inefficient excretion of an acid load from disturbed tubular function.

- Urine is acidic due to increased excretion of hydrogen ions to conserve potassium.

PEM AND DRUG DISPOSITION[11,12]

It is now well established that nutritional status of a child has significant effect on the bioprocesses involved in disposition of various drugs in the body. As a result, bioavailability of the drug(s) for therapeutic purposes is influenced, often warranting alteration in dose and frequency of administration.

The exact observations concerning different drugs in various studies are, however, far from uniform.

CLASSIFICATION

The time-honored classifications based on weight for age (e.g. Gomez's, Indian Academy of Pediatrics, Jeliffe's, Welcome) are now giving way to the classification put forward by WHO[13-17] (Table 29.1) which employs weight for height and height for age and highlights level of wasting and level of stunting.

Table 29.1: WHO classification of PEM

Criteria	*Moderate PEM*	*Severe PEM*
Symmetrical edema	No	Yes (Edematous PEM)
Weight for height (index of wasting)	70-79% of expected (Wasting)	< 70 % of expected (Severe wasting)
Height for age (index of stunting)	85-89% of expected (Stunting)	< 85% of expected (Severe stunting)

As per recommendations of the Indian Academy of Pediatrics, until acceptable Indian data become available, we should continue referring to the Western Standard for comparison. This recommendation has been in keeping with the World Health Organization (WHO) advocacy in favor of the data on north American children supplied by the National Center for Health Statistics (NCHS) as a single international reference standard. This recommendation was based on the observation that all children have the same genetic potential especially in early childhood, and their growth is more influenced by nutrition, illness and environment rather than by heredity. Secondly, it has been convincingly demonstrated that the growth of well-nourished children in the developing countries compares favorably with that of the developed world's children. Across the world, therefore, the old Harvard standards stood replaced by the NCHS/CDC standards. The NCHS/CDC standard has/now been replaced by the 2006-07 WHO standards.

Yet, it has been argued by some workers that since the average stature of Asian children fits about the 25th centile of the NCHS standards, there is need for availability of local standards that are based on well-nourished children and that are periodically upgraded.

SALIENT FEATURES OF SYNDROMAL STATES[18-20]

PEM should be viewed as "continuum", a sort of dynamic process with manifestations that depend on the severity of nutritional deprivation, its duration and associated conditions such as infections and infestations.

Kwashiorkor

The earliest description of kwashiorkor in the English medical literature was made in 1933 by Cicely Williams, a noted British physician. That time she did not really know how to christen the disease. Later, in 1935, she introduced the term "kwashiorkor", the local name for the disease in Ghana. It was said to mean the "red boy", because of the characteristic pigmentary changes. In 1950, the term was more aptly interpreted to apply to the mystique of the disease that affected the deprived child due to the arrival of yet another.

Clinical Features (Figs. 29.1 and 29.2)

The disease is chiefly encountered in infants and children in the preschool age group. A vast majority of the cases are in 1 to 4 years age group. No age is, however, exempt. Occasionally, it may be seen in infants aged few months, in adolescents and even in adults.

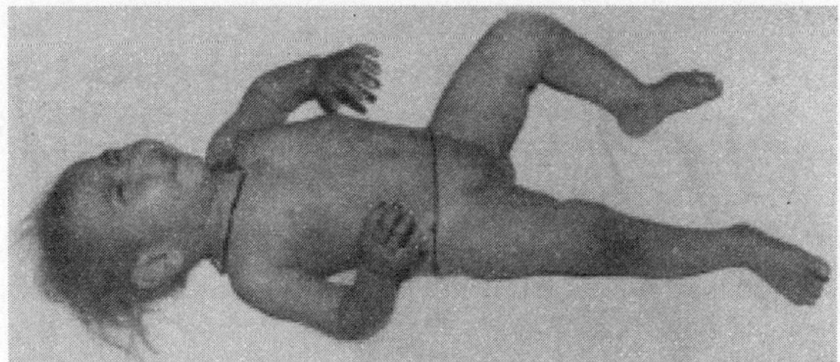

Fig. 29.1: Kwashiorkor: Note the characteristic features, including psychomotor change, oedema and hair changes (See for colour figure Plate 3)

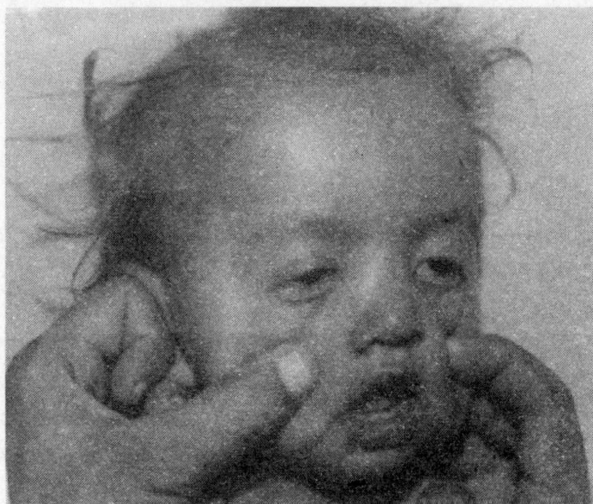

Fig. 29.2: Kwashiorkor: Note the hair changes and pallor. He had pedal edema with minimal ascitis (See for colour figure Plate 3)

A classical case of kwashiorkor is dull, apathetic and miserable, evincing hardly any interest in the surroundings. His growth is stunted and there is marked muscle wasting with some retention of subcutaneous fat. He has pitting edema over the legs and feet and perhaps over certain other parts of the body. There may be diarrhea, skin and hair changes, anemia and vitamin deficiency signs. Liver is, as a rule, enlarged due to fatty change.

Though this is the picture of full-blown kwashiorkor, it may be noted that only four signs growth failure, muscle wasting with retention of some subcutaneous fat, mental apathy and hypoalbuminemic edema (not of cardiac, renal or hepatic origin) taken together are sufficient by themselves to label a case as "kwashiorkor". The remaining elements may individually or collectively accompany the essential features, depending on the severity of the disease, dietary pattern and regional variations.

Biochemical Changes

These are striking. Serum proteins are always low, the maximum reduction being that of the albumin fraction; the globulins may often be found relatively elevated.

Anemia is usually moderate to severe and may be of variable morphology though iron-deficiency is a common denominator in most cases.

Low serum enzymes (esterase, amylase, lipase, cholinesterase and alkaline phosphatase), serum cholesterol, glucose, urea, certain vitamins, potassium and magnesium occur. The activity of pancreatic enzymes is considerably reduced. Total body potassium is diminished.

Imbalance of plasma amino acids and amines aciduria are common findings. Impaired cellular immunity is present.

Diagnosis

Dietetic enquiry reveals deficient intake of both proteins and calories, the protein lack being more predominant, over a prolonged period. Occurrence of an added stress like measles, whooping cough, diarrhea or bronchopneumonia often precipitates the overt picture, leading to development of pitting edema.

Diagnostic criteria may be divided into two major subdivisions: essential and nonessential.

A. **Essential Features** ***(Minimal Diagnostic Criteria)***
1. Growth retardation as evidenced by low weight and low height.
2. Muscle wasting with retention of some subcutaneous fat.
3. Psychomotor change as evidenced by mental apathy in the form of silent listless inertness, lack of interest in the surroundings.
4. Hypoalbuminemic pitting edema, at least over the pretibial region. Serum albumin should be less than 2.5 g/dL and cardiac, hepatic, renal and angioneurotic causes of edema should be led out. These essential features are to be considered the minimal diagnostic criteria for kwashiorkor.

B. **Nonessential Features**: These are variable features and may or may not be present in each and every case.
1. *Hair changes* in the form of hypochromotrichia (light-colored hair), sparseness (areas of alopecia), change in texture (coarseness, silkiness) and easy pluckability. Alternate bands of light and dark color have earned the name "flag sign" which signifies periods of inadequate, adequate and inadequate nutrition over a prolonged period. This fascinating sign is only occasionally encountered.
2. *Skin changes* include light-colored skin but the most classical dermatosis consists of areas of hyperpigmentation intervened by areas of raw red skin caused by shedding of the superficial skin flakes. This has been called *flaky-paint dermatosis*. Another similarly characteristic skin lesions of kwashiorkor is *crazy-pavement dermatosis*. Reticular pigmentation, mosaic dermatosis and pellagra-like lesions over the exposed parts (usually dorsal surfaces) may also be encountered.
   Besides the aforesaid dermatosis, kwashiorkor children may suffer from indolent sores and ulcers besides superadded skin infections like pyodermas and scabies.
3. *Gastrointestinal manifestations* include diarrhea, vomiting and anorexia. In spite of edema, the child may develop dehydration. Diarrhea may be due to:
   a. Superadded intestinal infections and parasitic infestations like Giardia lamblia.
   b. Effect of malnutrition *per se* on intestinal mucosa, causing reversible villous atrophy and malabsorption, inhibition of the activity of the enzyme disaccharidase (mainly lactase), causing disaccharide (mainly lactose) intolerance and damage to the pancreas, and
   c. Iron-deficiency anemia which can, on its own, lead to enteropathy by damaging the intestinal epithelium. Thus, it is obvious that diarrhea in children suffering from kwashiorkor has multifactorial etiology.
4. *Mineral and vitamin deficiencies* are common. Anemia is usually present and is moderate to severe in intensity. It is frequently iron-deficiency type though dimorphic and even pure megaloblastic morphology may be encountered. There is evidence that PEM may *per se* cause anemia. Accompanying factors such as intestinal parasitic infestations and systemic infections may also play a contributory role.

Other mineral deficiencies are those of potassium and magnesium.

Deficiency of vitamin A is frequent and may lead to serious problem of keratomalacia and irreversible blindness.

Deficiencies of vitamin B-complex, C, D and E may also complicate the picture.

5. *Hepatomegaly*, quite often fairly remarkable (liver may touch the umbilicus), is invariably present. The consistency is usually soft, the edge rounded and the surface smooth.
6. *Superadded infections* (say, tuberculosis, bronchopneumonia, enteritis, measles, pyodermas, etc.) and intestinal parasitic infestations (*L. giardia, Ent. histolytica*, roundworm, hookworm, threadworm, *H. nana,* etc.) are common. Infection by gram-negative organisms (usually enteritis and septicemia and occasionally urinary tract infection) are most troublesome to manage in such patients.
7. *Clubbing* may be encountered in a proportion of the children with kwashiorkor as a result of the accompanying steatorrhea.
8. *Nonspecific ECG changes* may be found in a small proportion of the cases. A significant cardiac involvement is seldom seen.

Nutritional Marasmus

Though kwashiorkor has received far greater attention from the researchers, nutritional marasmus is encountered more frequently in several parts of the world, particularly in north India. At times, the condition is referred to as *athrepsia or infantile atrophy*.

Clinical Features

Nutritional marasmus occurs usually in subjects less than 3 years of age; the peak incidence is seen during the first year of life. The disease may be encountered in later childhood.

A characteristic feature of the clinical picture is remarkable wasting of both muscles and subcutaneous fat (Figs 29.3 and 29.4). The face is wizened and shrivelled—just as in the case of a monkey. In the early stages, the child is irritable, hungry and craves for food. But, in the later stages, he may become miserable and apathetic, refusing to take anything. Edema is conspicuous by its absence. Significant hair changes, dermatosis and marked fatty liver are also absent. As in kwashiorkor, diarrhea, mineral and vitamin deficiencies, superadded infections and parasitic infestation are commonly seen.

Table 29.2 provides further grading of marasmus.

Table 29.2: Grading of nutritional marasmus

Grade	*Characteristic(s)*
1.	Loss of fat from axilla
2.	Loss of fat from abdominal wall and gluteal region
3.	Loss of fat from chest and back
4.	Loss of buccal pad of fat (which consists of fatty acids); it takes longer time to disappear

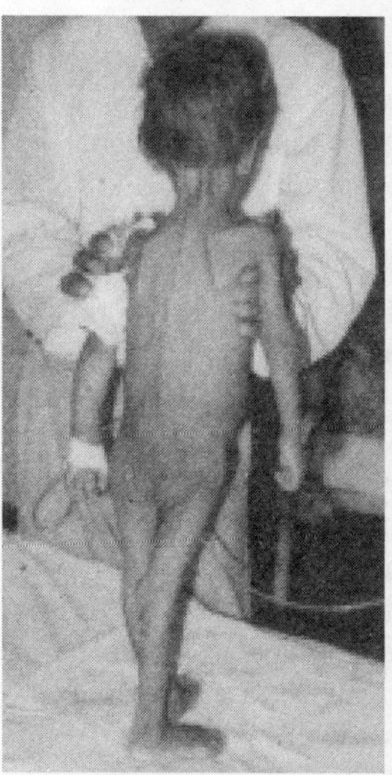

Fig. 29.3

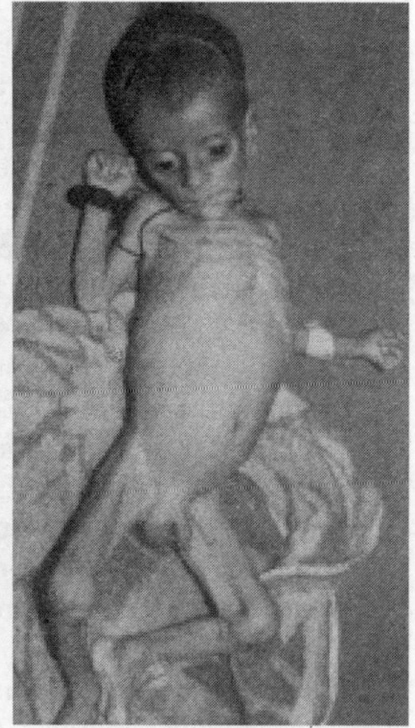

Fig. 29.4

Figs 29.3 and 29.4: Nutritional marasmus: Note the remarkable wasting (both muscle and subcutaneous fat) in two children who were hospitalized with severe PEM (See for colour figure Plate 3)

Biochemical Changes

These are slight until marasmus is of very advanced degree. The reason is that the amino acids liberated from child's own tissues make possible a continuing synthesis of serum enzymes, albumin and other essential metabolites.

Anemia is mild to moderate and may be of any morphologic type though iron-deficiency anemia undoubtedly dominates the picture.

Electrolyte disturbances may occur in the presence of diarrhea and vomiting. Blood urea is usually normal and blood sugar slightly raised. Duodenal enzymes show little or no reduction.

Diagnosis

Dietetic history suggests inadequacy of both proteins and calories (carbohydrates) in child's intake in the recent past. The predominant lack is of calories. Diagnostic criteria may be essential and nonessential as outlined below:

A. Essential Features
   1. *Growth retardation* as evidenced by marked loss of weight and subnormal height/length.
   2. Gross muscle as well as subcutaneous fat wasting;
   3. Absence of edema.

B. Nonessential Features
   1. Hair changes are usually not present.

2. Classical dermatosis of kwashiorkor is not seen. However, indolent sores and ulcers as also superadded skin infections occurs very frequently.
3. Gastrointestinal manifestations like diarrhea and vomiting occur as in kwashiorkor. A marasmic child is, however, hungry rather than anorexic though he may develop anorexia once marasmus has advanced to extreme degree.
4. Mineral and vitamin deficiencies occur fairly commonly. Anemia is usually mild to moderate and may be of varied morphology. Potassium and magnesium deficiencies occur in patients with diarrhea and vomiting. Vitamin deficiencies occur relatively less often compared to kwashiorkor.
5. Liver is rather shrunk which is in sharp contrast to the fatty, enlarged liver of kwashiorkor.
6. Superadded infections and infestations are nearly as common as in kwashiorkor.
7. Psychomotor change is usually in the form of irritability rather than listlessness. Advanced cases may, however, become apathetic as is seen in kwashiorkor.
8. Clubbing may be seen in a proportion of marasmic children. It seems to be related to the accompanying steatorrhea.

Salient features of Kwashiorkor and nutritional marasmus are given in Table 29.3.

Marasmic Kwashiorkor

Marasmic kwashiorkor refers to cases demonstrating a combination of features of kwashiorkor and marasmus. Presence of edema is essential for this diagnosis. For instance, an established case of nutritional marasmus may be mistakenly initiated on a diet consisting of lots of calories but very little proteins. Such a child is a candidate for developing hypoproteinemia and clinical edema. Remaining features of kwashiorkor may or may not be present.

Prekwashiorkor

Prekwashiorkor refers to a child who has quite poor nutritional status and certain other features of kwashiorkor such as hair changes minus edema. Such a child, unless taken care of at this very stage, may develop edema and other features of full-blown kwashiorkor.

Nutritional Dwarfing

If PEM starts fairly early in life and goes on and on over a number of years without causing overt picture of kwashiorkor or marasmus, child's height as well as weight may be significantly low for his age. This is what has been termed *nutritional dwarfing*.

Let us illustrate it through a specific example. An apparently healthy-looking child, appearing aged 4 years, is brought to a physician for a trivial medical problem. His height is 99 cm and weight 18.5 kg. Naturally, the physician forms an impression that the nutritional status of the child, including height and weight, is good enough for the age of 4 years. Right at this stage, the mother reveals that the actual age of the child is 8 years which indeed surprises the physician. The fact is that this child is quite stunted and underweight for his actual age.

Nutritional dwarfing is a common problem in developing countries but cases are not as frequently detected. It seems to be a kind of "adaptation" to poor diet (not as grave as to cause frank kwashiorkor or nutritional marasmus) over a prolonged period. These children are generally less active and less lively. They are more prone to diarrhea, pneumonia, tuberculosis or other infections prevalent in the region.

COMPLICATIONS OF PEM

These are given in Table 29.4. Vigilance and prompt remedial action is the cornerstone for their prevention and management.

Section 8

Table 29.3: Salient features of kwashiorkor and marasmus

Feature	*Kwashiorkor*	*Nutritional Marasmus*
Usual age group	1-3 years	0-3 years (mostly 0-1 year)
Essential Features		
Muscle wasting	Present though may be hidden by edema	Severe
Subcutaneous adiposity	Retained	Severe wasting
Edema	Present	Absent
Growth retardation (weight)	Low (may give erroneous impression because of edema)	Very low
Nonessential Features		
Psychomotor changes	Apathetic and listless	Usually irritable
Appetite	Poor	Usually hungry
Diarrhea	Present	Present
Characteristic dermatosis	Usually present	Absent
Hair changes	Sparse, light-colored, easily pluckable; at times flag sign	Usually absent
Hepatomegaly	Common (fatty change)	Rather shrunk

Table 29.4: Serious complications of severe PEM

Complication	*Remarks*
Superadded Infections	Both overt and hidden: Septicemia, pneumonia, UTI, tuberculosis.
Dehydration and dyslectrolytemia	Usually complicating accompanying diarrhea, often with lactose intolerance.
Hypothermia	An unattended rectal temperature of < 35 degree C may prove fatal (SIDS).
Hypoglycemia	It contributes to poor response to nutritional therapy and carries a poor prognosis.
CCF	It is usually precipitated by excessive intake of sodium and fluid or severe anemia. Since cardiac size is invariably small in PEM, even a normal sized heart in X-ray should arouse suspicion of CCF.
Anemia	Moderate to severe anemia may result from malnutrition as such or such factors as superadded infection(s), contributing to development of CCF.
Bleeding	DIC may complicate the clinical picture.
SIDS	Sudden death 4-7 days after admission. Usually, the cause remains unclear.

MANAGEMENT

Nutritional rehabilitation may be carried out:

- At home (domicilliary management) or in a nutrition rehabilitation center in case of mild to moderate PEM.
- In a hospital or health center in case of acute severe PEM.[21-23]

Domiciliary Management

Children with mild to moderate malnutrition are best managed in their own homes and kept under surveillance so as to find out improvement or deterioration in their nutritional status. The parents of such children are enlightened about the inadequacy in child's intake and guided how to correct it. The stress should be on the locally available economic foods rather than on expensive tinned protein preparations which should be reserved for special situations only. The parents must be apprised of the value of carbohydrates and the rationale of giving liberal amounts of semisolids and solids. They must understand why only milk will not be enough for the growing child. There is evidence that domiciliary treatment brings about gratifying results. It also reduces the unnecessary hospital load, is much less expensive, and, in addition, takes nutritional education to the family and the community.

Ours as well as many other workers' experience indicates that malnutrition relapse only infrequently when moderate PEM is treated at home. On the contrary, incidence of recurrences in hospital-treated cases is fairly high.

The management at home has got to be supervised and monitored by weekly visits of paramedicals (say an anganwadi worker), visits to a nearby nutrition rehabilitation center or OPD of a health centre/hospital.

A prerequisite to domiciliary treatment is absence of severe infection(s), fulminant gastroenteritis and electrolyte imbalance.

Good weight gain, as judged from the growth chart, is by and large the best yardstick of adequacy of response to nutritional rehabilitation.

Management in Nutrition Rehabilitation Center (NRC)

This concept, originally started in Southern America, aims at offering nutritional rehabilitation for mild to moderate PEM as a compromise between domiciliary and hospital managements. It offers a meeting point between classical treatment and prevention, embracing the positive points of both hospital and home management.

Two types of NRCs are: Day care center and residential center.

Day care NRC: It consists of a room for children, a kitchen, an examination room and a teaching space.

At least one good meal is provided to children. Around 20 to 40 malnourished children along with their mothers who are expected to involve themselves in various activities are taken care of. The center remains open from 8 AM to 6 PM daily.

Residential NRC: This is a larger and more organized NRC with a "housemother" as the fulltime head with responsibilities that include daily work schedule of the mothers, purchase of food, issuing the correct amount of food as decided by the nutritionist, and keeping stock and maintenance of cleanliness of the center. The supervisory staff is part time and includes a doctor, a medical assistant/nurse, a home economist/nutritionist, and an agriculture teacher/extension worker. The center is attached to a health center or the pediatric department of a teaching hospital, or an under-5-clinic. The criteria for admission to the NRC are:

- Children especially at risk.
- Children who fail to gain weight over a period of 3 months.
- Children who do not catch up in growth after serious illness (measles, whooping cough, diarrhea).
- Failure to breastfeeding.
- Mothers and children who find it difficult to cope with their problems in spite of the health teaching they receive at the under-5-clinic.
- Twins and triplets.

The stress in the NRC is on nutrition and health education, household budget teaching, homograft teaching and actual feeding, using locally available foodstuffs and local methods of cooking and preparation.

The successful rehabilitation at the NRC must be followed up at home so that the knowledge acquired during stay at the center continues to be applied at home.

Hospital Management

Acute severe PEM needs to be managed in hospital. The nutritional rehabilitation, the cornerstone of treatment, is carried by providing high protein and high energy diet. To begin with a daily intake of 100 kcal/kg/day of expected weight (150-200 kcal/kg/day of actual weight) and 3 g/kg of proteins calculated with reference to the actual weight should be achieved in very first week. This is vital for the much-needed catch-up growth. It is advisable to provide at least 10 percent of total calories from proteins of higher biological value. The choice of foodstuffs should be based on local resources. It is good to feed small amounts of food at more frequent intervals. In many cases, it may become necessary to initiate dietary therapy with tube feeding. Once the child is out of the acute phase, he may accept more and more food. Let him eat at liberty—of course, generously.

For details see Chapter 31.

Phenomena that May Occur During Nutritional Rehabilitation

Pseudotumor Cerebri

Overenergetic nutritional correction in malnourished infants may be accompanied by a transient rise of intracranial tension. The phenomenon is benign and self-limiting.

Nutritional Recovery Syndrome (Gomez Syndrome)

The term refers to an interesting sequelae of events seen in children who are being treated with very high quantity of proteins during the course of rehabilitation from gross malnutrition. The syndrome is characterized by increasing hepatomegaly, abdominal distention, ascites, prominent thoraco-abdominal venous network, hypertrichosis, parotid swelling, gynecomastia and eosinophilia. In some instances, splenomegaly also occurs. Though the syndrome was initially described in kwashiorkor from Africa, we have recorded its occurrence in both kwashiorkor and marasmus in north India.

Etiopathogenesis of this syndrome remains speculative. Our surmise is that its development may well be related to endocrinal disturbances. That in PEM the function of the pituitary and its target glands is set at a lower ebb is well known. This response of the pituitary to the state of poor dietary intake appears to be an adaptive mechanism that permits survival of the patient by reducing body activity and metabolic rate, and by retarding growth. During nutritional rehabilitation, the greater utilization of the hormone by the body stimulates the pituitary to produce its trophic hormones. This results in a response by the target glands. Thus, it appears that the nutritional recovery syndrome is caused by an increase in estrogen level and by a variety of trophic hormones produced by the recovering pituitary gland.

Encephalitis-like Syndrome

About one-fifth children with kwashiorkor become drowsy within 3 to 4 days after initiation of dietary therapy. Most often, the condition is self-limiting. Occasionally, it may be accompanied by progressive unconsciousness with fatal outcome. Even more rarely, a transient syndrome marked by coarse tremors, parkinsonian rigidity, bradykinesia and myoclonus (Kahn syndrome) may appear 6 to several days after starting the dietary rehabilitation. Sometimes, tremors (the so-called "kwashi-shakes") may occur during the recovery phase and may take even months to resolve.

These encephalitis-like states are considered to be the result of far too much of proteins in the diet.

Rickets

During nutritional recovery, as a result of rapid growth, vitamin D, calcium and phosphate consumption may fall short of the body needs, causing rickets. In some children, the pre-existing but hidden rickets become manifest following restoration of bone growth during nutritional rehabilitation.

Anemia/Micronutrient Deficiency

In addition to the pre-existing anemia as a part of malnutrition, the child may manifest further worsening in hemoglobin status if iron and folic acid supplements are not provided during nutritional rehabilitation. Likewise, deficiencies of micronutrients may too become manifest.

PROGNOSIS

With good hospital care, mortality rate in gross PEM has today considerably fallen. Against the alarmingly high figures of 20 to 50% in the older series, the recent reports indicate 5 to 20% mortality. In our experience, it is around 5-10%, kwashiorkor children dying more often than those suffering from nutritional marasmus.

Bad prognostic signs include severe dehydration, hypoglycemia, hypothermia, CCF, superimposed infections, xerophthalmia, bleeding diathesis, hepatic dysfunction, seizures, significant change in sensorium and cachexia (extreme weight loss).

The causes of mortality include dehydration and electrolyte imbalance (dyselectrolytemia), hypoglycemia, hypothermia, fulminant systemic infections and congestive cardiac failure. In our experience, dehydration and electrolyte imbalance due to diarrheal disease and fulminant systemic infections are the chief killers of malnourished children. Congestive cardiac failure, though uncommon, carries a very bad prognosis. In some cases hypoglycemia and hypothermia may prove fatal.

LONG-TERM SEQUELAE

Growth Retardation

Infants who suffer from significant PEM fairly early in life and over a prolonged period develop a permanent, irreversible stunting of growth. Today, studies from several parts of the world have established that the most common case of short stature is, in fact , chronic malnutrition (often mild-moderate) spread over a prolonged period. This concept has led to the widespread use of "height" in modern classifications (say Waterlow's, WHO) as an important tool for assessment and classification of PEM.

Mental Impairment[24-27]

Now a sort of consensus seems to have emerged concluding that IUGR and malnutrition in the first year of life, if severe enough to retard physical growth and to warrant hospitalization, causes retardation in mental performance, eventually leading to low intelligence and impaired learning skills. Recently, evidence has gathered to the effect that even mild-to-moderate malnutrition during any period of childhood harms cognitive development. As a consequence, their mental performance as adults is compromised.

It is of interest that effects on mental development are reversible following appropriate interventions early in life.

Malnutrition and Liver

The old belief that PEM causes cirrhosis in the long run is no longer tenable in the light of the epidemiologic studies spread over three decades or so. Longitudinal observations made on children suffering from severe PEM bear testimony to the current concept. Furthermore, it is significant that incidence of cirrhosis in Africa, the home of kwashiorkor, is very low.[28]

PREVENTIVE ASPECTS OF PEM

WHO has described malnutrition as a "global problem", having adverse effects on the survival, health performance and progress of population groups. The effects are of the highest order in the developing countries.

Fighting such a vital problem of tremendous dimension in the Third World, including India, is, therefore of paramount importance. The question is not of treating the individual cases suffering from overt picture of nutritional deficiencies or preventing the occurrence of malnutrition in the individuals. It is much more than that. And, that is prevention of malnutrition at a large scale. This can eventually be accomplished through improvement in the socio-economic status and coordinated as also well-planned efforts in the field of agriculture, education, social. Chapter 18 discusses this aspect in details.

REFERENCES

1. Alleyne GAO, Hay RW, Picou DI, Stanfield JP, Whitehead RG. *Protein-energy Malnutrition*. London: Edward Arnold 1989.
2. Gupte S, Gomez EM. Protein-energy malnutrition. In: Gupte S (ed): *The Short Textbook of Pediatrics,* 11th edn. New Delhi: Jaypee 2009:109-113.
3. Gupte S. Nutritional deficiency states. Quart Med Rev 1983:34:1-45.
4. Government of India. National Family Health Survey (NFHS-2), India, 1998-99. Mumbai: International Institute of Population Science/ORC Macro 1998-99.
5. Ghosh S. Current nutrition scenario. In: Gupte S, Gupte SB (eds): *Recent Advances in Pediatrics (Special Vol. 1: Nutrition, Growth and Development*). New Delhi: Jaypee 1997:1-17.
6. Gopalan C: Child care in India: Emerging challenges. *Indian Pediatr* 1993; 30:593-599.
7. Ghosh S. *Nutrition and Child Care: A Practical Guide,* 2nd edn. New Delhi: Jaypee 2004.
8. Jelliffe DB, Jelliffe EEP. Causation of kwashiorkor: Towards a multifactorial consensus. *Pediatrics* 1992; 4: 502.
9. Gupte S, Pal M: Some issues in protein-energy malnutrition. *Indian Pract* 1987;40:1037.
10. Seth V, Jain Y, Kabra S: Immunology of malnutrition: An overview. In: Gupte S (ed): Recent Advances in Pediatrics (Special Vol -1) *Nutrition, Growth and Development.* New Delhi: Jaypee 1997:240.
11. Gupte S: Diarrhea of malnutrition. *Indian Pract* 1975;28:255.
12. Samotra K, Gupte S, Raina RK: Effect of malnutrition on chloramphenicol kinetics in Indian children. *Acta Pharmacol Sinica* 1986;7:162-165.
13. Samotra K, Gupte S, Raina RK: Pharmacokinetics of gentamicin in protein-energy malnutrition. *Europ J Clin Pharmacol* 1985;29:255-259.
14. Gupte S. Samotra K, Raina RK: Nutrition and drug disposition. *Indian J Pediatr* 1987;54:462-463.
15. World Health Organization. WHO Global Database on Child Growth and Malnutrition. Geneva: WHO 1997.
16. World Health Organization (WHO) Working Group on Infant Growth. An evaluation of infant: The use and interpretation of anthropometry in Infants. Bull WHO 1995;73:165-174.
17. World Health Organization. Turning the Tide of Malnutrition: Responding to the challenge of 21st Century. Geneva: WHO 2000.
18. Inamdar S. Changing Trends in nutritional disorders: In: Gupte S (ed) *Recent Advances in Pediatrics* 4. New Delhi: Jaypee 1994:34-44.
19. Mathur GP, Kushwaha KP, Mathur S: Protein-energy malnutrition (PEM) updated. In: Gupte S, Gupte SB (eds): *Recent Advances in Pediatrics (Special Vol. 1) Nutrition, Growth and Development*). New Delhi: Jaypee 1997:94-122.

20. Reddy V. Child nutrition in India: Priorities for the coming decade. *Indian Pediatr* 1993;30:289-294.
21. Gupte S: Clubbing in protein-calorie malnutrition. *Indian Pract* 1974;27:501.
22. Gupte S: Nutritional recovery syndrome. *N Engl J Med* 1972; 291:501.
23. Gupte S: Nutritional rehabilitation. *Indian J Pediatr* 1983;50:97.
24. Hendarto SK: Nutrition and developing brain. In: Gupte S, Gupte SB (eds): *Recent Advances in Pediatrics, Vol. 2.* New Delhi: Jaypee 1991:201-212.
25. Udani PM: Protein-energy malnutrition (PEM), brain and various facets of child development. *Indian J Pediatr* 1992; 59:165-175.
26. Park K. Nutrition and health. In: *Park's Textbook of Preventive and Social Medicine*, 21st edn. Jabalpur: Banarsidas Bhanot 2011:438-487.
27. Martorell R. Long-term consequences of undernutrition on physical and cognitive development. *Annal* Nutr1999;57: 96-106.
28. Gupte S, Gomez EM. Nutrition and nutritional deficiency states. In: Gupte S (ed): *The Short Textbook of Pediatrics*, 11th edn. New Delhi: Jaypee 2009:129-153.

Suraj Gupte • EM Gomez

30 Various Classifications of Protein-Energy Malnutrition

INTRODUCTION

The clinical spectrum of PEM is wide, ranging from mild malnutrition with growth failure (often missed on account of difficulty in recognizing it or preoccupation with advanced malnutrition) through moderate malnutrition to overt syndromes of nutritional marasmus and kwashiorkor.

The aim and objective of classifying PEM is to identify children in need of nutritional intervention (of course, along with health intervention). To achieve this goal, a number of classifications of PEM over the past five decades or so have been introduced.

I. Syndromal Classification

This classification is based on presenting clinical features:

- Kwashiorkor.
- Nutritional marasmus.
- Marasmic kwashiorkor.
- Prekwashiorkor.
- Nutritional dwarfing.

This classification is useful for identifying acute severe categories of PEM and even for chronic PEM causing stunting. It fails to focus on mild-moderate PEM which does not have such overt clinical presentation as syndromes like kwashiorkor or nutritional marasmus.

II. Classifications Based on Weight for Age

These classifications are easy to compute but are not of much value when correct age is not known, a situation that is not infrequent in the Indian subcontinent. Secondly, by recording only weight for age, one cannot ascertain if the low weight is due to a sudden acute episode of PEM or chronic long-standing PEM.

Gomez's Classification

According to this classification, PEM is graded with reference to the weight for age as percentage of the expected weight as below:

First degree : Weight between 90 and 75% of expected
Second degree : Weight between 75 and 60% of expected
Third degree : Weight below 60% of expected.

Values between 90 to 110% indicate normal nutritional status. This was the first ever classification of PEM suggested in 1950s from Mexico by Gomez and coworkers.[1] The suggested reference standard was Harvard growth standards which commanded respect at that time and for several years to come until it was taken over by the United States NSCH norms.

The flaw in this classification is that the cutoff point of 90% is rather high. Thus, some normal children are likely to be erroneously categorized as "first degree PEM".

Welcome or International Classification

Weight between 80 and 60% of expected:
With edema — Kwashiorkor
Without edema — Undernutrition
Weight below 60% of expected:
With edema — Marasmic kwashiorkor
Without edema — Nutritional marasmus.

Indian Academy of Pediatrics (IAP) Classification

First degree : Weight between 80 and 70% of expected
Second degree : Weight between 70 and 60% of expected
Third degree : Weight between 60 and 50% of expected
Fourth degree : Weight below 50% of expected.

In case the patient has demonstrable pedal edema (suggesting "kwashiorkor), the letter "*K*" is placed in front of the evaluated grade as suffix.

This classification was proposed by the Nutritional Subcommittee of the Indian Academy of Pediatric (IAP) in 1972.[2] The cutoff point is 80% of expected rather than 90%. The suggested reference was Harvard growth standards.

Jelliffe's Classification

First degree : Weight between 90 and 80% of expected
Second degree : Weight between 80 and 70% of expected
Third degree : Weight between 70 and 60% of expected
Fourth degree : Weight below 60% of expected.

McLaren's Classification

Mild	Weight between 90 and 80% of expected
Moderate	Weight between 80 and 70% of expected
Severe	Weight below 70% of expected.

III. Classifications Based on Weight for Height and Height for Age

Waterlow's Classification

It is based on the principle that whereas weight for age assists in monitoring of growth, measurement of height assesses the effect of nutritional status on long-term growth. This classification focuses on two groups for PEM:

1. PEM with retarded growth in which a drop in the height/age ratio points to a chronic condition, say stunting or shortness.
2. PEM with a low weight for a normal height in which weight for height ratio is indicative of an acute condition of rapid weight loss or wasting.

Acute (wasted but not stunted)	Weight for height low, height for age normal
Acute/chronic (wasted and stunted)	Weight for height low, height for age low
Nutritional dwarfing (stunted but wasted)	Weight for height normal weight for age low, height for age not low

This classification, based on a combination of wasting and stunting, was proposed by, as the name suggests, Waterlow.[3]

WHO Classification

It is shown in Table 30.1.

Table 30.1: WHO classification of PEM[4]

Criteria	*Moderate PEM*	*Severe PEM*
Symmetrical edema	No	Yes
Weight for height (index of wasting)	70-79% of expected (wasting)	< 70% of expected (Severe wasting)
Height for age (index of stunting)	85-89% of expected (stunting)	< 85% of expected (Severe stunting)

IV. Classifications Employing other Parameters

Arnold Classification

It is based on midarm circumference (MAC) as follows:

Mild to moderate	MAC between 12.5 - 13.5 cm
Severe	MAC under 12.5 cm

Classification Based on Skinfold Thickness

Mild	80-90% of expected
Moderate	60-80%
Severe	Under 60%

Classification Based on Mid-upper-arm Circumference (MUAC)

Mild	< 13.5 cm
Moderate	12.5 – 13.5 cm
Severe	< 11.5

According to new recommendations of WH/UNICEF,[5] any one of the following parameters is good enough for labeling an under-5 as "acute severe malnutrition" (SAM), the term now preferred globally:

- Weight for height < 3 SD/Zscores of median WHO growth reference of 2006
- Visible severe wasting
- Bipedal edema, and
- MUAC < 11.5 cm

Here, the major deviation is in the form of not considering the earlier criteria of weight for height < 70% and employing 2006 standards rather than the old NCHS standards as recommended by the WHO earlier and later adapted by the Indian Academy of Pediatrics.[6,7]

REFERENCES

1. Gomez F, Ramos-Galvan R. Mortality in second and third degree malnutrition. *J Trop Pediatr* 1956;2:77-83.
2. Shah PM. Grading of malnutrition (Report of the Convenor, Nutrition Subcommittee, Indian Academy of Pediatrics). *Indian Pediatr* 1972;9:300-306.
3. Waterlow JC. Note on assessment and classification of protein-energy malnutrition in children. *Lancet* 1973;2:87-89.
4. World Health Organization. *Measuring Change in Nutritional Status.* Geneva: WHO 1983.
5. World Health Organization.WHO Child Growth Standards and the Identification of Severe Acute Malnutrition in Infants and Children. A Joint Statement by the WHO/UNICEF 2009. Available at: http://www.who. Int/nutrition/publications/severemalnutrition/9789241598163/en/index.html.Accessed on: 14 June 2011.
6. Bhatnagar S, Lodha R, Choudhury P. IAP guidelines 2006 on hospital based management of severely malnourished children (adapted from the WHO guidelines). *Indian Pediatr* 2007; 44: 443-461.
7. Gupte S, Gomez EM, Gomez EE, Gomez M. Protein-energy malnutrition: Changing trends in management. In: Gupte S, Gupte SB (eds): *Recent Advannces in Pediatrics (Special Vol. 20: Nutrition,Growth and Development).* New Delhi: Jaypee 2009: 91-120.

Ravinder K Gupta • Ritu Gupta

31 Mild-Moderate Protein-Energy Malnutrition: Nutritional Rehabilitation

INTRODUCTION

Nutritional deficiencies constitute a major public health problem in India and other countries of the third world. Protein-energy malnutrition (PEM) is a silent killer among children. Considerable morbidity (and at times mortality) accompanies others such as nutritional anemias and vitamin deficiencies. The calorie and protein requirements of young children are larger (in relation to their size) than in older children and adults. PEM is therefore seen more commonly among these groups and sometimes among women during pregnancy and lactation. These are called the "nutritionally vulnerable groups". Of these, infants and toddlers are the most commonly affected.[1,2]

In India, gross malnutrition is said to kill around 5,00,000 infants and children every year. This is quite understandable in view of the fact that around half of our pediatric population is suffering from one or another nutritional deficiency. About 75 to 80% of the hospitalized children suffer from some degree or type of malnutrition. Majority of infants and children suffering from PEM (60-70%) have mild to moderate degree of the problem. It is severe in only 2 to 5 percent of cases. As per the a National Family Health Survey, the most common age of PEM is between 6 months and 2 years. Around 50 to 60 percent of children are malnourished by 2 years.[1,3]

PRETREATMENT ASSESSMENT

This should aim at:

a. Evaluation of ecological and environmental factors.
b. Evaluation of growth and development.
c. Evaluation of associated conditions and complications, and
d. Minimum investigations necessary for management.

An attempt should be made to understand the conditioning influences like low birthweight and recurrent infections, cultural practices like food fads and dietary restrictions, socio-economic factors like illiteracy and poverty, dietary factors like breastfeeding and weaning practices, diet during illness, adequacy of present diet, etc. and availability and utilization of health and other facilities like immunization and medical care during illness. Micro-environment that includes the domestic and human influences like material attitude, child rearing skills, family harmony and support to the mother should also be included in the assessment.

Assessment of growth should include the various anthropometric measurements, computation of weight for age, height for age and weight for height and their interpretation. All those with acute PEM will have evidence of wasting and those with chronic PEM will have stunting. Many have both wasting and stunting due to acute on chronic PEM. Developmental evaluation should include developmental delay or arrest of developmental milestones due to acute illness. Associated infections, organ dysfunction and complications should also be carefully looked for.

Though, based on the pathological changes that can occur in PEM, a battery of biochemical tests and sepsis screen can be undertaken, in most cases for practical purposes, extensive investigations are unnecessary.

MANAGEMENT[3-5]

The management of PEM depends on nutritional status, degree of hypermetabolism, expected duration of illness and associated complications. The goals are to minimize weight loss, to maintain body mass and to encourage body mass repletion of growth.

The principles of management are as follows:

- The patient is evaluated with regard to severity of PEM, presence or absence of associated systemic infections, other nutritional deficits such as vitamin deficiencies or anemia and associated fluid and electrolyte disturbances.
- The intake of food is promoted by all available means. Locally available and culturally acceptable foods, which the family can afford are advised.

- Complications of malnutrition, sequelae and death are prevented by careful surveillance and prompt remedial action.
- Possible epidemiological factors for malnutrition are considered and attempt is made to eliminate these are as far as possible.

Nutritional rehabilitation may be carried out at home (domiciliary management), in a nutritional rehabilitation centre, or in a hospital or health centre.It is important to focus on a holistic approach, providing developmental stimulation.[6]

Domiciliary (Home) Management

It is for mild to moderate PEM and for those uncomplicated severe PEM who have fairly good appetite, normal body temperature, who are conscious and active and without evidence of serious infection. These children are managed at home by parents under observation and supervision.

The main goal of treatment is to provide adequate calories for dual purpose, to replace losses and to build-up nutrition and to promote growth. Caution must be taken to gradually build-up the calories and proteins.

The common foods advocated are double or triple mixes of cereals and pulses like dal, rice, khichdi, seasonal green leafy and yellow orange vegetables, root vegetables, sugar, jaggery, milk and milk products, if family could afford nuts like groundnuts. Emphasis must be laid on adding enough oil/vanaspati ghee/butter to the diet, to increase calories and palatability. Parents are educated to prepare suitable diets from these food sources, liquid semisolid or solid depending on the acceptability and appetite of the child. Frequent small feeds with calories and proteins distributed proportionately are encouraged rather than 1 or 2 major bulky meals. Non-vegetarian articles like egg, fish, meat, etc. are allowed for those whose cultural and religious practices permit them. Some of the isodense liquid diets ideal for nutritional rehabilitation are shown in Table 31.1.

Parents are educated about hygienic way of preparation and handling of food, use of safe and clean drinking water and importance of personal hygiene. Some basic advice is also given, for management of diarrhea by oral rehydration solution (ORS), immediate attention for treatment of common infestations and infections and appropriate management of anemia by oral iron and folic acid supplements and associated vitamin deficiencies. To promote growth, zinc supplements are given when positive nutrition balance starts occurring and child manifests with increase in weight gain. Due attention should be given to check and advise proper immunizations.

The aim of the dietary treatment is to restore weight for height.

The energy recommended is 120-150 kcal/kg/day, proteins 2 to 3 g/kg/day of high biological value and 150-165 ml fluid/kg. For this approach, the therapeutic calculations are based on the actual weight of the child irrespective of edema. The total calories can be divided into 8 feeds. During daytime 2 hourly feeds and during night, a late night feed and an early morning feed can be given to prevent hypoglycemia during night. This schedule will ensure adequate sleep to the child and the caretaker.

Children are monitored through weekly visits by paramedicals or visits to the hospital or at a nutritional rehabilitation center every week.

After the child passes through the initial phase, tolerates the prescribed diet and shows signs of improvement, one can gradually increase the calorie intake to approximately 150 to 180 kcal/kg/day. The amount of milk could be gradually decreased and the intake of semisolid/solids increased. Some of the high energy foods that can be offered are shown in Table 31.2.

Table 31.1: Isodense liquid diets

Item	*Composition*	*Calorie*
High energy Milk	½ glass milk 1 tsp sugar ½ tsp oil	100 Cal/100 ml
Cereal milk	½ glass milk 1 tsp sugar 11/2 tsp Cereal flour	100 Cal/100 ml
Cereal pulse-milk (SAT milk)	½ glass milk 2 tsp SAT mix*	100 Cal/100 ml
Fruit juice	1 orange 2 tsp sugar 2ater upto 100 ml	100 Cal/100 ml
Egg flip	One egg 2 tsp sugar 3/4 glass milk	200 Cal/200 ml
Sweet Yogurt/ Lassee	½ glass yogurt 2 tsp sugar	100 Cal/100 ml

* SAT mix–Precooked ready to mix palatable cereal pulse mixture prepared from rice: wheat: blackgram: sugar in the ratio 1:1:1:2.

Table 31.2: Energy-rich foods

Item	*Ingredients*	*Calories per 100 g*	*Proteins per 100 g*
1. Besan mix/ Laddoo/Panjiri	Bengal gram flour wheat flour	500	9
2. Sooji (Rawa) Red Kheer	Toned milk 750 ml Sugar 100 g Sooji 25 g Oil 5 g Water 1000 ml	1432	28.4
3. Hyderabad mix	Whole wheat 40 g Bengal gram 16 g Groundnuts 10 g Jaggery 20 g	330	11.3
4. Shakti Ahar	Roasted wheat 40 g Roasted gram 20 g Roasted peanut 10 g Jaggery 30 g	390	11.4

In lactose intolerance, breastfeeding can often be continued. The milk need not be omitted completely but the lactose content can be decreased by fortifying with other articles of diet like rice. Curd also have been very well tolerated by lactose intolerant children. Milk-free cereal based diets as shown in Table 31.3 can be tried.

Table 31.3: Milk free cereal based diets

Ingredients	*Suitable for infants 4-12 months* (Liquid diet)*			*Suitable for older children** (Semi-solid diet)*		
	Amount (g)	*KCal (%)*	*Protein (g)*	*Amount (g)*	*KCal (%)*	*Protein (g)*
Rice	10	34	0.8	15	48	1.2
Moong dal**	5.0	17	1.1	5.0	48	1.1
Sugar	2.5	10	—	2.5	10	—
Oil	2.5	22	—	2.5	22	—
Water q.s.	100 ml	—	—	100 ml	—	—
Total	100 ml	83	1.9	100 ml	97	2.3

- Liquid consistency; 0.8 Kcal/ml : volume 100 ml.
- Semi-solid consistency; approximately 1 Kcal/ml. Cook after mixing for 15 minutes and adjust final volume at 100 ml.
- Cooked moong dal for infants 4-12 months.

There is evidence that domiciliary treatment brings, about gratifying results. It also reduces the unnecessary pressure on hospital, is much less expensive and in addition, takes nutritional education to the family and the community.

It has been experienced by many workers that malnutrition relapse only infrequently when moderate PEM is treated at home. On the contrary, incidence of recurrences in hospital treated cases in fairly high.

Management in Nutrition Rehabilitation Centre (NRC)

This concept, originally started in Southern America, aims at offering nutritional rehabilitation for mild to moderate PEM as a compromise between domiciliary and hospital managements. It offers a meeting point between classical treatment and prevention, embracing the positive points of both hospital and home management.

Two types of NRCs are: Day care center and residential center.

Day care NRC: It consists of a room for children, a kitchen, an examination room and a teaching space. At least one good meal is provided to children. Around 20 to 40 malnourished children along with their mothers who are expected to involve themselves in various activities are taken care of. The center remains open from 8 A.M. to 6 P.M. daily.

Residential NRC: This is a larger and more organized NRC with a "housemother" as the fulltime head with responsibilities that include daily work schedule of the mothers, purchase of food, issuing the correct amount of food as decided by the nutritionist, and keeping stock and maintenance of cleanliness of the centre. The supervisory staff is part time and includes a doctor, a medical assistant/ nurse, a home economist/nutritionist, and an agriculture teacher/extension worker. The center is attached to a health center or the pediatric department of a teaching hospital, or an under-5-clinic. The criteria for admission to the NRC are:

- Children especially at risk.
- Children who fail to gain weight over a period of 3 months.
- Children who do not catch up in growth after serious illness (measles, whooping cough, diarrhea).
- Failure to breastfeeding.
- Mothers and children who find it difficult to cope with their problems in spite of the heath teaching they receive at the under-5-clinic.
- Twins and triplets.

The stress in the NRC is on nutrition and health education, household budget teaching, homecraft teaching and actual feeding, using locally available foodstuffs and local methods of cooking and preparation.

The successful rehabilitation at the NRC must be followed up at home so that the knowledge acquired during stay at the centre continues to be applied at home.

REHABILITATION PHASE[7-9]

Once the child is able to tolerate a high dose of therapeutic nutrition and has started gaining weight, he or she may be offered solid/semisolid family foods containing cereals, pulses, vegetables) rich in calories and quantitatively appropriate bengal gram, ground-nuts and dark green leafy vegetables should be added to regular family foods. Oils, sugar, and fruits should also be given and minerals and vitamins could be continued for 5 to 6 weeks. Parents could be given nutrition education with emphasis that nutritionally adequate diet need not be expensive and special foods need not be purchased or cooked. The diet prescribed for the child should be such that the family can provide within their limited income, can be easily cooked at home, does not perish easily, is culturally acceptable, as well as locally available.

Once weight for height is achieved, the aim should be to consolidate the cure, to prevent recurrence. Comprehensive rehabilitation aims at total care and total development of the child. This can be ensured by adopting NIMFES. In NIMFES, N stands for nutrition, I for immunization, M for medical care, F for family planning, E for education and S for developmental stimulation. Older children get stimulation by way of nonformal education from ICDS Programs. Younger children should also get developmental surveillance, developmental stimulation and tender loving care (TLC) in place of the nonformal education for the older children.

These interventions will help to improve quality of survival and will add life to years.

RECOVERY ASSESSMENT

Recovery can be assessed from:

- Improvement of general condition, alertness and smile.
- Return of appetite.
- Weight gain of 50-70 gm/kg/week in infants and 0.5 kg/ week in older children.
- Disappearance of edema.
- Disappearance of hepatomegaly and enteropathy.
- Restoration of weight for height may take upto 8-12 weeks.

PHENOMENA ENCOUNTERED DURING NUTRITIONAL REHABILITATION

Gupte and Gomez[3] have eminently summarized the various phenomenon encountered during nutritional rehabilitation/ recovery in a recent review. As emphasized by them, with rationalization in the amount of protein (around 3-4 g/kg/ day of expected weight), these phenomena are now only infrequently seen.

The indications for hospitalization are hypothermia, infection, fluid and electrolyte imbalance, conversions unconsciousness, xeropthalmia, severe dermatosis bleeding, be marked hepatomegaly, jaundice, anemia. Persistent vomiting, severe anorexia, distended tender abdomen etc.

IAP RECOMMENDATIONS ON INFANT FEEDING PRACTICES IN PREVENTION OF PEM[1]

Protein energy malnutrition being a social disease of multifactorial origin, its prevention requires a coordinated approach of many disciplines such as nutrition agriculture food technology, health administration, health education and strong political commitment. The Indian Academy of Pediatrics has come with recommendation on infant feeding which is crucial for optimum growth and health of our children. Following actions may be taken at family level to prevent PEM.

1. Protection, promotion and support for exclusive breastfeeding, right from birth to 6 months of life.
2. Correct infant and child rearing practices.
3. To impose no restriction on feeding during illness.
4. Supplementary feeding with energy dense semi-solid foods from 6 months, along with extended breastfeeding upto 2 years of age. Gradually, increasing the number, frequency and amount of family foods so that baby is able to take all by 1 year of age. Appetite is a central component in the decision-making process and skills used by care givers to determine when and how much to feed their infants. Chronic anorexia and illness related anorexia are important problems among infants and children in developing countries. Chronic anorexia is associated with parent-child interaction, characterized by unclear messages, premature termination of feeding, inconsistent meal times and limited food availability. This leads to poor and appetite behavior development in children. Similarly, a diet which is monotonous and non-nutritious of filling up by liquids, e.g. fruit juice leads to growth failure and poor appetite. An active parent-child interaction, motivation and response to queries of child, tasteful and diversified diet of good quality and quantity, good food hygiene, health care including breast-feeding and care during illness and adequate feeding time are some of the measures to enhance the acceptance of food by child.
5. Integrated health care package of appropriate feeding, immunization, ORS (Oral rehydration salt) for ADD (Acute diarrheal disorders), periodic deworming and early diagnosis and treatment of illnesses.
6. Special nutritional and health care to pregnant and lactating mothers. Following actions are required at community level:
   - Supplementary feeding program.
   - Agricultural development.
   - Education and environmental sanitation.
   - Population control.
   - Nutritional intervention programs.
   - Universal immunization program (UIP).
   - National control programs, e.g. control of diarrheal diseases (CDD), acute respiratory infections (ARI), malaria, anemia, etc.

REFERENCES

1. Mehta MN. Nutritional disorders in children. In: Parthasarathy A, Menon PSN, Nair MKC, *et al.* (eds): *IAP Textbook of Pediatrics*, 2nd edn. New Delhi: Jaypee 2006;120-134.
2. Mathur GP, Kushwaha KP, Mathur S. Protein-energy malnutrition updated. In: Gupte S, Gupte SB (ed): *Recent Advances in Pediatrics (Special Vol. 1: Nutrition, Growth and Development)*. New Delhi: Jaypee 1997; 94-122.
3. Gupte S, Gomez EM. Protein-energy malnutrition. In: Gupte S (eds): *The Short Textbook of Pediatrics*,11th edn. New Delhi: Jaypee 2009:129-154.
4. Elizabeth KD. Management of protein-energy malnutrition. *Indian J Pract Pediatr* 1998;6:339-344.
5. Kulkarni ML. Nutritional rehabilitation: In: Gupte S (ed): *Recent Advances in Pediatrics (Special Vol. 1 Nutrition,Growth and Development)*. New Delhi: Jaypee 1997:299-306.
6. Elizabeth KE, Sathy N. The role of development at stimulation in nutritional rehabilitation. *Indian Pediatr* 1997;34:681-695.
7. Singh S. Management of protein-energy malnutrition. In: Sachdev HPS, Choudhury P (eds): *Nutrition in Children: Developing Country Concerns*. New Delhi: BI 1994:206-216.
8. Government of India. *National Guidelines on Infant and Young Child Feeding*. New Delhi: Department of Women and Child Development/Food and Nutrition Board, Ministry of Human Resource Development 2004.
9. Kulkarni ML. Nutritional rehabilitation. In: Gupte S (ed): *Recent Advances in Pediatrics (Special Vol. 1: Nutrition, Growth and Development)*. New Delhi: Jaypee 1997;343-353.

Suraj Gupte, Mary Gomez

32 Severe Acute Malnutrition (SAM): State-of-the-art Management

INTRODUCTION

According to the World Health Organization (WHO) and United Nations Children Fund (UNICEF),[1] the diagnosis of acute severe malnutrition (SAM) in under-5s (6 months to 5 years) must satisfy any one of the following parameters:

- Weight for height <3 SD/Z scores of the median new WHO growth standards of 2006.
- Visible severe wasting.
- Bipedal edema; and
- Mid-upper-arm circumference (MUAC)< 11.5 cm.

Despite fall in the incidence of both severe and mild to moderate malnutrition, SAM (both primary and secondary) is still an important cause of mortality in the Indian subcontinent.[1-5] Notably, it seldom exists in its pure form. On the other hand, a multitude of conditions, particularly concomitant infections are, by and large, a rule rather than an exception.[6-10]

India harbors around half of the world's malnourished children. Furthermore, India is the home for nearly 9 million under-5 children suffering from SAM. Most cases of severe malnutrition without complications can be managed at home with medical inputs from the health-care providers. This, however, does not hold good for children with SAM with complications such as diarrheal dehydration, anemia, hypoglycemia, hypothermia, septic shock, etc. This group of children essentially need to be managed in a health facility, preferably a hospital.

No other condition qualifies for as holistic an approach as SAM. All evidence shows that the mortality rate in well-treated children with SAM is 8-10% compared to 50% in poorly managed complicated SAM.[7,8]

This chapter deliberates on the management of SAM in general and SAM with complications in particular.

ASSESSMENT

Initial Clinical Assessment

Initial clinical assessment of severe malnutrition is made as shown in Box 32.1. The main objective is to decide if the SAM is with complications or without complications.

Box 32.1: Initial clinical assessment of SAM

History

- Recent intake of food and fluids
- Usual diet before the current
- Type (watery or bloody), duration and frequency of diarrhea and vomiting
- Loss of appetite
- Fever
- Symptoms suggesting superimposed infection in different locations
- Family's social background
- Chronic cough and contact with tuberculous patient
- Recent contact with a measles patient
- Known or suspected HIV infection

Clinical Examination

- Anthropometry
  - Weight
  - Length/height
  - Mid-upper-arm circumference (abbreviated as MUAC or MAC)
- Signs of dehydration
- Shock
  - Cold hands
  - Slow capillary refill
  - Weak and rapid pulse
- Lethargy or unconsciousness
- Severe palmar pallor (whitening of creases)
- Localizing signs of infection, including:
  - Ear and throat infection
  - Skin infection
  - Pneumonia
- Fever
  - Temperature 37.5°C (95.9°C)
  - Rectal temperature < 35.5°C (95.9°C)-hypothermia
- Mouth ulcers
- Skin changes of kwashiorkor (flaky-paint, crazy-pavement or mosaic dermatosis)
- Eye signs of vitamin A deficiency (VAD)
- Signs of HIV infection

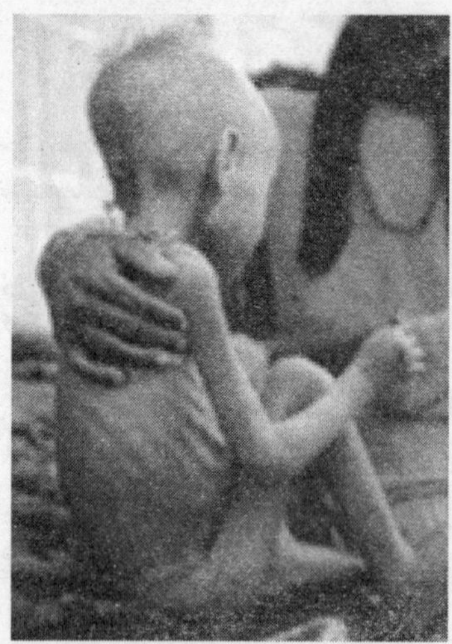

Fig. 32.1: Severe acute malnutrition: Note the obvious wasting with hair changes

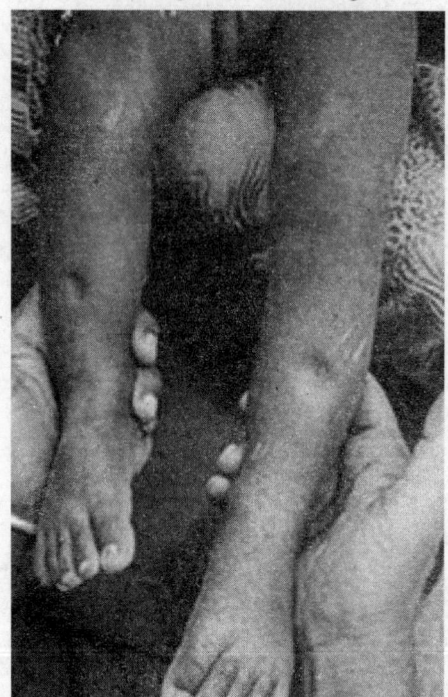

Fig. 32.2: Severe acute malnutrition: Note the demonstrable bipedal edema

Concurrently, usually some investigations (Table 32.1) are ordered.

Table 32.1: Initial investigations

Hemogram	
- Hemoglobin	Degree, type of anemia,
- Peripheral blood film	degree of dehydration,
- Hematocrit	malaria
- Malarial parasite	
Blood glucose	Hypoglycemia
Blood sodium	Type of dehydration
Blood potassium	Hypokalemia
Blood chloride bicarbonate, pH	Metabolic acidosis/alkalosis
Blood creatinine	Renal function status
C-reactive protein	Presence of infection
Stool microscopy	Ove, cysts, X-ray chest trophozoites
Mantoux test	Screening for tuberculous infection
Chest X-ray (CXR)	Pneumonia, pleural effusion, primary complex

MANAGEMENT: HOSPITAL OR DOMICILIARY

All SAM children with complications should be treated in a hospital or an alternative health facility. For uncomplicated SAM, earlier the WHO categorically insisted on hospital management. However, it has now fallen in line with such organizations as the Indian Academy of Pediatrics (IAP) that, since it is not practicable to accommodate them in a facility on account of the clinical load, they can be managed at home or in a nutritional rehabilitation center.

DOMICILIARY TREATMENT OF UNCOMPLICATED SAM

Box 32.2 summarizes the IAP guidelines on domiciliary treatment of SAM without complications.

Box 32.2: IAP guidelines on domiciliary treatment of uncomplicated SAM

Diet: Energy-dense therapeutic diet with low bulk in the initial phase:

- Home-based: Prepared/modified from the family pot; indigenously produced ready to use therapeutic food (RUTF)
- Cost-effective, easily available and acceptable
- Fed frequently (6-8 times/24 hours)

Supplements: Micronutrients, including vitamins and minerals

Oral Antibiotics: Usually cotrimoxazole or ampicillin for 7 days

Deworming: Single dose or a wormicidal like albendazole if even stools turn out to be negative for ova and cysts

Warming up: Hypothermia prevented by maintaining environmental temperature and covering the child well, especially during night

Immunization: Routine

Health education

Others: Family and community participation, nutrition counseling, household food security, etc.

HOSPITAL MANAGEMENT OF COMPLICATED SAM

According to current recommendations, management of complicated SAM is arbitrarily divided into three phases (Box 32.3).[7, 9-14]

Box 32.3: Three phases of management of SAM

Phase 1:	**Resuscitation/stabilizing phase,** extending from admission to 24-48 hours. The crux of its management is to resuscitate (stabilize) the seriously sick child who invariably has developed diarrheal dehydration plus other complications likely to prove fatal if left unattended (vide infra).
Phase 2:	**Acute (nutrition correction) phase,** extending from stabilization (2nd day) to 7th day. During this phase, focussed attention is given to nutritional correction, employing high energy and high protein diet (vide infra).
Phase 3:	**Rehabilitation phase,** after 7th day.

Ten essential steps under the umbrella of Phase 1, are:

Step 1 : Treatment/prevention of hypoglycemia
Step 2 : Treatment/prevention of hypothermia
Step 3 : Treatment/prevention of dehydration
Step 4 : Treatment/prevention of electrolyte balance
Step 5 : Treatment/prevention of infection
Step 6 : Treatment/prevention of micronutrient deficiencies
Step 7 : Initiation of cautious feeding
Step 8 : Achieving catchup growth
Step 9 : Provision of sensory stimulation and emotional support
Step 10 : Preparation for follow-up after recovery

Phase 1: Resuscitation (Stabilizing) Phase

(From admission to 24-48 hours)

During the first 6-24 hours, attempts are concentrated at stabilizing the acutely sick child through rehydration, treatment of hypoglycemia, thermoregulation, treatment of shock and treatment of severe anemia.

Rehydration

Assessment of Dehydration

Immediately on hospitalization, IV line must be started. The basic principles of assessing dehydration in malnourished children differ from healthy children in the following ways:

- A caution needs to be exercised in assessing dehydration in the presence of edema since the former is most likely to be erroneously missed or underdiagnosed because of waterlogging.
- In the presence of wasting, it is inclined to be over-estimated.
- Thirdly, some signs of dehydration may be encountered in septic shock which indeed may be frequently associated with severe PEM.

Box 32.4 lists the WHO recommended eight signs that are useful for assessing diarrheal dehydration in malnourished children. Out of these, the most useful and dependable criteria for assessing dehydration in acute severe malnutrition include:

- Dryness of buccal mucosa.
- Oliguria/anuria.
- Acidotic respiration, absence of tears.
- Shock (peripheral circulatory failure).

Box 32.4: WHO recommended eight signs for assessing dehydration in malnourished children

1. Watery diarrhea
2. Excessive thirst
3. Hypothermia
4. Sunken eyes
5. Weak or absent radial pulse
6. Cold hand and feet
7. Fall in urine output
8. Change in sensorium

Table 32.2 gives interpretation of these signs.

Table 32.2: Usefulness of WHO recommended signs for assessing dehydration and shock in malnourished children

Signs	*Some dehydration*	*Severe dehydration*	*Incipient septic shock*	*Overt septic shock*
Watery diarrhea	Yes	Yes	Yes/No	Yes/No
Thirst	Drinks eagerly	Drinks poorly	No	No
Hypothermia	No	No	Yes/No	Yes/No
Sunken eyes	Yes	Yes	No	No
Weak/absent radial pulse	No	Yes	Yes	Yes
Cold hand/feet	No	Yes	Yes	Yes
Urine output	Yes	No	No	Yes
Sensorium	Restless/ irritable	Lethargic/ comatose	Apathetic	Lethargic

For initial correction of dehydration, only 75% of calculated fluid and sodium requirements need be administered. IV fluid employed for this purpose should be hypotonic rather than hypertonic in view of the diminished water and sodium excretion capacity of the kidneys.

Oral Rehydration Therapy

This needs to be the first choice unless, of course, the malnourished child is severely dehydrated.

The malnourished child is known to have low potassium reserve and high sodium levels. With this background, ORS should be such as provides high potassium and low sodium. Such an ORS is available in the following two forms:

1. WHO recommended special rehydration solution for malnutrition (ReSoMal) with the composition shown in Table 32.3.

Table 32.3: ReSoMal vis-a-vis standard WHO ORS composition

Ingredient	*ReSoMal (mmol/L)*	*Standard WHO ORS (mmol/L)*
Glucose	125	111
Sodium	45	90
Potassium	40	20
Chloride	70	80
Citrate	7	10
Magnesium	3	0
Zinc	0.3	0
Copper	0.045	0
Osmolarity	300	311

2. Home-made ReSoMal can be prepared by diluting the standard WHO ORS in 2 liters of potable water rather than just one liter and adding 50 g sucrose (in place of 25 g) and 40 ml mineral mix. The composition of mineral mix is given in Table 32.4.

Table 32.4: Composition of mineral mix for ReSoMal

Ingredient	*Amount*
Potassium chloride	89.5 g
Tripotassium citrate	32.4 g
Magnesium chloride	30.5 g
Zin acetate	3.3 g
Copper sulfate	0.56g
Sodium selenate	10 mg
Potassium iodide	5
Water	1 L

ReSoMal is administered in a dose of 5 ml/kg every 30 minutes for 2 hours followed by 5-10 ml/kg/hour during the next 10 hours.

Intravenous Rehydration

In case of severely dehydrated malnourished child, this should be first option. Though the preferred fluid should be half-strength Darrow solution or half strength Ringer lactate with 5% dextrose, even half normal saline with 5% dextrose is suitable.

IV fluid is administered in a dose of 15 ml/kg over one hour. Side by side, ReSoMal is given in a dose of 10 ml/kg/hour by nasogastric tube. In case of unsatisfactory response, IV fluid is repeated and ReSoMal is continued for the next 10 hours.

Septic Shock

Poor response to this treatment points to presence of septic shock. Box 32.5 lists various features supporting diagnosis of septic shock.

Box 32.5: Features suggesting septic shock in acute severe PEM

- Failure of dehydration to respond to IV-cum-ORS (ReSoMal) regimen
- Such signs as limpness, apathy and anorexia without thirst or restlessness (incipient shock)
- Hypothermia
- Dilated superficial veins such as scalp veins
- Respiratory grunt or difficult breathing
- Gastrointestinal hemorrhage
- Abdominal distention

Once diagnosis of septic shock has been made, the child should be offered additional treatment with:

- Broad-spectrum antibiotics.
- Blood transfusion.
- Sympathomimetics (dopamine or dobutamine).
- Oxygen therapy and other supportive care.

Additional therapies aimed at modifying overexuberant host response, though of unconfirmed value, are listed in Box 32.6.

Box 32.6: Therapies aimed at modifying overexuberant response in septic shock

- Intravenous immunoglobulins (IVIG).
- Monoclonal antiendoxin anticore antibodies.
- Anti-TNF alpha IL-1 receptor antagonist.
- Granulocyte transfusions.

Treatment of Hypoglycemia

For asymptomatic hypoglycemia (blood sugar < 54 mg/dL or 3 mmol/L):

- Give 50 ml of 10% glucose or sucrose solution.
- Start feeding 2 hourly day and night (initially, 1/4th of the 2 hourly feed every 30 minutes till blood sugar stabilizes).
- Start appropriate antibiotics.

For symptomatic hypoglycemia:

- Give 10% dextrose IV, 5 ml/kg. If unavailable, give 50 ml 10% dextrose or sucrose solution by nasogastric tube.
- Follow with 50 ml of 10% dextrose or sucrose solution by nasogastric tube.
- Start feeding with the WHO's starter F-75 diet (Table 32.1) as quickly as possible and then continue the feeds 2-3 hourly day and night. Initially, give 1/4th of the 2 hourly feed every 30 minutes till the blood glucose stabilizes.
- Start appropriate antibiotics.

Treatment of Hypothermia (Thermoregulation)

Hypothermia is a known killer of malnourished children. It

may well be secondary to starvation, infection or hypoglycemia and, not infrequently, all these factors working in nexus. It should, therefore, be mandatory to keep the child in a warm environment covered with a blanket in order to combat hypothermia.

Treatment of Shock

The WHO guidelines for treatment of shock in acute severe malnutrition are as follows:

- Infuse IV fluids at 15 ml/kg over 1 hour. Use half normal saline with 5% dextrose or Ringer's lactate with 5% dextrose or, if unavailable, Ringer's lactate alone. Reassess after this.
  If child in shock is severely dehydrated, there should be improvement with IV treatment, manifested by fall in respiratory and pulse rates. In such a case:
- Repeat IV fluids 15 ml/kg over 1 hour once more and then switch to oral or nasogastric rehydration upto 10 hours (leave IV line in place in case required again). Then, initiate refeeding.
  If the subject fails to improve after 15 ml/kg/hour fluids, assume that he has septic shock. In this case:
- Maintenance IV fluids (4 ml/kg/hour) while waiting for blood. When blood is available, transfuse fresh whole blood at 10 ml/kg slowly over 3 hours. Then, initiate refeeding.

Treatment of Severe Anemia

According to the WHO, blood transfusion in severe anemia is warranted:

- When hemoglobin is < 4 g/dL.
- Respiratory distress with hemoglobin between 4-6 g/dL.

The WHO guidelines are as follows:

1. *Administration of Blood:* Administer whole blood 10 ml/kg slowly over 3 hours with frusemide 1 mg/kg IV at the start of transfusion. It is important that volume of 10 ml/kg is not exceeded. If the severely anemic child has signs of congestive cardiac failure (CCF), transfuse packed cells rather than whole blood.
2. *Monitoring for Transfusion Reactions:* Watch for signs of transfusion reactions, namely:
   - Fever.
   - Itchy rash.
   - Dark red urine.
   - Confusion and shock.

   In the presence of any of these signs, discontinue transfusion without loss of time.
3. *Monitoring for Respiratory and Pulse Rates:* While monitoring the respiratory rate and pulse rate every 15 minutes, if there is rise in any one, cut down the transfusion rate.
4. *Avoiding Repeat Transfusion:* If, despite blood transfusion, hemoglobin remains under 4 g/dL with continuing respiratory distress, do not jump at repeating the transfusion.

Treatment of Superimposed Infection(s)

Though empirical use of antimicrobials is believed to offer no advantage, broad spectrum antibiotic therapy should be given in children with ASPEM in the following situations without delay:

- In clearcut infection(s).
- Strongly suspected infections pending availability of culture and sensitivity report.

Phase 2: Acute (Nutritional Correction) Phase (From 2nd Day–7th Day)

Following stabilization of child's condition and his acceptance of oral feed in the stabilizing/resuscitation phase, nutritional rehabilitation should be initiated, preferably employing milk feeds.

Four important components (B-E-S-T) of this phase are:

1. **B**eginning of feeding.
2. **E**nergy dense feeds.
3. **S**timulation; and
4. **T**ransfer to home-based diet.

Nutritional rehabilitation is given by providing high protein and high energy diet. To begin with, a daily intake of 100 kcal/kg/day of expected weight or 150-200 kcal/kg/day of actual weight and 3 g/kg of protein calculated with reference to the actual weight should be the goal in the very first week. At least 10% of total calories should come from proteins of high biological value. This is important for the catch-up growth.

WHO's F-75 and F-100 (Box 32.7, Table 32.4) are the current recommendations. F-75 is for early dietary therapy when appetite is poor. F-100 is for subsequent dietary therapy when appetite improves and rapid weight gain is needed.

Box 32.7: Salient features of WHO's F-75 and F-100 diets

F-75 is the "starter" formula to use during initial management, beginning as soon as possible and continuing for 2-7 days until the child is stabilized. Severely malnourished children cannot tolerate usual amounts of protein and sodium at this stage, or high amounts of fat. They may die if given too much protein or sodium. They also need glucose, so they must be given a diet that is low in protein and sodium and high in carbohydrate. F-75 is specially made to meet the child's needs without overwhelming the body's systems in the initial stage of treatment. Use of F-75 prevents deaths. F-75 contains 75 kcal and 0.9 g protein per 100 ml.

As soon as the child is stabilized on F-75, F-100 is used as a "catch-up" formula to rebuild wasted tissues. F-100 contains more calories and protein: 100 kcal and 2.9 g protein per 100 ml. The choice of

Contd.

Contd.

recipe may depend on the availability of ingredients, particularly the type of milk, and the availability of cooking facilities.

The principle behind the recipes is to provide the energy and protein needed for stabilization and catch-up. For stabilization (F-75), it is important to provide a formula with the energy and protein as shown (no less and no more). For catch-up (F-100), the recipes show the minimum energy and protein contents needed.

The first three recipes given for F-75 include cereal flour and require cooking. The second part of the table shows recipes for F-75 that can be used if there is no cereal flour or no cooking facilities. However, the recipes with no cereal flour have a high osmolarity (415 mOsmol/l) and may not be tolerated well by some children with diarrhoea.

The F-100 recipes do not require cooking as they do not contain cereal flour.

In place of F-100, ready to use therapeutic food (RUTF) is a better option once the child is in a position to eat. Rather than a liquid form as is the case with F-100, it is precooked, moisture-free and oil-based. All this renders it microbiologically safe, readily available and yet nutritious. Ingredients of RUTF are: Peanut paste, milk powder, vegetable oil, sugar, potassium, magnesium, vitamins, minerals. Each 92 g packet provides 500 kcal.

Table 32.4: Composition of WHO's F-75 and F-100 diets

Ingredient	*Amount*	
	F-75[a-d]	*F-100*[e]
Dried skimmed milk	25 g	80 g
Sugar	70 g	50 g
Cereal flour	35 g	-
Vegetable oil	27 g	60 g
Mineral mix[f]	20 mL	20 mL
Vitamin mix[f]	140 mg	140 mg
Water to make	1000 mL	1000 mL

a. To prepare the F-75 diet, add the dried skimmed milk, sugar, cereal flour and oil to some water and mix. Boil for 5-7 minutes. Allow to cool, then add the mineral mix and vitamin mix and mix again. Make up the volume to 1000 mL with water.

b. A comparable formula can be made from 35 g of whole dried milk, 70 g of sugar, 35 g of cereal flour, 17 g of oil, 20 ml of mineral mix, 140 mg of vitamin mix and water to make 1000 mL.

c. Isotonic versions of F-75 (280 mOsmol/L), which contain maltodextrins instead of cereal flour and some of the sugar and which include all the necessary micronutrients, are available commercially.

d. If cereal flour is not available or there are no cooking facilities, a comparable formula can be made from 25 g of dried skimmed milk, 100 g of sugar, 27 g of oil, 20 mL of mineral mix, 140 mg of vitamin mix and water to make 1000 mL. However, this formula has a high osmolarity (415 mOsmol/L) and may not be well tolerated by all children, especially those with diarrhoea.

e. To prepare the F-100 diet, add the dried skimmed milk, sugar and oil to some warm boiled water and mix. Add the mineral mix and vitamin mix and mix again. Make up the volume to 1000 mL with water.

f. See "WHO Vitamin mix" and "WHO Mineral mix" tables. If only small amounts of feed are being prepared, it will not be feasible to prepare the vitamin mix because of the small amounts involved. In this case, give a proprietary multivitamin supplement. Alternatively, a combined mineral and vitamin mix for malnourished children is available commercially and can be used in the above diets.

It is advisable to avoid whole cow's milk in children < 1 year of age on account of risks of cow's milk protein (CMP) allergy, iron-deficiency anemia, and high osmolarity causing renal damage, especially in state of dehydration.

Local resources should always be borne in mind while making a choice of the foodstuffs. It is advisable to feed small amounts of food at frequent intervals.

At times, it may become necessary to initiate nutritional therapy through Ryle's tube (enteral feeding).

Too intensive nutritional therapy should be avoided in view of risk of occurrence of some adverse phenomena including refeeding syndrome and nutritional recovery (Gomez) syndrome, that can be counterproductive.

Phase 3: Rehabilitation Phase (After First Week – 2-6 Weeks)

Following the acute phase, the child usually accepts more and more food. This, in fact, should be encouraged. The employment of ready-to-use therapeutic food, the current recommendation by the WHO, may be taken into consideration. This paradigm shift in managing SAM is based on the observation that RUTF, being a ready-made oil-based food without water, is hygienically safe besides being nutritious. With its availability, the hospitalization for management of SAM may well be restricted to only children with complicated SAM.

According to the National Consensus Workshop on Management of SAM Children through Medical Nutrition Therapy,[15] product-based RUTF can be introduced on a pilot basis at district or state level, utilizing existing system for sustainability, provided that it is employed only:

- As a therapeutic and not supplementary feeding.
- Above 6 months of age.
- For a limited time (4-8 weeks) until the child recovers from SAM which should be defined in explicit treatment protocols.

Nutrition and Health Education During Hospital Stay: The hospital stay needs to be utilized to educate the parents (mother, in particular) about the value of high protein and high calorie diet of the family type so that it becomes easy to achieve consolidation of cure at home.

Follow-up Phase: An extension of this phase is the so-called "follow-up phase" (it may well be designated as the *Fourth phase*) in which it is ensured that the child's nutritional rehabilitation is consolidated at home as well for a complete recovery and to minimize risk of a relapse of SAM. The hallmark of this phase is consistent nutritional education together with periodic follow-up, including home visits by the health workers.

In view of the risk of death after discharge (since the child returns to the same environment in which he had developed SAM), follow-up is mandatory.

Each follow-up visit should be utilized:

- To record child's weight.

- For immunization; and
- For reinforcement of nutrition and health education.

At the same time, it is important to pay attention to child's immunization.

RESPONSE TO NUTRITIONAL REHABILITATION

Not all children respond to treatment according to our expectations.

Primary failure is indicated by failure of:

- Resumption of appetite by 4th day.
- Beginning of loss of edema by 4th day and its disappearance by 10th day.
- Weight gain: At least 5 g/kg/day by 10th day is mandatory.

Factors contributing to poor response to nutritional rehabilitation include:

- Feeding inadequacy.
- Failure to adequately treat accompanying infections.
- Failure to adequately treat accompanying dehydration and dyselectrolytemia.
- Failure to attend to accompanying nutritional deficiency states such as anemia.
- Poor facilities: Untrained and poorly motivated staff, inadequate environment.
- Serious underlying diseases: Malabsorption, immunodeficiency, inborn errors of metabolism, malignancy, etc.

DISCHARGE CRITERIA

The best time to discharge the child is when he has gained weight that is in keeping with his actual height (not age). That usually takes on an average about 6-8 weeks. But, then retaining the child so long is, as a rule, not workable on account of the increasing pressure on hospital beds. An acceptable way out is to discharge the child when he has achieved a weight that is 85-90% (preferably 90%) of the weight for height. This usually happens in 2 to 4 weeks time.

The following additional criteria should also be met:

- Absence of infection.
- Intake of at least 120-130 kcal/kg/day with adequate micronutrients.
- Consistent weight gain of at least 5 g/kg/day for 3 successive days on exclusive oral feedings.
- Absence of edema.
- Completed immunization appropriate for age.
- Sensitization of the care-providers to good home care.

Criteria for early discharge pertaining to the child are:

- > 12 months age.
- Antibiotic therapy completed.
- Appetite and weight gain good.
- Already received 2 weeks of vitamin/mineral supplement.

Or

Continuing such supplements at home is workable.

Criteria for early discharge pertaining to mother/care-provider.

- Not employed outside home.
- Specifically competent to give appropriate feeding.
- Financially resourceful to feed the child.
- Has a reachable hospital for urgent hospitalization if warranted.
- Can be visited weekly.
- Trained to give structured play therapy.
- Motivated to follow doctor's advice.

Criteria for early discharge pertaining to the local health worker:

- Trained to support home care.
- Specifically trained to examine child clinically at home, to take appropriate advice and to decide if the child needs referral back to the hospital.

In order that the child convalescing from SAM with nutritional rehabilitation continues to be appropriately looked after at home, the guidelines in respect of the care-providers are:

- Continuation of frequent feeding with energy and nutrient dense foods.
- Completion of leftover immunization shots.
- Vitamin A prophylaxis every 6 months.
- Provision of structured play therapy.
- Periodic regular follow-up checkups.

NUTRITIONAL REHABILITATION AT HOME

For complete recovery, another 2-4 months nutritional rehabilitation at home may be needed.

PROGNOSIS

A number of factors contribute to bad prognosis. Box 32.8 lists common causes of mortality in acute severe malnutrition. Timely and prompt attention to these conditions is crucial to cut down mortality. A high index of vigilance and suspicion plays a considerable role in their prevention, early diagnosis and treatment.

Box 32.8: Factors contributing to bad prognosis in SAM

- Severe dehydration, especially when accompanied by electrolyte and acid-base disturbances
- Hypoglycemia
- Hypothermia
- Fulminant infection
- Congestive cardiac failure
- Xerophthalmia
- Bleeding diathesis
- Grossly enlarged liver with deranged LFT
- Seizures
- Change in sensorium
- Cachexia
- Severe dermatosis

ADVERSE PHENOMENA ENCOUNTERED DURING OVERENTHUSIASTIC NUTRITIONAL CORRECTION

A. Protein Overload[13]

1. Pseudotumor Cerebri

Overenergetic nutritional correction in malnourished infants may be accompanied by a transient rise of intracranial tension. The phenomenon is benign and self-limiting.

2. Nutritional Recovery Syndrome (Gomez Syndrome)

The term refers to an interesting sequelae of events seen in children who are being treated with very high quantity of proteins during the course of rehabilitation from gross malnutrition. The syndrome is characterized by increasing hepatomegaly, abdominal distention, ascites, prominent thoracoabdominal venous network, hypertrichosis, parotid swelling, gynecomastia and eosinophilia. In some instances, splenomegaly also occurs. Though the syndrome was initially described in kwashiorkor from Africa, we have recorded its occurrence in both kwashiorkor and marasmus in India.

Etiopathogenesis of this syndrome remains speculative. Its development may well be related to endocrinal disturbances. That in PEM the function of the pituitary and its target glands is set at a lower ebb is well known. This response of the pituitary to the state of poor dietary intake appears to be an adaptive mechanism that permits survival of the patient by reducing body activity and metabolic rate, and by retarding growth. During nutritional rehabilitation, the greater utilization of the hormone by the body stimulates the pituitary to produce its trophic hormones. This results in a response by the target glands. Thus, it appears that the nutritional recovery syndrome is caused by an increase in estrogen level and by a variety of trophic hormones produced by the recovering pituitary gland.

3. Encephalitis-like Syndrome

About one-fifth children with kwashiorkor become drowsy within 3 to 4 days after initiation of dietary therapy. Most often, the condition is self-limiting. Occasionally, it may be accompanied by progressive unconsciousness with fatal outcome. Even more rarely, a transient syndrome marked by coarse tremors, parkinsonian rigidity, bradykinesia and myoclonus (Kahn syndrome) may appear 6 to 7 days after starting the dietary rehabilitation. Sometimes, tremors (the so-called "kwashi-shakes") may occur during the recovery phase and may take even months to resolve.

These encephalitis-like states are considered to be the result of far too much of proteins in the diet.

B. Energy Overload

Refeeding Syndrome

This is a complication of too intensive carbohydrate therapy.[16,17]

The syndrome is characterized by development of hemolytic anemia, seizures, muscle weakness and cardiac and respiratory failure in the first 1-3 days or sometime in the rest of the first week of nutritional correction with very high doses of carbohydrates, both orally and intravenously, given overenthusiastically, with high mortality.

It is hypothesized that when a child with SAM receives aggressive nutritional support, a sudden surge of insulin with a shift from protein to carbohydrate metabolism occurs, causing a massive intracellular move of phosphate, magnesium and potassium and a life-threatening depletion of these electrolytes in the blood. The lack of these three key electrolytes plus the target tissue hypoxemia causes the above-mentioned manifestations. Hemolytic anemia results since phosphate is needed in the RBCs for 2,3-diphosphaglycerate production used for easier release of oxygen into the target tissues.

Pathophysiology

Any child who has had negligible nutrient intake for 5 consecutive days is at risk of developing the refeeding syndrome. It occurs within four days of starting to feed. Patients who weigh less than 70% of ideal body weight or lose weight rapidly are at greatest risk for the syndrome. During prolonged starvation, the body conserves muscle and protein breakdown by switching to ketone bodies derived from fatty acids as the main energy source. The liver decreases its rate of gluconeogenesis thus conserving muscle and protein. Many intracellular minerals become severely depleted during this period, although serum levels remain normal. Insulin secretion is suppressed and glucagon secretion is increased.

During refeeding, the metabolism shifts from a catabolic to an anabolic state. Insulin is released on carbohydrate intake resulting in increased glycogen, fat and protein synthesis. Insulin release triggers cellular uptake of potassium, phosphate and magnesium, which are already depleted and the stores rapidly become used up. When the serum concentrations of these electrolytes are reduced, serious complications, such as irregular heart beat can occur. Patients can also develop fluid and electrolyte imbalance, low phosphate levels, neurologic, lung, heart, neuromuscular, and blood related complications. Refeeding increases the basal metabolic rate. Glucose and levels of the thiamine may also fall.

Irregular heart rhythm is the most common cause of death with other significant risks including confusion, coma and convulsions and cardiac failure. The diagnostic features are the presence of low phosphate, potassium, magnesium, vitamin B_1 levels and fluid overload with edema feet. Low phosphate level is the essential criterion for diagnosis.

Prevention

In order to safeguard from occurrence of this fatal syndrome, a multipronged strategy is needed (Box 32.9).

Box 32.9: Strategy to prevent refeeding syndrome

- Assessment of hydration status, serum electrolytes, magnesium and phosphate and electrolytes.
- Initiation of feeding by slowly increasing the volume and energy content, starting with about 70-75% of the calculated energy requirements.
- Provision of frequent, small meals consisting of proteins and lipids together with carbohydrates with an energy density of 1 kcal/ml to minimize the fluid load.
- Administration of supplement potassium 4 mmol/kg/day, magnesium 0.6 mmol/kg/day, sodium 1 mmol/kg/day, phosphate upto 1 mmol/kg/day (IV) or upto 100 mmol (O) for children > 5 years of age.
- Monitoring of electrolytes, phosphate, magnesium, glucose, calcium, urea and creatinine daily.
- Monitoring of hydration and cardiac status.
- Administration of supplements thiamine, riboflavin, folic acid, vitamin C, pyridoxine, vitamin A and D, and trace elements.
- Identification and omission (if feasible) of drugs that may further contribute to electrolyte imbalances.

Box 32.10 gives the approach in managing refeeding syndrome.

Box 32.10: Management of refeeding syndrome

- If the refeeding syndrome occurs, nutritional replenishment should be slowed down. Immediate correction of low levels of phosphates, potassium and magnesium, while monitoring the cardiovascular system is warranted.
- Before and during the first 10 days of feeding, it is important to give supplements of oral thiamine and a balanced multi-vitamin and mineral supplement each day.
  One should monitor and supplement oral, enteral, or intravenous potassium, phosphate and magnesium in such patients.
- On an average, patients should receive 2-4 mmol/kg/day potassium, 0.3-0.6 mmol/kg/day phosphate, and 0.2 mmol/kg/day IV or 0.4 mmol/kg/day oral magnesium. Moderately to severely ill patients with marked edema or a serum phosphorous <2 mg/dL should be hospitalized to intravenously correct electrolyte deficiencies.

Acknowledgements: Thanks are due to the WHO for permission to incorporate its data on F-75 and F-100. Thanks are also due to the Director, Principal and Medical Superintendent, Narayana Medical College and Hospitals for providing motivation and encouragement to complete this chapter for the book, ***Pediatric Nutrition***.

REFERENCES

1. World Health Organization.WHO Child Growth Standards and the Identification of Severe Acute Malnutrition in Infants and Children. A Joint Statement by the WHO/UNICEF 2009. Available at: http://www.who. Int/nutrition/publications/severemalnutrition/9789241598163/en/index.html.Accessed on: 14 June 2011.
2. Gupte S, Gomez EM, Gomez EE, Gomez M. Protein-energy malnutrition: Changing trends in management. In: Gupte S, Gupte SB (eds): *Recent Advances in Pediatrics (Special Vol 20: Nutrition, Growth and Development)*. New Delhi: Jaypee 2009: 91-120.
3. Kolacek S. Treatment methods and goals in pediatric malnutrition. Annales Nestle 2009; 67:85-93.
4. Gupte S, Padha V. Pitfalls in the treatment of advanced protein-energy malnutrition in a premier medical institute. *Int J Med Pediatr Pract* 1971; 6:231-236.
5. Elizabeth KE, George Jacob R. Nutritional support in the critically ill child. In: Gupte S, Gupte SB (eds): *Recent Advances in Pediatrics (Special Vol 14: Criticare Pediatrics)*. New Delhi: Jaypee 2004;546-565.
6. Ashworth A, Jackson A, Uauy R. Focusing on malnutrition management to improve child survival in India. *Indian Pediatr* 2007; 44:413-416.
7. Gupte S: Issues and controversies in rehabilitation of severely malnourished infants and children. *Hospital Rev* 2002; 21:112-115.
8. Gupte S. Acute severe protein-energy malnutrition (PEM). In: Gupte S, Gupte SB (eds): *Recent Advances in Pediatrics (Special Vol. 8: Emergency Pediatrics)*. New Delhi: Jaypee 2001;172-179.
9. Inamdar S. Changing trends in nutritional disorders. In: Gupte S, Gupte SB (eds): *Recent Advances in Pediatrics-4*. New Delhi: Jaypee 1994;9: 34-47.
10. Mathur GP, Kushwaha KP, Mathur S. Protein-energy malnutrition (PEM) updated. In: Gupte S, Gupte SB (eds): *Recent Advances in Pediatrics (Special Vol 6: Gastroenterology, Hepatology and Nutrition)*. New Delhi: Jaypee 2000;479-506.
11. Bhatnagar S, Lodha R, Choudhury P. IAP guidelines 2006 on hospital based management of severely malnourished children (adapted from the WHO guidelines). *Indian Pediatr* 2007;44:443-461.
12. Raju U. Nutritional support in the hospitalized children. In: Gupte S, Gupte SB (eds): *Recent Advances in Pediatrics (Special Vol 20: Nutrition, Growth and Development)*. New Delhi: Jaypee 2009:121-135.
13. Gupte S, Gomez EM. Protein-energy malnutrition. In: Gupte S (ed) *The Short Textbook of Pediatrics*, 11th edn., New Delhi: Jaypee 2009;128-154.
14. World Health Organization: WHO Guidelines for inpatient treatment of severely malnourished children. Available at: http:www.ishtm.ac.uk/eps/malnu,pdf. Accessed 4 June 2011.
15. Writing Committee: Sachdev HPS, Kapil U, Vir S. Consensus Statement: National Consensus Workshop on Management of SAM Children through Medical Nutrition Therapy. *Indian Pediatr* 2010;47:661-665.
16. Gupte S, Kumar R. Nutritional recovery syndrome Vs refeeding syndrome: Two different entities. *Asian Bull Nutr* 2008; 11: 45-49.
17. Afzal N, Addai S, Fagbemi A, *et al.* Refeeding syndrome with enteral nutrition in children: A case report, literature review and clinical guidelines. *Clin Nutr* 2002;21:515-520.

Novy Gupte • Suraj Gupte

33 Medical Nutrition Therapy in Severe Acute Malnutrition (SAM)

INTRODUCTION

Notwithstanding concerted remedial measures at various levels, severe acute malnutrition (SAM) in under-5s, though considerably fallen in incidence even in Sub-Saharan Africa,[1] continues to haunt us both in hospitals and other healthcare facilities and in the community.[2]

In India alone, almost 9 million under-5 children suffer from SAM (Fig. 33.1). The mortality too is colossal – 0.6 million. The DALYs stand at 24.6 million. This burden from SAM in India is perhaps highest in South-East Asian Region (SEAR), nay globally.

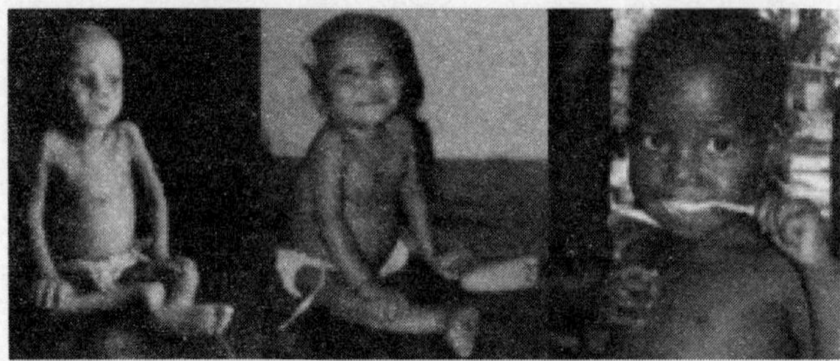

Fig. 33.1: SAM in under-5s: India has surpassed Sub-Saharan Africa as the home of SAM–a matter of serious concern for the policymakers

PROBLEM OF SAM MANAGEMENT

Ideally these children, especially with acute complications, need to be treated in a health facility.[2] After years of innovation, the World Health Organization (WHO) introduced special foods for nutritional rehabilitation of such children in the form of F-75 and F-100 (Table 33.1), the former for initial dietary correction when their appetite is poor and the latter for catchup/speedy weight gain after the recovery has begun. This is a liquid food meant for nutritional therapy in the healthcare facility.

The burden of SAM is large enough to be accommodated by the hospitals and other healthcare facilities regardless whether it is sub-Saharan Africa or the Indian subcontinent. At the same time, there is evidence that all the SAM children without acute complications can be treated in the domestic environments.

It has, therefore, been felt that ways and means to provide good, effective and practicable nutritional rehabilitation need to be searched to treat such children in their home environment. The modern nutritional therapies are based on the WHO-recommended F-75 formula for the sick without an appetite followed by F-100 formula for rapid weight gain.[3] The problem with these foods is that, being in a liquid form, these are vulnerable to bacterial contamination under routine environment such as at home.

The Way Out

The availability of medical nutrition therapy in the form of Ready-to-Use Therapeutic Food (RUTF) has opened up a promising avenue in this behalf. [4-6]

The RUTF has been shown to be efficacious in affecting complete recovery from childhood malnutrition in several studies, the most remarkable being from Chad and Senegal in hospital and Malayi and Ethiopia in the community.

The most well-known RUTF is available as a commercial product packed in oxygen-free foil sachets (Nutriset, Malaunay, France). The solid, peanut-butter based RUTF is an energy-dense lipid paste that resists bacterial contamination because of its low water content and does not require cooking before consumption. To make this therapy more widely available in the developing world where childhood malnutrition is rampant, local production is needed

This special therapeutic diet allows nutritional rehabilitation of a large number of children suffering from uncomplicated SAM at home, is preferred by parents, and dramatically improves the coverage. The candidates to receive treatment need to be screened in the community and treated before the child's SAM gets complicated. In the latter situation, hospitalization usually is required.

THE STORY OF RUTF IN A NUTSHELL

As far back as late 1990s, a private sector company, Nutriset, known for nutritional products for humanitarian relief, first introduced RUTF especially for treatment of

SAM in the nutritional rehabilitation phase. It is high in energy and protein with added electrolytes, vitamins and micronutrients. It is equivalent to WHO's F100 (Table 33.1) in terms of nutrients/100 kcal.

Table 33.1: Preparation of WHO-recommended F-75 and F-100 diets for nutritional rehabilitation

Ingredient	*Amount*	
	F-75[a-d]	*F-100*[e]
Dried skimmed milk	25 g	80 g
Sugar	70 g	50 g
Cereal flour	35 g	-
Vegetable oil	27 g	60 g
Mineral mix[f]	20 mL	20 mL
Vitamin mix[f]	140 mg	140 mg
Water to make	1000 mL	1000 mL

a. To prepare the F-75 diet, add the dried skimmed milk, sugar, cereal flour and oil to some water and mix. Boil for 5-7 minutes. Allow to cool, then add the mineral mix and vitamin mix and mix again. Make up the volume to 1000 mL with water.

b. A comparable formula can be made from 35 g of whole dried milk, 70 g of sugar, 35 g of cereal flour, 17 g of oil, 20 ml of mineral mix, 140 mg of vitamin mix and water to make 1000 mL.

c. Isotonic versions of F-75 (280 mOsmol/L), which contain maltodextrins instead of cereal flour and some of the sugar and which include all the necessary micronutrients, are available commercially.

d. If cereal flour is not available or there are no cooking facilities, a comparable formula can be made from 25 g of dried skimmed milk, 100 g of sugar, 27 g of oil, 20 mL of mineral mix, 140 mg of vitamin mix and water to make 1000 mL. However, this formula has a high osmolarity (415 mOsmol/L) and may not be well tolerated by all children, especially those with diarrhoea.

e. To prepare the F-100 diet, add the dried skimmed milk, sugar and oil to some warm boiled water and mix. Add the mineral mix and vitamin mix and mix again. Make up the volume to 1000 mL with water.

f. For preparing "WHO Vitamin mix" and "WHO Mineral mix", consult the recommended tables. If only small amounts of feed are being prepared, it will not be feasible to prepare the vitamin mix because of the small amounts involved. In this case, give a proprietary multivitamin supplement. Alternatively, a combined mineral and vitamin mix for malnourished children is available commercially and can be used in the above diets.

Adapted from: World Health Organization. *Management of Severe Malnutrition: A Manual for Physicians and other Senior Health Workers.* Geneva: WHO 1999.

Moreover, RUTF is precooked, needing no mixing with water. Thus, it is microbiologically safe and enables treatment in the community.

Currently, the most widely employed RUTF is Plumpy'nut. Its ingredients are:

- Peanut paste.
- Milk powder.
- Vegetable oil.
- Sugar.
- Potassium.
- Magnesium.
- Vitamins.
- Minerals.

Each 92 g pack provides 500 kcal.

According to WHO/UNICEF, RUTF is a medical nutrition therapy based on sound scientific principles with a balanced composition of type I and type II nutrients (Fig. 33.2). Extensive experience in Africa and some in the Indian subcontinent has shown that RUTF results in physiological

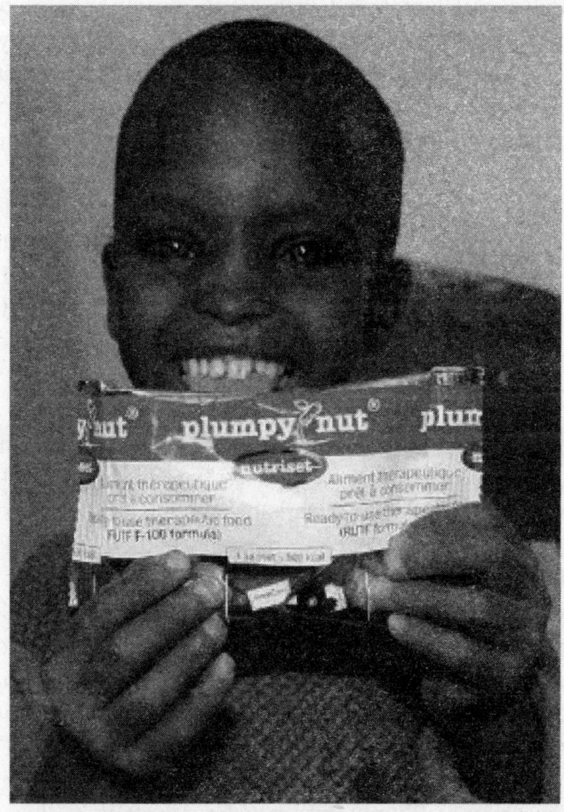

Fig. 33.2: RUTF as Plumy'Nut: The 'Plumpynut' is a ready-to-use therapeutic food (RUTF). It is nutrient-dense, basically made of peanut butter, powdered sugar, and is enriched with enough vitamins and minerals that could fulfill the needs of the children suffering from SAM. This dense therapeutic food can be produced and stored locally and transported easily, and requires no refrigeration, making it ideal for use in hot climates. Each serving is equivalent to a glass of milk and a multi-vitamin tablet and minerals. The international medical humanitarian organization 'Doctors Without Borders' hopes to eradicate the malnutrition deaths among children by addressing their needs with this nutritional breakthrough product

and functional (including immunological) recovery. Its specific composition has been tested and convincingly proved effective in functional recovery from SAM. What is noteworthy is that RUTF is of value both in the facility and home management of SAM. A rider is that in case of home-based rehabilitation, the SAM child should not be suffering from such medical complications as diarrheal dehydration, hypoglycemia, hypothermia, pneumonia, sepsis, bleeding diathesis, etc.

RUTF is a ready-made food that can be used by the child without the addition of water which otherwise in the given environment could well be a source of bacterial contamination of the food. The nutritional component is very close to the WHO-recommended F-100 diet. Such a diet is obtained by replacing in the original recipe about one-half of the dried skimmed milk with peanut butter, removing all water and increasing the amount of oil. Elimination of water from the RUTF recipe nearly removes the risk of bacterial contamination as bacteria need water to grow. This food is safe for use in the community, warranting no special storage facility and no cooking since it is precooked.

With the availability of RUTF, in patient management of SAM may well be restricted to complicated SAM only and that too only until medical complications exist. Once the child with SAMS is complication-free, he can be shifted to his home environment where RUTF should be continued.

PRODUCTION OF RUTF

Until recently, RUTF happened to be a monopoly of France that exported it to other countries. The high cost of the imported RUTF was a remarkable roadblock to its wide-scale usage. There were several other logistic difficulties in the wider use of the commercial product.

Mercifully, in Africa, the originator of the concept, RUTF of international standard (as good as from France) is now produced indigenously using local crops grown by small holder farmers, resulting in easy availability, and reduction in cost that is just one-half of the imported product. The locally produced RUTF in Malawi follows the same recipe as the original Plumpynut from France. It is packed in 250 g plastic jars. The shelf-life is up to 6 months. This RUTF is, in all ways, nutritionally equivalent to its imported version. A remarkable decline in mortality from SAM has resulted following the extensive use of the indigenous RUTF. Equally noteworthy is the fact that the strategy has also led to economic gains for the farmers.[1]

A recent study from Vellore, South India, has demonstrated that using a locally-made RUTF in the community-based treatment of childhood malnutrition is feasible and effective in rural South Indian setting.[4] The RUTF in this study differed from the standard RUTF in the micronutrient composition.

RUTF production is a simple process. All that is needed is grinding, mixing and packaging using widely available equipment. India is already manufacturing and exporting RUTF on commercial level. There is need to carry out work for production of safe, economic and effective RUTF at non-commercial level.

RUTF VIS-À-VIS FAMILY FOODS

A logical question arises: How does RUTF (which is more expensive) differ from the high energy mixtures of family foods fed to SAM infants and children? Unlike routine high-energy family foods, RUTF neither needs cooking nor mixing with water. This renders it microbiologically safer since high fat content and negligible moisture prevents bacterial growth. It has a shelf-life of several months in simple packaging. Furthermore whereas in family foods, electrolytes and micronutrients are added as supplements, in case of RUTF these are added during the process of production. In the light of all these plus points, the relatively high cost of RUTF appears to be easily nullified by its overriding benefits.

Nonetheless, well-planned studies exploring this aspect of RUTF are warranted.

RECOMMENDED INDICATIONS OF RUTF

RUTF needs to be employed as a therapeutic modality rather than as a supplementary feed in infants (>6 months) and children (up to 5 years) for a limited time period (say 4-8 weeks) until the child recovers from acute malnutrition in two settings:

1. Healthcare facility involving complicated SAM in which case it is continued after the child is discharged following recovery from complications of acute malnutrition and beginning of weight gain.
2. At home for children suffering from uncomplicated SAM and children rendered complication-free through initial treatment in a facility.

In order to safeguard from exploitation of the RUTF by the commercial companies, it has been suggested that RUTF should be operationalized by the Ministry of Health and Family Welfare through the IMNCI and ICDS in India.

GREY AREAS CONCERNING RUTF

Without any shadow of doubt, RUTF has proved its utility in medical nutritional therapy of SAM. Nevertheless, there remain certain aspects where we are yet not clear about RUTF. These aspects need further exploration.

For instance, it remains to be determined if RUTF, in any way, can adversely affect breastfeeding.

Secondly, what could its status be in comparison with home-based and locally-formulated products?

Thirdly, physiological/functional recovery and longer benefits of RUTF in comparison to home-based and locally-formulated products need to be determined.

Fourthly, operationalization and economic analysis in different settings is warranted.

Fifthly, it is mandatory to test RUTF for aflatoxin, microbials, heavy metals, pesticides, lipid oxidation, moisture content, fat and protein share, water activity and minerals and vitamin concentrations.[7]

Sixthly, it is very important to produce cost-effective RUTF that is effective and acceptable locally. The calculated expenditure for rehabilitation of a SAM child works out to be around US $ 55. It would double up if the child is also suffering from HIV/AIDS. This indeed is an exorbitant cost in the source-limited countries. Imagine, for instance, in India per capita healthcare expenditure on an average is just US $ 39 only.

Seventhly, there is need to establish cost-effectiveness of locally-produced RUTF as also similar locally-produced products in a non-emergency setting in the Indian context.[5, 6] This aspect has not yet been adequately studied.

RUTF IN INDIA

RUTF is a new concept for India. The experience to date has been very limited. As already pointed out, most of the studies demonstrating its efficacy and safety are from Africa and that too in emergency settings in a facility such as a hospital rather than the community-based. Only limited information is available on its usefulness and practicability in non-emergency settings. There is hardly any such study conducted in India in home/community setting.

Pilot studies conducted in Madhya Pradesh and Bihar vouch for the effectiveness of RUTF in SAM. Similar observations have been made from Maharashtra, Bengal and Gujarat employing locally-formulated products.[8]

A recently-held National Consensus Workshop has made favorable recommendations for promoting this strategy of managing SAM with RUTF in India (Box 33.1).[8]

Box 33.1: Highlights of the consensus statement of the National Consensus Workshop on Management of SAM children through medical nutrition therapy[8]

1. Upto 15% under-5 children with SAM require in patient management because of medical complications. The remaining 85% (without medical complications) can be managed through a community- and/or home-based care approach.
2. Medical nutrition therapy (MNT) in the form of Ready to Use Therapeutic Food (RUTF) has established its role in achieving physiological and functional (including immunological) recovery in SAM children between 6 months-5 years without complications primarily in studies from Africa for both facility and home-based management.

Contd.

Contd.

3. The limited Indian experience on the usefulness of RUTF supports the observations made from African countries.
4. The apprehension of commercialization in India can be obviated by:
   - Non-proprietary product.
   - Partially decentralized manufacture with public sector involvement.
   - Public health system, being the sole procurement agency with a specific strategy that ensures purchase from multiple producers; and
   - Prescribed product which is not freely available.
5. Product-based RUTF can be introduced on a pilot basis at scale (district or state level) utilizing existing system for sustainability, provided that it is employed only:
   - As a therapeutic and not supplementary feeding.
   - Above 6 months of age.
   - For a limited time (4-8 weeks) until the child recovers from SAM which should be defined in explicit treatment protocols.
6. MNT should be operationalized by the Health Ministry through the Integrated Management of Newborn and Childhood Illnesses (IMNCI) which also has a component for the management of SAM. The Integrated Child Development Service (ICDS) scheme could converge for the identification and referral of children with SAM and the follow-up of these children after their discharge from the therapeutic feeding.
7. To aid the evaluation process in an observational manner, outcome measures should be recorded after some time of operationalization of intervention program and include follow-up of rehabilitated children.
8. Regulatory issues need to be resolved between the 2 nodola authorities, i.e., Drug Controller General of India and Food Safety and Standards Authority of India, before MNT can be operationalized.
9. Food and nutrition security and preventive aspects should be ensured during treatment for and after recovery from SAM to prevent relapses.
10. Urgent research issues include:
    - Comparison of RUTF with home-based and locally-formulated products.
    - Physiological recovery and longer benefits of the above treatments.
    - Effects of introduction of RUTF on breast feeding.
    - Operationalization and economic analysis in different settings.

All said and done, RUTF is an important community-based medical therapeutic food for the management of SAM, both in hospital and at the domestic level. Its usage certainly needs encouragement and support from all stake-holders. The apprehension that it may in some way interrupt or undermine the activities aimed at promoting appropriate infant and young child feeding practices is not well founded in as much as that MNT using RUTF is only a short-term intervention to tide over the SAM.

Acknowledgements: Thanks are also due to the Director, Principal and Medical Superintendent, Narayana Medical College and Hospitals for providing motivation and encouragement to complete this chapter for the book, ***Pediatric Nutrition***.

REFERENCES

1. Briend A, Collins S. Therapeutic nutrition for children with severe acute malnutrition: Summary of African experience. *Indian Pediatr* 2010;47:655-659.
2. Gupte S, Gomez EM. Protein-energy malnutrition. In: Gupte S (ed): *The Short Textbook of Pediatrics*, 11th edn. New Delhi: Jaypee 2009: 129-153.
3. Golden MH. Review article: Evolution of nutritional management of acute malnutrition. *Indian Pediatr* 2010;47:667-678.
4. Singh AS, Kang G, Ramachandran A, Sarkar R, Peter P, Bose A. Locally made ready-to-use therapeutic food for treatment of malnutrition: A randomized controlled trial. *Indian Pediatr* 2010;47: 679-686.
5. Ashworth A. Efficacy and effectiveness of community-based treatment of severe malnutrition. *Food Nutr Bull* 2006;27: S24-48.
6. Gera T. Efficacy and safety of therapeutic nutrition products for home-based therapeutic nutrition for severe acute malnutrition: A systemic review. *Indian Pediatr* 2010;47:709-718.
7. Beesabathunt KN, Natchu UCM. Production and distribution of a therapeutic nutritional product for severe acute malnutrition in India: Opportunities and challenges. *Indian Pediatr* 2010;47:702-706.
8. Writing Committee: Sachdev HPS, Kapil U, Vir S. Consensus Statement: National Consensus Workshop on Management of SAM Children through Medical Nutrition Therapy. *Indian Pediatr* 2010;47:661-665.

Uday Bodhankar • Meenakshi Girish

34 The Child with Failure to Thrive

INTRODUCTION

The term, *failure to thrive (FTT),* was first coined to describe a syndrome of delayed growth and development that was also called the *maternal deprivation syndrome*. There is now consensus that FTT has a predominantly nutritional cause though the implication of an association with emotional and physical deprivation persists. However, all the early studies that emphasized the role of emotional and physical deprivation in this syndrome were of highly selected children referred to hospital. It is in only in the past 2 decades that population based studies have been conducted.

DEFINITION

Growth is a dynamic process. Any disorder of growth can best be appreciated in terms of abnormal velocity of growth as plotted on a *Road to Health Chart*. Unfortunately, most of the time we do not have any idea of growth velocity, simply because we don't have any past records of the child's weight. Therefore, all definitions of FTT are based primarily on attained weight or rate of weight gain. Although measurements of head circumference are important in the evaluation of infants and toddlers, failure of the head to grow is not part of the FTT entity. Assessment of length or height does help in the evaluation of FTT. For example, children who exhibit FTT usually have a weight age less than the height age whereas children who have growth hormone deficiency usually have a weight age equal to or greater than the height age.

Today, there are three distinct criteria to describe a child who has FTT, using standard NCHS charts:

- A child younger than 2 years of age, whose weight is below the 3rd or 5th percentile for age on more than one occasion.
- A child younger than 2 years of age, whose weight is less than 80% of the ideal weight for age.
- A child younger than 2 years of age, whose weight crosses two major percentiles downward on a standardized growth chart.

These criteria imply a disproportionately decreasing rate of weight gain compared with height growth, but in certain circumstances of FTT, height and head circumference as well as developmental skills may be affected. The criteria also include children under 2 years of age but can be extended upto 5 years of age in developing countries.[1]

There are several exceptions to the previously noted criteria:

1. Children of genetically short stature.
2. Small for gestational age infants.
3. Preterm infants.
4. Infants who are normally lean.
5. Overweight infants whose rate of height gain increases while the rate of weight gain decreases.

If no past record of weight is available, then the following algorithm may be useful for detecting FTT.

PATHOPHYSIOLOGY

Normal Growth in Term Infants

To recognize abnormal growth, one needs to understand normal growth. The average birth weight for an infant is 3.3 kg. Weight drops, as much as 10% in the first few days of life, probably, as a result of loss of excess fluids, however, birth weight should be regained within 2 weeks after birth. Breastfed infants tend to regain birth weight a little later than bottlefed infants.

The median increase in weight per day in children is summarized in Table 34.1. On average infants gain 1 kg/month for the first 3 months, 0.5 kg/mo from age 3-6 months, 0.33 kg/mo from age 6–9 months and 2.5 kg/mo from age 9-12 months. Term infants double their birth weight by age 4 months and triple their weight by age 12 months.

Table 34.1: Median daily weight

Age	Median Daily Weight Gain (g)
0 – 3 months	26-31
3 – 6 months	17-18
6 – 9 months	12-13
9 – 12 months	9
1 – 3 years	7-9
4 – 6 years	6

Term infants grow 25 cm in length during the first year, 12.5 cm in second year, and then slow down to approximately 5–6 cm, between age 4 years and the onset of puberty, at which time growth can increase upto 12 cm per day.

The average head circumference is 35 cm at birth and increases rapidly to 47 cm by age 1 year; the rate of the growth then slows, reaching an average of 55 cm by 6 years. Also, the upper/lower body segment ratio changes with growth. Normally, the ratio at birth is 1: 7; the ratio at age 3 years is 1: 3, and the ratio by age 7 years become 1: 0. The lower body segment is the measurement of the symphysis pubis to the floor.

In case of infants (premature), catchup growth is attained at approximately age 18 months for head circumference, age for weight and age for height; normal growth chart can be used. In some premature with very low birthweight, catchup growth does not occur until early school age. In the context of FTT, it is important to understand that some babies actually have a "catch-down" growth. Babies weight is determined by two factors: Its growth potential and maternal nutrition. Birthweight is largely influenced by good maternal nutrition and intrauterine environment in the antenatal period. If the baby's growth potential is actually on the lower percentile, then in the next few weeks or months, his growth velocity declines to its true potential. This may sometimes be falsely interpreted as FTT.

EPIDEMIOLOGY AND ETIOLOGY

FTT may be divided into three categories:

- **Organic FTT (OFTT)** involves infants with specific diagnosable disorders, and constitutes 20% to 40% of the children hospitalized with FTT.
- **Non-organic FTT (NOFTT)** is a category of FTT, which accounts for the majority of the FTT infants, although the percentage varies from institution to institution. NOFTT involves low rate of weight or length gain, delayed development, abnormal behavior, and distorted caretaker-infant interaction.[2]
- **Combined Organic and Nonorganic FTT** can result from the combination of both organic and non-organic reasons.[3] In one study, half of the cases with organic etiology had a psychosocial factor contributing to FTT. This is caused by a number of reasons. It is clear that illnesses in children, particular chronic illnesses, can take their toll on families. Stresses from coping with chronic illnesses may be lead to parental dysfunction, such as depression, alcohol or drug abuse, and divorce. Parental dysfunction and result negative atmosphere in which children are reared affect their food intake. In addition children suffering from chronic illnesses may undergo personality change. Medications (e.g. steroids) are well known to cause behavior changes but the mere presence of a chronic illness also can result in resistance or non-compliance in many aspects of the child's life, including consumption of proper energy intake. The important clue in evaluation of a child with suspected FTT is the modus operandi of development of malnutrition.

Diagnostic approach should be directed towards determining whether the patient is experiencing one or a combination of the following factors:

1. Inadequate caloric intake.
2. Inadequate caloric absorption.
3. Excessive caloric expenditure.

The first two factors have features of organic and psychosocial disorder; the third is due primarily to organic diseases.

The majority of children with FTT have nonorganic cause for their symptoms. In the Indian context, lack of parental (usually maternal) education is responsible for a large number of children with nonorganic FTT. In correct feeding technique, delayed weaning and misconception of the nutritional requirement of the infant are example of how a simple educational problem can lead to FTT. Severe complex patterns of deprivation, neglect and abuse, usually labelled 'environmental deprivation' is fortunately not common in India. Organic diseases are responsible for less than 20% of cases with FTT. Organic disorders causing FTT are mostly gastrointestinal or neurological. The following are the underlying causes of NOFTT:

Prenatal Causes of Nonorganic FTT

Mothers who are malnourished often have babies who are malnourished and small. Some evidence exists that, if mothers do not bond with their unborn babies, those babies undergo FTT *in utero* as well. Lower birth weights also are associated with teen pregnancies, lower socio-economic level, and multiple gestations. Maternal eating disorders (e.g. anorexia, bulimia) certainly can affect the growth of fetuses as well.

Postnatal Causes of Nonorganic FTT

Traditionally, it was thought that nonorganic postnatal causes of FTT were due to maternal rejection or neglect. In 1985, Skuse suggested that clinicians inquire about more than just the nutrition offered to children. He found behavior at meals and psychosocial issues to be important variables affecting whether children obtain sufficient energy. Poor family dysfunction can negatively affect the child's energy intake. Families characterized by less adaptive relationships, higher level of family conflict, and less emotional support for the mother have an increased percentage of children with FTT. The term psychosocial deprivation was created for these types of situations.

Other nonorganic reasons for FTT in younger children may be failure to signal hunger a poor suck difficulty in weaning, or refusal to eat, in older children, eating disorders including anorexia and bulimia, may lead to severe growth disturbances.

Nonorganic causes of FTT are summarized as follows:

- Poor feeding or feeding-skills disorder.
- Dysfunctional family interactions.
- Difficult parent-child interactions.
- Lack of support (e.g. no friends, no extended family).
- Lack of preparation for parenting.
- Family dysfunction (e.g. divorce, spouse abuse, chaotic family style).
- Difficult child.
- Child neglect.
- Emotional deprivation syndrome.
- Feeding disorders (e.g. anorexia, bulimia).

Causes of OFTT are numerous and almost every organ system is represented (Table 34.2).

Table 34.2: Organic causes of FTT

Prenatal causes	Prematurity with complications
	Maternal malnutrition
	Toxic exposure *in utero*
	Alcohol, smoking, medications, infections
	IUGR
	Chromosomal abnormalities
Postnatal causes	*Inadequate intake*
	Lack of appetite (e.g. iron deficiency anemia, CNS pathology, chronic infection)
	Inability to suck or swallow: CNS or muscular
	Vomiting (eg. CNS, metabolic, obstruction, renal)
	Gastro esophageal reflux and esophagitis.
	Poor absorption and/or use of nutrients
	GI disorder (e.g. CF, celiac disease, Schwachman—diamond syndrome, chronic diarrhea)
	Renal: renal failure, renal tubular acidosis
	Endocrine: hypothyroidism, diabetes mellitus, growth hormone deficiency
	Inborn error of metabolism
	Chronic infection (e.g. HIV, TB, Parasites)
	Increased metabolic demands
	Hyperthyroidism
	Chronic disease (e.g. heart failure, BPD)
	Chronic inflammatory conditions (e.g. inflammatory bowel disease lupus erythematosus)
	Renal failure
	Malignancy

There are many diseases that may not be detected by history and physical examination alone–these 'covert' causes are now listed separately.

Covert Causes of FTT

- Breastfeeding failure.
- Hypertension.
- Malabsorption.
- G. E. reflux.
- UTI/CRF/RTA.
- Inborn errors of metabolism.
- Anemia.
- Thyrotoxicosis/Cong. adrenal hyperplasia.
- Pediatric aids.
- Upper airway obstruction.
- Combined organic and nonorganic FTT.

DIAGNOSIS

FTT should be considered a sign or a symptom, not a disease state or a diagnosis. Clinical assessment of a child with FTT involved differentiating non-organic from organic causes. This is made possible by a detailed history and physical examination in most cases. This must not only exclude organic disease, but also help to establish a diagnosis nonorganic FTT. At the same time, it is important to recognize *normal children with short stature*. The following characteristics will distinguish this group of children from those who have chronic mild PEM and hence true FTT.

1. Low mid parental height (Table 34.3).
2. Born IUGR.
3. No lack of energy (very active and playful).
4. Nutritional history adequate.
5. No complaints indicating an illness.
6. Bone age = Chronologic age (BA = CA).

Children with *true FTT* generally are more listless and have a faulty nutritional intake. Their bone age is usually less than chronological age (BA < CA).

Table 34.3: Midparental height for calculating growth potential

1. Plot parents height on centile chart
2. Male child:
   Plot fathers' height
   Plot mothers' height after adding 12.5 cm.
3. Mid point, ± 8.5 cm is the normal range

History

The following points need attention: Ideally, both parents must be present during the interview and the examiner must critically assess parent-child and parent-parent interaction. Poor parent-child and parent-parent interaction suggests family pathology, which is often associated with emotional deprivation of the child.

Section 9

The educational status of the parents must be recorded. Illiterate and poorly educated parents may unknowingly deprive the nutritionally child.

History of preterm delivery must be recorded. Unless growth parameters are corrected for gestational age children born prematurely may be in appropriately labelled as failing to thrive. The age used to evaluate height and weight should be calculated by subtracting the number of weeks the child was preterm from the number of weeks since birth. Such corrections should be made for head circumference until 18 months after birth, for weight until 24 months and for height until 40 months.

A detailed social and family history provides the most useful clues to diagnose non-organic FTT. The following are the risk factors for family dysfunction, which usually lead to emotional deprivation of the child.

1. Lack of "support systems": relatives, friends, or neighbors.
2. Financial problems.
3. Psychiatric problems or drug abuse.
4. Prolong for frequent occupational absence of the father.
5. Marital problems: force marriage infidelity, marital friction, separation/ divorce, sexual dysfunction.
6. Frequent shifting of home.
7. Serious illness or death in the family.
8. Excessive crowding or lack of privacy.

The significance of the Road to Health card in patients with FTT cannot be overemphasized.

The growth curve can also help us in identifying a "constitutionally light child".

A detailed dietary history must be elicited in every child with FTT. The calorie and protein content of common Indian foods is given.

Physical Examination

While doing a detailed physical examination in a child with FTT, attention must be paid to the following points.

Detailed anthropometry: Length/height, weight, head circumference, upper segment/lower segment ratio. Remember that the measuring tape and the weighing machine are more useful than sophisticated investigations.

Growth should be plotted on a growth chart and the child should be followed up at regular intervals. It builds up the doctor's rapport with the child and instills confidence in the mother.

Laboratory Investigations

A few studies have reported that children with nutritional dwarfism tend to have decreased activity of erythrocyte Na+ - K+ - ATPase (ENKA), compared with those having familial short stature.[4] This enzyme is involved with the active transport of sugars and amino acids and with cellular thermogenesis. It usually accounts for one third of the basal energy requirements. A diminished energy intake further lowers basal metabolic rate and decreases the ENKA activity.

A battery of laboratory investigation for diagnosis of FTT is useless. If the diagnosis is not obvious on clinical examination then the investigation should be directed at detecting occult/covert causes.

The following investigations may be done:

- Urine routine and culture/sensitivity.
- Hb g%, peripheral smear.
- Stool examination.
- Serum Na^+/K^+, creatinine.
- T3, T4, TSH.
- ABG/urine pH.
- HIV Abs.

In this context, it is pertinent to quote a useful recommendation: "In case clinical workup suggests disturbance in a particular organ system, appropriate screening tests must be carried out. However, before resorting to sophisticated and cumbersome investigations, it is important to carry out meticulous microscopic examination of stools, at least on 3 successive days, treat intestinal parasitosis if detected in stools, and give a trial of feeding for at least 2 weeks in the hospital per se".[8]

TREATMENT

Hospital care of a child with FTT is recommended:

- When the patient has not responded to the outpatient management.
- The severity of malnutrition warrens it.
- For diagnostic and laboratory evaluation.
- When abuse, neglect or both are suspected.

Multidisciplinary team approach has resulted in improved weight gain compared with children in primary care setting.[5] The child's health and nutritional status, family issues and the parent-child interaction deserves the attention.

For children with organic FTT the underlying medical conditions should be identified and should be treated accordingly. This underlying condition should dictate the type of caloric supplementation (e.g. restricted protein diet in renal failure).[6]

Those children who are diagnosed as NOFTT need a specialized intervention of the dietician and pediatrician high calorie – adequate protein feeding with lower meal times of 20-30 minutes with minimal environmental distractions should be given, solid foods should be offered before liquids. The intake of water, juice and low calorie beverages should be limited. Emphasis should be on seasonal vegetables and culturally accepted recipes in the family. These foods need to be supplemented with adequate oil or ghee or butter and cheese to increase the calorie intake. The mother should be instructed to cook different dishes to give different taste palatability every day. The child should not be force-fed.

The mother should be the central member of the multidisciplinary team treating the child and should have a say in the management of the child. Her suggestions regarding change/modification of the child's menu should be taken.

Tube feeding is rarely indicated, except in those cases of severe malnutrition and failure to induce weight gain in the hospital.

Catch-up growth is defined as the acceleration in growth that occurs when a period of growth retardation ends and favorable conditions are restored.[1]

The goals of hospitalization are to obtain sustained catch up growth and educate the parents about appropriate foods and feeding styles.[6]

FOLLOW-UP

Continued treatment after discharge from the hospital is necessary and the infant should be followed at regular intervals for a long time. Growth, development and social behavior must be carefully and continuously monitored.

PROGNOSIS

The children with FTT in the past have been found to have lower height and weight ages compared to the controls.[7, 8]

Those children with NOFTT who have received intensive psychological or social intervention seemed to have greatest catch-up growth. Although FTT children may eventually reach normal size, they may ail to outgrow developmental deficits.[6, 9]

REFERENCES

1. Maggioni A, Lifeshitz F. Nutritional management of failure to thrive. *Ped Clin North Am* 1995;42:791-810.
2. Barbero GJ, Shaheen E. Environmental failure to thrive. *Pediatrics* 1967;71:639-642.
3. Casey PH.: Failure to thrive: A reconceptualization. *J Dev Behav Pediatr* 1983; 4:63-66.
4. Lifshitz F, Moses N. Nutritional dwarfing growth dieting and fear of obesity. *J Am Coll Nutr* 1988;7:367-370.
5. Bithoney WG, Dubowitz H, Egan H.: Failure to thrive: Growth deficiency. *Pediatr Rev* 1992;13:453-457.
6. Bauchner H: Failure to thrive. In Behrman RE, Kleigme RM, Jenson HB (eds): *Nelson Textbook of Pediatrics*, 18th edn. Philadelphia: Saunders 2004:120-121.
7. Oates RK, Yu JS. : Children with nonorganic failure to thrive: A community problem. *Med J Aust* 1971;2:199-201.
8. Gupte S. Failure to thrive (FTT). In: *Differential Diagnosis in Pediatrics*, 5th edn. New Delhi: Jaypee 2009:195-232-242.
9. Gupte S, Gomez EM. Growth and development. In: Gupte S (ed) *The Short Textbook of Pediatrics,* 11th edn. New Delhi: Jaypee 2009:25-39.

Novy Gupte, Suraj Gupte, EW Christopher, EM Gomez

35 The Child with Short Stature

INTRODUCTION

In resource-limited countries such as India, short stature is a common problem. The most important cause of short stature in these countries is chronic malnutrition which slowly results in adaptation by the body by undergoing diminished growth velocity.

Generally, 95% of the normal infants and children have the length/height ranging between 3rd to 97th percentiles or within 2 standard deviations (SDs) around the mean for age as per the standard.

Strictly speaking, the term, *short stature*, denotes length/height:

- < 3rd percentile for age, or
- < more than 2 SDs of mean for age and sex.[1-6]

Over and above this, the length/height velocity during observation period of 6-12 months is usually < 25th percentile for age and/or he falls considerably short of the target height {midparental height (MPH)}. In the presence of one or both of these observations, he should be considered "short statured" even though the actual height is within normal range. Sometime the term dwarfing is employed. Conventionally, it denotes severe short stature, the height falling at least < 3 or 4 SD of the mean.

Most relevant to the discussion on short stature is the paradigm shift that has occurred as regards the growth standards – varying from Harvard through NCHS and CDC/NCHS to the new standards in second half of first decade of the 21st century. With the release of World Health Organization (WHO) growth standards in 2006, what is being universally recommended is these standards which are based on data on breastfed children from diverse ethnic background and cultural settings, including India.[7-9] The rationale behind this recommendation is that differences in children's growth upto 5 years of age are more influenced by feeding practices, environments and health care rather than genetic or ethnic factor. In other words, children born anywhere in the world and given the optimum start in life have the potential to grow within the same range of height and weight.

The child with short stature needs to be evaluated fully, bearing in mind that, though a large number of etiologic factors can lead to short stature, quite a proportion of them are either treatable (provided that adequate measures are taken well in time) or do not need any intervention.

PATHOPHYSIOLOGY

Short stature (sometime termed "under-stature") is a common pediatric problem. It may be the result of:

- *Primary*, i.e., intrinsic growth defects. The intrinsic defect in the skeletal system is as a result of some genetic or prenatal damage such as IUGR. The potential for normal bone growth is retarded though skeletal age is not affected. The dominant effect is on diaphyseal growth.
- *Acquired*, i.e., extrinsic factors which impair growth. It is characterized by impairment of bone age and height to the same extent. Here, the potential for reaching the adult height is subject to availability of proper treatment.[10,11]

ETIOLOGY

A large number of conditions may contribute to development of short stature (Box 35.1).[10,11] It is useful to classify it into two parts:

- Proportionate short stature which is responsible for a large majority of the cases.
- Disproportionate short stature which is further of two types:
  - Short-limb short stature; and
  - Short-trunk short stature.

IMPORTANT TYPES OF SHORT STATURE

Genetic/Familial Short Stature

Short stature may run in the family members of varied generations on account of certain genetic factors. This, a

Box 35.1: Etiologic classification of short stature

A. Proportionate Short Stature

Normal Variants

Constitutional.

Familial/Genetic.

Prenatal Origin

Intrauterine growth retardation (IUGR): Maternal diabetes, toxemias, infections, teratogens (alcohol, nicotine, etc.).

Dysmorphic syndromes: Silver-Rousell syndrome.

Chromosomal anomalies: Turner's syndrome, Down's syndrome.

Postnatal Origin

Nutritional

- Chronic malnutrition spread over a prolonged period.

Organic Diseases

- *Gastrointestinal:* Malabsorption syndrome in the form of celiac disease, endemic tropical sprue or cystic fibrosis, heavy intestinal parasitism, cirrhosis of liver, congenital megacolon.
- *Cardiovascular:* Congenital heart disease, rheumatic heart disease.
- *Respiratory*: Pulmonary tuberculosis, bronchial asthma, bronchiectasis, cystic fibrosis.
- *Hematologic:* Chronic iron deficiency anemia (IDA), thalassemia, sickle-cell anemia.
- *Endocrinal*: Pituitary dwarfism, hypothyroidism, hypogonadism, dysmorphic syndromes, precocious puberty, pseudohypoparathyroidism, diabetes mellitus, Cushing's syndrome, Laurence-Moon-Biedl's syndrome, Frohlich's syndrome.
- *Renal*: Renal rickets from chronic renal failure and tubular disorders.
- *Chronic Infection:* Tuberculosis, malaria, syphilis, heavy parasitic infestation, *H. pylori* infection.

Drug Induced

- Prolonged use of anabolic steroids or corticosteroids.

Psychosocial

- Emotional deprivation, parental neglect, child abuse and neglect (CAN).

B. Disproportionate Short Stature

Short Limbs

Congenital hypothyroidism, achondroplasia, hypochondroplasia, osteogenesis imperfecta, amelia, rickets.*

Short Trunk

Mucopolysaccharidosis (Morquio's disease), spondyloepiphyseal dysplasia, Turner's syndrome, mucolipidosis, caries spine, hemivertebrae, rickets.*

* Notably, rickets figures in both since it may cause gross deformities (shortening) of trunk and legs.

leading cause of short stature universally, runs as a familial trait with one or both parents and sibling(s) being short. Bone age is consistent with chronological age. The child is usually small right at birth. Growth occurs at the genetic potential which is, indeed less than average. In other words, growth velocity is subnormal though not as poor as in hypopituitarism or hypothyroidism. Eventually, the child attains a height that is consistent with the midparental height (vide infra) but less than that of the normal peers. Another noteworthy feature is that sexual maturation, i.e. the larches (breast development) in girls and pubarche in boys, is not delayed. In fact, it may be precocious in some.

Its hallmarks, therefore, are:

- Bone age appropriate for chronologic age;
- Normal growth velocity; and
- Predicted adult height appropriate to the familial pattern.

This type of short stature needs to be differentiated from constitutional growth delay which is characterized by delayed bone age, normal growth velocity, and predicted adult height appropriate to the familial pattern (Fig. 35.1).

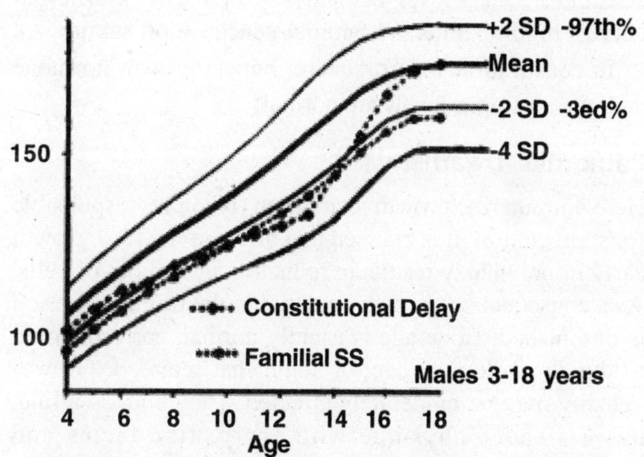

Fig. 35.1: Constitutional vis-à-vis familial (genetic) short stature. Note that in constitutional short stature, growth curve slows down towards the end of first year, remaining below 2SD until puberty when it catches up to reach the mean for age. That does not happen in familial short stature where the curve consistently remains below 2SD

These children have normal human growth hormone and gonadotrophin levels.

Response to improved nutrition may help in marginally improving the height which, however, is finally dependent on parents' heights, i.e., the genetic factor.

Constitutional Short Stature

This type of short stature is characterized by delayed skeletal growth (bone age), "less height" for chronologic age (child looks all right for his weight, however) and delayed puberty. Facial features may be somewhat immature. These children, once they cross the early childhood, finally reach normal adult height.

This condition should be regarded as a sheer variant of normal growth and is, therefore, more appropriately termed *constitutional growth delay*. Here, bone age is consistent with height age but less than the chronological age. Onset of puberty is delayed. Eventually, however, adult height and sexual maturation are normal.

Persistence of the relatively hypogonadotrophic state of childhood is believed to be responsible for this kind of short stature. Frequently, one or both parents or other close family members have a history of short stature in childhood, delayed puberty and finally, normal stature.

Classically, such a child is born with normal weight and length. Growth remains normal for the first 4 to 12 months. Then, it slows down until 2 to 3 years age when it becomes normal but at a relatively lower level of normal (5 cm or little more per year). Puberty too is delayed. Nevertheless, final outcome is satisfactory as normal adult height as well as sexual development are attained.

Figure 35.1 shows comparison of the length/height curves in idiopathic and familial/genetic short stature.

In constitutional short stature, human growth hormone and gonadotropin levels are normal.

Primordial Dwarfism[12-14]

Here, intrauterine growth retardation (IUGR) is responsible for short stature. It is claimed that arrest of the fetal growth early in pregnancy results in reduction in number of cells. As a consequence, growth potential in the postnatal period is diminished. Bone age is usually normal, corresponding to the chronological age, or somewhat retarded. Growth velocity may be moderately affected. The child, as a rule, has a slender physique with sharp, fine facies and craniofacial disproportion. Associated learning disabilities are common. Usually, prognosis for adult height is poor, particularly in the subjects who are small for gestational age.

There is evidence that most of the short children with history of low birthweight secondary to IUGR have growth hormone deficiency.

Russel-Silver syndrome (also called Silver-Russel syndrome) is characterized by short stature, small triangular facies, frontal bossing, scanty subcutaneous fat, and short and incurved fifth finger with or without hemihypertrophy in a child who had low birth weight for gestational age. It was first described by Silver and co-workers in 1953, then independently by Russell in 1954. This is rare. Reported cases since the discovery of the syndrome number in the hundreds but it may be underdiagnosed. Estimates of incidence vary from 1 in 3,000 births to 1 in 100,000.

Differential diagnosis includes fetal alcohol syndrome and Fanconi syndrome.

Nutritional Dwarfing/Dwarfism

Chronic protein-energy malnutrition or iron-deficiency anemia (IDA) of long-standing, particularly when it is not gross enough to cause overt disease, leads to stunting in height as an adaptation reaction. The child often appears to be all right since wasting may not be present and stunting is appreciated only once the actual age is revealed. Bone age is, as a rule, less than the chronological age.

Catch-up growth, though incomplete, is expected in these children once nutritional rehabilitation is satisfactorily achieved.

Emotional Deprivation

The so-called "psychosocial dwarfism", "deprivation dwarfism" or "reversible hyposomatotropism", it is believed, causes short stature through functional hypopituitarism. These children have perverted appetite, enuresis, encopresis, insomnia, crying spasms and sudden tantrums. They may be passive or aggressive. History of upset mother-child or family relations provides clue to the diagnosis. Bone age is little delayed or just normal. Body proportions are normal.

With the provision of adequate emotional warmth and security, these children show catch-up growth.

Chronic Systemic/Visceral Diseases

Short stature is a feature of most chronic visceral diseases (malabsorption syndrome, inflammatory bowel disease, congenital heart disease, renal tubular acidosis, chronic renal failure, occult renal disease, diabetes mellitus, thalassemia, bronchial asthma) as also chronic infections (tuberculosis, chronic intestinal parasitosis, malaria, kala-azar, syphilis, pyelonephritis). As a matter of fact, the retardation is in total growth.

Recently, it is being increasingly recognized that short stature may be the solitary manifestation in certain cases of celiac disease. The implication of this observation, particularly in areas where this disease occurs, is significant.

Endocrinopathies

Short stature accompanying endocrinal disorders is conspicuous by presence of remarkable delay in bone age.

Growth hormone deficiency (*pituitary dwarfism*) should be suspected if the subject's appearance is infantile, bone age is considerably retarded and the growth velocity is less than 4 cm per year. Diagnosis is confirmed by testing growth hormone levels after provocative stimulation (say: exercise, insulin, propranolol, arginine, L-dopa).

Remember that growth hormone deficiency is an uncommon cause of short stature. It may occur in isolation or in association with other pituitary hormones when the condition is termed panhypopituitarism.

Hypothyroidism is easily recognized when the clinical profile of a full-blown case is classical. What needs to be especially borne in mind is that hypothyroidism can present with short stature and growth retardation alone. Body proportions remain infantile. Bone age shows remarkable retardation. Diagnosis must be confirmed by demonstrating low T_4 and high TSH levels.

Cushing's syndrome may result from exogenous steroid therapy or secondary to a pituitary or adrenal tumor. Despite being overweight, the child has growth retardation, short stature and delayed epiphyseal maturation. Remaining features of the syndrome such as moon facies, abdominal striae, plethora, hypertension and reduced glucose tolerance may be present.

Diabetes mellitus is usually accompanied by growth retardation, particularly when it is poorly controlled. There may be history of polyuria, nocturnal enuresis, polydipsia and polyphagia. Urine and blood sugar clinch the diagnosis.

Skeletal Disorders

Disproportionate short stature should arouse suspicion of chondrodystrophies such as achondroplasia, pseudoachondroplasia, osteogenesis imperfecta, spondyloepiphyseal dysplasia, profound rickets, hemivertebrae or caries spine.

Chromosomal Disorders

It is important to consider Turner's syndrome (classical pattern XO) in the differential diagnosis of short stature in girls. Remaining features of the condition include webbing of neck, edema of lower limbs, widely-placed nipples, cubitus valgus, coarctation of aorta and a short fourth metacarpal as also absence of secondary sex characters.

Noonan's syndrome is just the prototype of Turner's syndrome in girls as well as boys with the exception that chromosomal count is normal, and in place of coarctation of aorta, pulmonary stenosis with or without ASD is more common.

Genetic Disorders

Several genetic disorders, e.g., mucopolysaccharidosis, aminacidura, galactosemia, glycogen-storage disease, renal tubular acidosis, etc. may be accompanied by short sature. Figure 35.2 demonstrates the pattern of height for age in four general causes of short stature, namely:

1. Postnatal-onset pathologic short stature.
2. Constitutional short stature/growth delay.
3. Familial short stature.
4. Prenatal-onset short stature.[9]

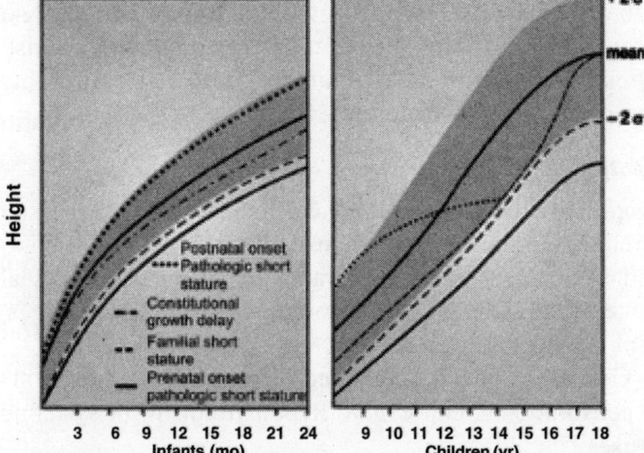

Fig. 35.2: Growth (length/height for age) curves in four general types of short stature in infancy and childhood[9]

CASE WORKUP/EVALUATION[4-8]

Generally speaking, the evaluation should be based on:

- Good history and physical examination.
- Routine investigations.
- Bone age and study of growth rate.
- Hormonal studies, karyotyping and other special investigations (in selected cases).

Appearance

The very look of the child often points to the likely diagnostic probabilities (Table 35.1).

Table 35.1: Appearance as a clue to diagnosis in short stature

Appearance	*Likely probabilities*
Short limb	Chondrodystrophy Multiple epiphyseal dysplasia Achondroplasia Congenital hypothyroidism Turner's syndrome
Short trunk	Spondyloepiphyseal dysplasia Mucopolysaccharidosis (Morquio's syndrome) Severe anomalies of the vertebral column Congenital: Kyphosis, scoliosis, lordosis Acquired: Advanced rickets
Frontal bossing, small triangular facies, sparse subcutaneous issue, short and incurved fifth finger, hemihypertrophy, history of LBW	Silver-Russell syndrome
Large head with dysmorphic facies, arms failing to reach upper thighs	Achondroplasia
Mental retardation with repulsive, dull facies, sluggishness, hypotonia	Hypothyroidism
Proportionate short stature with nearly normal intelligence, round head, short and broad face, small, saddle-shaped and depressed nose, infantile mandible and chin	Congenital hypopituitarism (pituitary dwarfism)

Anthropometry

Growth Velocity (GV)

In anthropometry, *growth/height velocity* is more useful than a single recording of the height. It is calculated from at least two accurate readings at a gap of 6 months (preferably one year).

Growth velocity (GV) in cm

$$= \frac{\text{Present height (cm) – initial height (cm)}}{\text{Time period between two measurements (years)}}$$

Table 35.2 lists the cutoff line for subnormal growth velocity indicating short stature.

Table 35.2: Cutoff line for subnormal growth velocity indicating short stature

0 – 6 months	15 cm
6 months – 4 years	7 cm
4 years – 6 years	6 cm
6 years – puberty	5 cm

Body Proportions

Body proportions are considered to be most accurate index of height.

Table 35.3 gives the normal upper segment lower segment ratio at various ages.

Table 35.3: Normal upper and lower segment ratio at different ages

Age	*Ratio*
Birth	1.7 : 1
6 months	1.6 : 1
1 year	1.5 : 1
2 years	1.4 : 1
3 years	1.3 : 1
4 years	1.2 : 1
5 years	1.1 : 1
7 years	1.0 : 1

Upper segment/lower segment ratio is increased in hypothyroidism, short-limb dwarfism (achondroplasia), Turner's syndrome and in most cases of mucopolysaccharidosis (Morquio's disease is a noteworthy exception in which it is decreased). Box 35.2 gives the significance of this ratio in arriving at certain diagnoses in children with short stature.

Box 35.2: Significance of upper and lower segment ratio

Increased Ratio (Short-limb short stature)
- Achondroplasia
- Congenital hypothyroidism
- Turner's syndrome
- Mucopolysaccharidosis (most)

Decreased (Short trunk short stature)
- Spondiloepiphyseal dysplasia*
- Morquio's disease
- Abnormalities of spine (severe kyphosis, scoliosis, lordosis, severe rickets)

Normal
- GHD
- Chronic malnutrition
- Malabsorption syndrome

Contd.

Contd.

- Chronic systemic disease
- Familial
- Constitutional

* Spondyloepiphyseal dysplasia is a group of heterogeneous disorders characterized by shortening of the trunk and, to a lesser extent, the extremities and the radiologic hallmarks like abnormal development of the vertebral bodies and epiphyses. Lethal, congenital, Kniest and late-onset types are known.

Measurement from midfinger tip to midfinger tip (span) is case of fully outstretched arms and hands is increased (it is significantly more than height) in spondyloepiphyseal dysplasia (Morquio disease).

Midparental (Target Height)

Measuring parents' height is of value. The so-called *midparental height*, a genetic component, gives the subject's target height. It is determined as mean of father and mother's heights plus 13 in case of boys and minus 13 in case of girls. Other words, mean of parents' heights plus/minus 6.5 (cm) gives target height of the boy/girl.

$$\text{In boys : Midparental (target) height in cm} = \frac{\text{Father's height + Mother's height + 13}}{2}$$

$$\text{In girls: Midparental (target) height in cm} = \frac{\text{Father's height + Mother's height –13}}{2}$$

If weight is less proportionally reduced in relation to height, nutritional deprivation must be seriously considered. On the contrary, if weight is nearly normal but height is significantly less, hypothyroidism must be seriously considered. Growth hormone deficiency and hypercorticism also figure in the differential diagnosis.

Pubertal Staging

Pubertal staging is done by Tanner's classification (Box 35.3).

Box 35.4 gives sequence of events in normal puberty.

Children with delayed puberty and short stature should arouse suspicion of sex chromosomal anomalies such as Turner's syndrome. Here, stature, despite timely onset of puberty, is likely to end up with short stature. In "late maturers", both short stature and delayed puberty coexist. These late-maturers ultimately attain better heights compared to early-maturers.

Bone Age

Bone age, meaning epiphyseal development, assessed through radiologic examination of certain bones (Table 35.4) and then comparing the appearance and fusion of epiphyseal centers with standard normal radiographs for different ages, is of considerable value.

Generally speaking, retarded (delayed) bone age points to constitutional, endocrinal (hypothyroidism) or systemic causes.

Normal bone age is suggestive of genetic cartilage dysplasia or growth plate disorder.

Box 35.3: Tanner's sexual maturity rating (SMR)

Pubic hair stages for boys and girls

PH-1 Preadolescent, no pubic hair

PH-2 Sparse growth of long, pigmented hair at base of penis (boys) and bilaterally along medial border of labia (girls)

PH-3 Hair, which begin to curl and develop increased pigmentation, spread laterally in boys and over mons pubis in girls

PH-4 Hair become coarse and involve more area

PH-5 Hair spread to medial side of thigh

Genitalia stages for boys

G-1 Testes, scrotum and penis of small size

G-2 Testes and penis slightly enlarged, scrotum develops red hue

G-3 Testes, scrotum and penis further enlarge

G-4 Penis enlarged in breadth and develop glands; scrotal skin become dark

G-5 Mature adult sized penis, testes and penis

Breast development stages in girls

B-1 Preadolescent, elevated papilla

B-2 Breast bud forms, elevated breast and papilla, increased areolar diameter

B-3 Further enlargement of breast and areola without separation of the contours

B-4 Well-defined breast contour with areola and papilla forming a secondary mound above the contour

B-5 Mature breast with areola receding into general contour of breast and papilla projecting as nipple

Box 35.4: Sequence of events in normal puberty

Girls
- Thelarche
- Pubarche
- Peak growth velocity
- Menarche

Boys
- Testis growth
- Penis growth
- Pubic hair
- Axillary hair

Table 35.4: Recommended sites for X-rays for bone age*

Age group	*X-rays*
Neonate	Knee, ankle, foot
3-12 months	Shoulder
1-12 years	Wrist and hand
12-14 years	Elbow and hip

* As a convention, X-rays are taken of the left side of the body.

Box 35.5 lists causes of delayed bone age and advanced bone age in children with short stature.

Box 35.5: Bone age in short stature

Normal bone age
- Familial short stature

Delayed (Retarded) bone age
- Constitutional short stature
- Hypothyroidism (grossly retarded)
- Hypopituitarism (grossly retarded)
- Cushing's syndrome
- Chronic diseases (moderately retarded)
- Chronic malnutrition (moderately retarded)
- Delayed adolescence

Advanced bone age
- Genetic and chromosomal disorders: Down's, Turner's, Sickel's syndrome
- Sexual precocious puberty
- Obesity (frequently, though not always)
- Hyperthyroidism
- Adrenal hyperplasia

Interpretation of Clinical Information

With the availability of assessment mentioned so far, the guidelines for interpretation are as per Box 35.6.[4]

Box 35.6: Guidelines for interpretation of information/data

- If height age falls within 2 years of the chronologic age, the subject need not be considered to have short stature.
- If height age is less than the chronologic age and the bone age equal to height age, slow growth, in other words constitutional delay, is the likely cause of short stature. In this situation, the child may well attain his normal height subsequently.
- If the height age is less than the chronologic age and the bone age equal to chronologic age, genetic short stature is the diagnosis. Such a child has short parents and is likely to remain short.
- If bone age is less than chronologic age, one should consider constitutional growth retardation, hypothyroidism, malnutrition, growth hormone deficiency and chronic systemic disease as the cause of short stature.

Besides radiology and routine investigations, including meticulous stool examination on at least 3 successive days, it should be ascertained if there is need for intensive workup.

The major indications for such a workup are listed in Table.

Table 35.5 gives major differences between familial (genetic) and constitutional short stature.

Table 35.5: Major differences between familial, constitutional, pituitary (growth hormone deficiency) and hypothyroid short stature

Feature	*Familial/ Genetic SS*	*Constitutional SS*	*Pituitary SS*	*Hypothyroid SS*
Bone age	Normal (consistent with chronologic age)	Delayed (<chronologic age)	Grossly delayed	Grossly delayed Low
Growth velocity	Normal	Normal	Low	Slow from birth
Growth pattern	Slow from birth	Slow from infancy	Slow from infancy	Remains short
Adult height	Predictable	Attained late	Remains short	Absent
History of constitutional delay in family	Absent	Present	Absent	Absent
History of familial short stature	Present	Absent	Absent	Absent
Birth weight/length	Low	Normal	Normal	Normal
Puberty	Normal	Delayed	Delayed	Delayed
GH	Normal	Normal	Low	Normal
Gonadotropin	Normal	Normal	Low	Variable
Treatment	NA	Not needed	Replacement therapy	Replacement therapy

Investigations

In addition to routine tests (Box 35.7), specific investigations may be warranted (Box 35.8) depending on the individual merits of the case.

Box 35.7: Routine screening tests in short stature

Blood
- Hemoglobin, PBF, hematocrit, TLC, DLC, ESR
- Blood sugar, urea, creatinine, cholesterol, proteins, calcium, phosphorus, sodium, potassium, alkaline phosphatase, venous blood gases

Urine

Microscopy, biochemistry for sugar and proteins, pH, specific gravity

Stool

Multiple examination for ova and cysts; screening for fat, blood
Tuberculin (Mantoux) test
Chest X-ray

Box 35.8: Specific (special) investigations in short stature

- Buccal smears
- Thyroid function tests to exclude hypothyroidism
- Insulin-like growth factor-1 (IGF-1)(Somatomedin-C) and insulin-like growth factor-binding protein-3 (IGFBP-3) measurement
  - Growth hormone (GH) levels
- Cortisol, LH, FSH, PRL, testosterone, estrogen levels
- Urinary iodine levels
- Complete karyotyping
- Malabsorption studies to exclude celiac disease, cystic fibrosis, tropical sprue, etc.
- Renal acidification test
  Urinary aminoacidogram
- Imaging studies like:
  - Radiographs for bone age
  - Ultrasound, especially in Turner's syndrome, to exclude

Contd.

Contd.

anomalies such as horse-shoe kidney and bicuspid aortic valve
  - CT scan (pituitary, adrenals, pelvic organs)
  - MRI to exclude pituitary pathology

Provocative growth hormone deficiency (GHD) tests
Propranolol, levodopa, insulin-induced hypoglycemia

MANAGEMENT [4,15-18]

Management depends on the underlying cause (Table 35.6). Even if no treatable cause is found, the situation should be explained to the parents.

Table 35.6: Guidelines about treatment in short stature

Situation	*Treatment*
General	Good balanced diet, wormicidals, hematinics, zinc
Growth hormone deficiency	Replacement therapy
Hypothyroidism	Replacement therapy
Turner's syndrome	Low dose estrogens, anabolic steroids, growth hormone
Systemic diseases	Specific therapy
Idiopathic (ISS)*	Zinc supplementation, growth hormone
Skeletal dysplasia	Limb lengthening surgery possible though expensive and vulnerable to morbidity
Familial	No treatment
IUGR (primordial dwarfism/ Russell-Silver syndrome	Growth hormone (if growth failure continues beyond 3 years)

* Idiopathic short stature (ISS) refers to a group of causes which may not be recognised clinically as well as on investigations. Some of these cases may have growth hormone deficiency which somehow is not demonstrable.

Box 35.9 gives salient information about use of growth hormone in short stature.[19,20]

Box 35.9: Growth hormone therapy in short stature

Established Indications

Growth hormone responsiveness in cases of:

- Biochemical GH deficiency supported by stimulation test(s), after thyroid function has been shown to be normal, plus slow growth velocity, and
- Slow growth velocity in idiopathic short stature.

Equivocal Indications

- Turner's syndrome
- Primordial dwarfism (IUGR), say Silver-Russell syndrome, if growth fails to occur by 3 years
- Prader-Willi syndrome
- End-stage chronic renal disease

Administration and Dosage

Genetically-engineered GH [recombinant human GH (rhGH)] therapy is costly. Such a therapy must begin before 11 years of age for attaining the optimal height. Dose is 0.18-0.3 with an average of 0.1 unit/kg/day (SC), preferably at night, in 6 or 7 divided doses until near final adult height is attained. Usually height gain is 10-12 cm in first year and 6-8 cm every year subsequently.

Monitoring

More recently, it has been advocated that GH therapy should preferably be monitored by insulin-like growth factor-1 (IGF-1) to ensure safety and efficacy of GH.

Criteria for Stopping GH Therapy

- Growth rate < 2.5 cm/year
- Bone age > 14 years in girls and > 16 years in boys

Adverse Effects

- Malignancy, including leukemia
- Pseudotumor cerebri
- Gynecomastia
- Slipped capital femoral epiphysis
- Worsening of scoliosis
- Reversible hypothyroidism
- Diabetes mellitus (rare)

The use of growth hormone has been criticized by some authorities in view of its high cost which is considered far beyond the benefit.[21]

Aromatase inhibitors (anastrozole, letrozole), which are known to delay premature closure of ossification centers and thus reduce acceleration of bone age, have, of late, given gratifying results in short adolescent boys.

Limb-lengthening procedures are useful in selected cases. Nevertheless, the risk of morbity undermines their role.

Surgical intervention may be warranted in an occasional case of short stature secondary to brain tumor causing hyposomatotropism.

COMPLICATIONS

One usually does not think of complications in a chronic state like short stature.

Nevertheless, it is important to bear in mind that:

- Short stature may be a manifestation of a hidden chronic disease that may have its own complications.
- Psychological trauma, including inferiority complex, proving a roadblock in attaining full potentials of the individual, is common in children with short height.
- Reduced bone density/osteoporosis may be encountered sooner or later in these children.

PROGNOSIS

Children with bone age appropriate or advanced for chronologic age have less growth potential than in children with delayed bone age. In a recent study conducted by Gomez and Christopher,[19] this significant point has been further substantiated.

SUMMARY AND CONCLUSIONS

The term, *short stature*, denotes length/height below 3rd percentile for age, or below more than 2 SDs of mean for age in context of new (2006) WHO standards. A large number of conditions, classified under short-limb SS and short-trunk SS, may contribute to development of short stature. Proportionate short stature which is responsible for a large majority of the cases. Disproportionate short staure which is furher of two types. Evaluation should be based on a good history and physical examination, routine investigations, bone age and study of growth rate. In addition to routine tests, specific investigations (hormonal studies, karyotyping and other special investigations) may be warranted depending on the individual merits of the case. Management depends on the underlying cause; even if no treatable cause is found, the situation should be explained to the parents. Only established indication for growth hormone therapy is GH responsiveness, i.e., pituitary dwarfism; GH must be started early enough for good results.

Children with bone age appropriate for chronologic age or advanced bone age have less growth potential than in children with delayed bone age.

ACKNOWLEDGEMENTS

The authors record their indebtedness to the Principal, Government Medical College and Hospitals, Jammu, India, Administration, Narayana Medical College and Hospitals, Nellore, India, and Medical Director, Institute of Child and Adolescent Health, London, UK, for permission to publish this update.

REFERENCES

1. Zargar AH. Short stature. In Gupte S, Gupte SB (eds): *Recent Advances in Pediatrics (Special Vol 13: Pediatric Endocrinology).* New Delhi: Jaypee 2004: 49-58.
2. Gupte S, Gomez E. Growth disorders. In Gupte S (ed): *The Short Textbook of Pediatrics*, 11th edn. New Delhi: Jaypee 2009: 40-45.
3. Gupte S. Short stature. In Gupte S (ed): *Differential Diagnosis in Pediatrics*, 5th edn. New Delhi: Jaypee 2009.
4. Green M. *Pediatric Diagnosis*, 6th edn. Philadelphia: Saunders 1998.
5. Rosenfeld RG. Short stature. In Green M, Haggerty RJ (eds): *Ambulatory Pediatrics.* Philadelphia: Saunders 1990:481-484.
6. Mahoney CP. Evaluating the child with short stature. *Pediatr Clin North Am* 1987; 34:825-847.
7. World Health Organization. WHO Child Growth Standards. Geneva: WHO 2006.
8. Reddy V. New WHO growth standards for young children. *Indian Pediatr* 2006;43:851-853.
9. Needlman RD. Assessment of growth. In Behrman RE, Kliegman RM, Jenson HB (eds): *Nelson Textbook of Pediatrics*, 18th edn. Philadelphia: Saunders 2008:58-62.
10. Gomez EM, Christopher EW, Gupte S. Chronic malnutrition: The leading cause of short stature among the underprivileged. *Asian Med Bull* 2001; 2:145-152.
11. Gupte S, Gomez EM. Changing concepts in short stature. *Asian Med Bull* 2002; 3:54-58.
12. Ferry RJ. Short stature. Medscape. Available at: http://emedicine.medscape.com/article/924411-overview. Accessed on: 18 June 2011.
13. Silver HK, Kiyasu W, George J, *et al.*, Syndrome of congenital hemihypertrophy, shortness of stature, and elevated urinary gonadotropins. *Pediatrics* 1953;12:368-376.
14. Russell A. A syndrome of intrauterine dwarfism recognizable at birth with cranio-facial dysostosis, disproportionately short arms, and other anomalies (5 examples). *Proc R Soc Med* 1954;47:1040-1044.
15. Medical Informaion on Dwarfism. Available at: http// www.Ipaonline.org/resources/html. Accessed: 6 June 2011.
16. Spranger JW, Brill PW, Poznansk A. *An Atlas of Genetic Disorders of Skeletal Development,* 2nd edn. New York: Oxford University Press 2002.
17. Palwlikowska-Haddal A, Cohen P. Editorial: Advances in pediatric growth hormone therapy: IGF-1-based dosing. *Indian Pediatr* 2006;43:577-581.
18. Park P, Cohen P. The role of insulin-like growth factor-1 monitoring in growth hormone-treated children. *Horm Res* 2004; 62:59-65.
19. Gomez EM, Christopher EW. Newer trends in managing understature. *Eur Chron Pediatr* 2007; 21:345-348.
20. Gupte S, Gupte N. The child with short stature. *J Clin Pediatric* 2008; 2:12-17.
21. Allen DB. Growth hormone therapy for short stature: Is the benefit worth the burden? *Pediatrics* 2006;118:343-348.

EAS Nelson • Louise A Baur

36 The Child with Obesity

INTRODUCTION

While obesity is a very common problem in industrialized countries, it is being increasingly recognized as a major health problem in developing countries with fast growing economies.[1-5] What is noteworthy, notwithstanding the overwhelming problem of malnutrition, it is being increasingly seen even in children in India and rest of the developing world, especially in infants, children and adults of the elite families who ape the western lifestyle.

OBESITY AFFECTS CHILDREN AND ADOLESCENTS

Table 36.1 shows prevalence rates for several countries, all using the same internationally agreed definition of overweight and obesity.[6] Rates vary greatly, reflecting environmental (lifestyle) and ethnic variations between countries, as well as differences in the timing of studies (secular trends). There has also been a rise in obesity prevalence rates in many industrialized countries in recent years. For example, over the ten years from 1985, the prevalence of overweight in Australian children and adolescents almost doubled and the prevalence of obesity more than tripled.[7] Thus, obesity is one of the most common chronic diseases in childhood and adolescence and is becoming even more common.

CONSEQUENCES OF OBESITY IN CHILDHOOD AND ADOLESCENCE

Overweight and obese children and adolescents are at risk of a range of health problems and have an increased risk of premature death in adulthood.[8] Psychosocial problems, including social isolation, decreased self-esteem and social discrimination, are common. Orthopedic and gastrointestinal problems, obstructive sleep apnea, metabolic abnormalities (e.g. hypertension, abnormal lipid profile, insulin resistance) and cardiovascular risk factors are also complications of obesity in this age group. Obesity in childhood and adolescence is also a major risk factor for obesity in adulthood, with at least 1 in 3 obese children becoming an obese adult. In turn, adult obesity is a significant risk factor in global morbidity and mortality due to cardiovascular disease, hypertension, type 2 diabetes, stroke, some cancers, gallbladder disease and accidents. Preventing or effectively managing overweight and obesity in childhood may prove highly strategic for tackling these prevalent non-communicable diseases of adulthood.

Table 36.1: Percentage of overweight and obese children and adolescents in selected countries*

Country	*Year*	*Boys*		*Girls*	
		overweight & obese %	*obese %*	*overweight & obese %*	*obese%*
Brazil	1989	4.7	0.1	15.2	2.0
Great Britain	1978-93	9.6	0.9	11.7	1.2
Hong Kong	1993	11.7	3.1	9.8	1.8
Netherlands	1980	5.5	0.3	6.5	0.3
Singapore	1993	10.5	1.7	7.0	1.0
United States	1963-80	18.1	3.3	16.5	4.0
Australia	1985	10.7	1.4	11.8	1.2
Australia	1995	19.5	4.5	21.1	5.3

* % overweight and % obese determined according to criteria of Cole and colleagues[6] data adapted from Cole *et al.*[6] and Magarey *et al.*[7]

DEFINITION OF OBESITY IN CHILDREN

Distribution and amount of fat may be directly assessed with such techniques as magnetic resonance imaging (MRI) and dual energy X-ray absorptiometry (DXA) but these methods are not suitable for routine screening or clinical work. Therefore anthropometric measurements are commonly used to define obesity despite the fact that these measures have limitations. For many years, the median weight-for-height was commonly used, with a value greater than 120% being used to define the cut-off between overweight and obesity.[9] Body Mass Index (BMI; weight in kg/height in metres squared), has been accepted as a reasonable index of adiposity in children and adolescents. Because BMI changes substantially with age and gender, values are presented as percentiles or SD scores. Until very recently, arbitrary population distribution cut-offs have been used to define 'at risk of overweight' and overweight/ obese.[10] Thus, the prevalence of overweight and obesity depended on the reference population used and led to variable estimates of prevalence, and difficulties in interpretation and comparison of study outcomes. This difficulty has to some extent been overcome with the recent publication of the international standard cut-offs to define overweight and obesity in childhood (Table 36.2).[6] Although these cut-offs are designed for research and epidemiological use, rather than routine clinical use, there are currently no alternative internationally accepted criteria. If BMI charts are used within the clinical setting it is important that their limitations are recognized and serial measurements used.

Skinfold thickness measurements have been another popular technique that can be applied to large populations but unfortunately subcutaneous fatness is not necessarily strongly correlated with deeper lying fat deposits and skinfold thickness measurements in obese individuals can be technically difficult.[11] Wells suggests that accurate assessment of excess fatness requires that both fat mass (FM) and fat free mass (FFM) be normalized for height, i.e., FM in kg/height in metres squared and FFM in kg/ height in metres squared.[11]

Assessment of fat distribution is also useful in clinical assessment as a central fat distribution (visceral or intra abdominal fat) is associated with an increased metabolic risk, even in childhood. In clinical practice a central fat distribution is indicated by a high waist circumference. There are no reference values for waist circumference in childhood or adolescence. However, they are useful measurements for following an individual child's clinical progress.

Table 36.2: Proposed international BMI cutoffs for overweight and obesity

	BMI 25 kg/m²		*BMI 30 kg/m²*	
Age (years)	*Male*	*Female*	*Male*	*Female*
2	18.4	18.0	20.1	19.8
2.5	18.1	17.8	19.8	19.6
3	17.9	17.6	19.6	19.4
3.5	17.7	17.4	19.4	19.2
4	17.6	17.3	19.3	19.2
4.5	17.5	17.2	19.3	19.1
5	17.4	17.2	19.3	19.2
5.5	17.5	17.2	19.5	19.3
6	17.6	17.3	19.8	19.7
6.5	17.7	17.5	20.2	20.1
7	17.9	17.8	20.6	20.5
7.5	18.2	18.0	21.1	21.0
8	18.4	18.4	21.6	21.6
8.5	18.8	18.7	22.2	22.2
9	19.1	19.1	22.8	22.8
9.5	19.5	19.5	23.4	23.5
10	19.8	19.9	24.0	24.1
10.5	20.2	20.3	24.6	24.8
11	20.6	20.7	25.1	25.4
11.5	20.9	21.2	25.6	26.1
12	21.2	21.7	26.0	26.7
12.5	21.6	22.1	26.4	27.2
13	21.9	22.6	26.8	27.8
13.5	22.3	23.0	27.3	28.2
14	22.6	23.3	27.6	28.6
14.5	23.0	23.7	28.0	28.9
15	23.3	23.9	28.3	29.1
15.5	23.6	24.2	28.6	29.3
16	23.9	24.4	28.9	29.4
16.5	24.2	24.5	29.1	29.6
17	24.5	24.7	29.4	29.7
17.5	24.7	24.9	29.7	29.8
18	25.0	25.0	30.0	30.0

International cutoff points for body mass index for overweight and obesity by sex between 2 and 18 years, defined to pass through body mass index of 25 and 30 kg/m² at age 18, obtained by averaging data from Brazil, Great Britain, Hong Kong, Netherlands, Singapore and United States.[6]

CAUSE OF THE EPIDEMIC OF OBESITY

To tackle the problem of obesity we need to understand the cause. The primary causes of the rapid global rise in obesity are believed to be the result of environmental and societal changes (modernization, urbanization and changing occupational structures), i.e. increased intake of high fat, energy dense foods and low physical activity. During the past few decades significant changes in lifestyles have influenced children and adults alike. Thus, the rise of sedentary pursuits (e.g. television viewing, video games, computer use), an increase in the use of the motor car for transport, a decrease in physical activity and an increase in the consumption of high fat and energy dense foods are the major factors in this epidemic.[3] The early 21st century in westernized communities provides the most obesity conducive environment known in the history of humankind. Yet it is clear from case-control, longitudinal studies and twin/adoption studies that genetic predisposition also plays a very important part in the development of obesity. Despite these associations, obesity due to single gene defects are rare and tendency to overweight is considered to be the result of combination of major and minor genes. Genes that control the functions of adipose tissue may be of particular importance in understanding these associations.[12] However as genetic predisposition cannot explain the obesity epidemic, it is likely that there is a complex interaction between the various environmental factors and the underlying genetic make up of populations and individuals.

RECOMMENDED DIETARY ALLOWANCES, DIETARY GUIDELINES AND FOOD PYRAMIDS

In 1979 in the United Kingdom "recommended daily amounts" of nutrients were defined as "the average amount of nutrients which should be provided per head in a group of people if the needs of *practically all* members of the group are to be met". In 1980 in the USA "recommended dietary allowances" of nutrients were defined as "the level of intake of essential nutrients considered to be adequate to meet the known nutritional needs of *practically all* healthy persons". Three years later Canada defined "recommended nutrient intake" (RNI) as "the level of dietary intake thought to be sufficiently high to meet the requirements of *almost all* the individuals in a group".[13] All these recommendations assume nutrient requirements are normally distributed and, to ensure that deficiency does not occur for most individuals in the population, recommendations are set at high levels (2 standard deviations above the mean). In other words, the assumption is made that too many nutrients are better than not enough. However in terms of obesity this is clearly not the case. Thus in more affluent countries and communities we are moving from concerns of malnutrition to concerns of obesity, and the focus is changing from preventing deficiency to preventing excess. A number of countries have developed dietary guidelines, although we need to be aware that some guidelines may still overestimate requirements. Examples of dietary guidelines include those published in Australia and the US (Tables 36.3 and 36.4).

A practical way to implement dietary guidelines is to follow the Food Guide Pyramid and use nutrition facts labels. The Food Guide Pyramid intends to describe food choices to enable people to consume recommended dietary allowances. For example, the American Food Pyramid has 6 food groups from the base up with suggested servings for adults in brackets: bread, cereal, rice, pasta (6-11); vegetable group (3-5); fruit (2-4); meat, poultry, fish, dry beans, eggs, nuts (2-3); milk, yoghurt, cheese (2-3); fats, oils, sweets (sparingly). It is also advised that growing children, teenage girls and women need more calcium and iron-rich foods. Other countries have similarly adapted the Food Guide Pyramid concept to suit their local needs. For example Hong Kong has proposed a pyramid with four food groups: cereals, rice, bread, grains (eat most); vegetables and fruits (eat more); fish, poultry, lean meat, dried beans, nuts, eggs, milk, cheese, yoghurt (eat moderately); fats, oils, salt and sugar (eat less).

Table 36.3: Australian dietary guidelines for children and adolescents (1995)

- Encourage and support breastfeeding
- Children need appropriate food and physical activity for normal growth and development —check growth regularly
- Enjoy a wide variety of nutritious foods
- Eat plenty of breads and cereals, vegetables and fruits
- Low fat diets are not suitable for children–for older children, a diet low in fat and in particular, low in saturated fat, is appropriate
- Encourage water as a drink–alcohol is not recommended for children
- Eat only a moderate amount of sugars and foods containing added sugars
- Choose low salt foods
- Eat foods containing calcium
- Eat foods containing iron

The National Health and Medical Research Council of Australia 1995

Table 36.4: Dietary guidelines for Americans

AIM FOR FITNESS ...

- Aim for healthy weight
- Be physically active each day

BUILD A HEALTHY BASE ...

- Let the pyramid guide your food choices
- Choose a variety of grains daily, especially whole grains
- Choose variety of fruits and vegetables daily
- Keep food safe to eat

CHOOSE SENSIBLY...

- Choose a diet low in saturated fat and cholesterol and moderate in total fat
- Choose beverages and foods to moderate your intake of sugars
- Choose and prepare foods with less salt
- If you drink alcoholic beverages, do so in moderation

The United States Department of Agriculture and Department of Health and Human Services

ROLE OF DIETARY FAT IN A HEALTHY DIET

There is some epidemiological evidence to suggest a positive association between dietary fat intake and obesity.[14,15] In addition, a recent meta analysis has concluded that a reduction in dietary fat without intentional energy restriction is effective in producing weight loss in overweight adult subjects.[16] There are several metabolic reasons why a high fat diet may compromise regulation of energy balance, particularly in those with a genetic predisposition to obesity and low levels of activity. For example, fat is more than twice as energy dense as carbohydrate or protein, it is less satiating than carbohydrate and excess fat is readily stored, whereas the body has a limited capacity to store excess carbohydrate or protein. Focussing on fat and hence eating habits and the type of food, rather than quantity and strict dietary restriction may also be an important strategy to support the development of the child's capacity to self-regulate intake.

Despite these negative messages about fat it is increasingly recognized that there are "good" fats as well as "bad" fats. Although saturated fatty acids have been linked to coronary heart disease, there are other fats (linoleic [C18:2, omega 6] and alpha-linolenic [C18:3, omega 3]) that are essential for humans. These fats are elongated into long chain poly-unsaturated fatty acids such as arachidonic acid (C20:4 omega 6) and docosahexaenoic acid (C22:6 omega 3). Omega 6 and omega 3 fatty acids compete for synthesis and incorporation into cell membranes and have different functional roles. Linoleic acid (omega 6) is important for growth, dermal integrity, wound healing and immunity whereas alpha-linolenic acid (omega 3) is important for sensory and neurally based behaviors and development. Linoleic acid lowers both LDL-cholesterol and HDL-cholesterol, whereas alpha-linolenic acid lowers triglyceride levels and decreases coronary heart disease risk. This suggests that an overemphasis of the need to reduce fat intake has the potential to produce negative effects on health.

GLYCEMIC INDEX

Conventional wisdom tells us that the body works like a "boiler" i.e. calorie intake = calorie expenditure. We therefore believe that weight loss requires that we follow the simple equation of diet (calorie reduction especially fats) and exercise (calorie expenditure). Yet the body's metabolic processes may be more complex than this. Supporting this viewpoint is the paradox that the percentage energy from fat in US diets have declined significantly in recent years and yet the rate of obesity has escalated, albeit that other authors suggest this apparent reduction in fat intake may be misleading.[17;18] It has been suggested that the amount and type of carbohydrate may also help to explain the obesity epidemic. The glycemic index (GI) is the property of a carbohydrate food that describes the rise of blood glucose occurring after a meal. Rapidly digested and absorbed foods have high-GI values and this includes most western carbohydrates with refined grains and potatoes. Vegetables, legumes and fruits have low GI values. Fat can slow gastric emptying and therefore low fat meals may accelerate carbohydrate absorption and increase the overall GI of a meal and it is likely that the GI of western diets has risen in recent years. It is possible that the rapid absorption of glucose after consumption of high-GI meals induces a sequence of hormonal and metabolic changes that promote excessive food intake in obese subjects.[19] Although more research is needed, it is possible that GI has a role to play in long-term weight regulation. We may find that the food pyramid and dietary advice that we are giving today may change in the future.

PHYSICAL ACTIVITY, SEDENTARY BEHAVIOR AND OBESITY

Obesity is a chronic disorder of energy balance, with both sides of the energy balance equation being important in its development. Nevertheless, food intake has traditionally been seen as the major factor in the evolution of obesity. However, Prentice and Jebb have pointed out that proxy measures of physical inactivity such as car ownership and television viewing seem more closely related to changes in obesity at a population level than are measures of dietary intake.[20] Indeed, the association between television viewing and obesity in children and adolescents has been demonstrated in both cross-sectional and longitudinal studies.[21-23] Of particular interest is the finding in the prospective studies that television viewing is associated with an increased incidence of new cases of obesity, as well as a decrease in remission rates of established obesity.[22]

Measuring physical activity levels in childhood is difficult. Despite this there is some evidence that pre-school children at high risk of the development of obesity have spent less time in total physical activity and more time in sedentary activity than do children from low-risk families. This suggests a pattern of activity that may predispose the at-risk child to the development of obesity.[24]

MANAGEMENT OF CHILDHOOD OBESITY

Management of established obesity is challenging. The basics of therapy include:

a. Behavioral change.
b. Lifestyle modifications (a decrease in sedentary behavior, an increase in physical activity and a decrease in energy/fat intake).
c. A family focus (especially for the pre-adolescent), and
d. A developmentally appropriate approach. In tackling the problem of obesity, it is important that effective management of overweight and established obesity is addressed. However, a public health approach (primary prevention) is vital if any sustained change in the prevalence of overweight and obesity is to be achieved.

An expert committee of the American Academy of Pediatrics reviewed obesity evaluation and treatment[25] and made a number of recommendations. However it was emphasized that as there are so few studies on assessment and treatment of childhood obesity, many recommendations are rarely evidence based.

Initial Assessment

The initial assessment of the obese child or adolescent should focus on medical and therapeutic aspects. Medically it is important to identify exogenous causes and complications of obesity and to determine the degree of obesity. The following *may* suggest underlying exogenous causes or complications: developmental delay (genetic disorders); poor linear growth (hypothyroidism, Cushing's syndrome, Prader-Willi syndrome); headaches (pseudotumor cerebri); nighttime breathing difficulty or daytime somnolence (sleep apnea, hypoventilation syndrome); abdominal pain (gall bladder disease); hip or knee pain (slipped capital femoral epiphysis, Blount disease); oligomenorrhea or amenorrhea (polycystic ovary syndrome). It is also important to determine if there is a family history of obesity, type 2 diabetes, cardiovascular disease, hypertension, dyslipidemia or gall bladder disease. Evidence for depression, eating disorders or tobacco use should be sought. Physical examination should include height and weight (to calculate BMI), waist circumference and blood pressure. Evidence of exogenous causes and complications should be looked for during the examination: truncal obesity (cardiovascular risk; Cushing's); dysmorphic features (genetic disorders, e.g. Prader-Willi syndrome); acanthosis nigricans (type 2 diabetes, insulin resistance); hirsutism (polycystic ovary syndrome, Cushing's); violaceous striae (Cushing's); hepatomegaly (fatty liver); optic disk abnormalities (pseudotumor cerebri); tonsillar hypertrophy (sleep apnea); abdominal tenderness (gall bladder disease); undescended testis (Prader-Willi syndrome); limited hip range of motion (slipped femoral epiphysis); lower leg bowing (Blount disease). Useful investigations may include fasting blood sugar, fasting insulin, fasting cholesterol (HDL/LDL) and trigylcerides to assess coronary heart disease risk; thyroid function tests; liver function tests and possibly assessment for obstructive sleep apnea. Note that there may be no need for specific investigations in otherwise well children with mild obesity.

Approach to Behavior Change

Goals of therapy include: (a) behavior goals, with the primary goal of treatment being the establishment of healthy eating and activity patterns, (b) medical goals such as resolution of any secondary complications e.g. abnormal blood pressure or lipid profile, and (c) weight goals (usually weight maintenance rather than weight loss unless there are complications of obesity or unless the child is over 7 years old with a BMI above the 95th percentile).

Facilitating change is difficult but success can be increased if intervention begins early and if the family is ready for change. It is important to educate families about the complications of obesity and to involve all family members and caregivers. Indeed, when dealing with preadolescent children, the focus should be on the parents/caretakers as the agents of change, rather than expecting young children to be responsible for any lifestyle change.[26] The family should be told that the aim is achieve permanent changes and not to focus on short-term diets or exercise programs for rapid weight loss. The family needs to learn how to monitor eating and activity and the intervention program should help the family to make small gradual changes. It is important for the doctor to encourage and empathize, and not to criticize. Depending on resources it is beneficial to involve a variety of experienced professionals. Parenting skills advice may help to bring about change and this can be placed in a prominent place in the home (Table 36.5). Advice needs to be tailored to the age of the child.

Table 36.5: Parenting skills advice

- Find reasons to praise the child's behavior
- Never use food as a reward
- Establish daily family meal and snack times
- Offer only healthy options
- Remove temptations
- Be a role model
- Be consistent
- Parents/caregivers determine what food is offered and when–child decides whether to eat or not

Dietary Change and Food Intake

The family should be given advice on reducing calorie intake. The goal should be the provision of well-balanced, healthy meals without an emphasis on a "diet". It is recommended that the Food Guide Pyramid is helpful in selecting foods and that the family should try to eliminate 1 or 2 high-calorie foods at a time. A "Stoplight diet" (green/orange/red) can also be useful. These diets do not forbid foods but stress the appropriate balance between of high-, medium- and low-calorie foods. Dieticians can work with families but counting calories is not recommended as this is tedious, difficult, inaccurate and may unwittingly promote the development of an eating disorder.

Involvement of the entire family in making a change to a sustainable and healthy food intake is usually vital. This is because changes in shopping and cooking practices, and altered attitudes to snacking and meal-times, may all be required. Essentially, the focus should be on behavior change and moderate fat restriction, rather than calorie restriction or a diet prescription. Families can be helped to become aware of some at risk features in their usual dietary intake, such as the following:

- Skipping breakfast or lunch.
- Having regular high fat or high energy snacks.
- Snacking frequently in the after-school period.
- Having take away meals, or eating out, on a frequent basis.

- Stocking tempting high fat or high energy foods (e.g. cookies) in the cupboards.

A more healthy food intake may include some of the following elements:

- Use low fat dairy products.
- Stock a range of low fat snacks that the child enjoys eating.
- Make time to eat breakfast.
- Eat together as a family most days of the week.

Physical Activity

An increase in the level of physical activity during treatment is a long-term predictor of maintained non-obesity. The type of activity employed (i.e. "lifestyle" exercise versus programmed aerobic exercise) also appears to be important for sustained weight loss. For example, while both forms of exercise help promote weight loss in the initial phase, the child or adolescent is more likely to continue long-term with the "lifestyle" form of activity. These include the sort of activities that can be incorporated readily into child or adolescent's lifestyle, e.g. walking, cycling, dancing to music, playing outside, etc.

Obese children may not enjoy group physical activities, such as school sports, because their performance may not be as good as their leaner peers. However, they, or their families, need to be encouraged to incorporate some opportunities for activity into their everyday lifestyle. The following suggestions may be helpful:

- Is it possible to walk part or all of the way to or from school?
- Does the family car need to be used for small chores in the neighborhood? Is it possible to walk instead?
- Can some of the family go for a walk together at least once a week?
- Are there safe parks or cycle-ways nearby where young children can play?

Targeting Sedentary Behavior

Interestingly, targeting a decrease in sedentary behavior may be more effective than targeting an increase in physical activity. If families and young people are encouraged to be aware of situations when they are being sedentary, then they may more readily choose to be active. Families or young people should be encouraged to consider the following:

- How is television used in the household? Is it continually turned on, or does the family use it more discerningly?
- How many hours of television, videos, video games or computers are watched per day?
- Is the remote control used to change television channels?
- Is the family car used to take children to and from school?

When to Refer?

The vast majority of children and adolescents with overweight or obesity can be managed in the community by their family doctors or dietitians. However, those with significant metabolic complications of obesity, or with growth failure or other signs suggestive of endocrine or genetic disease, will need referral to a pediatrician or specialist clinic for more specific management. In a very small proportion of obese children and their families significant psychosocial disturbance may be present—this warrants referral to a specialist child and adolescent psychiatric service.

Drug Therapy

There is no ideal weight-reducing drug. To date, all have had significant side-effects and all have only been useful in long-term weight-management when used in conjunction with a well-managed behavioral management program. There are few reports of the effect of weight-reducing drug therapy in children or adolescents.

PREVENTION

The magnitude of the problem of obesity in many industrialized countries means that, to prevent further increases in prevalence, population-level strategies must be applied. Interventions focussing on simply educating individuals and communities about behavior change have had limited or no success. Instead, there is an urgent need to produce an environment, which supports healthy eating and physical activity throughout the community.[3,8] This requires a commitment from many sectors of society. Potential environmental strategies could include:

- Creating opportunities for planned and incidental activity in community environments (pedestrian-friendly environments, more public space available for recreational use, safe bike paths, improved street lighting, modified building design to encourage the use of stairs).
- Encouraging private sector and public sector food services (childcare centers, take away food outlets, lunch bars, school canteens) to provide healthy food choices.
- Improving the labelling of food products.
- Encouraging schools to include physical activity opportunities as part of their usual program.
- Providing economic incentives for the production and distribution of fruits and vegetables.
- Limiting and regulating advertising directed at children.

RESEARCH PRIORITIES RELEVANT TO CHILD AND ADOLESCENT OBESITY

These include:

- Regular population monitoring in order to track trends in the prevalence of overweight and obesity.
- Improved understanding of the forces promoting the development of obesity in different communities (e.g. the rise of sedentary pursuits and the changing food culture).
- Effective clinical management of overweight and obesity in childhood and adolescence.
- Effective population level strategies for the prevention of overweight and obesity.

CONCLUSIONS

The severity of obesity epidemic is now well-established although the exact mechanisms causing the epidemic may not be as clearcut as we believe. Although current dietary guidelines provide reasonable recommendations for families to follow, there is the possibility that modifications to these guidelines may occur in the future. The management of the individual with obesity is difficult and resource intensive. Public health and government policy interventions are essential for the ultimate control and prevention of obesity in populations.

REFERENCES

1. World Health Organization: Nutrition. http://www.who.int/nut/obs.htm. 6-1-2001.
2. World Health Organization: Global database on obesity and body mass index. http://www.who.int/nut/db bmi.htm. 6-1-2001.
3. World Health Organization. *Preventing and Managing the Global Epidemic. Report of a WHO Consultation on Obesity*. Geneva: World Health Organization (WHO/NUT/NCD/98.1), 1998.
4. Birmingham CL, Muller JL, Palepu A, *et al.* The cost of obesity in Canada. *CMAJ* 1999;160:483-488.
5. Colditz GA: Economic costs of obesity and inactivity. *Med Sci Sports Exercise* 1999;31:663-667.
6. Cole TJ, Bellizzi MC, Flegal KM, *et al.* Establishing a standard definition for child overweight and obesity worldwide: International survey. *BMJ* 2000;320:1240-1243.
7. Magarey AM, Daniels LA, Boulton TJ: Prevalence of overweight and obesity in Australian children and adolescents: Reassessment of 1985 and 1995 data against new standard international definitions. *Med J Australia* 2001;174:561-564.
8. Must A, Strauss RS: Risks and consequences of childhood and adolescent obesity. *Int J of Obesity Related Metabol Disorders* 1999;23 Suppl 2:S2-11.
9. Leung SS, Lau JT, Tse LY, *et al.* Weight-for-age and weight-for-height references for Hong Kong children from birth to 18 years. *J Pediatr Child Health* 1996;32:103-109.
10. Dietz WH, Bellizzi MC: Introduction: The use of body mass index to assess obesity in children. *Am J Clinl Nutr* 1999;70:123S-125S.
11. Wells JC: A critique of the expression of pediatric body composition data. *Arch Dis Child* 2001;85:67-72.
12. Arner P: Hunting for human obesity genes? Look in the adipose tissue! *Int J Obesity Related Metabol Disorders* 2000;24 Suppl 4:S57-S62.
13. Weaver LT: Nutrition. In: Campbell AGM, McIntosh N (eds.) *Forar and Arneil's Textbook of Pediatrics*. New York: Churchill Livingstone, 1998;1179-1185.
14. Bray GA, Popkin BM: Dietary fat intake does affect obesity! *Am J Clinl Nutr* 1998;68:1157-1173.
15. Lissner L, Heitmann BL: Dietary fat and obesity: Evidence from epidemiology. *Europ J Clin Nutr* 1995;49:79-90.
16. Astrup A, Grunwald GK, Melanson EL, *et al.* The role of low-fat diets in body weight control: A meta-analysis of ad libitum dietary intervention studies. *Int J Obesity Related Metabol Disorders* 2000;24:1545-1552.
17. Heitmann BL, Lissner L, Osler M: Do we eat less fat, or just report so? *Int J Obesity Related Metabol Disorders* 2000;24:435-442.
18. Harnack LJ, Jeffery RW, Boutelle KN: Temporal trends in energy intake in the United States: An ecologic perspective. *Am J Clin Nutr* 2000;71:1478-1484.
19. Ludwig DS, Majzoub JA, Al Zahrani A, *et al.* High glycemic index foods, overeating, and obesity. *Pediatrics* 1999;103:E26.
20. Prentice AM, Jebb SA: Obesity in Britain: Gluttony or sloth? *BMJ* 1995;311:437-439.
21. Dietz WH, Gortmaker SL: Do we fatten our children at the television set? Obesity and television viewing in children and adolescents. *Pediatrics* 1985;75:807-812.
22. Gortmaker SL, Dietz WH Jr, Cheung LW: Inactivity, diet and the fattening of America. *J Am Dietet Assoc* 1990;90:1247-1252.
23. Locard E, Mamelle N, Billette A, *et al.* Risk factors of obesity in a five-year-old population. Parental versus environmental factors. *Int J Obesity Related Metabol Disorders* 1992; 16:721-729.
24. Eck LH, Klesges RC, Hanson CL, *et al.* Children at familial risk for obesity: An examination of dietary intake, physical activity and weight status. *Int J Obesity Related Metabol Disorders* 1992;16:71-78.
25. Barlow SE, Dietz WH: Obesity evaluation and treatment: Expert Committee recommendations. The Maternal and Child Health Bureau, Health Resources and Services Administration and the Department of Health and Human Services. *Pediatrics* 1998;102:E29.
26. Golan M, Weizman A, Apter A, *et al.* Parents as the exclusive agents of change in the treatment of childhood obesity. *Am J Clin Nutr* 1998; 67:1130-1135.

KE Elizabeth

37 Nutrition in Health and Illness

Food is the most primitive form of comfort.

—Sheila Graham

INTRODUCTION

By definition, nutrition is the process by which the organism utilizes food. The term, *malnutrition*, refers to the clinical condition in which there is a disequilibrium between nutrient intake and requirements. This can mean overnutrition, undernutrition or micronutrient malnutrition. Often, it is the result of insufficient intake, exaggerated loss of nutrients or increased catabolism. It has been estimated that in India, 65 per cent of the under five children suffer from varying degrees of undernutrition.[1] Obesity is the other end of the spectrum, which is emerging as a global pandemic among all age groups.[2-7]

Nutritional factors like breast-feeding practices, weaning practices and diet during illness influence the growth and development of children. It has been rightly said that "malnutrition may start in the womb and end in the tomb." The triad of genetic, nutritional and environmental factors influences total development of the children. Nutrition of the child is important in both health and disease, it may be difficult to show that nutritional support alters the outcome of many disease processes, but it helps in restoring the nutritional status of the patient and it plays an adjunctive role in the disease and immune process. It improves physical and mental function. It decreases the effects of catabolism. It prevents further weight loss and death from cachexia. Identifying patients who are malnourished or at risk for malnutrition that may benefit from nutritional therapy is the first step in nutritional support.

BASAL METABOLISM

Basal metabolic rate (BMR) is the number of calories used by the body when it is at rest. BMR accounts for 50 per cent of the calories that a person utilizes. A person's basal metabolic rate is based on body functions such as respiration, digestion, heart rate and brain and other organs function. One's age, sex, body weight, and level of physical activity have an impact on basal metabolism. Basal metabolic rate increases with the amount of muscle tissue a person has and it reduces with age. Energy expenditure in a normal child is given in Table 37.1. Specific dynamic action (SDA) is the energy spent on digestion and assimilation.

Table 37.1: Energy expenditure in a normal child

Basal metabolism	50 %
Activity	25 %
Growth	12 %
Specific dynamic action (SDA)	5 %
Fecal loss	8 %

NUTRITIONAL REQUIREMENT IN HEALTH[2]

Energy

The recommended dietary allowances (RDA) for the age is used to calculate the nutritional requirement. According to American Food and Nutrition Board, 'RDAs are levels of intake of essential nutrients that on the basis of scientific knowledge and adequate to meet the known nutrient needs of all healthy persons'. The minimum RDA can be easily calculated using the bedside calculation (Table 37.2) and the ideal or maximum as per the ICMR guidelines (Table 37.3). Under no circumstances, the intake should go beyond 150% of the RDA.

Table 37.2: Bedside calculation of RDA among children

Age	*Energy (Kcal)*
1	1000
2	1100
3	1200
4	1300
5	1400
6	1500
7	1600
8	1700
9	1800
10	1900
11	2000
12	2100
Adolescent boy	2400
Adolescent girl	2100

Table 37.3: RDA as per the ICMR recommendations

Age	*Energy (Kcal)*	*Protein (g)*
0 – 6 months	118/kg	2.05/kg
6 – 12 months	108/kg	1.65/kg
1 – 3 years	1240	22
4 – 6 years	1690	30
7 – 9 years	1950	41
10 – 12 years (Boys)	2190	54
10 – 12 years (Girls)	1970	51

Fluid

Fluid requirement can be calculated using Holliday-Segar Formula, which was originally designed to calculate the energy requirement. As energy and fluid requirements tally, this clinical application is justified. The Holliday-Segar formula, as generally applied, does not address deviations from normal activity. While applying this formula for energy calculation, many clinicians tend to prescribe more calories for the overweight and less calories for the underweight as they use the observed weight for the calculation. RDA is for the age and the physiological status and so this fallacy can be overcome by taking into account the ideal weight. But it is used most frequently because of the ease with which the formula can be remembered and applied. It is very useful to use this for fluid calculation using the observed weight without causing fluid overload (Table 37.4). Fluid requirement can be increased to 165-200 ml/kg in special situations in young children.

Table 37.4: The Holliday and Segar formula as applied for fluid calculation

Weight (kg)	*Fluid (ml/day)*
0 to 10	100 ml/kg
10 to 20	1,000 + (50 ml/each kg > 10
>20	1,500 + (20 ml/each kg > 20

Carbohydrate

As much as 50 to 55% of the total energy can be derived from carbohydrate. Complex carbohydrate like starch and glucose polymers keep the osmolarity low and prevent wide variations in blood sugar. The SDA for carbohydrate is as low as 5%.

Protein

The protein requirement is assessed as per the ICMR recommendations (Table 37.3). Roughly it is 0.7-1g /kg/ day. In no circumstance it should go beyond 7 g/kg/ day, which is around 15% of the total calories. The SDA for protein is as high as 30%.

Lipids

Average Indian diet is low in fat upto 25% of the energy being derived from lipids. It may be increased upto 40-45% in special circumstances. 3% of the calories should be derived from essential fatty acids (EFA). The polyunsaturated: monounsaturated: saturated fatty acid ratio may be kept as 1:1:1. Among the polyunsaturated fatty acids (PUFA), the ratio of Omega 6: Omega 3 ratio may be kept as 5:1. In some of the PUFA oils like sunflower oil, it is as high as 56:1, with absolute deficiency of Omega 3 fatty acids. Omega 6 fatty acid is linoleic acid (LA) and the Long Chain Polyunsaturated (LCP) fat derived from it is arachidonic acid (ArA) and adrenic acid (AdA). Omega 3 is alpha linolenic acid (ALA) and the LCP derived from it is eicosa pentaenoic acid (EPA) and docosa hexaenoic acid (DHA). These are 'heart friendly LCPs' and are present in fish, greens and grams.

Fiber

These are non-absorbable carbohydrates like cellulose, hemicellulose, gums, pectins, lignins, mucilages etc. these increase the bulk of the food, prevent constipation, hold a lot of water and increase GI transit time. It also lowers cholesterol, blood sugar and the chance for colon cancer. Excess fiber may bind trace elements. The recommended intake is 20-40 g /day or up to 200-400 mg/kg/day.

Micronutrients

These refer to substances that are needed in small quantities to the body like vitamins and minerals that is to the tune of 'milligrams per day' in contrast to the major nutrients, which are required in 'grams per day'.[3] Micronutrients are cofactors of enzymes, gene activators and scavengers of free radicals. **Trace elements or micro minerals** are those minerals present in traces or small concentration in the body, <0.01% of body weight, i.e., < 0.1 mg/g or 100 mcg/g. The requirements of vitamins and minerals are given in Tables 37.5 and 37.6.

Table 37.5: RDA of vitamins

Vitamin	*Infants*	*Children*
Thiamine	0.3–0.4 mg	0.5 – 1.5 mg / day
Riboflavin	0.4–0.5 mg	0.5 – 1.5 mg / day
Niacin	5–6 mg (niacin equivalent)	5 – 15 mg / day
Folic acid	25–35 mcg	50 – 150 mcg / day
Pantothenic acid	2–3 mg	5 mg
Vitamin B-6	0.3–0.6 mg	0.5 – 1.5 mg / day
Vitamin B-12	0.3–0.5 mcg	0.5 – 1.5 mcg / day
Biotin	10–15 mcg	10–15 mcg
Ascorbic acid	30–35 mg	40 mg
Vitamin A	375 mcg	400 mcg / day or 1500 IU / day
Vitamin E	3–4 mg	5 – 15 mg
Vitamin K	5–10 mcg	5–10 mcg

Table 37.6: RDA of minerals and electrolytes

Item	*Enteral*
Chromium	2.5 mcg/kg
Copper	No RDA
Iodine	40–50 mcg
Iron	6–10 mg
Sodium	2.0 – 3.0 mEq/kg/day
Potassium	2.0 – 3.0 mEq/kg/day
Chloride	2.0 – 4.0 mEq/kg/day
Calcium	0.5 – 3.0 mEq/kg/day
Magnesium	0.25 – 0.5 mEq/kg/day
Phosphorous	1.0 – 2.0 mEq/kg/day

Antioxidants[4]

Free radicals are constantly formed endogenously during mitochondrial respiratory chain metabolism, detoxification and phagocytosis and also due to trauma, inflammation, sepsis, intake of drugs, chemicals and exposure to radiation. These lead to tissue damage, degeneration and are implicated in hundreds of conditions ranging from malnutrition to immunodeficiency and arthritis to cancer. The antioxidant defenses in the body consist of endogenous and exogenous enzymes, nutrients and certain drugs. These are summarized in Table 37.7.

Table 37.7: Classification of antioxidants

Intracellular Antioxidants	Superoxide dismutase, Catalase, Glutathione peroxidase
Extracellular Antioxidants	Transferrin, Haptoglobin, Albumin, Extracellular Superoxide dismutase and Catalase, Bilirubin, Mucus, Glucose, Vitamin C, Urate
Lipoprotein Antioxidants	Vitamin E, Beta carotene, Retinyl stearate, Lycopene
Membrane Antioxidants	Vitamin E, Beta carotene, Coenzyme Q
Nutritional Antioxidants	Vitamin E (tocopherols and tocotrienols) Beta carotene, Vitamin C, Phytochemicals like flavanoids, flavones, flavanols, cinnamic acid, cumarin derivatives, phytoalexane derivatives, Selenium as a Co-factor for Glutathione peroxidase, Cysteine, Taurine
Synthetic Antioxidants	Selenium compound like Glutathione peroxidase, Food additives like propyl gallate, Butylated hydroxy anisole, Antioxidant drugs like Allopurinol, Desferrioxamine, N-acetyl cysteine

Carotenoids are a group of yellow, orange and orange-red fat soluble pigments present in vegetables and fruits and that impart color to them. **Beta-carotene** is most popular among them and is the provitamin A compound. The less understood **lycopene** is now found to be much more abundant in human blood and tissues and a more potent antioxidant than beta-carotene. It is rich in red tomatoes, watermelon, guava, papaya and pink grapes. It is twice as effective as beta-carotene in limiting cell membrane tissue damage by free radicals. It is reported to inhibit proliferation of cancer cells in cell culture studies. The 'rainbow revolution', which envisages the cultivation and consumption of green, yellow, orange and red (GYOR) vegetables and fruits, is a positive approach in this respect.

NUTRITIONAL REQUIREMENT IN ILLNESS

Energy Expenditure in Critically Ill Children[8]

The nutritional requirements and the nature of fuel utilization in critically ill children have not yet been well defined. Overfeeding can lead to many side- effects, including diet-induced thermogenesis, increased carbon dioxide production and fatty deposition in the liver. Underfeeding, on the other hand, may result in depletion of fat and protein stores and malnutrition.16% to 20% of critically ill hospitalized children have been reported to develop significant acute protein-energy malnutrition (A/c PEM), some within 48 hours of admission to a pediatric intensive care unit. Nutrient store deficiencies and A/c PEM have been reported to be common early in the course of critical illnesses in children, especially in those <2 yrs of age. Many children also may develop acute fluid and electrolyte malnutrition (A/c FEM).

Numerous equations have been used to estimate the energy needs of the critically ill child. They calculate the predicted basal metabolic rate (PBMR) and then add the correction factor for the illness to calculate the predicted energy expenditure (PEE). There are many formulas that estimate PBMR in children, the most common being the Harris-Benedict and the Food and Agriculture Organization and World Health Organization[9,10] (Table 37.8).

Table 37.8: Calculation of predicted basal metabolic rate (PBMR)

Harris-Benedict equation (Kcal/day)	
Males: 66.473 + (13.7516 × Wt) + (5.0033 × Ht) - (6.755 × age)	
Females: 665.0955 + (9.5634 × Wt) + (1.8496 × Ht)- (4.6756 × age)	
WHO equation (Kcal/day)	
<3 yrs:	Boy: (60.9 × Wt) – 54
	Girl: (61 × Wt) – 51
3-10 yrs:	Boy: (22.7 × Wt) + 495
	Girl: (22.5 × Wt) + 499
10-18 yrs:	Boy: (17.5 × Wt) + 651
	Girl: (12.2 × Wt) + 746
Correction factors (% of PBMR to be added)	
Elevated temperature	+12% per °C above 37°C (98.6°F)
ARDS	+20%
Sepsis	+10% to 30% depending on severity
Trauma	+10% to 30% depending on severity
Surgery	+10% to 30% depending on severity

Nutritional Requirements

Children differ from adults, as they require nutrients for growth in addition to basal metabolism activity and so on. The energy requirements for the child can be calculated using the RDA. In general, they require more enteral calories than parenteral calories because a portion of the former is lost in stool and expended for the digestive process, represented as SDA.

Carbohydrates

Glucose is the carbohydrate of choice and is readily metabolized by the body. Current recommendation is that 50% of the total calories may be derived from carbohydrate. Hyper metabolic patients may require slightly more. Excess carbohydrate supplementation can result in increased carbon dioxide production, fever, hepatic steatosis, hyperosmolarity and osmotic diuresis. Carbohydrates are given in a stepwise method by slowly increasing the concentration of dextrose solution to allow the body to increase its endogenous insulin production and thus prevent glycosuria. In children upto 15-30 g / kg / day of glucose can be given. Glucose intolerance is uncommon and in infants should be regarded as an early sign of sepsis, however insulin is rarely indicated. Maintenance fluid containing 5% dextrose can supply upto 20% of energy requirements and is just enough to prevent extreme catabolism.

Lipids

The goals of lipid supplementation includes providing of essential fatty acids (EFA), promoting nitrogen sparing, and offering a balanced approach to fulfilling energy requirements. To prevent EFA deficiency children require 0.5 g/kg/d of lipids. Parenteral lipid solutions are calorie dense, isotonic and rich in EFA and are metabolized in a similar manner as chylomicrons. 25-45% of the energy can be given as fat. In general 3% of the calories should come from EFA. Parenteral lipids should be introduced at a dose of 0.5-1.0 g / kg / day and increased by 0.5g / kg / day to a maximum of 2.0-3.0 g / kg / day. Altered lipid metabolism in stressed patients may result in increased levels of triglycerides and free fatty acids. Hence, monitoring is particularly important in hyper metabolic patient.

Proteins

The goal of supplemental protein is to provide substrate for cellular protein synthesis and the maintenance of lean body mass. The common clinical practice is to give hospitalized children, who are presumed to be under metabolic stress, 1.5 g/kg per day of protein. The administration of protein in a range higher than 4 g/kg per day may result in abnormal amino acid profiles. Histidine is a conditionally essential amino acid for neonates and infants upto 6 months of age and should be specifically supplemented. 10-15% of the total calories must come from proteins.

Fluids

Parenteral fluid therapy is a basic component of the care of hospitalized infants and children. Maintenance fluid and electrolyte can be given as per the Holliday and Segar formula.

Immunonutrition

Increasing research in the field of nutrition is directed towards nutrition providing more than simply the needed nutrients. Nutrients can be used to provide pharmacotherapy that may improve the health of the patient and the function of gastrointestinal tract. Different agents are under trial in animal and humans with some initial success. This new approach is called **immunonutrition or nutritional pharmacology**. Glutamine supplementation has been the best studied.[11] Glutamine is found to be deficient in trauma, infection, and starvation, so that the use of supplemental dietary glutamine has been suggested to reverse the deficient state in the enterocyte in these diseases.

ENTERAL NUTRITION (EN)[12-14]

The golden rule in nutrition is that **"if the gut works, use it"**. Enteral nutrition is indicated for patients with a functional gastrointestinal tract whose oral nutrient intake is insufficient to meet estimated needs. Selection of the proper enteral access device is based on the patients' gastrointestinal anatomy and function, anticipated duration of enteral nutrition, and the potential for aspiration. Nasoenteric feeding is preferred because of its ease of administration and simple technique of insertion. Among all nasoenteric routes, nasogastric is the preferred one. If there is increased risk of aspiration, feeding can be administered into distal duodenum or jejunum. Tubes can be passed beyond the pylorus, i.e., nasoduodenal or naso-jejunal, along with peristaltic movements or under endoscopic / fluoroscopic guidance.

The only absolute **contraindications** are intestinal obstruction, intestinal anatomic disruption, abdominal distension, and severe intestinal ischemia. Relative but not absolute contraindications include continued and unexplained vomiting or diarrhea, intestinal dysmotility, high-output enteric fistula, gastrointestinal bleeding, and a greater than 90% resection of small bowel.

Modes of Enteral Feeding

The delivery method can be by bolus, gravity, or pump-controlled techniques based on the patient's activity level and underlying illness. Bolus feed should be allowed to fall by gravity using the syringe based system. It mimics normal feeding, but is less tolerated. It has advantages of requiring fewer amounts of time and equipment and also reduced risk of contamination. However, there are more chances of vomiting and aspiration after a bolus feed. Continuous drip can be given using IV drip set. This type of feeding has the advantage of leaving smallest residual volume, has least potential for aspiration, bloating and diarrhea. However, it requires close monitoring and has danger of causing bacterial overgrowth. Intermittent feeding is given as 2 ml/kg every 4-6 hourly, each time over a period of half an hour. This type of feed is usually well tolerated. The desired calories can be given as 6-8 feeds/day. Two hourly feeds during daytime and one late night and one early morning feed can be planned. Isodense formulas that give 100 Kcals/100ml are preferred and well tolerated. Kitchen based preparations are given in Table 37.9 and commercial preparations in Table 37.10.

Table 37.9: Kitchen-based isodense preparations

Item	*Composition*	*Energy*
High energy milk	½ glass milk, 1 tsp sugar ½ tsp oil	100 Kcal/100ml
Cereal milk	½ glass milk, 1 tsp sugar 1 ½ tsp cereal flour	100 Kcal/100ml
Cereal pulse	½ glass milk 2 tsp SAT mix*	100 Kcal/100ml
Fruit juice	1 orange, 2 tsp sugar ½ glass water	100 Kcal/100ml
Egg Flip	One egg, 2 tsp sugar, ¾ glass milk	200 Kcal/200ml
Curd/Lasses	½ glass curd, 2 tsp sugar	100 Kcal/ 100ml

Note: * SAT mix is a precooked ready to mix cereal pulse sugar mixture (Rice, Wheat, Black gram and Sugar in the ratio of 1:1:1:2).

Table 37.10: Commercial enteral preparations

1. Pepeti –2000 Elemental Diet 500 ml Liquid or 5 sachets	Osmolarity –40 mOsm/L Renal Solute load-334mOsm/L Energy 100 Kcals
2. Bonvit Liquid and Powder	Osmolarity 250 mOsm/L Renal solute load 330 mOsm/L Energy 100 Kcals
3. Recupex 500g sachet	Low lactose, low residue Energy 220 Kcals
4. ToCal 100g packet	Lactose free, residue free Energy 500 Kcals
5. Renocare I	For pre-dialysis state 4 sachets=1000 Kcals
6. Renocare II	4 sachets=1016 Kcals
7. Ten-O-Lip	6 sachets=1800 Kcals
8. Ten-O-Lip-LF	Lactose free 1 sachet=250 Kcals
11. Pramilac	Skimmed Milk Powder
12. Portal M	25g Pack = 86 Kcals
13. Nusobee	480 Kcals / 100 g
14. Pediasure	100 Kcals / 100 g

The feeds may be started in half dilution especially in children who have been nil per oral for more than 3 days and then gradually they should be made isotonic. Feeding tolerance should be monitored closely. Poor tolerance is indicated by vomiting, abdominal cramping, worsening diarrhea, or measured residuals greater than 50% of the given volume in the previous 4 hours. If intolerance is encountered measures like decreasing the rate, changing the delivery method, or searching for the causes of the feeding intolerance should be undertaken. If all interventions fail to identify and correct the source of feeding tube intolerance and nutrition is definitely needed, parenteral therapy should be considered.

Complications

Problems directly due to or associated with enteral feeding can be divided into four major categories: mechanical, gastrointestinal, infectious, most notably aspiration pneumonia and metabolic. Gastrointestinal complications most commonly encountered with enteral feeding are feeding intolerance and feeding-related diarrhea. The most serious infectious complication of enteral nutrition is aspiration pneumonia, which can occur frequently (1% to 70%) and can be associated with a reported mortality of 41% to 100%. The most effective approach to prevent enteral formula aspiration is to reduce gastric residual volume. Increased gastric residual volume is associated with vomiting; pneumonia, reduced feeding tolerance, prolonged ICU stay, and increased ICU mortality. Currently the most effective approach to reducing gastric residual volume is with jejunal feeding. The most common nutritional complication of tube feeding is failure to meet the nutritional goal. Overzealous initiation of feeding leads to **refeeding syndrome** in 25% of patients. It is manifested by glucose intolerance, fluid retention and electrolyte imbalance, including hypophosphatemia, hypomagnesemia, and hypokalemia. In particular, hypophosphatemia is considered as the hallmark of refeeding syndrome. These manifestations are usually observed during the first few days after initiation of feeding. It may be delayed until enteral feeding reaches nutritional goals, because the syndrome is primarily associated with anabolism. Daily monitoring of electrolyte concentrations should continue until nutritional goals are achieved, and appropriate correction should be made as needed. If refeeding syndrome is recognized and treated expeditiously, consequences will be minimal. If the condition is left untreated complications like paralysis, respiratory failure, and even death can occur. Table 37.11 outlines the guidelines for monitoring a patient on enteral nutrition.

PARENTERAL NUTRITION (PN)[15,16]

Parenteral nutrition is the other modality by which artificial nutrition is provided to patients. Parenteral nutrition usually

Table 37.11: Parameters to be monitored during enteral nutrition

Parameter	*Critical Illness*	*Stable*
Weight	Daily	1-2/wk
Intake and output	Daily	Daily
Urine or blood glucose	2/d	Weekly
Electrolytes, urea, creatinine	Daily to 3/wk	3/wk
Magnesium, phosphorus, calcium	Daily to 3/wk	Weekly
Liver function tests	1-2/wk	Weekly
Albumin	Weekly	Weekly
Prealbumin	Weekly	Weekly

is provided systemically usually through the central veins. It is primarily indicated in malnourished patients when there is a contraindication to enteral feeding or when enteral feedings are not providing satisfactory quantities of nutrients to the patient. Peripheral parenteral nutrition (PPN) provides nutrition through peripheral veins in diluted solutions of protein and carbohydrates with lipids as the major amount of calories in the solution. The solutions are usually 5% amino acids, 10% dextrose, and 2% lipid emulsion. PPN solutions, to be administered safely through peripheral veins must have a low caloric density. In order to provide calories, large volumes of fluid are required and hence in most of the patients the caloric need is not met and also in those cases where fluid restriction is needed it cannot play a role.

Total parenteral nutrition (TPN) allows infusion of large amounts of fluid volume through a central vein necessary to deliver the greater and required caloric density and protein amounts. Central parenteral nutrition (CPN) in comparison with enteral nutrition has an equal ability to provide protein synthesis, maintain nitrogen balance, maintain weight, and meet caloric needs. Catheterization of the infraclavicular subclavian vein with placement of the catheter tip in the superior vena cava is the most commonly used location. The internal jugular, basilic, saphenous, and femoral veins can be used. Central venous solutions come premixed to contain the three major nutrients—carbohydrates, proteins, and fat. Protein requirements usually are met with a 10% amino acid mixture, which contains approximately 50% essential and 50% nonessential amino acids. Energy stores are supplied by 50% dextrose solutions. Fat emulsions provide energy and usually are supplied as soybean oil or soybean with sunflower oil and egg yolk phospholipids. Fats can be given separately on a weekly basis, added to the daily solution, or come in a pre-added mixture.

Complications

Four major categories of complications exist:

1. Mechanical.
2. Infectious.
3. Metabolic; and
4. Nutritional.

Primary and secondary catheter infection and catheter-related sepsis remain critical problems, with catheter-related sepsis arising in at least 4% of all patients per year receiving TPN. Primary catheter infection is defined as occurring in a patient who has evidence of infection, such as fever or leukocytosis, and the catheter is the only focus of sepsis. Secondary catheter infection results from an infectious source elsewhere in the body that leads to bacteremia and then seeds the catheter. Metabolic complications and problems are common with the use of TPN, but generally are prevented by close monitoring, early treatment and by altering the type and amount of nutrients that are given to the patient. Glucose should be monitored daily, hyperglycemia being a common problem in the critically ill patient, which may be an early sign of sepsis. Laboratory monitoring of children receiving long-term parenteral nutrition is routine. The frequency depends on the individual patient and disease state and the duration of therapy. Monitoring includes testing of electrolytes, renal and hepatic function, glucose, triglycerides, and cholesterol. Depending upon the clinical context and the facilities available periodic monitoring of trace elements level should also be considered. Some practical guidelines regarding parenteral nutrition are given in Table 37.12 and some of the commercial preparations available in India are outlined in Table 37.13.

Table 37.12: Practical guideline for pediatric PN

Day	*CHO (g/kg)*	*Fat (g/kg)*	*Amino acid (g/kg)*
a. Newborns (per 24 hrs)			
1	10	1.0	0.75
2	12	2.0	1.50
3	12	3.0	2.00
4	14	3.5	2.50
b. Infants, <10 kg (per 24 hrs)			
1	10	1	1.0
2	12	2	1.5
3	13	2	2.0
4	14	3	2.5
c. Children between 10-30 kg (per 24 hrs)			
1	4.5	1.5	1.5
2	7.5	2.0	2.0
d. Children over 30 kg (per 24 hrs)			
1	2	1	1
2	5	2	1.5

CONCLUSION

Nutritional support is a very powerful tool that can maintain health, protect from illness and modulate the outcome of any illness.[17] The right nutrition at the right time can buy time for appropriate intervention, save lives and achieve quality of survival.

Table 37.13: PN products available in Indian market

1. Aminoplasmal (B.Braun)	
a. 5% Solution	500 ml, 250 ml and 100 ml
b. 10% Solution	500 ml, 250 ml and 100 ml
2. Proteinsteril (Fresenius)	
a. Proteinsteril	10%
b. Proteinsteril Hepa (42% branched chain amino acids)	8% and 5%
c. Proteinsteril Nephro (Rich in Arginine)	
3. Vitamin-G (Pharmacia and Upjohn)	500 ml, 100 ml
4. Aminocore (Core Parenterals) 5%	500 ml, 10%-500 ml
5. Celecel 4,5,7 (Claris)—Parenteral trace elements	
6. Celepid MCT-LCT (Claris) 20%, 10%	50 ml, 100 ml, 200 ml, 500 ml
7. Celemin (Claris) 5%, 10% —amino acids	

REFERENCES

1. UNICEF. Focus on nutrition. *The State of World Children*. New York: UNICEF 1998.
2. WHO. *Energy and Protein Requirements*: Report of a joint FAO/WHO/UNU expert consultation. Geneva: World Health Organization. WHO Technical Report Series No.724, 1985.
3. Elizabeth KE. Micronutrients in child nutrition. *Proceedings of the South Zone Conference of IAP*, Vellore 2003: 9-15.
4. Elizabeth KE. Micronutrient deficiency disorders (MDDs). In: Gupte S (ed): *Recent Advances in Pediatrics*, Vol 14. New Delhi: Jaypee 2004: 33-50.
5. Elizabeth KE. Protein-energy malnutrition. In: *Nutrition and Child Development, 3rd edn.* Hyderabad: Paras 2004: 133-182.
6. Elizabeth KE, Jacob RG. Nutritional support in the critically ill child. In: Gupte S, Gupte SB (eds): *Recent Advances in Pediatrics (Special Vol. 14: Criticare Pediatrics)*. New Delhi: Jaypee 2004: 546-566.
7. Butterworth CW, Blackburn GL. Hospital malnutrition and how to assess the nutritional status of a patient. *Nutr Today* 1975;10:10-18.
8. Apelgren RN, Rombeau JL, Towmey PL, *et al.* Comparison of nutritional indices and outcome in critically ill children. *Crit Care Med.* 2000;28: 28-32.
9. Briassoulis G, Venkataraman S, Thompson AE. Energy expenditure in critically ill children. *Crit Care Med.* 2000, 28:1166-1172.
10. Fung EB. Estimating energy expenditure in critically ill adults and children. *AACN Clin Issues.* 2000;11:480-497.
11. Frantisek Novak, Daren K. Heyland, Alison Avenell, Glutamine supplementation in serious illness: A systematic review of the evidence: *Crit Care Med* 2002;30: 2022-209.
12. Torres D, Pat Wiggins P. Nutrition in the pediatric ICU patients. *Pediatr Crit Care* 2000; 311-331.
13. Salaria M, Singhi S. Enteral nutrition for critically ill patients. *Indian Pediatr* 2001;38:256-263.
14. Bhagawati AM. Nutrition in critical care. Proceeding of the APICON, 2002.
15. Vani S, Chowdhary J, Gupte S. Neonatology In: Gupte S (ed): *The Short Textbook of Pediatrics,* 11th edn, New Delhi: Jaypee 2009: 185-244.
16. Iyer PU. Nutritional support in critically ill child. *Indian J Pediatr* 2002;69:405-410.
17. Pfau PR, Rombeau JL. Advances in gastroenterology. *Med Clin North Am* 2002; 84:1209-1230.

Sandeep B Bavdekar • Jyoti Suvarna

38 Immunonutrition

INTRODUCTION

Nutrition has been used to complement the healing process from times immemorial. Even without the scientific backup of double blinded randomized studies, grandmother's remedies, herbal teas and a host of other remedies have been used to augment and complement the healing processes in various medical conditions. An avalanche of nutritional products available in the market (claiming to promote health and to cure various diseases) bears testimony to man's faith in the nutrition as a mode of therapy. A number of individuals unhappy with the effects of modern medicines are also looking upon this modality as a natural way to combat various disorders.

The medical fraternity has also used nutritional therapy to complement the treatment of various disorders. Nutrient enemas to provide nutritional support have been used as far back as 3500 years ago.[1] This field has grown by leaps and bounds since then. Nutrition was originally visualized as a modality to provide energy, proteins, and essential micronutrients, to offset muscle wasting and starvation induced immune depletion in patients.[2] Dudrick and co-workers flagged off the modern era of clinical nutrition with the development of intra-venous hyper-alimentation, followed by the development of chemically defined diet by Greenstein and co-workers.[1] Total parenteral nutrition was considered as an all purpose panacea. But soon the scientific fraternity realized that there are certain nutrients that can have pharmacological effects on the immune system which can be used to the patient's advantage. Thus apart from providing calories and essential nutrients, one could also use nutrients to modulate the immune and the inflammatory response.[3] The role of several specific nutrients including macronutrients, vitamins and trace elements in augmenting or modulating the immune system has been the focus of studies for the last 20 years.[3,4] The mode of action could be through their effects on the mucosal barrier, cellular defense mechanism, local / systemic inflammatory response.[5] The need of the hour is to study and identify nutrients as primary treatment agents.

This communication offers an overview of work done in the field of immunonutrition, the factors that determine its efficacy and provides a peek at the current status of knowledge in this evolving field. It should, however be conceded that the vast majority of work has been carried out in adults and that there is a need to check if it could be applied to infants and children.

CONCEPT OF IMMUNONUTRITION

Immunonutrition is the process of studying the potential of specific nutrients to modulate the activity of the immune system and the use of diets for enhancing immune function.[2,6] Certain molecular compounds, while being dietary components also have a favorable influence on some aspects of immune response. They are added to standard nutritional support solutions for deriving immunological benefits and are termed as immunonutrients. These immunonutrients may be given in supranormal doses enterally or parenterally, to achieve a pharmacological effect for modulating the response to surgery, trauma or infection.[7] Although many nutrients are potential immunonutrients, the most commonly used and researched upon immunonutrients are arginine, glutamine, omega-3 polyunsaturated fatty acids and nucleotides.[8]

HOST RESPONSE TO INJURY AND INFECTION

In response to challenges like injury or infection, the body recruits the immunological system to induce an array of metabolic and chemical changes. The chief among them is the activation of the T- and B-lymphocytes, and the systemic inflammatory response engineered by the pro-inflammatory cytokines- interleukin-1, interleukin-6 and tumor necrosis factor- alpha. Cytokines increase the catabolism of the body proteins and fat to provide nutrients for the immune system.[7] Other mediators like the chemokines, anti-inflammatory cytokines, growth factors, nitric oxide, eicosanoids and free radicals are also released. The timing of the mediator release and the amount of these mediators available in circulation or at the site, determine the inflammatory response and ensuing effects.[7]

Central to the inflammatory changes is the activation of the nuclear transcription factors such as nuclear factor kappa B (NFkB) and activator protein-1 (AP-1). NFkB plays a key role in inflammation (promoted by oxidant molecules) and AP-1 in cellular immune function.[7] Increased NFkB activation in patients with sepsis is associated with increased mortality rates.[9] Prevention of NFkB activation can thus be exploited for treatment. Anti-oxidants prevent the activation of the NFkB activation by decreasing the oxidative stress and omega-3 fatty acids decrease the activation by stabilization of the transcription factor complex.[7]

ENTERAL FEEDING, IMMUNITY AND IMMUNONUTRITION

The gastrointestinal tract, besides being an organ for digestion, absorption and utilization of nutrients, is an important immunological organ.[6] Patients with gastro-intestinal diseases are at an increased risk for immunological problems not only due to the disease process itself but also because of therapeutic interventions undertaken. Several gastro-intestinal diseases are associated with a breach in the mucosal lining and often manifest with anorexia and altered nutritional requirements,[6] which further compromise the tract's immune function. Many patients, especially if they are very sick, are treated with limitation or even proscription of enteral feeding resulting in mucosal atrophy.[6] Mucosal lesions whether suffered as a consequence of disease process or due to therapeutic or diagnostic interventions (including withholding enteral feeds), lead to a breach in the mucosal lining, which in turn, results in an increased permeability to bacteria and bacterial exotoxins. The resultant endotoxemia and bacteremia can trigger off a local and/or systemic inflammatory response syndrome (SIRS) that carries the risk of multiple organ failure and high mortality.[6,10,11]

The clinicians should be aware of this vital relationship between gastrointestinal mucosal integrity and future course of illness. They should maximize their efforts at maintaining the gastrointestinal mucosal integrity in critically ill or other patients to allow the host immunity to be maintained or enhanced.[6] One of the principal ways of doing this is through continuation of enteral feeds. The goal of enteral therapy is not only to provide adequate caloric and protein requirements, but also to continue to stimulate the mucosal lining so as to prevent gut mucosal atrophy,[10] and thereby prevent all the consequent complications related to breach in the gut integrity. In addition to the obvious benefits stated above, enteral feeding is available at a much lower cost, is more physiological and is associated with lower incidence of complications as compared to parenteral nutrition.[11,12] TPN should be resorted to only when a true contraindication to enteral feeding exists[12] like perforation, total obstruction, proven mesenteric ischemia and toxic megacolon. It could also be employed in conjunction with enteral nutrition when nutritional requirements cannot be met fully by enteral administration alone.[12]

Immunonutrients such as arginine, glutamine, omega-3 fatty acids, RNA nucleotides and fiber exert their effect by helping maintain gut integrity, by stimulating the immune system and by preventing bacterial translocation from the gut into the circulation.[12]

The immune system is profoundly affected by poor nutritional status[13,14] illnesses and states with hypercatabolism such as sepsis, surgery and trauma. The latter group of diseases is associated with malnutrition and this complication further adds to the adverse effects on the immune system.[13] Protein energy malnutrition (PEM) can suppress essentially all arms of the immune system, including B-cell, T-cell, macrophage, neutrophil functions and complement activation.[14] It also adversely affects regeneration processes and compromises host's position in his fight against infection.[15] The associated deficiency of specific trace elements and vitamins also contributes to derangement of the immune status.[13] It should be remembered that even over-nutrition and obesity are associated with altered immune status.[13]

APPLICATION OF IMMUNONUTRITION IN VARIOUS DISORDERS

Sepsis

Sepsis is a complex syndrome characterized by hyper-catabolism and an initial hyperinflammatory response that is followed by immune suppression.[14] Hyperinflammatory response leads to a simultaneous activation of pro-inflammatory and pro-coagulant processes in response to microbial insult.[16] The syndrome is associated with release of pro-inflammatory cytokines and pro-coagulant substances and formation of reactive oxygen and nitrogen species[17] and adhesion molecules from the immune cells or damaged endothelium. These processes and events can cause severe tissue damage and immunesuppression[18] and are responsible for the increased morbidity and delayed recovery associated with sepsis. It is being postulated that immunonutrition provides a means of modulating the inflammatory response to injury and infection, and thereby helps in improving the clinical outcome.[18] Early institution of therapy with immunonutrition is aimed at decreasing the pro-inflammatory responses, abolishing or decreasing hyper-inflammation and preventing the occurrence of compensatory immunosupression subsequently.[14] Studies have shown that although immunonutrition may not decrease mortality, it does decrease infection rates, duration of hospital stay and requirement of ventilatory support.[18] Omega-3 polyunsaturated fatty acids have a direct immuno-enhancing effect, glutamine acts by influencing the anti-oxidant status and suppressing the inflammation, and nucleotides exert direct effects on lymphocyte proliferation.[18]

The effects of immunonutrition in critically ill patients may be different from those in patients undergoing elective surgery. Studies have shown conflicting results (Table 38.1).

Table 38.1: Summary of selected trials and reviews regarding use of immunonutrition in subjects with sepsis

Investigators	*Significant findings*
Atkinson, *et al.*[19]	Randomized controlled double blind trial enrolling 398 critically ill subjects demonstrated that the group receiving immunity-enhancing formula showed a significant reduction in requirement for mechanical ventilation and reduced duration of hospital stay.
Tugrul, *et al.*[20]	Mechanically ventilated patients receiving immunonutrition exhibited better nutritional status and improved scores.
Bower, *et al.*[21]	Prospective randomized multi-center clinical trial carried out in ICU patients demonstrated that patients receiving enteral formula supplemented with arginine, nucleotides and fish oil had shorter duration of hospital stay. However, the group also demonstrated significant higher mortality.
Bertolini, *et al.*[22]	Study done in 39 critically ill patients with severe sepsis showed an increased mortality amongst patients receiving enteral immunonutrition as compared to those on parenteral nutrition.
Galban, *et al.*[23]	Study showed significant lower mortality and lower number of episodes of bacteremia amongst ICU patients in the immunonutrition group. These effects were seen in the least sick patients (APACHE II< 15), whereas there was no effect on mortality in more sick patients
Heyland, *et al.*[24,25]	The authors concluded that immunonutrition may decrease the incidence of infectious complications in critically ill patients based on the review of 326 titles, abstracts and articles. No beneficial effect in terms of reduction in mortality was observed.

Trauma

Trauma and sepsis share a similar pathophysiology. Severe trauma threatens the life of victims directly and indirectly via immunological deregulation that follows severe trauma and results in sepsis and multi-organ failure.[26] Early Immunomodulation, in the form of institution of immunonutrition in patients with severe trauma,[26] has been undertaken in anticipation of beneficial effects such as amelioration of the early hyper-inflammatory phase, reduced incidence of SIRS and multiple organ failure and reduction in the use of antibiotics and in duration of hospital stay. Results of some of these studies are summarized in Table 38.2.

Table 38.2: Summary of selected studies regarding use of immunonutrition in subjects with severe trauma

Investigators	*Salient findings*
Kudsk, *et al.*[27]	Patients with trauma receiving immune enhancing diet experienced reduced number of septic complications compared to those receiving iso-nitrogenous enteral diets.
Engel JM, *et al.*[28]	Early enteral nutrition stabilizes the immunosuppression associated with poly-trauma. There was no advantage with immunonutrition.
Chuntrasakul C, *et al.*[29,30]	The study demonstrated that institution of immunonutrition in patients with severe trauma showed significant improvement in the nutritional and immunological parameters, with shorter ICU stay, lesser number of days on the respirator, but without any improvement in the mortality rate.

Surgery

Major surgery is followed by a period of immune-suppression that increases the risk of morbidity and mortality due to infection.[14] Gastrointestinal tract surgery is followed by formation of micro-vascular thrombi, gut hypoperfusion and mucosal lesions[10,11,31] that disrupt the mucosal barrier. Improving the immune function with immunonutrition before and during this period may reduce the incidence of infectious complications,[14] especially if the patient is malnourished, as well.

Many studies have shown that early pre-operative and/or post-operative enteral immunonutrition is associated with beneficial immunological effects. Senkel *et al.*[32,33] in their study on patients with upper gastrointestinal malignancy undergoing surgery demonstrated that early enteral immunonutrition was well tolerated and was associated with reduced incidence of late post-operative infections, lesser wound-related complications and lowered costs. They also showed that peri-operative immunonutrition decreases the probability of developing early postoperative infections, in addition to reducing the treatment costs. Although immunonutrition is per se expensive, it is cost-effective considering the savings made in terms of expenditure incurred on prolonged hospital stay related to infectious complications and resources spent on treating these complications[32, 34] Studies done on patients with cancer undergoing surgery by Gianotti *et al.*[35] showed that immunonutrition modulates. cytokine production, enhances cell mediated immunity, boosts the synthesis of short half-life proteins, decreases the incidence of post-operative infections and shortens length of stay in the hospital.[36] It is associated with better immune response, better gut oxygenation and improved micro-perfusion, better immuno-metabolic response and reduced infection rate.[37] The same investigators also carried a study in a subgroup of malnourished patients and showed a decreased rate of complications and shortened post-operative stay in those receiving peri-operative immunonutrition.[38]

Inflammatory Bowel Disease

Chronic gastrointestinal inflammatory diseases like ulcerative colitis or Crohn's disease are associated with decreased oral intake, malabsorption, accelerated nutrient losses, increased nutritional requirements and drug-nutrient interactions. These result in nutritional and functional deficiencies. It has been postulated that correction of nutritional deficiencies and steps aimed at modulation of inflammatory response could exert a positive influence on the disease activity.[39] Although the first aim of nutritional rehabilitation could be achieved through institution of feeding either by enteral and parenteral route, the former carries the advantages of lower complication rate and lower costs in patients who can tolerate enteral feeds. Immunonutrition is an important therapeutic alternative, modulating inflammatory processes and changing the eicosanoid synthesis profile.[33, 39] It induces remission in adult subjects and promotes growth in children[39] with inflammatory bowel disease. Early reports suggest that enteric-coated sustained release fish oil capsules may help sustain remission in patients with Crohn's disease.[40]

IMMUNONUTRITION AND PREVENTION OF CANCERS

As early as 1863, Rudolf Virchow observed the presence of leucocytes in tumor tissues and suggested a role for chronic inflammation in the origin of cancers.[41] This postulation has been confirmed by our understanding of the pathogenesis of cancers in the recent years.[17] Inflammatory processes result in release of pro-inflammatory cytokines and formation of reactive oxygen and nitrogen species. Although anti-inflammatory effects usually follow such actions rapidly, excessive production of pro-inflammatory cytokines, or their production in the wrong biological context may lead to perpetuation of inflammation over time.[17] In certain situations, chronic inflammation increases the risk of developing cancer, for e.g. colo-rectal cancer in inflammatory bowel disease, esophageal cancers in Barrett's esophagus, pancreatic cancer in chronic pancreatitis.[17]

Chronic inflammation occurs either when the perpetuating factor remains or when the process of resolution fails. The reactive oxygen and nitrogen species produced can damage DNA and contribute to tumorogenesis. The inflammatory response activates the transcriptor factor NFkB, which regulates many pro-inflammatory cytokines, adhesion molecules, chemokines, growth factors, and other inflammatory mediators like cyclooxygenase-2 (COX-2).[17] NFkB also promotes cellular proliferation of the tumor cells and protects them from apoptosis.[17] Activation of NFkB has been reported in cancers of breast, colon, pancreas, thyroid, bladder and skin.[17] COX-2 leads to release of prostaglandins, which favour cancer development and progression.[17] Thus inflammatory responses may play a decisive role in the initiation, progression (cell division, neo-vascularization and angiogenesis), and perpetuation of the tumor.[17] A multitude of avenues like pharmacotherapy and immunotherapy have been tried, to temper down the inflammation and in turn, restrict or destroy the tumor. Immunonutrition may provide a less invasive alternative to immunotherapy and pharmacotherapy, for prevention of cancers associated with chronic inflammation.[17]

A number of nutrients zinc, epigallacatechin gallate (EGCG), omega-3 polyunsaturated fatty acids, probiotics and prebiotics, all act differently to modulate the immune response, but all seem to have the potential to protect the host from the development of cancer and its progression.[17] A better understanding of the innate or adaptive immunity and its regulation, may pave the path to better dietary management of cancer for cancer patients and the general public.[17]

IMMUNONUTRITION AND FACTORS AFFECTING ITS EFFICACY

Type of Immunonutrient

The requirement of adequate nutrition and specific immunomodulating nutrients, to maintain the gut integrity and function, would be common to all sick patients. But the extent of gut failure, bacterial translocation, failure of cellular defense mechanisms, balance between inflammation and anti-inflammatory actions, regional and systemic generation of reactive oxygen species (ROS), would vary from patient to patient, and from time to time in the same patient.[42] The use of a cocktail of multiple nutrients in a heterogenous group of patients may lead to the loss of any benefit (or harm) achieved from the therapy. Tailoring the immunonutrient use as per the underlying pathophysiological processes in a given individual would help yield better results. For example a patient undergoing elective surgery demonstrates minimum cytokine activation and some postsurgery immunosuppression leading to infections and morbidity. In such a scenario arginine that stimulates the cellular defense mechanism, may fit the bill.[42] However, in a critically ill patient, the process is much more complex with an exaggerated inflammatory response (with excess of reactive oxygen species, lipid mediators and nitric oxide), and cellular immune dysfunction. Here we require immunonutrients that will augment the cellular defense, ameliorate the reactive oxygen species and the oxidative stress, without increasing the inflammatory response. In such a situation glutamine and anti-oxidant strategies could prove more useful.[43] Use of immunonutrients like arginine that will augment the inflammatory process could prove deleterious in such cases.[44] Studies focusing on single nutrients tested in homogenous populations would chart a more definite path for the use of specific immunonutrients.[42]

Dose of Immunonutrient

There is a dearth of literature on the dosage requirements. At least some of the treatment failures in immunonutrition could be related to inadequate doses. Meta-analysis has shown that a higher dose of glutamine showed a greater response.[43] Clinical benefits with arginine were seen in patients receiving an arginine concentration of at least 12 g/L.[2] Immunonutrients are at present being added to voluminous amounts of standard enteral nutrition solutions. Sick patients, many a times, have problems with tolerating the enteral feeds. These factors may result in sub-optimal intake of nutrient supplement with consequent sub-optimal therapeutic benefit or even failure. Providing immunonutrient separately would simplify its administration and would ensure its intake even food tolerance is a problem.[42, 45]

Route of Administration

The debate of enteral versus parenteral immunonutrition continues. Although parenteral therapy can be resorted to when enteral administration is not possible, enteral immunonutrition can be given to all intensive care patients with a fully functioning gastrointestinal tract.[11, 12]

Timing of Immunonutrition

Studies have shown that pre and peri-operative immunonutrition is more advantageous than only post operative immunonutrition.[14, 32, 33]

Nutritional Status

Pre-operative enteral nutrition benefits malnourished patients more than well nourished patients and the benefit is increased by using immunoenhancing diets which reduce the duration of the hospital stay and complication rates.[38]

Genetic Variability

Different genotypes differ in their response to immunonutrition. Many genes have single base variations in their promoter regions (single nucleotide polymorphism—SNP), which decide the amount of gene produced when the activation occurs. These SNP for the cytokines and other inflammatory chemicals would decide the outcome of the disease of the patient and hence the response to the immunonutrition.[7] More studies are warranted to decide the genotype suitability for immunonutrition and specific immunonutrients.

Gender Variability

Gender seems to affect the response to immunonutrition. For example, critically ill female patients in ICU have a better prognosis than their male counterparts.[46] However in ICU patients receiving immunonutrition, the frequency of infectious complications and duration of ICU stay are decreased in such a manner that male patients seem to fare better than female patients admitted in the ICU.[46] The reason for this phenomenon remains to be elucidated. It is thought that arginine load leads to relatively much higher levels of growth hormone in females, which in turn is responsible for hyperglycemia. It is believed that hyperglycemia has a negative effect on the clinical outcome.[47] In addition increased levels of interleukin-1 and arginine may lead to excessive amounts of nitric oxide production, and exacerbation of the inflammatory process and systemic inflammatory response syndrome.[46]

IMMUNONUTRIENTS

Glutamine

Glutamine is a precursor for nucleotide synthesis, a substrate for liver gluconeogenesis and an important fuel source for cells with rapid turnover (such as gastrointestinal epithelia, lymphocytes, fibroblasts and reticulocytes).[48] It is a precursor for nucleotide synthesis and for glutathione synthesis, which is a major link in the anti-oxidative defense mechanism.[49] It is a non-essential amino acid under normal circumstances.

Under catabolic stress, humans show an increased efflux of glutamine from the skeletal muscle, where it is normally stored. Visceral organs, enterocytes, T lymphocytes and macrophages utilize glutamine mobilized from muscle and plasma as a source of fuel.[50] Catabolic states are also characterized by increased metabolic demand for glutamine. To make the matters worse, most parenteral solutions do not contain glutamine, as the amino acid is highly unstable in standard protein solutions.[48] Thus, severely ill patients whose nutrition is supported solely by parenteral route are at risk of developing glutamine deficiency state due to inadequate supply of glutamine, mobilization of the amino acid from the stores and increased needs. Hence in catabolic states, glutamine is regarded as "a conditionally essential nutrient". [48] Considering the fact that glutamine is vital for the rapidly dividing cells like lymphocytes and gastrointestinal mucosal cells, it is not surprising that its depletion contributes to the development of immunosuppression in critically ill patients.[51] Studies have documented that:

- Use of glutamine results in amelioration of mucosal atrophy,[48] enhanced healing of gastro-intestinal mucosa damaged due to radiotherapy or chemotherapy[48] and reduction in the number of episodes of bacterial translocation from the gut to the systemic circulation.[52] Glutamine decreases negative nitrogen balance and maintains muscle mass and gut integrity in very low weight babies[53] and in patients after major surgery.[54] Glutamine-enriched TPN improves net nitrogen balance, reduces third space fluid accumulation and shortens the length of hospital stay in bone marrow transplant recipients.[55, 56] Enterally administered glutamine decreases the incidence of sepsis in premature neonates and reduces the incidence of pneumonia, bacteremia and severe sepsis in critically ill patients.[57] Parenteral glutamine administration reduces the incidence of infections in bone marrow transplant recipients and induces a change in the pattern of mortality in patients in intensive care units.[57] These clinical benefits seem to be related to improvements in intestinal integrity and cellular immune function.[57] Use of glutamine is associated with better survival rates, lowered incidence of intra-abdominal abscesses, lesser infection rates, reduced hospital costs and decrease in the duration of antibiotic usage.[27,51,58] Novak *et al.*[43] conducted a systematic review and meta-analysis of studies to determine the role of glutamine in surgical and critically ill patients. Eight trials in surgical patients showed a decrease in the infection rates and length of hospital stay, without an effect on the mortality. Six trials in critically ill patients (three with parenteral and three with enteral glutamine) showed better survival and fewer infectious complications. When the enteral and parenteral trials were considered separately, parenteral therapy seemed to result in better survival and shorter ICU stay; however the data was inadequate to evaluate the effect on infections.

- Although many in-vitro and in-vivo studies suggest an important role for glutamine in the maintenance and repair of gastrointestinal mucosa; larger well-designed randomized trials are needed[48] to confirm this finding. The use of glutamine supplementation in conditions like prematurity, short bowel syndrome, immunocompromised status secondary to HIV infection or chemotherapy/radiotherapy, and the efficacy of parenteral versus enteral glutamine need to be investigated with larger number of well-controlled studies.[59]

Arginine

Arginine is a non-essential amino acid[50,60] that has a wide range of biological actions that are beneficial to the body. Like glutamine, arginine becomes a "conditionally essential amino acid" during catabolic states like sepsis and trauma.[48] For many mammals, arginine is essential for normal growth and development of the young ones and is regarded as non-essential only in the fully-grown adults.[60]

Arginine owes it immunomodulatory functions to two major metabolic pathways: the arginase pathway and the nitric oxide synthesis pathway. In the arginase pathway, arginine is converted to urea and ornithine. This pathway generates polyamines, which are known to augment lymphocyte mitogenesis, enhance cell division and DNA replication and regulate cell cycle.[60] In addition, the arginine-dependant macrophage-mediated tumor cell cytotoxicity is mediated through induction of arginase.[60]

Arginine is the sole substrate for nitric oxide synthesis. This pathway is mediated by nitric oxide synthetase and results in the formation of nitric oxide and citrulline. Nitric oxide is one of the most versatile molecules. It plays an important role in smooth muscle relaxation and in regulation of blood flow,[48,59] coagulation pathway, immune function[48,60] and intestinal secretions.[59] It plays a vital role in disease states such as gastro-esophageal reflux,[59] pyloric stenosis,[59] sepsis, hypertension and cirrhosis.[60] In addition, nitric oxide produced by human intestinal epithelial cells inhibits the growth, encystation, and excystation of *Giardia lamblia*.[48] Nitric oxide can have both anti- and pro-inflammatory effects. Anti-inflammatory and homeostatic effects are observed with small amounts of nitric oxide, whereas pro-inflammatory effects are seen with large amounts of nitric oxide.[48] The use of inhaled nitric oxide especially in the management of post-operative pulmonary hypertension,[59] respiratory distress syndrome[59] and other cardiopulmonary problems in pediatric ICUs is gaining momentum. Reduced serum levels of arginine[61,62] and glutamine[61] have been documented in premature infants with necrotizing enterocolitis. Arginine supplementation is also associated with a dramatic decrease in the incidence of necrotizing enterocolitis in low birth babies.[63]

Supplementation with arginine in post-operative patients results in beneficial effects on T-cells: It increases the mitotic response of peripheral lymphocytes to standard stimuli and accelerates wound healing with increase in wound tensile strength and collagen deposition.[60] Arginine supplementation also inhibits the growth of tumors by up-regulating natural killer and lymphokine-activated killer function.[60,64] Supplementary dietary arginine enhances lymphocyte cytotoxic mechanisms and acts synergistically with interleukin-2 (IL-2) immunotherapy in the treatment of certain tumors.[65] Tumor response to arginine appears to depend on the immunogenecity of the particular tumor and on the requirements of arginine by that tumor as a growth substrate.[60] Clinical benefits with arginine immunonutrition is seen only when the arginine concentration is at least 12 g/l.[2] Addition of arginine as the lone supplement in the enteral solution did not provide any beneficial effects to ICU patients.[66]

Two groups have provided a meta-analysis of studies of supplementation with commercial formulas containing arginine and other additives. One analysis of 12 trials with 1557 patients showed shorter hospital stay, lower infection rates, and shorter duration of ventilator care in those fed with the formula.[47, 48] However, there was no effect on the mortality. The second analysis of 22 trials involving 2419 patients showed lesser infectious complications and decrease in the length of hospital stay.[60] Patients undergoing surgery did better than the critically ill patients. A higher mortality was seen in patients who were very sick, although they were shown to have fewer infectious complications.[68] Data that is available today suggests that arginine has a great potential as an immunomodulator, especially in catabolic conditions like post-operative stress, sepsis, trauma, and certain tumors. More number of well controlled trials is required to define the use of arginine in different clinical conditions.

Nucleotides

Dietary nucleotides play a vital role in T-cell function and cell mediated immunity. RNA appears to have immunostimulatory properties[50] and RNA-enriched enteral diets increase the maturation and phenotypic expression of T-cells.[50] Studies in rodents have shown that addition of nucleotides to the diet augments immune responses to fungal infection.[69] Nucleotide-deficient diets are associated with reduced cell mediated immunity and hampered T-cell activation, the defects that are reversed with addition of nucleotides to the diets.[50]

Studies in cancer patients undergoing surgery showed an enhancement of natural killer (NK) cell cyto-toxicity and increased disease-free duration in patients supplemented with polyadenylic and polyuridylic acid.[51] Nucleotides are in abundance in the breast milk and are perhaps play an immunomodulatory role in infants. Data showing the effects of nucleotide supplementation in children is limited. Carver *et al.*[70] demonstrated that breastfed infants and infants receiving diet supplemented with nucleotides have higher levels of NK cell cytotoxicity and IL-2 production by macrophages as compared to unsupplemented controls. It may, however, be conceded that the clinical extrapolations in terms of higher growth or reduced frequency of infections could not be demonstrated. Sanchez-Pozo and co-workers showed that lecithin cholesterol acyl transferase and apoprotein A-4 concentrations rise following nucleotide supplementation in pre-term infants. This suggests that nucleotides play a role in the postnatal maturational changes in the hepatic handling of cholesterol and lipids. The role of nucleotides as semi-essential nutrients in infants (especially the premature infants) needs to be evaluated. Early studies indicate that they may have an important role to play in intermediate metabolism, in modulation of immune response and in gut maturation.[59]

Omega-3 Fatty Acids

Two essential fatty acids, linoleic acid (omega-6 fatty acid, found in cooking oils—safflower, soy, corn, sunflower oil, lean meat and fish, and lipid emulsions of parenteral solutions) and linolenic acid (omega-3 fatty acid, found in fatty fish oils—salmon, tuna, herring fish oil) have a significant impact on the immune system.[50] Linoleic acid (omega-6 fatty acid) is a precursor of arachidonic acid, which forms 4-series leukotrienes, 2-series eicosanoids, thromboxane A2 and prostaglandin E2. Leukotriene B4 is a potent neutrophil chemotactic agent and helps in neutrophil adhesion.[50] Thromboxane A2 is a potent bronchoconstrictor and promotes platelet aggregation.[50] Prostaglandin E2 contributes to superoxide generation and increases suppressor T-cell activity, reducing cell mediated immunity.[50] Thus omega-6 fatty acids are pro-inflammatory, but limit the immune system's ability to clear the insult. Linolenic acid (omega-3 fatty acid) is a precursor for docosahexaenoic acid and eicosapentaenoic acid, which form the 3-series prostaglandins and thromboxanes, and 5-series leukotrienes. These products have much lesser biological activity than the omega-6 products. They are less effective in promoting inflammation and immunosuppression as compared to omega-6 fatty acids.[70] Omega-3 fatty acids may also have an indirect action through the inhibition of the activation of the tumor necrosis factor-alpha and nuclear factor—k B, which mediate inflammation.[17]

Studies in stressed animals receiving omega-3 fatty acids have shown increased survival and improved cell mediated immunity.[50] Gadek *et al.*[72] showed that ICU patients with acute respiratory syndrome demonstrated reduced incidence of infections and shorter duration of ventilation if they received fish oil in addition to nutritional formulas. Gogos *et al.*[73] in his study of cancer patients receiving omega-3 supplements or placebo, showed improved T-helper to T-suppressor cell ratio and normalization of lowered tumor necrosis factor-alpha concentrations in the malnourished subgroup receiving fish oil. Recent trials done using parenteral omega-3 fatty acids showed immunological benefits and anti-inflammatory effects,[74] but their use was not associated with better infection rate or mortality rate. The post-operative stay in the intensive care units and hospital were shorter in the fish oil group.[74] It has been suggested that the provision of omega-3 fatty acids to immunonutrition solutions may be important for dampening the pro-inflammatory effects of arginine added to these solutions.[2] Fish oils may be useful in the treatment of atopic dermatitis[45] and they slow down the process of IgA nephropathy[75] and prolong the survival in patients with untreatable cancers.[45] Several studies have shown that addition of medium chain triglycerides to TPN achieves more reduction in the production of TNF by stimulating monocytes as compared to what addition of long chain triglycerides to TPN is able to achieve.[51]

Taurine

Taurine plays an important part in membrane stabilization, osmoregulation, anti-oxidation, calcium homeostasis, apoptosis, bile salt formation, stimulation of glycolysis and glycogenesis, growth modulation and vision.[76] Along with glutamine and arginine it has intestinal protective effects during periods of stress.[14] It is present in high concentrations in most tissues especially in the pro-inflammatory cells like the neutrophils and the lymphocytes and is regarded as a semi-essential amino acid. Normally humans have an inherent capacity to maintain endogenous taurine levels from dietary methionine and cysteine. However during various stressful conditions like cancer, sepsis and post-operative states, decreased levels have been observed.

Taurine constitutes 76% of the free amino acid pool in the neutrophils. The neutrophil modulating action of taurine is mediated through its interaction with the respiratory burst enzyme, myeloperoxidase. The hydrogen peroxide–myeloperoxidase–chloride system generates HOCL. Taurine combines with this HOCL, to form taurine chloramine, which has the following functions:

a. It has bactericidal activity.
b. It modulates the HOCL induced tissue damage.
c. It is an immunomodulator.
d. It regulates the pro-inflammatory mediator release by the macrophage.
e. It behaves as a neutrophil derived signalling molecule which puts the brakes on the production of inflammatory mediators by the macrophages and the neutrophils, and stalls the perpetuation of the inflammatory process.
f. It has cyto-protective function by virtue of its bactericidal action and preservation of cellular function in the face of physiologic stress.
g. It maintains the phagocytic and microbicidal activity in aged neutrophils due to its membrane stabilizing effects and its anti-oxidant effects.
h. It inhibits neutrophil apoptosis via the maintenance of calcium homeostasis.

More than 50% of the free amino acid pool of the lymphocytes is composed of taurine. It has a protective role in the lymphocytes due to its membrane stabilizing effect and prevention of calcium influx. T-Lymphocytes are more susceptible to age related decline in the proliferation compared to B- lymphocytes. Taurine tones down the age related decline in the T-cell proliferation and modulates the macrophage mediated T-cell activation via its action on class 2 Major Histocompatibility Antigen.

Role of taurine in sepsis and surgical trauma: The initial host response to sepsis or surgical trauma is mediated through the activated neutrophil. Therefore the advantages of taurine are through its myriad actions on the neutrophils, and taurochloramine formation, as already stated above. In the immediate post-operative period, a spurt in the release of free radicals in the neutrophils, translates into an increase in the levels of taurine in the neutrophils. The taurochloramine among its other actions confers microbicidal action and limits the host cytotoxicity. Gray *et al.* has shown a decrease in taurine levels in cancer patients and post-operative patients. Further studies with pre-operative taurine supplementation and corresponding effect on the septic outcome needs to be investigated.

In a post ischemia set-up, activated neutrophils and pro-inflammatory cytokines mainly constitute the post ischemic reperfusate, which give rise to localized, and distal endothelial injury and distant organ injury like Adult Respiratory Distress Syndrome (ARDS), and Multiple Organ Dysfunction Syndrome (MODS). Taurine modifies this through the actions already stated. It decreases the lipid per-oxidation and cell damage during the reperfusion period.

Taurine is capable of influencing programmed cell death depending on the apoptic stimulus. It has been shown to decrease the bleomycin induced pulmonary fibrosis and reduce cyto-toxicity induced by various poisons. Thus apart from a plethora of medical conditions in which taurine is used, like congestive cardiac failure, psoriasis, pulmonary fibrosis, cholestasis associated with total parenteral nutrition and post operatively, taurine can be used as an immunonutrient by virtue of its action on various limbs of the immune system. Taurine is regarded as a conditionally semi-essential amino acid in preterms and neonates and is currently used to supplement most infant foods.

Vitamins and Minerals

Anti-oxidants play an important role in cytokine production, phagocyte function, cell-mediated responses and immunoglobulin production.[59] These minerals and vitamins interact and complement each other facilitating immune-competence at all levels.[59]

Zinc

Zinc is required as a catalytic, structural and regulatory ion for enzymes, proteins and transcription factors.[17] It is an important component of the cell membrane structure and function, and being an anti-oxidant, it protects from lipid peroxidation.[48] It is a component of several metalloenzymes like alkaline phosphatase, carboxypeptidases, thymidine kinase, and DNA- and RNA- polymerases. It plays a role in DNA synthesis and repair, maintenance of red cell integrity and in bone and liver metabolism. Its role in DNA synthesis and in regulating gene expression makes it especially important for cells having a rapid turnover like hemopoietic cells, thymic tissue, gastrointestinal mucosal cells and cells of the immune system. Matrix metalloproteinases (MMPs) are a family of zinc dependant proteinases that perform the degradation of the extracellular matrix which play a key role in the invasiveness and metastasis of beast cancer. These MMPs play a role in tumor invasion, migration, host immune escape, extravasations, angiogenesis and the tumor growth.[17] Zinc deficiency has detrimental effects on B- and T-cell function, efficiency of phagocytosis, cytokine production, chemotactic function of neutrophils, monocytes, macrophages and delayed cutaneous hypersensitivity reactions.[48,77] It is, therefore, not surprising that acrodermatitis enteropathica, a congenital disorder of zinc metabolism related to its defective absorption and transport, manifests with recurrent infections especially with candida albicans[78] as one of its features.

Zinc is important for the conversion of pre-thymulin to thymulin, in the thymus. A low level of functionally active thymulin in Down's syndrome causing thymic dysfunction was postulated to be due to deficiency of zinc. Prolonged zinc deficiency results in a substantial decrease in the thymus size, depletion of the T-cells from spleen and lymph nodes and reduced pre-B and immature B-cells in the bone marrow.[17] Licastro *et al.*[59] showed that, after four months of zinc supplementation, there was normalization of zinc and thymulin levels, normalization of lymphocyte proliferation and neutrophil function, and improved DNA repair in patients with Down's syndrome. However other studies have failed to substantiate these findings.[59] Many clinical trials showed improved outcomes in children with gastrointestinal diseases, when supplemented with zinc. The benefits are especially noteworthy in children with low levels of zinc or in those with high dietary phytate intake. Zinc supplementation has been shown to decrease the number of watery stools[79] and duration of acute diarrhea,[79] improve intestinal permeability,[48] reduce duration of illness in children with persistent diarrhea,[80] and lower the probability of continuing diarrhea, treatment failure and death.[48] There are ongoing studies that are examining the role of zinc supplementation in preventing childhood mortality in developing countries. The aspect of combining zinc with standard oral rehydration solutions in the treatment of acute diarrhea is also under scrutiny. Further studies are needed to find the mechanism behind this and to identify patient population whose dietary requirements are higher than expected. It is important to realize that excessive zinc can lead to copper deficiency, anemia, growth retardation and depressed immunity.[17]

Selenium

Selenium is a trace element that plays an important role in maintaining the integrity of muscles and nervous system.[59] It also has anti-oxidant activity by virtue of being a part of the glutathione-peroxidase complex, though its role in immuno-competence is less well-defined. It has synergistic actions with vitamin C and vitamin E. Selenium deficiency was noticed in children receiving long-term intravenous nutrition, when it was not a routine practice to add trace minerals to intravenous nutrition fluids.[59]

Vitamin A

Vitamin A plays an important role in cellular differentiation and immune modulation[81] and has anti-tumorogenic capabilities. The extensive involvement of body epithelial surfaces in diseases like measles and protein calorie malnutrition leads to a fast depletion of this vitamin.[59] Administration of vitamin A increases IgG production and lymphocyte counts, without any changes in the complement activity or interleukin-2 production.[59] Children with even mild deficiency of vitamin A are at an increased risk for diarrhea, respiratory infections and death.[48] A large number of clinical trials carried out in various parts of the world have demonstrated the therapeutic efficacy of vitamin A supplementation. Vitamin A supplementation reduces mortality amongst children with diarrhea or respiratory diseases.[48] A meta-analysis of trials showed that vitamin A supplementation helped achieve a 30% decrease in the mortality in infants and young children.[82] A study conducted in Bangladesh showed that vitamin A supplemented group showed a significantly enhanced improvement in clinical recovery from acute shigella infection.[48] A study in Brazil showed improvements in the number of episodes of diarrhea (especially severe episodes) in the vitamin A-supplemented group.[48] A study carried out in India showed that the supplemented children aged less than 23 months suffered from lesser number of episodes of measles and older children when supplemented with vitamin A had lesser episodes of diarrhea and fever.[48] Children with pneumonia receiving vitamin A had fewer episodes of diarrhea in the one-year follow-up in a study conducted in Tanzania.[48] A decrease in all-cause mortality and diarrhea-specific mortality was seen in HIV-infected children after vitamin A supplementation.[48] Vitamin A deficient status was shown to be associated with impaired gastrointestinal barrier function,[48] which could be reversed with administration of a large dose of vitamin A in a study carried out in Indian infants.[48] There is sufficient data to indicate that vitamin A supplementation is of paramount importance for decreasing the morbidity and mortality associated with certain clinical conditions in developing countries.

Vitamin E

Vitamin E is the main membrane-bound anti-oxidant and free radical scavenger, which prevents lipid peroxidation damage.[59] Excessive tissue damage related to local inflammatory reactions and excessive production of free oxygen radicals is known to occur in various disorders such as necrotizing enterocolitis (NEC),[59] ulcerative colitis and Crohn's disease.[59] There have been some reports that indicate that anti-oxidants and recombinant dismutase are able to modulate these inflammatory reactions.[59] Larger controlled studies are needed to confirm these preliminary findings.

Iron

Iron prevents anemia and helps in normal somatic growth and normal neurophysiologic development. It also plays an important role in immune function, as demonstrated by the increased susceptibility to infections in children with iron deficiency anemia.[59] Animal studies indicate that iron deficiency affects the immune system at various levels (impaired bactericidal activity and cell mediated immunity, decreased NK cell function, decreased B-cell responses).[59] Young children with iron deficiency showed T-cell dysfunction, decreased IL-2 levels and impaired cell-mediated immunity.[59] However, paradoxically excessive iron induces tissue damage through its oxidant potential. Increased levels of free iron are associated with a risk of overwhelming sepsis, as iron a factor essential for bacterial growth, becomes easily available to them.[59]

Polyphenols: EGCG

Polyphenols are a group of chemicals that are not essential for human health. However they may play a beneficial role in human nutrition by virtue of their anti-oxidant, anti-mutagenic and anti-inflammatory properties.[17] Certain polyphenols may decrease the expression of the pro-inflammatory cytokines and adhesion molecules from the endothelial cells and reduce monocyte adhesion.[17] One of the polyphenols popularly used is the Epigallocatechin-3-gallate (EGCG), which is found in green teas.[17] They are known to possess significant anti-inflammatory and chemopreventive properties. EGCG inhibits the tumor necrosis factor-alpha and blocks the activation of the nuclear factor-kB.[17]

Probiotics

Probiotics are live microorganisms in fermented foods that promote good health, through establishing an improved balance in intestinal micro-flora.[48, 83] They have been used for their health promoting benefits for times immemorial. The use of probiotics in the modern era was sparked off by the Nobel Prize-winning scientist Elie Metchnikoff's observation that the long life span of Bulgarian peasants was a result of consumption of fermented milk products.[48] Since probiotics do not permanently colonize the intestine they should be in sufficient quantities to maintain adequate levels in the colon. They should also be of human origin and be able to adhere to the intestinal enterocytes.[48] The commonly used microorganisms include various species of lactobacilli (L. acidophilus, L. bulgaricus, L. casei), bifidobacterium, streptococcus thermophilus and saccharomyces boulardii.

Several general mechanisms have been cited to explain the beneficial effects of these organisms. They probably enhance the mucosal immune defenses[48] and also protect the host from colonization by pathogenic microorganisms. They also probably reduce the chances of microbial translocation by competing with them for receptor sites on the intestinal surface. Their ability to reduce colonization could be related to competition for intra-luminal nutritive substances, crowding out effect, production of antibiotic substances and enhancement of host immune defenses (by means of adjuvant effect, increased polymeric immunoglobulin A production and cytokine stimulus).[84] They can also exert beneficial effects on non-immunological host defenses by strengthening intestinal tight junctions, increasing mucous secretions, enhancing motility and producing metabolic products (amino acids such as arginine and glutamine and short chain fatty acids) that secondarily function as protective nutrients,[85] generating hydrogen peroxide and by decreasing luminal pH and redox potential making it difficult for the pathogenic bacteria to colonize and grow.[59]

Several well-controlled studies have shown encouraging results, but there are methodological difficulties in demonstrating actual colonization by the added live bacteria directly. Reports suggest that the human derived GG strain of lactobacillus casei is able to shorten the duration of diarrhea and help eradicate recurrent clostridim difficile colitis unresponsive to multiple courses of conventional antibiotics in children.[59] Saavedra *et al.* showed that supplementation with bifidobacterium bifidum and *sreptococcus* thermophilus shortened the duration of shedding of rotavirus in chronically hospitalized children[86] Majamaa and co-workers demonstrated that use of Lactobacillus GG was associated with an enhanced rotavirus-specific immune response.[59] In a pediatric intensive care unit with a high incidence of NEC, premature infants given probiotics had a lower incidence of disease as compared to the controls.[48] A clinical trial with non-pathogenic E. coli in patients with ulcerative colitis showed that the clinical outcome with its use was comparable with that associated with the use of anti-inflammatory agent mesalamine.[48] Probiotics also improve lactose tolerance when added to ferment dairy products like yoghurt, thereby decreasing gas and cramping and decrease in the exhaled hydrogen levels. This enables patients to consume calcium and protein-rich food, which they would otherwise avoid.[59]

Recent clinical studies suggest that probiotics may provide beneficial effects for patients with inflammatory bowel disease.[48] A study in Finland showed that probiotics used along with protein hydrolysate (hypoallergenic formula) can decrease intestinal inflammation, mucosal barrier permeability and clinical symptoms in infants with allergic dermatitis.[48] These findings need to be confirmed with larger studies.

Although probiotics are generally recognized as safe, the possibility of overloading the ability of the intestinal barrier to contain the added yeast should be kept in mind. The case of a one-year-old immunocompetent infant, who developed fungemia and septicemia with saccharomyces boulardii, while receiving this probiotic for the treatment of severe gastroenteritis and dehydration, is an eye opener.[59] Eight patients in Mayo Clinic have showed positive blood cultures for lactobacilli following liver transplantation and Imunosuppression.[59] Factors like bowel decontamination routines, bile stasis, drastic changes in the colonic flora, intravenous vancomycin, biliary anastomosis can result in translocation and dissemination of these organisms that are usually considered as non-pathogenic.

Prebiotics

Prebiotics are non-digestible food ingredients that provide beneficial effects to the host by selectively stimulating the growth and activity of one species or a limited number of species of bacteria in the colon.[83] Unlike the probiotics, which introduce exogenous bacteria into the human colon, prebiotics stimulate the preferential growth of a limited number of health-promoting commensal floras already residing in the colon. For example, oligosaccharides in the human milk facilitate the growth of bifidobacteria and lactobacilli in the colon.

The use of fructose oligosaccharides[83] and inulin-type fructans[87] provide bifidogenic action on the human endogenous flora. Both inulin (group of fructose polymers-fructans) and fructose oligosaccharides are found in many plant foods like wheat, onion and banana.[48] Prebiotics act through the following mechanisms: They are preferred as substrates by the bifidobacteria. They also bring about changes in the luminal pH and other factors that preferentially favour the growth of bifidogenic activity.[48] Their use in infants with NEC or short bowel syndrome and in older patients with colitis or Crohn's disease needs to be probed. Pierre *et al.* found in their study that addition of fructo-oligosaccharides to food reduced the incidence of colonic tumors associated with multiple intestinal neoplasia.[17] Prebiotics have been added to yogurt in an effort to combine the prebiotic and probiotic effects (termed as a synbiotic effect).[87] Prebiotics by virtue of their chemical structure are not absorbed in the small intestines, but are fermented into gases, combustible gases and short chain fatty acids in the colon. This makes them a preferred sugar replacement in diabetics.[48]

Breastmilk

Any discussion on immunonutrition would be grossly inadequate if one fails to mention the immunonutritive role of breastmilk. The breastmilk has numerous nutrients and other substances that assume an immunonutritive role. These include secretory IgA, IgG, IgM, IgE, IgD, lactoferrin, macrophages, bifidus factor, T- and B-lymphocytes, anti-adherence substances, lysozymes, interferon, epidermal growth factor, nerve growth factor, insulin-like growth factor, amino sugars, fatty acids, taurine, glutamine, cortisol and thyroxine.[59]

No wonder then that breastfeeding is associated with decreased incidence of gastrointestinal and respiratory infections in the first two years of life.[59] Oligosaccharides in the breastmilk inhibit the adhesion of pneumococci and Hemophilus influenzae to the pharyngeal and buccal epithelial cells. This protects breastfed infants from infections caused by these pathogens.[59]

Iron is an essential element required for the growth of gram-negative bacteria. These organisms require the element for their multiplication, metabolic pathways and virulence. Lactoferrin in the breastmilk binds with iron making it unavailable to these potentially pathogenic bacteria.[59] This favours the growth of lactobacilli and bifidobacteria, which foster an acidic environment in the gut, further inhibiting the growth of enteropathogens.[59]

In addition, breastmilk shows lymphocyte transforming activity resulting in the production of alpha-interferon.[59] The decrease in the levels of the myeloperoxidase and beta-glucuronidase activity induced by breastmilk tends to help modulate the inflammatory reactions mediated by neutrophils. The milk contains a multimeric alpha-lactalbumin complex that binds with potential pathogens offering protection to the babies.[59]

IMMUNONUTRITION IN FUTURE

On the basis of available data, immunonutrition seems to have immense potential for decreasing the morbidity and mortality amongst critically ill individuals, those with gastro-intestinal diseases, immune deficiency disorders, polytrauma, sepsis or severe infections.[60-71] It could be of great importance in cancer prevention as well. Carbohydrates especially the complex or slowly absorbed ones, seem to have a role in immunomodulation. They have been shown to alter the flora of the small bowel and colon through stimulation of the short chain fatty acids production.[88] More studies are required to elucidate the clinical relevance of these findings. During periods of stress, like post-operative states, severe trauma, gastrointestinal disorders etc. there is a possibility of restriction and at times proscription of diet. It has been postulated that this deprives the normal bacteria in the gut of a secure environment and a regular supply of food. As a result of this, these bacteria may show virulent characteristics for self-preservation, which may harm the host. This further lends support to the need for enteral nutrition.[89]

It should, however, be conceded that although the idea of immunonutrition is not new, a lot of work needs to be done for establishing its efficacy and safety. The scientific data available regarding the use of immunonutrition for individual disorders, and the use/efficacy of individual immunonutrients, is scanty at its best and more prospective controlled studies may have to be undertaken to get the correct picture. It is also important to note that most of the data pertains to use of immunonutrition in adults and there is hardly any data about its use in children and infants. Young infants and children have diseases that are peculiar to their age group. They also have metabolic, physiological and immunological processes that are unique. Hence, it may be inappropriate to extrapolate data obtained from studies carried out in adults to infants and children. This makes it imperative for researchers to take special interest in studying the use of immunonutrition in infants and children. Here a mention of needs and priorities of children in developing countries would not be out of place. Infectious diseases in the background of widespread malnutrition continue to besiege children in the developing countries. As immunonutrition has been shown to be effective in these very processes, it is of great significance to children here. More work is needed to identify the nutrients that would help in specific conditions.

Preliminary data also suggests that all genotypes might not be equally sensitive to the effects of immunonutrition. This phenomenon offers a fascinating prospect for research: identifying the genotype and phenotype (response to injury, degree of inflammation, etc.) that would derive the maximum benefit from these interventions. This would bring in strategies tailor-made based on gene polymorphism.[1] In the interim period it is necessary to disseminate information available to healthcare providers so that they can start using simple and affordable interventions straightaway.

Acknowledgements

The authors thank Dr Nilima A Kshirsagar, Dean, Seth GS Medical College and KEM Hospital, Mumbai, for permission to publish this chapter.

Annexure I: Immunonutrient preparations available

Reconvan (Fresenius–Kabi)

Constituents:
- ***Calories:*** 420 KJ / 100 Kcal / 100 ml
- ***Protein:*** 5.5 g (22 %)
  Glutamine: 1 g; Arginine L: 0.6 g
- ***Carbohydrates:*** 12 g (48 %)
  Sugars: 0.7 g; Lactose: <0.01 g
- ***Fats:*** 3.3 g (30 %)
  Saturated fatty acids: 2 g; Mono-saturated fatty acids: 0.2 g; Cholesterol: < 6 mg;
  Polyunsaturated fatty acids: 1.2 g Medium chain triglycerides: 1.9 g
- ***EPA:*** 0.15 g
- ***DHA:*** 0.1 g
- ***Fiber:*** 0 g
- ***Vitamins:*** A, D, E, K, B_1, B_2, B_6, B_{12}, C, Niacin, Pantothenic acid, Biotin, Folic acid, beta-carotene and Choline
- ***Minerals:*** Zinc, Selenium, Iron, Sodium, Potassium, Chloride, Calcium, Magnesium, Phosphorus, Copper, Manganese, Iodide, Fluoride and Chromium
- ***Essential amino acids:*** Lysine, Threonine, Methionine, Phenylalanine, Tryptophan, Valine, Leucine and Isoleucine
- ***Conditionally essential amino acids:*** Glutamine, Arginine,
- Tyrosine, Cysteine and Histidine
- ***Non-essential amino acids:*** Glycine, Alanine, Proline, Serine, Glutamic acid, Aspartic acid and Aspargine

Adult doses:
Complete nutrition: 1.5 lit/day
Critically ill patients: 10 ml/hour and increase every hour by 10 ml/hour

Cost:
Rs. 495 for 500 ml

REFERENCES

1. Iwasaki T, Ohyanagi H. Advance and perspective of clinical nutrition. *Nippon Geka Gakkai Zasshi* 2004; 105:196-199 (Abstract).
2. McCowen KC, Bistrian BR. Immunonutrition: Problematic or problem solving. *Am J of Clin Nutr* 2003; 77:764-770.
3. Alvarez W, Mobarhan S. Finding a place for immunonutrition. *Nutr Rev* 2003; 61: 214-218 (Abstract).
4. Davidson A. The pharmacological effects of novel nutrients on the immune system. *Nurs Times* 2004; 100: 62-63 (Abstract).
5. Suchner U, Senftleben U, Felbinger TW. Immune function and organ failure, immunomodulation with nutritional support—An update. *Anaesthetist* 2000;49:460-465 (Abstract).
6. Baik HW. Nutritional therapy in gastrointestinal disease. *Korean J Gastroenterol* 2004; 43: 331-340 (Abstract).
7. Grimble RF. Immunonutrition. Curr Opin Gastroenterol 2005; 21: 216-222.
8. Koretz RL. Immunonutrition: Fact fantasy and future. *Curr Gastroenterol* Rep 2002; 4: 332-337 (Abstract).
9. Parson RL, Galley HF, Dhillon JK, Webster NR. Increased nuclear factor kappa B activation in critically ill patients who die. *Crit Care Med* 2000; 28: 1047-1051.
10. Bastian L, Weimann A. Practical aspects of early enteral feeding. *Anesthesiol Recanim* 1999; 24: 95-100 (Abstract).
11. Grotz M, Regel G, Bastian L, Weimann A, Neuhoff K, Stalp M, Tscherne H. The intestine as the central organ in the development of multiple organ failure after severe trauma-pathophysiology and therapeutic approaches. *Zentralbl Chir* 1998; 123: 205-217 (Abstract).
12. Mc Clave SA, Lowen CC, Snide HL. Immunonutrition and enteral hyperalimentation of critically ill patients. *Dig Dis Sci* 1992; 37: 1153-1161 (Abstract).
13. Keith ME, Jeejeebhoy KN. Immunonutrition. *Baillieres Clin Endocrinol Metab* 1997; 11: 709-738 (Abstract).
14. Calder PC. Immunonutrition. *BMJ* 2003; 327: 117-118.

Omegaven (Fresenius-Kabi)

Constituents:

- ***Calories:*** 470 KJ /112 Kcal / 100 ml

  Highly refined fish-oil comprising;

Eicosapentaenoic acid: 1.25- 2.82 g;	Docosahexaenoic acid: 1.44-3.09 g
Myristic acid: 0.1- 0.6 g;	Palmitic acid: 0.25-1 g
Palmitoleic acid: 0.3-0.9 g;	Stearic acid: 0.05-0.2 g
Oleic acid: 0.6- 1.3 g;	Linoleic acid: 0.1-0.7 g
Linolenic acid: 0.2 g;	Octadecatetraenoic acid: 0.15-0.45 g
Eicosaenoic acid: 0.05-0.3 g;	Arachidonic acid: 0.1-0.4 g
Docosaenoic acid: 0.15 g;	Docosapentaenoic acid: 0.15-0.45 g
Alpha-tocopherol: 0.015-0.0296 g;	Glycerol: 2.5 g

Adult Dose:

10-20 % of total lipid intake, 1-2 ml/kg with an infusion rate of not more than 0.5 ml/kg/hour

Cost:

Rs. 695 for 50 ml (5 g)

Dipeptiven (20%) (Fresenius–Kabi)

Constituents: N2- L- Alanayl-L-Glutamine: 20 g/100 ml

Dose: 0.3 g / kg for all age groups

Cost: Rs. 1590 for100 ml (parenteral solution).

Glutammune (Fresenius-Kabi)

Constituents:

L-Glutamine: 10 g/satchet.

Dose: 2-40 g/day in 3-6 divided doses (adult)

Impact (Novartis)

Constituents:

- ***Calories:*** 420 KJ / 100 Kcal / 100 ml
- ***Protein:*** 5.6 g (22 %)
- ***Carbohydrates:*** 13.16 g (53 %)

  Low Lactose: <0.01 g
- ***Fats:*** 2.82 g (25 %)

  Saturated fatty acids: 60 % of the fats

EPA: Eicosapentaenoic acid; DHA: Docosahexaenoic acid.

Vitamins: A, D, E, K, B_1, B_2, B_6, B_{12}, C, Niacin, Pantothenic acid, Biotin, Folic acid, beta-carotene and Choline

Minerals: Zinc, Selenium, Iron, Sodium, Potassium, Chloride, Calcium, Magnesium, Phosphorus, Copper, Manganese, Iodide, Fluoride and Chromium

Essential amino acids: Lysine, Threonine, Methionine, Phenylalanine, Tryptophan, Valine, Leucine and Isoleucine

Conditionally essential amino acids: Glutamine, Arginine, Tyrosine, Cysteine and Histidine

Non-essential amino acids: Glycine, Alanine, Proline, Serine, Glutamic acid, Aspartic acid and Aspargine

Contains:

L- Arginine	1.35 gm/100 ml
L-glutamine	0.36 gm/ 100 ml
Omega 3 fatty acids	0.34 gm/100 ml i.e. 12.4 % of the fat
Omega 6 fatty acids	0.25 gm/100 ml i.e. 9.92 % of the fat
RNA nucleotides	
Gluten Free	

Adult doses:

1 sachet (61 g) to be dissolved in 206 ml of boiled and cooled water.

3 sachets per day for 3 days pre-op and 3 sachets per day post-op. For ICU cases 3 sachets per day

Critically ill patients: 10 ml /hour and increase every hour by 10 ml /hour

Cost:

Rs. 89 per sachet. Available as 4 sachets per pack costing Rs. 356.

15. Culebras FJM, de Paz Arias R, Jorquera PF, Garcia de Lorenzo A. Nutrition in the surgical patient: Immunonutrition. *Nutr Hosp 2001*; 16: 67-77 (Abstract).
16. Cunneen J, Cartwright M. The puzzle of sepsis: Fitting the pieces of the inflammatory response with treatment. *AACN Clin Issues* 2004; 15: 18-44 (Abstract).
17. Philpott M, Ferguson LR. Immunonutrition and cancer. Mutat Res 2004; 551:29-42.
18. Grimble RF. Nutritional modulation of immune system. *Proc Nutr Soc* 2001; 60: 389-397 (Abstract).
19. Atkinson S, Sieffert E, Bihari D. A prospective randomized, double blind, controlled, clinical trial of enteral immunonutrition in the critically ill. *Crit Care Med* 1998; 26: 1164-1172.
20. Tugrul S, Ozcan PE, Akinei IO, Ismailov M, Cagatay A, Cakar N, Esen F. Effect of immunonutrition on the development of nosocomial infection and on clinical outcome in critically ill patients. *Ulus Trauma Derg* 2004; 10: 89-96 (Abstract).
21. Bower RH, Cerra FB, Bershadsky B, Licari JJ, Hoyt DB, Jensen GL *et al.* Early enteral administration of a formula (Impact) supplemented with arginine, nucleotides and fish oil in intensive care unit patients: Results in a multicentric, prospective, randomized, clinical trial. *Crit Care Med* 1995; 23: 436-449.
22. Bertolini G, Iapichino G, Radrizzani D, Facchini R, Simini B, Bruzone P, Zanforlin G, Lognoni G. Early enteral immunonutrition in patients with severe sepsis: results of an interim analysis of a randomized multicentre clinical trial. *Intensive care Med* 2003; 29: 669-671 (Abstract).
23. Galban C, Montejo JC Mesejo A, Marco P, Colaya S, Sanchez-Segura JM *et al.* An Immune enhancing enteral diet reduces the mortality rate and episodes of bacteremia in septic intensive care unit patients. *Crit Care Med* 2000; 28: 643-648.
24. Heyland DK, Novak F, Drover JW, Jain M, Su X, Suchner U. Should immunonutrition become routine in critically ill patients? A systematic review of the evidence. *JAMA* 2001;286:944-953.
25. Heyland DK, Novak F. Immunonutrition in critically ill patients: More harm than good? *J Parenter Enteral Nutr* 2001; 25(2S): 51-57 (Abstract).
26. Bastian L, Weimann A. Immuonutrition in patients after multiple traumas. *Br J Nutr* 2002; 87: S133-S134 (Abstract).
27. Kudsk KA, Minard G, Croce MA, Brown RO, Lowrey TS, Pritchard FE, *et al.* A randomized trial of iso-nitrogenous enteral diets after severe trauma: An immune enhancing diet reduces septic complications. *Ann Surg* 1996; 224: 531-543 (Abstract).
28. Engel JM, Menges T, Neuhauser C, Schaefer B, Hempelmann G. Effects of various feeding regimens in multiple trauma patients on septic complications and immune parameters. *Anesthesiol Intensivmed Notfallmed Schmerzther* 1997; 32: 234-239 (Abstract).
29. Chuntrasakul C, Siltham S, Sarasombath S, Sittapairochana C, Leowattana W, Chockvivatanavanit S, Bunnak A. Metabolic and immune effects of dietary arginine, glutamine, and omega-3 fatty acids supplementation in immunocompromised patients. *J Med Assoc Thai* 1998; 81: 334-343 (Abstract).
30. Chuntrasakul C, Siltham S, Sarasombath S, Sittapairochana C, Leowattana W, Chockvivatanavanit S, Bunnak A. Comparison of an immunonutrition formula enriched with arginine, glutamine and omega-3 fatty acids with currently high enriched enteral nutrition for trauma patients. *J Med Assoc Thai* 2003; 86: 552-561 (Abstract).
31. Chieveley WS, Hamilton DC. The role of the gut in major surgical postoperative morbidity. *Int Anesthesiol Clin* 1999; 37: 81-110 (Abstract).
32. Senkal M, Zumtobel V, Bauer KH, Marpe B, Wolfram G, Frei A *et al.* Outcome and cost effectiveness of peri-operative enteral immunonutrition in patients undergoing elective upper gastro-intestinal surgery: A prospective randomized study. *Arch Surg* 1999; 134: 1309-1316 (Abstract).
33. Senkal M, Mumme A, Eickhoff U, Geier B, Spath G, Wulfert D, Toosten U, Frei A, Kemen M. Early post-operative enteral immunonutrition: Clinical outcome and cost comparison analysis in surgical patients. *Crit Care Med* 2000; 28: 1255-1256.
34. Gianotti L, Braga H, Frei A, Greiner RD, Di Carlo V. Health care resources consumed to treat post-operative infections: Cost saving by peri-operative immunonutrition. *Shock* 2000; 14: 325-330 (Abstract).
35. Gianotti L, Braga M, Fortis C, Soldini L, Vignali A, Colombo S, Radaelli G, Di Carlo V. A prospective randomized clinical trial on peri-operative feeding with an arginine, omega-3 fatty acids and RNA enriched enteral diet: Effect on host response and nutritional status. *J Parenter Enteral Nutr* 1999; 23: 314-320 (Abstract).
36. Braga M, Gianotti L, Radaelli G, Vignali A, Mari G, Gentilini O, Di Carlo V. Perioperative Immunonutrition in patients undergoing cancer surgery: Results of a randomized double blinded phase 3 trial. *Arch Surg* 1999; 134: 428-433 (Abstract).
37. Braga M, Gianotti L, Vignali A, Di Carlo V. Pre-operative oral arginine and omega-3 fatty acids supplementation improves the immunometabolic host response and outcome after colorectal resection for cancer. *Surgery* 2002; 132: 805-814 (Abstract).
38. Braga M, Gianotti L, Nespoli L, Radaelli G, Di Carlo V. Nutritional approach in malnourished surgical patients: A prospective randomized study. *Arch Surg* 2002; 137: 174-180 (Abstract).
39. Campos FG, Waitzberg DL, Teixeira MG, Mucorino DR, Habr-Gama A, Kiss DR. Inflammatory bowel diseases: Principles of nutritional therapy. *Rev Hosp Clin Fac Med Sao Paulo* 2002; 57: 187-198 (Abstract).
40. Belluzi A, Brignola C, Campieri M, Pera A, Boschi S, Miglioli M. Effect of an enteric coated fish oil preparation on relapses in Crohn's disease. *N Eng J Med* 1996; 334: 1557-1560.
41. F Balkwill, A Mantovani. Inflammation and cancer: Back to Virchow? *Lancet* 2001; 357: 539-545.
42. Heyland D, Dhaliwal R. Immunonutrition in the critically ill: From old approaches to new paradigms. *Intensive Care Med* 2005; 31: 501-503.
43. Novak F, Heyland DK, Avenell A, Drover JW, Su X. Glutamine supplementation in serious illness: A systematic review of the evidence. *Crit Care Med* 2002; 30: 2022-2029.
44. Stechmiller JK, Childress B, Porter T. Arginine immunonutrition in critically ill patients: A clinical dilemma. *Am J Crit Care* 2004; 13: 17-23 (Abstract).
45. Koretz RL. Immunonutrition: Can you be what you eat? *Curr Opin Gastroenterol* 2003; 19: 134-139.
46. Kieft Hans, Roos AN, van Drunen JDE, Bindels AJGH, Bindels JG, Hofman Z. Clinical outcome of immunonutrition in a heterogenous intensive care population. *Intensive Care Med* 2005; 31: 524-532.
47. van den Berghe G, Wouters P, Weekers F *et al.* Intensive insulin therapy in critically ill patients. *N Engl J Med* 2001; 345: 1359-1367.
48. Duggan C, Gannon J, Walker AW. Protective nutrients and functional foods for the gastrointestinal tract. *Am J Clin Nutr.* 2002; 75: 789-808.

49. Chen da W, Wei Fei Z, Zhang YC, Ou JM, Xu J. Role of enteral immunonutrition in patients with gastric carcinoma undergoing major surgery. *Asian J Surg* 2005; 28:121-124.
50. Schears GJ, Deutschman CS. Common nutritional issues in pediatric and adult critical care medicine. *Crit Care Clin* 1997; 13: 669-690.
51. Singh R, Gopalan S, Sibal A. Immunonutrition. Indian J Pediatr 2002; 69: 417-419.
52. Gianotti L, Alexander J, Gennari R, Pyles T, Babcock G. Oral glutamine decreases bacterial translocation and improves survival in experimental gut origin sepsis. *J Parenter Enteral Nutr* 1995; 19: 69-74 (Abstract).
53. Neu J, Rio JC, Meetze WH, Veerman M, Carter C, Millsaps M, *et al*. Enteral glutamine supplementation for very low birth weight infants decreases morbidity. *J Pediatr* 1993;13:691-699.
54. Hammerquist F, Wernerman J, Vander DA, Vinnars E. Alanylglutamine counteracts the depletion of free glutamine and the post-operative decline in skeletal muscle. *Ann Surg* 1990; 213: 637-642 (Abstract).
55. Schloerb PR, Amare M. Total parenteral nutrition with glutamine in bone marrow transplant and other clinical applications. *J Parenter Enteral Nutr* 1993; 17: 407-413 (Abstract).
56. Ziegler TR, Young LS, Benfell K, Scheltinga M, Hortos K, Bye R *et al*. Clinical and metabolic efficacy of glutamine supplemented parenteral nutrition after bone marrow transplantation. *Ann Intern Med* 1992; 116: 821-28 (Abstract).
57. Andrews J, Griffiths RD. Glutamine: Essential for immune nutrition in the critically ill. *Brit J Nutr* 2002; 87 (suppl): S3-S8 (Abstract).
58. Griffiths RD, Jones C, Palmer TEA. Six-month outcome of critically ill patients given glutamine supplemented parenteral nutrition. *Nutrition* 1997; 13: 295-302.
59. Levy J. Immunonutrition. The pediatric experience. Nutrition 1998; 14: 627-633.
60. Evoy D, Lieberman MD, Fahey TJ, Daly JM. Immunonutrition: The role of arginine. *Nutrition* 1998; 14: 611-617.
61. Becker RM, Wu G, Galanko JA, Chen W, Maynor AR, Bose CL, Rhoads JM, *et al*. Reduced serum amino acid concentrations in infants with necrotizing enterocolitis. *J Pediatr* 2000; 137: 785-793.
62. Zamora SA, Amin HJ, Mc Millan DD, Kubes P, Fick GH, Butzner JD. Plasma L-arginine concentrations in premature infants with necrotizing enterocolitis. *J Pediatr* 1997;131:226-232.
63. Amin HK, Zamora SA, Mc Millan DD *et al*. Arginine supplementation prevents necrotizing enterocolitis in the premature infant. *J Pediatr* 2002; 140: 425-431.
64. Brittenden J, Park KG, Heys SD, Ross C, Ashby J, Ah-see A, Eremin O.L-Arginine stimulates host defences in patients with breast cancer. *Surgery* 1994; 115: 205-212 (Abstract).
65. Lieberman MD, Nishioka K, Redmond BP, Daly JM. Enhancement of interleukin-immunotherapy with L-arginine. *Ann Surg* 1992; 215: 157 (Abstract).
66. Caparros T, Lopez J, Grau T. Early enteral nutrition in critically ill patients with a high protein diet enriched with arginine, fibre, and anti-oxidants compared with a standard high protein diet: The effect on nosocomial infections and outcome. *J Parenter Enteral Nutr* 2001; 25: 299-308 (Abstract).
67. Beale RJ, Bryg DJ, Bihari DJ. Immunonutrition in the critically ill: A systematic review of clinical outcome. *Crit Care Med* 1999; 27: 2799-2805.
68. Stechmiller JK, Childress B, Porter T. Arginine immunonutrition in critically ill patients: A clinical dilemma. *Am J Crit Care* 2004; 13: 17-23 (Abstract).
69. Fans Fourlow WC, Kulkarni AD, Van Buren CT, Rudolph FB. Effect of nucleotide restriction and supplementation on resistance to murine candidiasis. *J Parenter Enteral Nutr* 1988; 12: 49-52 (Abstract).
70. Carver JD, Pimentel B, Cox WI, Barness LA. Dietary nucleotides effects upon immune function in infants. *Pediatrics* 1991; 88: 359-363.
71. Alexander JW. Immunonutrition: Role of omega-3 fatty acids. *Nutrition* 1998; 14: 627-633.
72. Gadek JE, De Michele SJ, Karlstad MD, Pacht ER, Donahoe M, Albertson TE, *et al*. Effect of enteral feeding with eicosapentaenoic acid, anti-oxidants in patients with acute respiratory distress syndrome. *Crit Care Med* 1999; 27: 1409-1420.
73. Gogos CA, Ginopoulos P, Salsa B, Apostolidou E, Zoumbos NC, Kalfarentzos F. Dietary omega-3 polyunsaturated fatty acids plus vitamin E restore immunodeficiency and prolong survival for severely ill patients with general malignancy: A randomized control trial. *Cancer* 1998; 82: 395-402 (Abstract).
74. Weiss G, Meyer F, Mathiess B, Pros M, Koenig W, Tippert H. Immunomodulation by peri-operative administration of omega-3 fatty acids. *Br J Nutr* 2002; 87 (suppl): S89-S94.
75. Donadia JV, Berstralh EJ, Offord KP, *et al*. A controlled trial of fish oil in Ig Nephropathy. *N Engl J Med* 1994; 331: 1194-1199.
76. Redmond HP, Stableton PP, Neary P, Bouchier HD. Immunonutrition: The role of taurine. *Nutrition* 1998;14:599-604.
77. Shankar AH, Prasad AS. Zinc and immune function: The biological basis of altered resistance to infection. *Am J Clin Nutr* 1998; 68 (suppl): S447-S463.
78. Moynahan E. Acrodermatitis Enteropathica: A lethal inherited human zinc deficiency disorder. *Lancet* 1974; 1: 399-400.
79. Sazawal S, Black RE, Bhan MK, Bhandari N, Sinha A, Jalla S. Zinc supplementation in young children with acute diarrhoea in India. *N Eng J Med* 1995; 333: 839-844.
80. Penny ME, Peerson JM, Marin RM *et al*. Randomized, community based trial of the effect of zinc supplementation with and without other micronutrients on the duration of persistent childhood diarrhea in Lima, Peru. *J Pediatr* 1999; 135: 208-217.
81. Bates CJ. Vitamin A. *Lancet* 1995; 345: 351.
82. Fawzi W, Chalmers T, Herrera M, Mosfeller F. Vitamin A Supplementation and child mortality: A meta analysis. *JAMA* 1993; 269: 898-903.
83. Gibson GR, Roberfroid MB. Dietary modulation of the human colonic microbiota: Introducing the concept of prebiotics. *J Nutr* 1995; 125: 1401-1412 (Abstract).
84. Lu L, Walker WA. Pathologic and physiologic interactions of bacteria with the gastrointestinal epithelium. *Am J Clin Nutr* 2001; 73 (suppl): S1124-S1130.
85. Vanderhoof JA. Probiotics: Future directions. *Am J Clin Nutr* 2001; 73 (suppl): S1552-S1555.
86. Saavedra JM, Bauman NA, Oung I, Perman JA, Yolken RH. Feeding of Bifidobacterium bifidum and streptococcus thermophillus to infants in hospital for prevention of diarrhea and shedding of rotavirus. *Lancet* 1994; 344: 1046-1049.
87. Roberfroid MB. Prebiotics and synbiotics: Concept and nutritional properties. *Br J Nutr* 1998; 80 (suppl): S197-S202 (Abstract).
88. Vanderhoof JA. Immunonutrition: The role of carbohydrates. *Nutrition* 1998; 14: 595-598.
89. Alverdy J, Stern E. Effect of immunonutrition on virulence strategies in bacteria. *Nutrition* 1998; 14: 580-584.

Ajay Gaur

39 Nutrition of the High-Risk Neonate

INTRODUCTION

Nutrition in the high-risk neonate is quite different from feeding healthy babies. Most of the high-risk babies are sick and often not well enough to breastfeed. If the high-risk neonate is preterm and very low birthweight (VLBW), the problems are doubled up, as prematures may not be able to suck effectively and their gastrointestinal tract maturity and digestibility may be questionable. On the other hand, high-risk premature infants have greater nutritional needs to achieve optimal growth than at any time of life. The condition of these infants also imposes additional burdens on nutrient supply. Impediments to growth include the stress of common pathophysiologic events (hypoxia, acidosis, infection), therapies (corticosteroids) and physiological immaturity (decreased gastrointestinal mortality and delayed enzyme expression). There is also the fear that aggressive feeding may produce pathologic conditions such as feeding intolerance and necrotizing enterocolitis (NEC). Babies who are metabolically and hemodynamically unstable are often unable to take regular feelings. High-risk newborns with umbilical catheters and those on mechanical ventilators may not be able to feed because of the risk of aspiration.

Over the last 20 years, in the management of high-risk sick neonate, the focus of attention was the drug management in most of the NICU. But, with recent advances in critical care and evidence-based medicine, there has been an increasing attention focused on the subject of nutritional support of the "high-risk neonate". Evidence suggest that optimal nutritional support is related to a better outcome—both improved overall survival as well as decreased NICU stay.[1]

AIMS OF NUTRITIONAL SUPPORT

Nutritional support in the "high-risk neonate" addresses two facts: first that the newborn is growing and developing and, secondly, newborns rapidly adapts from a relatively constant intrauterine supply of nutrients to intermittent feeding of milk. The full-term newborn infant grows at a rate of 25 to 30 g/day. However, preterm infants or those with medical or surgical conditions commonly exhibit impaired sucking or absorption or may have increased nutritional needs. High-risk neonates, including those in shock often present with extreme degrees of metabolic derangement in protein and energy metabolism characterized by increased protein breakdown which is not entirely suppressed by protein or energy intake, reprioritization of protein synthesis with increased synthesis of acute phase proteins, decreased production of structural body proteins and thus a very high protein turn over.[2] In addition there is also an extreme degrees of glucose and lipid intolerance.[3,4]

An adequate, optimal and intense support is needed to correct growth restrictions present at birth in order to continue appropriate weight gain thereby constituting the mainstay in managing the high-risk and sick neonate (Table 39.1).

Table 39.1: Who are at risk

- Birthweight of < 1800 g or gestation of < 34 weeks.
- Delayed passage of meconium (> 24 hours) and urine (> 48 hours).
- Inability to such or swallow.
- Reduced activity or excessive inconsolable crying.
- Marked changes in color: Pale, blue, yellow.
- Cold and febrile baby.
- Rapid breathing (respiratory rate > 60 per mintue, alae nasi moving, chest retractions).
- Superficial infections (purulent conjunctivitis, thrush, umbilical sepsis, pyoderma, abscess).
- Persistent vomiting or watery diarrhea.
- Abdominal distention.
- Bleeding from any site.
- Seizures.

PRINCIPLE AND GOALS OF NUTRITIONAL SUPPORT

Most of the time, high-risk neonates receive nutritional requirements just like healthy neonates, despite the fact that illness deranged their physiological and metabolic demand. Similarly our targeted goals should not only focus on physiological and/or pharmacological support but one must fix goals for nutritional support (Table 39.2).

Table 39.2: Growth guidelines

Weight gain	> 15 g/kg/day for infants < 2.0 kg > 20 g/day for infants > 2.0 kg
Length gain	0.7—1.0 cm/wk
Head circumference gain	0.7—1.0 cm/wk

Early concepts in critical care nutrition were to maximize caloric delivery with the idea of "more calories the better", based on predicated energy expenditure (PEE) extrapolated from nonograms of well newborn. Recent studies on resting energy expenditure (REE) using indirect calorimeter have clearly documented that predicted energy expenditure or "PEE" is a considerable overestimation and a reduction in the calorie requirement has proven optimal for the sick neonate.[5] Few years ago, 50-70 cal/kg per day was routinely being delivered during critical illness and currently this has been decreased to 22-30 cal/kg per day or even less. This appears to be optimal level caloric delivery in the hypermetabolic setting. This reduction in calorie delivery has occurred for a number of reasons, including. Newborns during hypermetabolic stress are unable to utilize excess calories. Despite of providing adequate nutritional endogenous glucose production is not reversed; in fact, it continues.

Understandably, excess calorie delivery results in numerous metabolic complications like hyperglycemia, hyperinsulinemia and hepatic steatosis.[6-8] Severe hyperglycemia (blood sugar even greater than 600 mg/dl) is associated with glycosuria and hyperosmolar dehydration leading to a grave disturbances of fluid and electrolyte homeostasis in the unstable neonate. In addition, hyperglycemia has also been shown to result in significant reduction in neutrophil cell function, including decreased chemotaxis, bacterial adherence, oxidative burst and phagocytosis. The secondary inefficient hyperinsulinemia leads to increased sodium and water retention with resultant greatly increased ventilatory requirements in the unstable neonate due to impaired lung. This leads to inhibition of endogenous lipolysis causing greater carbohydrate utilization, increased carbon dioxide production and impairment of respiratory function in a borderline reserves neonate (Fig. 39.1). These observations have led to a significant reduction in calorie delivery and a patient-tailored calorie regime.

A concept now gradually developing in the neonatal intensive care setting is the delivery of "eucaloric nutrition" or permissive hypocaloric nutritional support during the early unstable resuscitation phase of the critical neonate. As the neonate improves and the hypermetabolic state reverses caloric supply may be increased to even hypercaloric nutritional support, once it is clear that inefficient metabolism has ceased and that calorie and nutrient delivery will indeed support grow and tissue healing.[10] The purpose of "nutrition in high-risk neonates" is to stabilize the neonate,

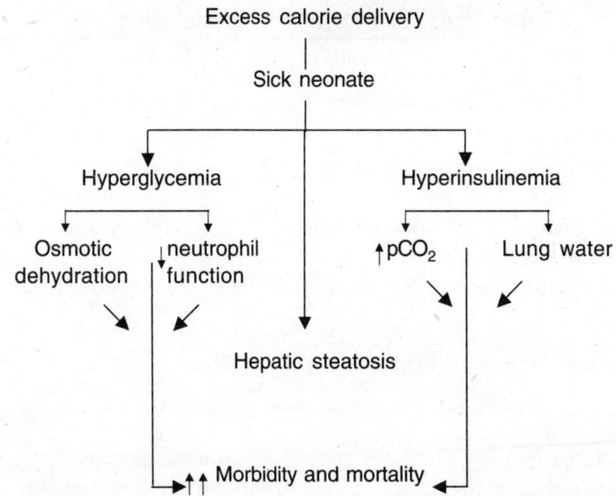

Fig. 39.1: Effect of excess calorie delivery on sick neonate

repair injured tissues, to restore organ function, to resist infection and to respond to stress.

In the initial phase of management, "parenteral nutrition" (PN) fulfills these criteria but the prerequisite to starting PN is first to rule out any metabolic disturbances and secondly to correct any fluid-electrolyte/acid-base imbalances.[11,12]

NUTRITIONAL NEEDS

Fluids

Fluid management is important because most high-risk neonates require IV fluids. Appropriate fluid therapy ensures maintenance of homeostasis and assist recovery. After birth there is an increase in renal perfusion and glomerular filtration followed by diuresis. These results in loss of extracellular water and weight. The two main areas of fluid loss are the kidneys and transepidermal water loss. Thus preterm sick are more prone to lose water and weight. In high-risk neonates fluids loss can be multifactorial as shown in Figure 39.2. The fluid requirements are lowest soon after birth and rise subsequently. There are some variations as shown in Tables 39.3 and 39.4.[13]

Table 39.3: Daily fluid requirements during first week of life (ml/kg/day)

Birth weight	Day 1	Day 2	Day 3	Day 4	Day 5	Day 6	Day 7
> 1000 g	80	100	120	130	140	150	160
1000-1500 g	80	95	110	120	130	140	150
> 1500 g	60	75	90	105	120	135	150

Note: i. 1500 to 2500 and term: 60-80 day 1-2, 100-150 day 3-7.
ii. After day 7: term babies with BW > 1500 g: 150-160 ml/kg/day: preterm babies with BW 1000-1500 g: 50-160 ml/kg/day.
iii. Sodium supplementation at 3-5 mEq/kg continue till 32-34 weeks corrected gestational age.
iv. Add 20 ml/kg of extra fluid if newborn is under phototherapy and radiant warmer.

Table 39.4: Fluid therapy in special situations

Situation	*Total fluids*	*Watch for signs of*
Patent ductus arteriosus	120 ml/kg/day	Heart failure
Bronchopulmonary dysplasia	120-140 ml/kg/day	Worsening oxygenation
Necrotising enterocolitis	200 ml/kg/day	Hypotension, shock
Acute renal failure	400 ml/m^2/day + UOP	Fluid overload

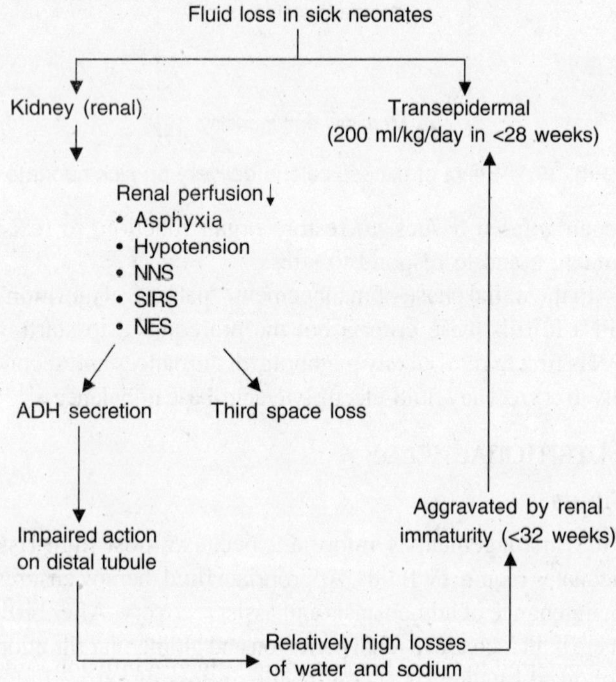

Fig. 39.2: Fluid loss in sick neonates

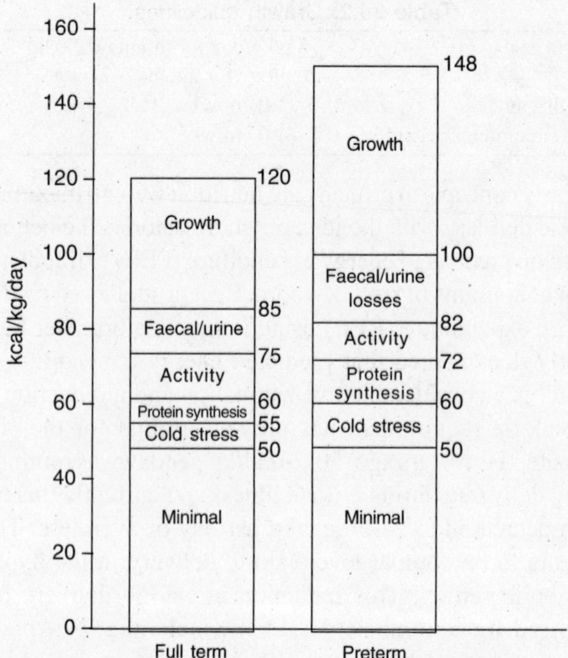

Fig. 39.3: Energy requirement for full-term and preterm broken down into the actual distribution of energy usage

Energy

The energy needs of the neonate are derived from a computation of the energy expenditure, energy storage (growth), and energy loses.[14] Energy is required for the maintenance of body metabolism as well as for the growth. The energy needs and reserved of infants are unique (Figure 39.3). In general, infants require more calories enterally than parenterally.[15] More simply, energy needs can be viewed as being nearly equivalent to the infants daily water requirements. When newborns are fed intravenously no fat and carbohydrate intakes are unabsorbed. They also expend less energy in physical activity because of the impediment to mobility. Average energy requirements are, therefore, at least 7% lower in newborn fed intravenously, and the decrease in activity probably increase this figure to a total reduction of 10-15%. Though a caloric intake of 121 kcal/kg/day is recommended for growth of preterm.[16] Studies have demonstrated that on parenteral nutrition, a calorie intake of 50 kcal/kg/day prevent catabolism and 80 kcal/kg/day is sufficient, if adequate protein is concurrently provided.[17]

A multitude of factors can significantly increase the energy requirement, including exposure to a cold environment, fever, sepsis, burns, trauma, cardiac or pulmonary diseases. With few exceptions e.g. some cases of respiratory insufficiency, at least 60% of energy requirements are provided as glucose. Upto 40% of calories may be provided by intravenous fat emulsions. During the acute phase of the disease, aim is to avoid catabolism and not growth. This is difficult in VLBW sick neonate due to higher requirements, poor stores and reduced intake. There should be positive energy balance to initiate and sustain growth.[18,19]

It is evident that to achieve a weight gains of 15 g/kg/day an estimated energy intake of ~120-130 kcal/kg/day is required. Rate of energy expenditure is ~60 kcal/kg/day and accretion is ~50 kcal/kg/day. Although fetus needs about 30 kcal/kg/day for accretion but this extra calorie is required for catch up growth of low birthweight neonate who has different significant post natal malnutrition or for intrauterine growth retarded fetus due to their higher energy maintenance needs and more energy costs of new tissue growth.

The most common method of measuring energy expenditure is indirect calorimetry. In this method, the amount of oxygen absorbed across the lung is assumed to be exactly equal to the amount of oxygen consumed in metabolic processes. Commonly used nomograms may significantly underestimate or often overestimate energy expenditure determined by calorimeter.[20-23]

Macronutrients

The proportion of nutrients delivered to high-risk neonate has also undergone change in the last 10-15 years. The appropriate protein intake for premature infants has been defined further from evaluations of weight gain, nitrogen retention, and serum biochemical indicators of protein nutritional status. Protein now appears optimal at 2.0-2.5 g/kg/day depending on renal and hepatic functional status.[24] In sick VLBW, for optimal achievement in weight gain, a total protein of 3.5-4.0 g/kg/day daily loss 1 g + accretion 2 g + 80 to 90% of protein retention).[25]

Proteins are needed for growth and wound healing. It is seen that, in infants weighing < 1000 g, more than 1% of endogenous proteins was lost on a daily basis if only glucose was given, a finding that provides impetus for giving early proteins and calories. When newborns were given as little as 60 kcal/kg/day, but including 2.5 g/kg/day of amino acids, a positive nitrogen balance was achieved. It is essential to note that protein needs should be considered in conjunction with energy. Protein synthesis requires energy. If energy intake is inadequate, protein synthesis may be depressed and amino acid oxidation increased. Hence, protein intakes of 2.7-3.5 g/kg/day stimulated fetal nitrogen accretion rates. This daily requirement of 3.0-3.5 g/kg/day (preterm and term both) is achieved initially with 0.5 g/kg/day with increments of 0.5 g/kg/day to a maximum of 3-3.5 g/kg/day.

Carbohydrate is supplied as dextrose, which provide 3.4 cal/g. Ideally 50-70% of the total calories should come from dextrose. The goal of glucose administration is to provide energy particularly to tissues dependent on glucose for energy (e.g. brain). A glucose infusion rate of upto 7 mg/kg/min is associated with increased glucose utilization for energy and a rate of more than 7 mg/kg/min with fat synthesis. Initiate glucose infusion at 6-8 mg/kg/min is increased at increments of 3 mg/kg/min (not to exceed 15 mg/kg/min). It is always helpful to consider dextrose infusion in terms of milligrams of glucose per kilogram per minute (mg/kg/min), which expresses to total glucose load and accounts for infusion rate, dextrose concentration and patient weight (Fig. 39.4).Glucose infusions are best guided by periodic blood sugar measurements. The signs of glucose intolerance are hyperglycemia, hyperosmolality and secondary glucosuria and osmotic dieresis. Hyperglycemia is often encountered in the stressed neonate.[4,9,26-28] Blood sugars should be retained ideally below 200 mg/day in the critically ill stressed neonate. Blood sugars > 300 mg/day are associated with osmotic dieresis and > 250 mg/day need some intervention. Blood sugar < 200 mg/day often need no intervention (Fig. 39.5).

Glucose tolerance is related to gestational age. Preterms have decreased peripheral glucose utilization, and because of hepatic insensitivity to insulin, may have persistent hepatic glucose production in the setting of hyperglycemia. Low birthweights usually tolerate an initial infusion rate of 6-8 mg/kg/min, while VLBW may develop significant and persistent hyperglycemia if infusion rates exceeds 6-7 mg/kg/min, which is equivalent to 10% D/W infused at about 100 ml/kg/day. The increased rate of glucose infusion in sick neonate increases both metabolic rate (oxygen consumption) and carbon dioxide production (carbohydrate is converted to fat). Thus, very high glucose infusion rates may compromise infants with lung disease by increasing oxygen consumption and carbon dioxide production; these effects can be limited by replacing some carbohydrate with fat.

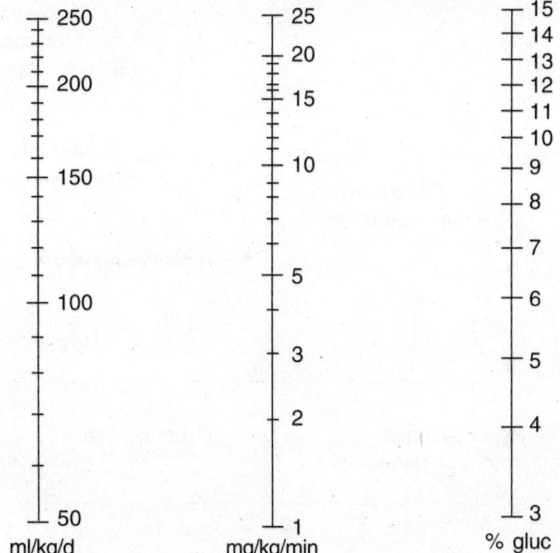

Fig. 39.4: Interconversion of glucose infusion units

Recent data suggest that fructose may perhaps be more efficiently metabolized in the hypermetabolized in the hyermetabolic state and will be used in future as source of carbohydrate in critical and sick neonates.[2]

Fat Requirements

Intravenous fats have the highest caloric density of the three major nutrients (9 kcal/day) and allow delivery of high calorie density in comparatively low volumes. In addition, the ideal R/Q (respiratory quotient) of lipids makes it an attractive substitute for carbohydrates as an energy source in children with borderline respiratory reserves. In general 2 to 4% dietary energy should come from linoleic acid, the essential fatty acid. Deficiencies of linoliec acid may occur rapidly in neonates. With holding of lipids from a neonate's parenteral nutrition for as little as 2 days may lead to fatty acid deficiency.[29] Manifestations of fatty acid deficiency include scaly skin, diarrhea are impaired wound healing.[30]

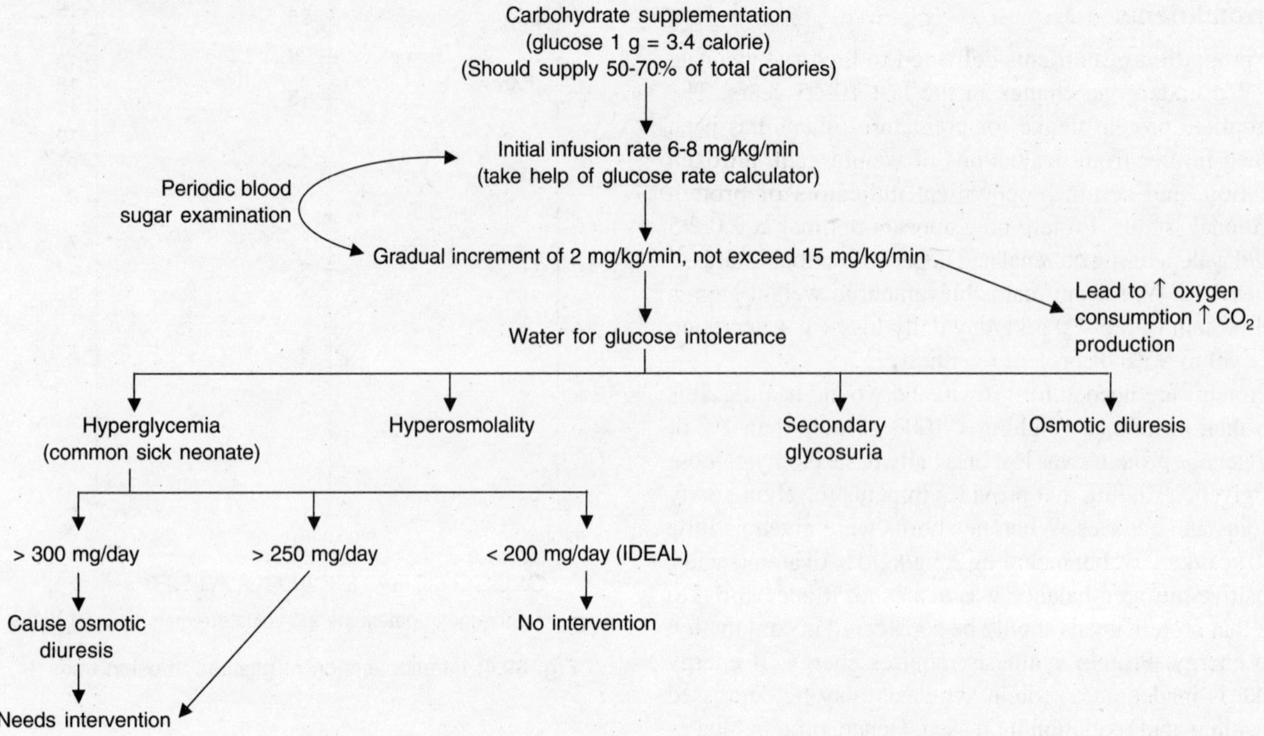

Fig. 39.5: Suggested protocol for carbohydrate supplementation

The advantages of using fat emulsions provide upto 40% of caloric intake include the following:[31]

1. The energy density, which is 2 kcal/ml for 20% emulsions, allows more energy to be provided when fluid volume is restricted.
2. The low osmolality is (280 mOsm/kgH_2O) is of special value when using a peripheral line.
3. Deficiencies in essential fatty acids can be prevented.
4. The production of CO_2 is 40% lower per unit of energy, an important consideration in cases of pulmonary insufficiency.
5. The energy cost of fat storage is negligible.
6. The risk of fatty liver is decreased because of decreased hepatic lipogenesis from dextrose.

There are some potential disadvantages of fat emulsions including:

1. Impairment of function of lymphocytes, neutrophils, macrophages, and reticulo endothelial system.
2. Coagulation defects, including thrombocytopenia, elevated prothrombin time (PT), and partial thromboplastin time (PTT).
3. Decrease in pulmonary oxygen diffusion.
4. Competition with bilirubin and drugs for albumin binding site.
5. Increase in LDL cholesterol.

Several commercial fat emulsions are now available. All consist of more than 50% linoleic acid and 4-9% linoleic acid. The particle size is approximately that of chylomicrons (0.5 µm), but the particle contains no protein. Thus the infused fat emulsion must acquire apolipoprotein C-II from HDL particles before it can be acted on by endothelium-bound Lipoprotein Lipase (LPL) a hepatic triglyceride lipase. LPL activity is inhibited or decreased in prematurity and enhanced by glucose, insulin, lipid and catecholamines. Among 10% and 20% lipid emulsions, a 10% solution delivers more phospholipids per gram of lipid than a 20% solution, 10% solutions are less suitable for neonatal use and 20% are preferred for all patients.

In case of severe sepsis, special caution is required to ensure that the lipid is effectively metabolized. Continuous monitoring with long-term use is also essential. Start with 1 g/kg/day, advance every 1-2 days by 0.5-1 g/kg/day upto 2.5 g/kg/day. Check serum triglycerides before starting and before and after increasing dose. Request results the same day. As a general rule, do not increase dose if serum triglycerides are greater than 150 mg/dl during infusion. Now-a-days, in some parts of Asia, lipid emulsions which include medium chain triglycerides (MCT) and omega-3 fatty acids are available and are being increasingly used. It is recognized that long chain fatty acids (LCT) are potentially immuno suppressive when either administered rapidly or in large quantities. Likewise, the amount of lipid administered in the septic or immuno suppressed child has been reduced to 15-20% if total caloric intake as opposed to the traditional 30 percent.[14,26,32,33]

Thus, current practice is to commence a low-dose lipid in the septic neonate, preferably combinations of MCT and LCT instead of only LCT. Likewise, peripheral preparations of omega-3 fatty acids have also been introduced into Indian market recently.

Essential Amino Acids

Of the twenty standard amino acids, eight are classically essential in that no enzymatic pathways are available in humans to synthesize them (Table 39.5). Unique to the neonate are three additional essential amino acids (phenylalanine, cystine and taurine) which because of immature amino acid synthetic mechanisms are not formed in sufficient amounts[34-36] (Fig. 39.6). Recently proline has been suggested as an essential amino acid although this has yet to be confirmed by others.[37] The administration of a specially designed pediatric formulation leads to a normalization of the neonate's plasma amino gram levels[38-40] and prevention of retinal degeneration changes.[41] Two additional amino acids, glutamine and arginine, although not defined as essential, appear to have special functions relevant to metabolism and may be classified as relatively essential.

Table 39.5: Essential amino acids

Threonine	Methionine	Cystine †
Leucine	Phenylalanine	Proline †
Isoleucine	Tryptophan	Glutamine ++
Valine	Histidine *	Arginine ++
Lysine	Tyrosine †	

* Essential only in infancy.
† May be essential in the premature baby.
++ May be essential in times of excess stress and energy demands.

Glutamine is a vital source of protein and energy for several organs.[42] It is the most abundant amino acid in whole tissues and in blood and is the most important vehicle for the transfer of nitrogen for renal ammoniagenesis and hepatic ureagenesis. Glutamine is an essential precursor for nucleic acid biosynthesis and is, therefore, essential for the proliferation of cells that are rapidly turning over, such as the intestinal mucosa and lymphocytes. The gastrointestinal tract is the principle organ of glutamine utilization.[42-44] Glutamine plays multiple role in intestinal metabolism, structure and function. Gut mucosal cells have high glutaminase activity, and the human gastrointestinal tract extracts 12-13% of circulating glutamine.[45] Glutamine is a major energy source and appears to be more important than glucose for enterocyst and colonocytes. Although glutamine is readily available in healthy individuals, in pathophysiologic states this carefully balanced homeostasis may be lost. In neonatal sepsis, shock or after surgery blood glutamine levels are fall, primary insult to the gut causes increased gastrointestinal permeability, which results in the passage of bacterial endotoxin into the portal venous system, causing macrophages to release the cytokines tumor necrosis factor and interleukin-1. These cytokines act on multiple end organs to stimulate the production of

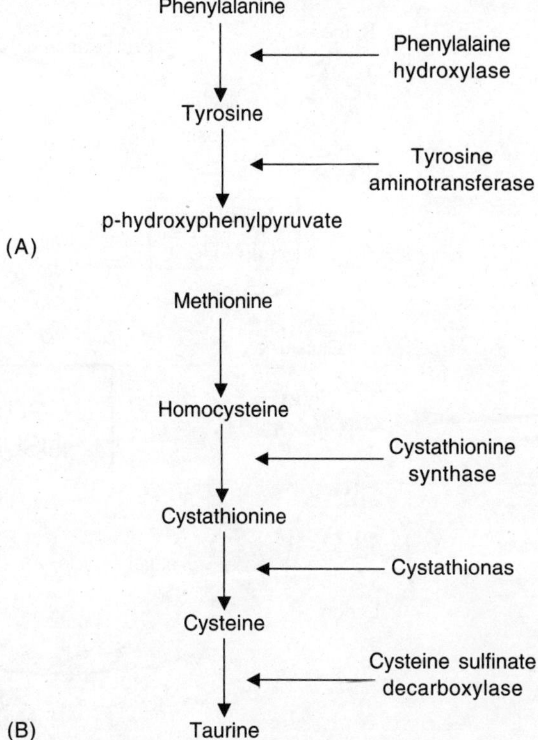

Fig. 39.6: Metabolic pathways demonstrating two enzymes that are deficient in neonates: (A) Metabolic pathways for the formation of tyrosine and p-hydroxyphenylpyruvate (B) Metabolic pathways for the formation of cysteine and taurine

glutamine, with a resultant replenishment of the glutamine pool. This increase in glutamine is needed for the removal of acid through the kidney and for the generation of new lymphocytes and enterocytes. During periods of increased stress, the circulating pool of glutamine may drop, despite this mechanism, causing a relative dependency on exogenous sources. ACTH, adrenocorticotropic hormone; GLN, glutamine; TNF, tumor necrosis factor (Fig. 39.7). Evidence is available that supplemental glutamine enhances glutathione synthesis—the human body's most potent endogenous antioxidant.[15,46]

Arginine, which may be essential in times of excess stress and energy demand, is a dibasic amino acid.[47] Arginine supplementation improves nitrogen retention and would healing in sick neonates.[48,49] The mechanism of arginine's actions has not been fully demonstrated, although its function appears to require an intact hypothalamic-pituitary axis.[50] Arginine is present in all commercially available amino acid mixtures, with higher concentrations found in pediatric formulation (approximately 123 mg/g of amino acid) compared with adult formulations (95 to 99 mg/g).

All standard preparations arc equally good source of amino acids and the final infusate contains 2.3% amino acids. In the very low birthweight, the initial amount should be 1 g/kg/day. Because of the high osmolality of amino

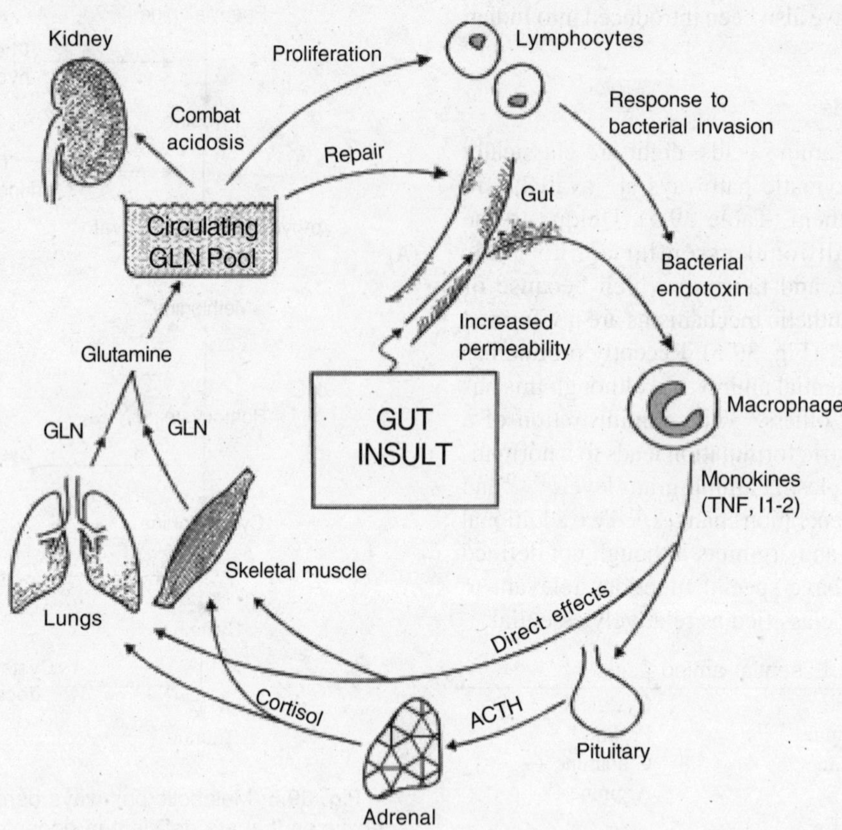

Fig. 39.7: Metabolic routes in which glutamine is utilized during a septic event

acid solutions, the concentration should not be advanced beyond 2% in peripheral vein infusates. Monitoring for tolerance of the intravenous amino acid solutions should include routine blood urea nitrogen (BUN).

Vitamin, Minerals and Electrolytes

The current evidence and emerging data indicate that increased antioxidant vitamins may be beneficial in these circumstances. The newborns that have undergone ischemia reperfusion injuries or have very high oxygen demand (ARDS, chronic lung disease) benefit from increasing antioxidant vitamins (vitamin A, C and E). Recommendations for intravenous vitamin intakes are given in Table 39.6. Pediatric MVI ampoule meets the guidelines for term infants. The recommended dose of MVI Pediatric for premature infants is 2 ml (40%) of a single dose vial per kilogram per day. This formulation is not optimal as it contains too little vitamin A, excessive amounts of water-soluble vitamins, but it is currently the best available.

For vitamin D, 40 IU/kg/day (maximum 400 IU/day) is adequate for both term and preterm infants. The higher dose of 160 IU/kg/day has not been associated with any complication and continues to be recommended.

Table 39.6: Suggested intakes of vitamins

Vitamins	*Premature infants (per kg/d)*	*Term infants (per day)*
Thiamine (mg)	0.35	12
Riboflavin (mg)	0.2	0.5
Pyridoxine (mg)	0.2	0.6
Niacin (mg NE)*	7	17 (NE)
Pantothenic acid (mg)	2	5
Biotin (µg)	6	20
Folic acid (µg)	50	140
Cobalamine (µg)	0.3	1
Vitamin A (µg RE)**	500	700
Vitamin C (mg)	25	80
Vitamin D (µg) (Cholecalciferol)	4 (160 IU)	10 (400 IU)
Vitamin E (mg) (α-tocopherol)	3	7
Vitamin K (µg)	80	20

* NE = Niacin equivalents.
** RE = Retinol equivalents. 1 RE = 1 µg retinol or 6 mg β-carotene.

Calcium Phosphorus and Magnesium

Recent studies have indicated that the intravenously-fed premature and term infants should be given relatively high

Section 10

amounts of calcium and phosphorus. Current recommendations are to supply calcium 500-600 mg/l, phosphorus 400-450 mg/l and magnesium 50-70 mg/l. The calcium phosphorus ratio should be 1.3:1 by weight or 1:1 by molar ratio.[31] These recommendations assume an average fluid intake of 120-150 ml/kg/day and an infusate of 25 g of amino acid per litre. With lower amino acid concentrations, the concentrations of calcium and phosphorus should be decreased.

Electrolytes

Standard recommendations are given in Table 39.7. The required concentrations of electrolytes depend on the flow rate of the infusate and must be modified if flow rates are unusually high and low. Replacement electrolytes and fluids should be delivered via a separate infusate.

Trace Elements

When intravenous nutrition is only supplemental or limited to less than 2 weeks, only zinc need routinely be added. Before considering for copper and manganese, monitoring is must, particularly in the presence of cholestatic liver disease. If monitoring is not feasible, temporary withdrawal is advisable. As selenium, chromium and molybdenum are excreted primarily in the urine, therefore these trace elements should be administered with caution in the presence of renal failure.

Iodine 1 μg/kg/day is advisable if newborn is on long-term parenteral nutrition. Iron added to the infusate should be in a diluted form of iron dextrose in a concentration of 1 mg/l. There are few concerns of adding iron; one is risk of iron over load particularly if the newborn has received blood transfusions, second is potential increase in the free iron because of low transferrin levels. Excess iron is thought to enhance the risk of gram-negative septicemia. Iron has powerful oxidant properties and can enhance the demand for antioxidants, especially vitamin E.

Additional Growth Factors and Nutrients

Carnitine is synthesized from lysine and methionine and serves as an important effector of fatty acid oxidation in the mitochondria. Although the liver is able to synthesize this factor, it is felt that the newborn, and particularly the preterm, may not be able to manufacture sufficient amount of carnitine although human milk contains abundant carnitine.[51] Provision of carnitine in the diet results in improved fatty acid oxidation. In general 5 to 10 mg/kg/day should supplies in neonates but it is difficult to determine about the supplementation.[52] A variety of growth factors have a beneficial effect on intestinal growth, and their absence prevents normal growth of an organism. They may needed in sick neonates on TPN. Some of these factors are found in breast milk and appear to play a major role in the transition of a neonate's intestine from one that is maternally supported to one that must actively absorbs nutrients.

INTRAVENOUS NUTRITION

In India, the technique of PN has not developed in keeping with other advances in neonatal critical care. Non-availability of nutrients, inadequate pharmacy support, lack of know-how, high costs and the potential risk of infection are the main reasons for non-utilization of PN in care of neonates.[12]

PN should be reserved for infants in whom an adequate enteral diet is not possible, or unable to meet the demand. The other indications are:

- Weight less than 1800 g and the neonate not expected to receive significant enteral nutrition for more than 3 days.

Table 39.7: Routine monitoring

Variables	*Acute stage*	*Long-term*
Growth		
Weight	Daily	Weekly
Length	Weekly	
Head circumference	Weekly	
Urine		
Glucose (dipstick)	Void	Twice weekly
Specific gravity	Void	
Volume	Daily	
Blood		
Glucose	4 hours after changes,[1] then daily for 2 days	Twice weekly
Na^+, K^+, Cl^-, CO_2, BUN	Daily for 2 days after changes,[1] then twice weekly	Twice weekly
Ca^{2+}, Mg^{2+}, P	Initially, then twice weekly	Weekly
Total protein, albumin, bilirubin, AST, and Alkaline phosphate	Initially, then weekly	Weekly
Zinc and copper	Initially, then weekly	Monthly
Triglycerides	Initially, 1 day after changes,[1] then weekly	Weekly
CBC	Initially, then twice weekly; according to clinical indications	Twice weekly

[1]Changes include alterations in concentrations or flow rate.

- Weight more than or equal to 1800 g and not expected to receive significant enteral nutrition for more than 5 to 7 days.
- Premature infants who weighs less than 1500 and who has respiratory distress or other contraindications to enteral feeding should be started on intravenous glucose during the first hours of life.
- Larger premature and sick term newborns may be maintained on only glucose and electrolyte solutions, if is anticipated that full enteral feedings will be tolerated by 5 to 7 days of age.

PN solutions can be infused into peripheral veins or a central vein, usually the vena cava. Central PN allows the use of more hypertonic solutions but have greater risks. It is possible to support growth by the use of peripheral PN with a fat emulsion, thereby avoiding the complications associated with prolonged use of central venous catheters. However peripherals PN may not support adequate growth in extremely premature infants with high metabolic demands.

Placement of a central venous is indicated under the following circumstances:

- An extended period (e.g. > 1 week) of bowel rest in some postoperative conditions and in NEC.
- Nutritional requirements exceeding the capabilities of peripheral PN, require dextrose concentrations higher than 10 to 12.5%.
- Imminent lack of peripheral venous access.

Goals of Parenteral Nutrition

1. To promote nitrogen retention and protein sparing.
2. To provide energy for metabolic processes.
3. To establish growth and maturation during the critical postnatal period.

The Broviac is the catheter of choice for long-term intravenous nutrition. For periods of upto 3-4 weeks, a percutaneous central venous catheter threaded into the superior vena cava from a peripheral vein can be used. For the infusion of dextrose concentration higher than 12.5%, the tip of the catheter should be located in the superior vena cava or right atrium. After placement, a chest X-ray must be obtained to check this position. If the catheter is to be used for nutrition and medications, a double line catheter should be inserted.

Complications of PN are:

a. *Complications Related to Catheter Insertion and Use*
Thrombosis, superior vena cava syndrome, perforation of central vessel, infiltration with tissue injury, pneumothorax, hydrothorax, hemothorax, hydropericardium and hemopericardium, catheter sepsis.

b. *Metabolic Complications*
Electrolyte imbalance, hypoglycemia and hyperglycemia, abnormal plasma aminogram, hyperammonemia, azotemia, hyperchloremic metabolic acidosis, hyperlipidemia, essential fatty acid deficiency, osteopenia, cholestatic liver disease, trace mineral deficiencies, vitamin deficiency.

c. *Hematologic complications*
Thrombocytopenia, fat overload syndrome/DIC, bilirubin displacement from albumin, iron deficiency anemia.

d. *Pulmonary Complication*
Oxygen diffusion block, lipid deposition, pulmonary artery hypertension, malasezia furfur vasculitis.

An example of order form[31] is given as Figure 39.8. Order should be revised daily or as per need in the sick neonates.

Vital signs should be checked at each shift. Routine monitoring guidelines[31] are given in Table 39.8. These are minimum requirements except in the very long-term stable patients. Individual variables should be monitored more frequently as indicated.

ENTERAL NUTRITION

Since the discovery of TPN nearly three decades ago, early concepts in critical care nutrition were to maximize TPN use and defer enteral feeding till fairly late. But in recent years the optimal route of feeding has undergone tremendous scrutiny and this concept has undergone fairly radical change. With the enteral route being the preferred route today, even in very sick neonate on assisted ventilation or requiring multiple inotropes.[53,54] Documented advantages of enteral feeding includes:

- Ease of administration.
- Feasibility of use.

Table 39.8: Suggested dietary intakes of minerals and trace elements*

Nutrient	*Preterm infant***	*Term infant*
Sodium		50 mg/kg/d (2 mmol/kg/d)
Potassium		80 mg/kg/d (2 mmol/kg/d)
Chloride		70 mg/kg/d (2 mmol/kg/d)
Calcium	180	400 (200)***
Phosphorus	150	300 (100)***
Magnesium	15	40
Iron	2 (after first 1-2 mo)	1 mg/kg/d (≤ 0.1)*** (after 2 mo)
Zinc	1.5	4→2 (2→0.75)
Copper	0.12	0.2–0.4
Selenium	0.003	0.01-0.03
Iodine	0.01	0.05

* Amounts expressed in mg/d unless otherwise indicated.
** The figures in this column indicate mg/kg/d.
*** Amounts in parenthesis are for the fully breast-fed infant aged loss than 4-6 months.

Section 10

ORDER FORM

Name ___________

Weight of patient_____kg | Central line _________ | Age _____

Peripheral line _________ | Bed No. _____

Rate ___________

	Standard Order	Modifications To Standard Order	*Adjustment for Neonates and Premature Infants (Circle these when required and cross out corresponding items* under "Standard order").
Protein (as amino acid)*		g%	
Dextrose		g%	*Use trophamine and cysteine for patients in level II and III nurseries who have a central line or are on day 6 of peripheral therapy.
Na		30 meq/L	
K		25 meq/L	
Cl		20 meq/L	
Acetate		45 meq/L	
Ca (as gluconate) (10 mM Ca/L)		20 meq/L	
Mg (as sulfate)		3 meq/L	
P		10 meq/L	*2 mL/kg/d for patients < 2.5 kg *Zn: 400 μg/kg/d < 2 kg body weight 250 μg/kg/d others < 3 mo old
MVI Pediatric		*5.0 meq/L	
Zinc		*1.0 meq/L	
Copper		200 μg/L	
Manganese		5.0 μg/L	
Chromium		2.0 μg/L	
Selenium		20.0 μg/L	
Iodide		10 μg/L	*Use only with trophamine
Heparine		1000 Units/L	
Cysteine (40 mg/g trophamine)*		mg/L	

Pharmacy will automatically account for electrolytes provided in amino acid preparation.
Changes in Na or K to be made as Cl only __, or Cl acetate 1:1 __, or other
Cl: Acetate ratio (specify________________________).

Date: Signature:

Fig. 39.8: An example of order form

- Decreased incidence of infections.
- Better overall survival.
- Decreased morbidity.
- Less NICU stay; and
- Relatively lower cost saving of resources.

MINIMAL ENTERAL NUTRITION (MEN)

The concept of minimal enteral nutrition (MEN) or minimal enteral feeding (MEF) is defined as starting small amount of enteral feeding, with a vide range of 5-25 ml/kg depending upon the circumstances, as soon as possible after birth.[23] Early enteral feeding has been shown to attenuate the hypermetabolic response to stress. Even small amounts of enteral feeding preserved normal intestinal villus and microvillus structure, which helps in normal absorptive processes and maintains epithelial barrier function,[55] by preventing gut from injurious luminal factors, such as endotoxins. It appears that loss of enteral feeding, with TPN administration, leads to an increased expression of interferon-γ in the mucosal epithelium, which may mediate the observed loss of epithelial barrier function.[56] Septic complications are far more common in patients on PN than in patients on enteral nutrition.[57-60]

But, the major concern in feeding of high-risk neonate particularly VLBW and sick neonate is high incidence of feed intolerance and narcotizing enterocolitis (NEC) though there is no evidence that delayed feeding prevents NEC. The gut hormone and enzymes are not fully functional, there is delayed gastric emptying and quite often these are associated with respiratory distress and perinatal asphyxia. Small for gestational age (SGA) babies can have in addition abnormal umbilical artery flow leading to significant gut ischemia. This makes them more prone for feed intolerance and NEC. However, it has been found that by 24 weeks

GI tract is anatomically well developed and most of the digestive enzymes are present in sufficient amount to metabolize oral feeds though immature gastric motility remains a limiting factor for effective feeding as organized gut motility starts only at 32-34 weeks of gestation.

The "gut priming" with MEN has numerous positive impacts on development and maturation of gut function, hormonal and digestive enzyme surge.[61,62] This early hypocaloric minimal enteral feeding has also been shown to diminish the incidence of SIRS (systemic inflammatory response syndrome) and MOFS (multiorgan failure syndrome) in critically ill, hemodynamically unstable newbonrs.[53,63] The decrease in infectious complications associated with MEF is believed to be at least partially a result of enhancement of gut-associated lymphoid tissue (GALT) and maintenance of GI mucosal integrity. It significantly increases GI hormones like enteroglucagon and gastrin that in turn improves mucosal growth and development.[64-65] Low level of enteral feeding or "trophic feeds" have also been shown to reverse GI mucosal ischemic changes, secondary to shunting away of visceral blood flow that occurs in the critically ill stressed neonate. Even very low levels of enteral feeding have been shown to increase the mucosal blood flow protecting the GI mucosa from ischemia. Feeds are usually administered by different routes[53,66] and methods.[67,68]

There are no consensus guidelines on how to progress, how long to continue and when to shift to full nutritive feeding. It may be advisable to commence at a very low rate 10-15% of usual daily requirement and advanced only very gradually as tolerated by the neonate. If tolerance is not the issue than ~10 ml/kg/day is advisable in hemodynamically stable neonate. Majority of the neonate's usually attaining full eucaloric (permissively low) requirement by 72-96 hours for better weight gain. The decision for advancement of feeding is made after clinical stability is achieved.

IMMUNONUTRITION

The recent trend in the nutritional support of the high-risk sick neonate is the concept of "immunonutrition". The use of various immunonutrients like glutamine, arginine, omega-3 fatty acids and various nucleic acids have shown positive benefit with a decreased rate of infection as well as decrease in length of hospital stay.[33,69-71] These immunonutrients along with MEN have also been shown to have synergistic effect in attenuating the "pro-inflammatory cascade" which is believed to lead to SIRS, ADRS and MOFS, the usual causes of mortality in critically ill and hemodynamically unstable neonate. Thus, the practice of combining minimal enteral nutrition (MEN) with immune enhancement based on the concept of "total splanchnic resuscitation" is a practice that is slowly gaining popularity in the nutrition support of sick neonate[2] (Figs 39.9 and 39.10).

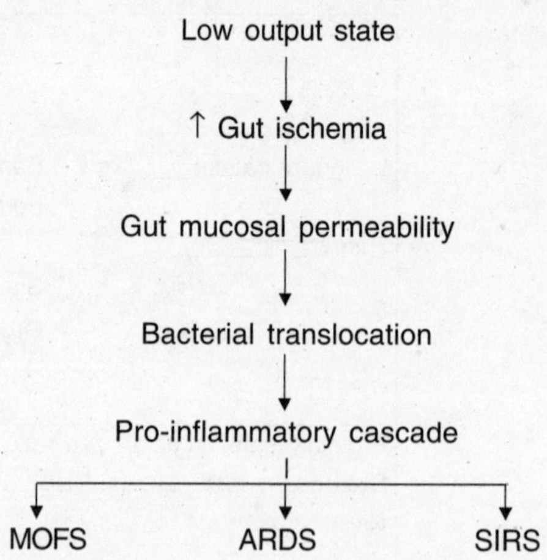

Fig. 39.9: Gut and the critically sick neonate

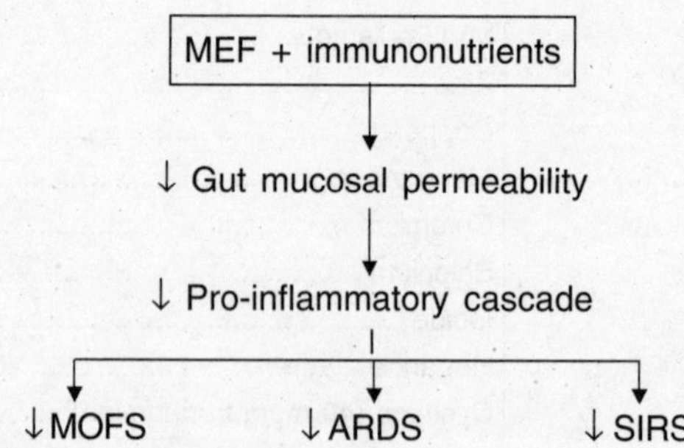

Fig. 39.10: The concept of "total splanchnic resuscitation"

NUTRITIONAL DEMAND IN SPECIFIC SITUATIONS

Nutrient needs to be adjusted according to clinical, biochemical and hemodynamic situations in conditions like ARDS, cardiac, renal and hepatic failure.[1] Fluid restriction needs to be employed in all these conditions. Fluid requirement is best monitored by serum Na^+, osmolality, BUN, creatinine and strict fluid intake and output record. Likewise, nutrient needs like protein needs to be adjusted as per renal functions, dialysis is indicated or not. Traditionally, in renal failure protein intake was restricted to nil or 0.25 g/kg/day, to 0.5 to 1.0 g/kg/day to prevent catabolism and in dialyzed neonate, protein may be liberalized to 1.5 to 2.0 g/kg/day. The branched chain amino acids have been shown to be of therapeutic benefit in ARDS and in liver failure. Thus, the current practice of "protein liberalization" is based on the belief that deliberate protein restriction in renal or hepatic failure is unjustified in the presence of such extreme protein catabolism.

All other macronutrients in these specific situation needs to be tailored and adjusted according to periodic trends in biochemical parameters but restriction may be liberalized as the clinical conditions improve.

Practice Guidelines

Necrotizing Enterocolitis (NEC)

a. Cautions introduction of MEN (minimal enteral nutrition) should be considered for low infants.
b. Enteral feeding must be immediately discontinued if NEC is suspected.
c. PN (parenteral nutrition) should be provided when enteral nutrition is discontinued because of suspected or proven NEC.
d. Parenteral amino acid concentration should be increased by 10% to 30% for proven cases of NEC.
e. Protein and mineral status should be monitored frequently to assess additional needs during PN interval.
f. In NEC stage II or III; increased fluid intake is often required to maintain hemodynamic stability. Isotonic saline (crystalloid) is as effective as 5% albumin (colloid) in treating hypotensive preterm, and causes less fluid retention.[72]
g. If there is no improvement with multiple fluid infusions (upto 40 cc/kg), inotropes such as dopamine are usually added.[72]
h. Enteral nutrition should be reintroduced gradually only when the NEC has resolved, as evidenced by heme test-negative stool.[1]

Renal Failure

a. If along with AFR, gastrointestinal tract functions are impaired then parenteral support should be considered.
b. The strategy in renal decompensation is to provide minimal requirements of the essential amino acids and should contain arginine in the formulation.

Liver Failure

a. Enteral feeding should always be attempted particularly with formulas containing MCTs.
b. Those who fail to grow with enteral support, likely to be benefit from TPN.
c. Hepatic amino acids (Hepat Amine) can be used when liver disease is associated with hyperammonemia.

VLBW Infants

i. Infants less than 1200 g/30 weeks
- Start IV fluid at birth.
- Start 10 ml/kg/day feed by gavage as soon as stable, continue if tolerance is borderline.
- Advance by 10 ml/kg/day if tolerance is good.
- Frequency of feeding 2 hourly, intermittent bollus.

ii. 1200-1500 g/30-32 weeks
- No IV fluid if the baby is stable.
- Start with 60 ml/kg/day by gavage.
- Advanced by 20 ml/kg/day.
- Frequency of feeding 2 hourly.

iii. 1500-2000 g/32-34 weeks
- Total enteral feeds should be started for non-distressed infants, graduating soon to spoon and breast feeds as assessed by such, swallow and respiratory coordination.
- In sick babies on IVF, feeds are advanced at a rate of 30 ml/kg/day after stabilization.

iv. > 2000 g/> 34 weeks
- Start breast-feeds from day 1 if asymptomatic.
- Rapid enhancement of more than 30 ml/kg/day may be associated with higher risk of NEC and hence one should monitor closely all babies who are on enteral feeds. Pre-feed aspirates (NEC alert if > 25% pre-feed aspirate) and abdominal girth should be checked 4-6 hourly. Altered aspirates should be viewed with caution and investigated.
- Non-nutritive sucking should always be tried while on gavage feeds from 30-32 weeks of gestation.

Choice of Milk

Breast milk remains the choice of feeding of all neonates with more than one hundred advantages. The beneficial effects generally relate to improvements in host defenses, digestion and absorption of nutrients, gastrointestinal function, neurodevelopment, and maternal psychological well being. However, the special needs of these infants that arise as a result of metabolic and gastrointestinal immaturity, immunologic compromise, and associated medical conditions must be considered so that adequate nutrition can be provided to meet the needs for intrauterine rates of growth and nutrient accretion. Human milk is capable of satisfying most of the needs of premature at risk neonates if careful attention is given to nutritional status.

Limitations in the Use of Unfortified Human Milk

A major impediment to advocating human milk for premature infants is the difficulty many mothers experience in providing sufficient quantities of milk. Another reason of concerns is that nutrient intake is limited by the milk volume restrictions because of fluid restriction. The most compelling reason for concern is that nutrient intake is adequate to meet the very great needs of the premature infant. Unfortified human milk may not supply sufficient quantities of nutrients because of differences in methods of milk expression and storage, the quality feeding samples, use of feeding tubes, the differences in length of lactation and the macronutrient composition of human milk used in feeding premature infants varies greatly, particularly of fat, sodium, calcium, phosphorus, vitamin C, A and riboflavin. Thus, the exclusive feeding of unfortified milk in premature infants (bw < 1500 g) has been associated with poorer rates of growth and nutritional deficit, during beyond the period of hospitalization.[73]

Apart from human milk, external nutrition products include,[74,75] human milk + calcium phosphate and vitamin supplements, human milk + fortifier, human milk + preterm formulas, preterm discharge formula, cow milk based formulas includes iron-fortified formulas, lactose free formulas, low mineral/electrolyte formula, high (86%) medium chain triglyceride (MCT) formula, follow-up formula, soy-based formula (milk-free, lactose-free), soy-based formula with fiber, casein-hydrolysate formulas, amino acid-based formulas and modified amino acid formulas.

Human Milk Fortifiers

Human milk fortifiers are designed to be mixed with human milk. Most fortifiers are powered nutrient preparations that contain protein, carbohydrate, calcium, phosphorus, magnesium and sodium; the contents of zinc, copper and vitamins are variable. If there is an inadequate amount of mother's milk, two options are currentlly available. One option is to alternate the feeding of fortified human milk with preterm formula, and a second option is to mix mother's milk with preterm formula.

Contraindications

Contraindications to enteral feeding are very few and include persistent emesis, upper GI bleeding, GI obstruction or GI perforation. Enteral feeding in the "hemodynamically unstable" neonate remains a significant potential problem. It is probably prudent to commence only after adequate hemodynamic resuscitation and advance gently as tolerated individually.

Feeding Tolerance

Limitations in the ability to tolerate feedings constitute a major problem for premature infants. The feeding tolerance is always a primary concern because it affects the decision to initiate, advance and discontinue feedings. Clinical criteria's of feeding intolerance (Table 39.9) generally include physical findings on examination, gastric residual volume and other associated signs. Unfortunately, the afore-mentioned criteria have little prognostic significance, but careful assessment and examination prior to the next feeding generally aid the decision to continue feeding.

Converting Gavage to Oral Feeds

Once baby's condition is stable, readiness for feedings is checked by signs of sucking, active bowel sounds, passage of meconium and signs of abdominal distention or infection.

Transition should be slow. First a single supervised breast-feeding or spoon feed is given and if the baby accepts well i.e., without any sign of fatigue then the number of feeds gradually increased over next few days. If the advancements are too fast, the baby may show signs of fatigue in the form of apnea, poor weight gain, colour changes and vomiting. The goal or oral feeding is that the baby should gain weight. If a sick neonate is having poor weight gain during stable and growing period other causes like inadequate calorie provided/consumed, anemia, cold stress, underlying systemic illlness, late hyponatremia, late metabolic acidosis and urinary tract infection should come in differential diagnosis.

Table 39.9: Potential criteria used to assess feeding tolerance

Abdominal distention
With visible bowel loops
Without visible bowel loops
Abdominal tenderness
Emesis
Gastric residual volume
> 2 mL/kg
> 50% of 3 hours of feeding
Any change from previous pattern
Gastric residual characteristics
Green, bilious
Red, blood-tinged
Stool output
Incresed frequency
Decresaed frequency
Feeding withheld
Document reasons feedings withheld
Assess number of feedings withheld
Clinical condition
Any worsening in previous medical condition

Post Discharge Feeding

Though the current feeding policies concentrate only on feeding practices during hospital stay, there is a need to have adequate calorie, protein and other mineral intake after discharge also. Nutrition should be discussed at all times when discharge planning is done. Most common specific nutrient deficiencies are calcium and phosphate and it has been found that babies with evidence of metabolic bone disease (MBD) are significantly shorter on follow-up. VLBW babies also need higher protein and calorie to have adequate catch up growth. There are certain guidelines indicating the length of continuing supplements.

1. If the baby is on HMF or preterm formula, these should be stopped when the baby reaches 2 kg or starts accepting full breast feeds. These babies should be started on calcium-phosphate and vitamin supplements once HMF/formula are stopped.
2. If the baby was only on breast milk, calcium-phosphate supplements are continued till the baby reaches corrected age of term (wt~3-3.5 kg). One should check serum calcium, phosphate and alkaline phosphatase periodically and before stopping calcium

supplements especially in ELBW babies to rule out any osteopenia of prematurity.

3. Multivitamins are stopped when the baby reaches 6 to 7 months or 4.5 kg.
4. Iron is continued for at least 1 year, and if weaning is not adequate then it should be continued till 2-3 years of age.

SUMMARY

To summarize, appropriate goal-oriented nutritional support is of paramount importance in both decreasing morbidity and mortality in the hypermetabolic and stressed critically ill neonate. The concept of permissive hypocaloric feeding combined with an aggressive approach to obtain better euglycemic control is gaining wider acceptance in the NICU. The systemic immunosuppressive effects of TPN restrict its use to only situations when absolutely indicated. The philosophy of "gut priming" with MEN (minimal enteral nutrition) or "trophic feeds" is an attractive one, with the current tendency to initiate enteral feeds as soon as possible. The approach is multifaceted, beginning with minimal enteral or trophic feeding to enteral nutrition, and continuing to full enteral feeding and hospital discharge.

Future directions will involve the routine use of immunonutrition, with glutamine and other additional growth factors and nutrients. More and more refinements are expected in this area in the form of better modulation and fine-tunning of goal-oriented approach towards the better nutritional management of high-risk neonate.

REFERENCES

1. Kler N, Soni A. Parenteral nutrition in the critically ill neonate and special situations. *J Neonatal* 2002;16:27-32.
2. Iyer PU. Nutritional support in the critically ill child. *IJP* 2002;69:405-409.
3. Curley MA, Castillo L. Nutrition and shock in pediatric patients. *New Horiz* 1998;6:121-225.
4. Huddleston KC, Ferraro MC, Duffie A, Wolff-Small T. Nutritional support of the critically ill child. *Crit Care Nurs Clin North Am* 1993;5:65-78.
5. Persis A. *Neonatal Intensive Care*. London: Smithson 2005.
6. Witte MK. Metabolic measurements during mechanical ventilation in the pediatric intensive care unit. *Respir Care Clin North Am* 1996;2:573-586.
7. Klen CJ, Stanek GS, Wiles CE. Overfeeding macronutrients to critically ill adults: Metabolic complications *J Am Diet Assoc* 1998;98:795-806.
8. Chwals WJ. Overfeeding the critically ill child: Fact or fantasy. *New Horiz* 1994;2:145-155.
9. Liposky JM, Nelson LD. Ventilatory response to high caloric loads in critically ill patients. *Crit Care Med* 1994;22:796-802.
10. Baltglia FC, Meschia G. Fetal nutrition *Annu Reve Nutr* 1998;8:43-50.
11. Gilberto R, Pereira, Georgief MK. *Clinicis in Perinatology* 1995;22:30.
12. Anderson TL, Muttart CR, Beiber MA. A controlled trial of glucose versus glucose and amino acids in premature infants. *J Pediatr* 1979;94:947.
13. Sandesh Kiran PS, Shenoi A. Neonatal fluid and electrolyte therapy. *IJPP* 2004;6920:32-42.
14. Spiekerman M. Protein used in nutritional assessment. *Clin Lab Med* 1993;13:353-369.
15. Reichman B, Chessex P, Putel G. Diet, fat accretion and growth in premature infants. *N Engl J Med* 1981;305:1945-1950.
16. Brans YW, Andrew DS, Carrillo DW. Tolerance of fat emulsions in very low birthweight neonates. *Am J Dis Child* 1998;142:145-149.
17. Aggett PJ. Trace elements of the micropremie. *Clin Perinat* 2000;27:119-127.
18. Denne SC, Point dexter BB, Leitch CA. Nutrition and metabolism in the high risk neonate. In: Fanaroff AA Martin RJ (eds) *Neonatal Perinatal Medicine-Disease of the Fetus and Infant*, 7th edn. Missouri, Mosby, 2002;578-617.
19. Zuegler EE, O' Donnell AM, Nelson SE. Body composition of reference fetus, *Growth* 1976;40:329-341.
20. Kalpan AS, Zemel BS, Neiswender KM, Stallings VA. Resting energy expenditure in clinical pediatrics: Measured versus prediction equation. *J Pediatr* 1995;127:200-205.
21. Mendeloff E, Wesley J, Deckert R. Comparison of measured resting energy expenditure (REE) versus estimated energy expenditure (EEE) in infants. *J Parenter Enteral Nutr* 1986;10:65-69.
22. Mitchlel IM, Davies PSW, Day JME. Energy expenditure in children with congenital heart disease, before and after surgery. J Thorac Cardiovasc Surg 1994;107:374-380.
23. Mukhopadhyay K, Narang A. Enteral nutrition of very low birthweight neonates. *J Neonatal* 2004;18:30-38.
24. Thureen PJ, Hay WW. Intravenous nutrition and postnatal growth of the micro premie. *Clin Peinat* 2004;27:197-219.
25. Wimck M, Rosso P. The effect of severe early malnutrition on cellular growth of human brain. *Pediatr Res* 1969;3:181-184.
26. Joosten KF, Verhoeven JJ, Hazelzet JA. Energy expenditure and substrate utilization in mechanically ventilated children. *Nutrition* 1999;15:444-448.
27. Coss BUJA, Jefferson LS. Walding D, David Y, Smith EO, Klish WJ. Resting energy expenditure and nitrogen balance in critically ill pediatric patients on mechanical ventilation. *Nutrition* 1998;14:649-652.
28. Binder ND, Raschko PK, Benda GI. Insulin infusion with parenteral nutrition in extremely low birthweight infants with hyperglycemia. *J Pediatr* 1989;114:273-277.
29. Friedmanz, Danm A, Stablman MT. Oates JA. Rapid onset of essential fatty acid deficiency in the newborn. *Pediatrics* 1976;58:640-649.
30. Feuerstein G, Hallenbeek JM. Leukotrienes in health and disease *FASEBJ* 1987;1:186-192.
31. Hambridge KM, Krebs NF. Normal childhood nutrition and its disorders. In: Hathway W, Groothnis JR, Hay JRWW, Paisley JW (eds) *Current Pediatric Diagnosis and Treatment:* 11th edn. Prentice-Hall International 1993;236-261.
32. Patino JF, Deplumiento SE, Vergara A, Savino P, Rodrigeez M, Escalo J. Hypocaloric support in the critically ill. *World J Surg* 1999;98:795-806.
33. Gadek JE, DeMichele SJ, Karlstad MD, Pacht ER, Donahoe M, Albertson TE, *et al*. The enteral nutrition in ARDS study

group. Effect of enteral feeding with elcosapentaenoic acid, linolenic acid and anti-oxidants in patients with acute respiratory distress syndrome. *Crit Care Med* 1999;27:1409-1420.
34. Duffy B, Pencharz P. The effect of surgery on the nitrogen metabolism of parenterally fed human neonates. *Pediatr Res* 1986;20:32-35.
35. Dahlstrom KA, Amennt ME, Laidlaw SA, Kople JD. Plasma amino acid concentrations in children receiving long-term parenteral nutrition. *J Pediatr Gastroenterol Nutr* 1988;7:748-754.
36. Zlotkin SH, Andrson SH. The development of cystathionase activity during the first year of life. *Pediatr Res* 1982;16:65-66.
37. Miller R, Jahoor F, Jaksic T. Decreased cysteire and proline synthesis in parenterally fed, premature infants. *J Pediatr Surg* 1995;30:953-958.
38. Heird WC, Dell RB, Helms RA. Amino acid mixture designed to maintain normal plasma amino acid patterns in infants and children requiring parenteral nutrition. *Pediatrics* 1998;81:41-50.
39. Das JB, Filler PM. Amino acid utilization during total parenteral nutrition in the surgical neonate. *J Pediatr Surg* 1973;8:793-799.
40. Okamoto E, Rassin DK, Zucker CL. Role of taurine in feeding the low birthweight infant. *J Pediatr* 1984;104:936-940.
41. Tyson JE, Lasky R, Flood D. Randomized trial of taurine supplementation for infants less than or equal to 1300 g birthweight: Effect on auditory brain stress-evoked responses. *Pediatrcs* 1989;83:406-415.
42. Souba WW, Herskowitz K, Austgen TR. Glutamine nutrition: Theoretical considerations and therapeutic impact. *J Parenter Enteral Nutr* 1990;14:2375-2435.
43. O' Dwyer A, Smith R, Hwang T, Wilmore D. Maintenance of small bowel mucosa with glutamine-enriched parenteral nutrition. *J Parenter Enteral Nutr* 1989;13:579-585.
44. Alverdyl JC. Effects of glutamine supptamted diets on immunology of the gut. *J Parentr Enteral Nutr* 1990;14:109-113.
45. Loch H, Hubl W. Metabolic basis for selecting glutamine-containing substrates for parenteral nutrition. *J Parentr Enteral Nutr* 1990;14:114s-117s.
46. Treme IH, Kiefe B, Neilemann LS. Glutamine dipeptide supplemented parenteral nutrition maintains intestinal function in the critically ill. *Gastroenterology* 1994;107:1595-1601.
47. Rose J, Gibbons K, Carlson SE, Koowwk. Nutrient needs of the preterm infant. *Nutr Clin* Pract 1993;8:226-232.
48. Barbul A, Arginine; Biochemistry, physiology and therapeutic implications. *J Parenter Enteral Nutr* 1986;10:227-238.
49. Hibbs JB, Vavrin Z, Taintor RR, L-arginine is required for expression of the activated macrophage effector mechanism causing selective metabolic inhibition in target cells. *J Immunol* 1987;138:550-565.
50. Daly JM, Reynolds J, Thom A. Immunie and metabolic effects of orginine in the surgical patient. *Ann Surg* 1998;208:512-518.
51. Senkal M, Mymme A, Eickhoff U. Early postoperative enteral immunonutrition: Clinical outcome and cost-comparison analysis in surgical patients. *Crit Care Med* 1997;25:1489-1496.
52. Roe C. Clinical experience with carnitine deficiency. *J Rore Dis* 1997;111:S-11.
53. Delucas C, Moreno M, Lopez-Herce J, Ruizt, Perez-Palencis M, Carillo A. Transpyloric enteral nutrition reduces the complication rate and cost in the critically ill child. *J Pediatr Gastroenterol Nutr* 2000; 30:175-180.
54. Vanderhoff JA, Matya SM. Enteral and parenteral nutrition in patients with short bowel syndrome. *Eur J Pediatr Surg* 1999;9:214-219.
55. Pang KY, Bresson JL, Nalker WA. Development of the gastrointestinal barrier. Evidence for structural differences in microvillus membranes from newborn and adult rabbits. *Biochim Biophys Acta* 1983;727:201-208.
56. Kiristioglu I, Teitelbaum DH. Attention of intestinal intraepithelial lymphocytes during total parenteral nutrition. *J Surg Res* 1998;79:91-96.
57. Kudskk, Croce M, Favian T. Enteral versus parenteral feeding. Effects on septic morbidity after blunt and penetrating abdominal trauma. *Ann Surg* 1992;215:503-511.
58. Moore FA, Moore EE, Kudsk KA. Clinical benefits of an immune enhancing die for early post injury enteral feeding. *J Trauma* 1994;37:607-615.
59. Alverdy J, Aoys E, Moss G. Total parenteral nutrition promotes bacterial translocation from the gut. *Surgery* 1988;104:185-190.
60. Cummins A, Chu G, Faust L. Malabsorption and villous atrophy in patients receiving enteral feeding *J Parenter Enteral Nutr* 1995;19:193-198.
61. Lucas A, Bloom S, Aynsley A. Gut hormones and "minimal enteral feeding". *Acta Paediatr Scand* 1986;75:719-723.
62. Aynsley Green A, Adrian T, Bloom S. Feeding and the development enteroinsular hormones secretion in the preterm infant: Effects of continuous gastric infusions of human milk compared with intermittent boluses. *Acta Paediatr Scand* 1982;71:379-383.
63. Adam D, La Gamma EF, Browne LE. Nutritional management and the multisystem organ failure/systemic in inflammatory response syndrome in critically ill preterm neonates. *Crit Care Clin* 1995;11:751-784.
64. Berseth CL, Nordyke C. Enteral nutrients promote postnatal maturation of intestinal motor activity in preterm infants. *Am J Physiol* 1993;264:G1046-G1051.
65. Klagsburn M. Human milk stimulates DNA synthesis and cellular proliferation in cultured fibroblasts. *Proc Natl Acad Sci* USA 1978;75:5057-5061.
66. Smith HG, Orlando R. Enteral nutrition: Should we feed the stomach? *Crit Care Med* 1999;27:1652-53.
67. Gharpure V, Maert KL, Sarnaik AP, Metheny NA. Indicators of post pyloric feeding tube placement in children. *Crit Care Med* 2000;28:2962-2966.
68. Spalding HC, Sullivan KJ, Soremi O, Gonzalez F, Goodwin SR, Bed side placement of transpyloric feeding tubes in the pediatric intensive care unit using gastric insufflation. *Crit Care Med* 2000;28:2041-2044.
69. Ray Duncan. *Neonatology on the Web*. CSSM teaching files.
70. Berard MP, Zazzo JF, Condat P, Vassm MP, Cynober L. Total parenteral nutrition enriched with arginine and glutamate generates glutamine and limits protein catabolism in surgical

patients hospitalized in intensive care units. *Crit Care Med* 2000;28:2627-2644.

71. Mendez C, Jurkovich CJ, Wener MH, carcial, Mays M, Maier RV. Effects of supplemental dietary arginine, canola oil and trace elements on cellular immune function in critically injured patients. *Shock* 1996;6:7-12.
72. Avery ME, Tooley WH, Keller JB, Hurd SS, Bryane MH, Cotton RB. Is chronic lung disease in low birthweight preventable? A survey of eight centers. *Pediatrics* 1987;79:26-30.
73. Kashyap S, Schulze KF, Forsyth M, *et al*. Growth, nutrient retention and metabolic response of low-birth-weight infant fed supplemented and unsupplemented preterm human milk. *Am J Clin Nutr* 1990;52:254-262.
74. National guideline http/www.guideline.gov. Administration of specialized nutrition support issues unique to pediatrics. *J Parenter Enteral Nutr* 2002;26:97 SA-110 SA.
75. Clinical algorithms of the Nutrition Care Process and Route of Administration of Specialized Nutrition Support are provided in the companion document: Nutrition care process. Section II: Nutrition Care Process. *JPEN K Parenter Enteral Nutr* 2002 Jan-Feb; 26 (1 Suppl): 7SA-8SA.

Karoly Horvath

40 Nutrition in Celiac Disease

INTRODUCTION

Celiac disease (CD), also termed "gluten-sensitive enteropathy", is the destruction of absorptive surface as the consequence of immune response to the ingested gluten in the small intestine. Essentially, three components are present in the pathogenesis of CD, namely:

- Genetic background.
- Immune system reacting to gluten; and
- Ingestion of the gluten containing foods (Fig. 40.1).

There are known HLA haplotypes, which predispose an individual to gluten-induced intestinal and/or skin disease. CD is the results of the combined effect of normally functioning gene products. The genes predisposing to CD involve both HLA and non-HLA genes. The primary HLA-haplotypes associated with CD are the HLA-DQA1* 0501, DQB1*0201 genes encoding the DQ2 molecule, and to a lesser extent, the DQA1* 0301, DQB*0302 genes encoding the DQ8 molecule. These HLA haplotypes found in 80-90% of patients with CD in Northern Europe as compared to 20-30% of non celiac patients in the same region.[1] These HLA genes code the synthesis of the gluten binding sites on the antigen presenting cells.

The second condition is the immune system, which should be able react to gluten. The intestinal damage starts when unknown environmental trigger(s) changes the status of immunological tolerance to immune reaction. The triggering factor(s) is not known.

The third and crucial component is the ingestion of gluten. If gluten is not present in the diet, there is no intestinal damage. This fact determines the main management of the disease, which is the elimination of gluten from the diet.

WHAT IS GLUTEN?

Gluten is the collective name for specific alcohol-soluble storage proteins called prolamins present in wheat (gliadin),

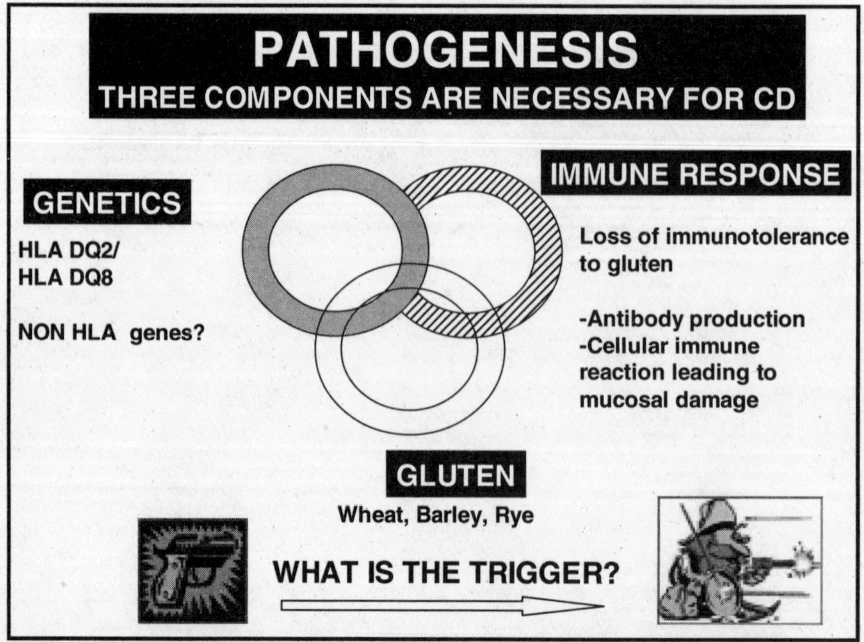

Fig. 40.1: The three key elements of the celiac disease pathogenesis

barley (hordein) and rye (secalin). The protein content of wheat consists of four fractions (Box 40.1).

Box 40.1: Four fractions in gluten

- Prolamins (soluble in ethanol).
- Glutenins (partially soluble in dilute acid or alkali solutions.
- Globulins (soluble in 10 percent NaCl).
- Minor albumins (soluble in water).

Based upon their electrophoretic mobility the gliadins can be separated into four major fractions (alpha, beta, gamma and omega). The amino acid sequence of an alpha gliadin called A-gliadin is known.[2]

The three main grains containing prolamins belong to the family of triticeae (Fig. 40.2). However, it should be emphasized that there are other grains with gluten content with different names.

Gluten is a large complex molecule, which has peptide segment(s) inducing the immunoreactions. There are controversial data regarding the amino acid sequence of the possible toxic peptide fragments.

TREATMENT OF CELIAC DISEASE

A consensus panel convened by the National Institutes of Health gave a mnemonics for the treatment of CD (Fig. 40.3). The initial management typically dietary but occasionally includes drug therapy.

The nutritional management of CD includes:

1. Gluten-free diet, and
2. Management of complications due to the malabsorption.

A gluten-free diet requires the elimination of all foods that contain gluten. This diet demands a significant lifestyle

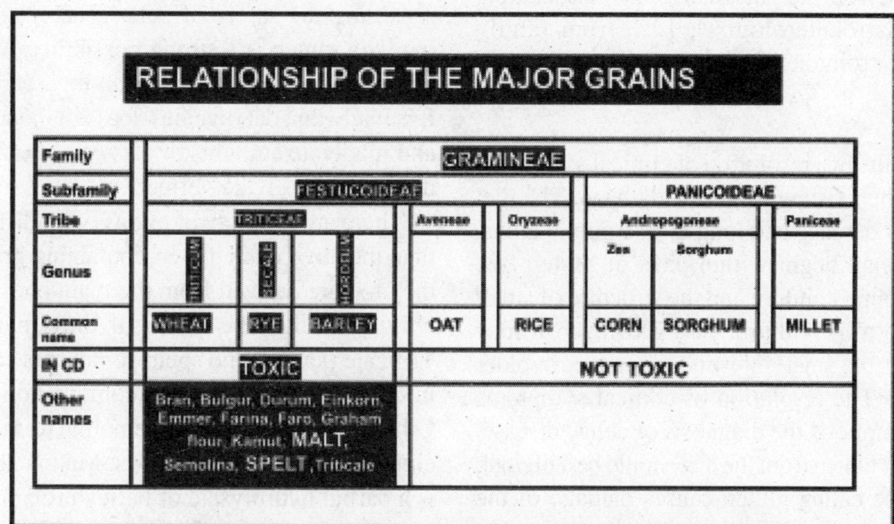

Fig. 40.2: The main toxic and non-toxic grains in celiac disease

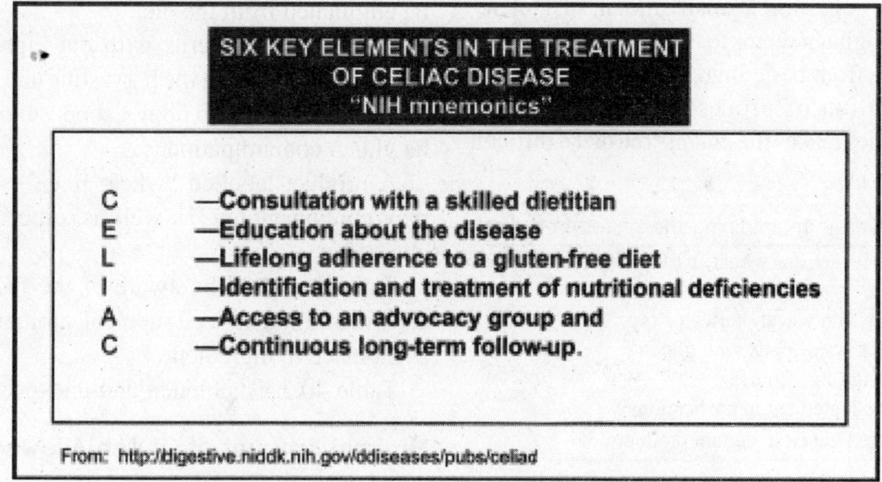

Fig. 40.3: The NIH celiac disease treatment mnemonics

change. School children should learn to select proper lunch at school, on parties, and what snack they can eat. Family eating out can be a challenge and it requires questioning of the waiter or chef about possible hidden sources of gluten. If there is no food labelling policy for gluten in a country parents continuously should call the manufacturers of the processed foods. In the US there are patients' support groups publishing booklets every year after the members verifying with the manufacturers that which products are gluten-free in their region.

Celiac support groups in many countries are the most useful education/teaching sources for the newly diagnosed patients. A recent United States survey on 1,600 patients with celiac disease 88% stated that the patients obtained most of their information about CD from celiac groups. Only 10% received information from their primary care physician and 39% from their gastroenterologist.[3] Another survey from Canada reported that 83% of patients received excellent information from the Canadian Celiac Association, 35% from their gastroenterologists, 12% from family physicians and 29% from dietitians.[4]

Gluten-Free Diet

Gluten-free diet results in a resolution of clinical symptoms and the healing of the existing intestinal damage. The diet also prevents further damage and long-term complications. The improvement may begin within days of gluten-free diet, especially in young children and the structure of small intestine usually recovers within a year. However, it may take upto 2 years for the small intestine to recover in older children and adults. The resolution of clinical symptoms on gluten-free diet supports the diagnosis of celiac disease.

The elimination of gluten from the diet should be a lifelong commitment because eating gluten causes damage of the small intestine. The gluten ingestion does not cause immediate symptoms in the majority of patients after the gut healed. However, a small portion of patients report symptoms even after ingesting a small amount of gluten.

The elimination of gluten seems to be easy if all the meals are prepared at home from basic ingredients. However, the worldwide distribution of processed foods by large international companies makes the gluten-free diet a difficult daily task (Table 40.1).

Table 40.1: Difficulties in maintaining the gluten-free diet

- There are grains derived from wheat, barley and rye but have different names
- Contamination of oat with wheat, barley or rye
- Contamination of processed foods with gluten
- Contamination of gluten-free flours
- Gluten use as inactive ingredient in medications
- Hidden and unexpected gluten in certain products

The diet requires an ongoing education of patients and their families by both doctors and dieticians. Once the diagnosis is made, it is important to refer the patient to a dietitian with experience in CD for diet education, assistance in meal planning, and social and emotional adaptation to a radically new lifestyle. Gluten-free diet influences the diet and lifestyle of the whole family and it is useful if family members attend the initial educational sessions with the nutritionist and the support group meetings. The advantage of the support groups of children is not only that they may offer resource materials and updated product research, but provide emotional and social support.

Despite the restrictions of gluten containing foods, children with CD are able to eat a well-balanced diet with a variety of foods, including even bread and pasta made from gluten-free flours, e.g. potato, rice, soy, or bean flour. There are special food companies producing gluten-free bread, pasta, and other products.

Many published reports support that oats are not toxic in CD.[5, 6] However, a recent challenge study raised concern regarding the safety of oats.[7] The cross-contamination of oat with gluten is a strong possibility. Many experts agree that oat from clear sources can be used in treated patients. It is likely that oat (avenin) does not induce immunoreaction and moderate amounts of oats can be included in the celiac diet without adverse effects.

There are a variety of grains (with different names) other than the three main gluten-containing grains. Undoubtedly, they too are derived from the main ones. Parents and older children should be aware of these names. (Table 40.2) Triticale (kamut, and spelt; sometimes called farro) is toxic in celiac patients as it is a combination of wheat and rye. Other forms of wheat are semolina (durum wheat), emmer, einkorn, bulgur and couscous. Malt is also toxic because it is a partial hydrolysate of barley prolamins. It may contain 100-200 mg of barley prolamins/100 g of malt.[8] In general an ingredient with malt in its name (barley malt, malt syrup, malt extract, malt flavorings) is made from barley and should be eliminated from the diet.

One of the concerns with oat ingestion is a possible contamination during the harvesting and milling procedures. In other foods, which do not suppose to contain gluten can be gluten contamination.

A product labelled "wheat free," is not gluten-free. It may contain gluten, as well as, other grains that are not allowed.

Patients should be aware of the fact that medications and vitamin and mineral supplements may also contain gluten as an inactive ingredient.

Table 40.3 lists hidden and unexpected gluten sources.

Minimal Amount of Gluten Allowed

The stringency of gluten restriction is an issue, which is far from being resolved, as the opinions differ among

Table 40.2: Grains, flours and extracts, which have to be eliminated and allowed in the celiac diet

Not allowed	*Allowed*
Barley	Arrowroot
Bran	Amaranth
Bulgur	Bean flours (garfava, romano)
Couscous	Buckwheat
Durum flour	Flax
Einkorn*	Corn (maize)
Emmer*	Legume flours (garbanzo/ chickpea, lentil, pea)
Farina	Millet
Farro*	Montina™ (Indian Rice Grass)
Gluten, gluten flour	Nut flours (almond, hazelnut, pecan)
Graham flour	Quinoa
Kamut*	Rice—brown, white, wild, Basmati, etc.
Malt, malt extract, malt flavoring	Rice bran
Oats**, oat bran**, oat syrup**	Potato starch, potato flour, sweet potato flour
Orzo	Sago
Panko	Seed flours (sesame)
Rye	Sorghum
Seitan	Soy
Semolina (durum wheat)	Tapioca
Spelt	Teff
Triticale	
Udon	
Word with **wheat** in its name, e.g. wheat germ, wheat starch, wheat bran	

* Types of wheat

** Moderate amount of oat ingestion is probably safe; however, there is concern over the contamination of oats by wheat and/or barley. Therefore, commercial oats are not recommended on the GF diet in North America.

Table 40.3: Not evident gluten sources

Possible Gluten Sources	*Hidden gluten*
Brown rice syrup	Broth
Caramel color	Candy
Dextrin	Imitation bacon/seafood
Malt/malt extract/flavoring	Marinades
Modified food starch	Processed meats
Modified hop extract	Self-basting poultry
Seasonings and spice blends	Soy Sauce
"Starch" in pharmaceuticals	Thickeners
Yeast-malt sprout extract	

scientists and celiac support groups worldwide. There is lack of scientific evidence for what constitutes a safe amount of gluten ingestion. There are no published studies establishing the daily minimum amount of gluten, which does not cause evident damage in the majority of patients. Furthermore, there is no easy and accurate method to detect gluten in food products.

The long-term complications of CD are reported in untreated or non-compliant patients and there is no study on the long-term consequence of small amount (e.g. 0.1-1g) of daily gluten ingestion. Therefore, the recommended minimum gluten content in foods reflects expert opinion rather than evidence based fact.

In the past products containing less than 200 ppm (<200 mg/kg) were considered as gluten free. Recently a value less than 20 ppm (<20 mg/kg) was proposed by the Codex Alimentarius Guidelines as gluten free. The National Food Authority has recently re-defined their term for gluten-free. By their definition gluten-free now refers to no gluten and <200 ppm is regarded as low gluten.

Safe Foods in the Celiac Diet

Plain meat, fish, beans, legumes, eggs, nuts, plain vegetables, fruits, milk and butter are allowed in the gluten-free diet. While dairy products and cheeses are allowed, the coating of certain cheeses might contain gluten.[9]

Rice is the basis of many safe cereals and pastas. Different rice flours are often used in gluten-free baking and are usually combined with other gluten-free flours or baking ingredients. Rice can be ingested in all of its varieties including white rice, brown rice, rice bran, rice polish, sweet rice and wild rice.

Corn is safe in all of its varieties including corn flour, corn starch and corn meal. Corn is the basis of many cereals, pastas and some tortillas.

Sorghum and millet are closely related to corn and can be used as a cereal.

Potato also can be part of the celiac diet.

Quinoa can be used in the diet of celiac patients as a cereal, pasta or flour.

Amaranth is a gluten-free grain-like plant used in cereals, pastas, baked goods and other foods.

Teff flour is used for different baked goods.

Soy flour has a strong tasting but it can be used in combination with other flours.

Several other gluten-free ingredients are used in baking, such as, *tapioca,* tapioca flour, tapioca starch, potato flour, potato starch and *arrowroot* (Table 40.1).

Tests for the Dietary Compliance

Repeat serologic testing is recommended in children to assess the initial response to treatment. It may take upto 6-12 months to have normal test results. Persistence of positive serological tests is suggestive of the lack of adherence to the gluten-free diet or due to unintended gluten ingestion.

Children who do not respond to a gluten-free diet require reevaluation. One explanation can be the presence of other food allergies. A small study showed that 12% of the children with proven celiac disease had food or environmental allergies based on skin tests.[10]

After the full clinical and histological recovery, the serological tests used for the diagnosis of celiac disease are not sensitive enough to detect dietary non-compliance. Troncone *et al.*[11] reported that an endomysium antibody test was not a reliable marker of slight dietary problems.

Other Dietary Therapies in Celiac Disease

In addition to the gluten-free diet, secondary consequences of malabsorption such as vitamin and mineral deficiencies, including iron, calcium, phosphorus, folate, B_{12} and fat-soluble vitamins should be treated. It can be beneficial to take multivitamins with mineral at the beginning of the diet.

Lactose Malabsorption

The most frequent disaccharidase deficiency associated with untreated CD is a low intestinal lactase activity. This deficit typically resolves on diet within a few months unless the patient has permanent adult-type hypolactasia. In our practice we routinely obtain biopsy tissue for disaccharidase measurement in children undergoing upper gastrointestinal endoscopy with the suspicion of celiac disease.

Roggero *et al.*[12] performed lactose breath hydrogen test on 42 infants and children who had flat small intestinal mucosa. All patients had positive tests with the standard challenge dose of 2 g/kg body weight. However, most of the children tolerated lower, 0.5-1.5 g/kg doses.

These data support that the necessity of a lactose-free diet should be assessed individually. If bloating, diarrhea and abdominal pain do not resolve on gluten-free diet the patient probably has lactose intolerance and needs to be treated with lactase enzyme supplements. The full elimination of milk is not recommended unless someone has concomitant milk protein allergy.

Anemia

Iron-deficiency anemia (IDA) represents one of the most frequent extraintestinal symptoms of subclinical CD.[13] The majority (51-84%) of children experience iron deficiency at the time of diagnosis.[14,15] Iron replacement therapy should be considered.

Osteopenia

Children with CD may develop low bone-mineral density. Persistent villous atrophy is associated with low bone mineral density. However, in children it seems to be a temporary problem and resolves in gluten-free diet. Studies in children with CD have shown complete reversal of low bone mineral density following introduction of a GFD.[16, 17]

Transient Pancreatic Insufficiency

Twenty-four to 40 percent of patients with untreated CD have temporary pancreatic hypofunction.[18,19] Carrocio *et al.*[19] performed a double blinded, placebo controlled study on 40 patients. Half of the patients received an enzyme substitution preparation. The control group was treated with a placebo. After 30 days of treatment, the increase in height Z score, weight for height, arm circumference, and subscapular and triceps fold measurements were greater in the enzyme treated group.

Pharmacological Treatments in CD

Lymphocytic Gastritis and Colitis

Lymphocytic gastritis (LG) is associated with CD and has been reported in asmuch as 33% of adult patients. Lymphocytic colitis is also more common (38%) in CD patients affected by LG.[20] The treatment of lymphocytic colitis requires the use of anti-inflammatory medications or steroids.

Refractory Sprue

The most likely cause of non-responsiveness to the diet is continued gluten ingestion, which can be voluntary or inadvertent. Other causes include food allergies (e.g. milk, soy), lactose intolerance, infestation with *L giardia*, or pancreatic insufficiency.

Refractory sprue is uncommon in children. A review of the published reports revealed that the youngest patient was above 20 years of age. Celiac patients in whom the noncompliance to a gluten-free diet has been ruled out belong to the refractory sprue category. These patients typically undergo pharmacological therapies, including steroids,[21] immunosuppressants, such as, azathioprine[22] and cyclosporin.[23] If patients do not respond to these managements, the ultimate treatment is total parenteral nutrition. However, none of these therapies have been subjected to rigorous controlled studies.

REFERENCES

1. Kagnoff MF. Celiac disease. A gastrointestinal disease with environmental, genetic, and immunologic components. *Gastroenterol Clin North Am* 1992;21:405-425.
2. Kasarda D, Okita T, Bernardin J, Baecker P, Nimmo C, Lew E, *et al.* Nucleic acid (cDNA) and amino acid sequences of alpha-type gliadins from wheat (Triticum aestivum). *Proc Natl Acad Sci U S A* 1984;81:4712-4716.
3. Green P, Stavropoulos S, Panagi S, Goldstein S, Mcmahon D, Absan H, *et al.* Characteristics of adult celiac disease in the USA: Results of a national survey. *Am J Gastroenterol* 2001;96:126-131.
4. Cranney A, Zarkadas M, Graham ID, Switzer C. The Canadian celiac health survey—The Ottawa chapter pilot 2003;3:8.
5. Janatuinen EK, Kemppainen TA, Julkunen RJ, Kosma VM, Maki M, Heikkinen M, *et al.* No harm from five year ingestion of oats in coeliac disease. *Gut* 2002;50:332-335.
6. Storsrud S, Olsson M, Arvidsson Lenner R, Nilsson LA, Nilsson O, Kilander A. Adult coeliac patients do tolerate large amounts of oats. *European Journal of Clinical Nutrition* 2003;57:163-169.

7. Lundin KE, Nilsen EM, Scott HG, Loberg EM, Gjoen A, Bratlie J, *et al.* Oats induced villous atrophy in coeliac disease. *Gut* 2003;52:1649-1652.
8. Ellis HJ, Doyle AP, Day P, Wieser H, Ciclitira PJ. Demonstration of the presence of coeliac-activating gliadin-like epitopes in malted barley. *Int Arch Allergy Immunol* 1994;104:308-310.
9. Friederich P, Mulder CJ, Mearin ML, Beerling G, Schalekamp G. [Gluten as food additive in The Netherlands: Cheese forbidden for celiac patients? *Ned Tijdschr Geneeskd* 1997;141:393-394.
10. Szaflarska-Szczepanik A, Adamska I, Swincow G, Sobkowiak E, Czerwionka-Szaflarska M. Occurrence of allergy symptoms in celiac disease children—Preliminary report. *Med Sci Monit* 1998;4:942-944.
11. Troncone R, Mayer M, Spagnuolo F, Maiuri L, Greco L. Endomysial antibodies as unreliable markers for slight dietary transgressions in adolescents with celiac disease. *J Pediatr Gastroenterol Nutr* 1995;21:69-72.
12. Roggero P, Ceccatelli MP, Volpe C, Donattini T, Giuliani MG, Lambri A, *et al.* Extent of lactose absorption in children with active celiac disease. *J Pediatr Gastroenterol Nutr* 1989;9:290-294.
13. Bottaro G, Cataldo F, Rotolo N, Spina M, Corazza GR. The clinical pattern of subclinical/silent celiac disease: An analysis on 1026 consecutive cases. *Am J Gastroenterol* 1999;94:691-696.
14. Carroccio A, Iannitto E, Cavataio F, Montalto G, Tumminello M, Campagna P, *et al.* Sideropenic anemia and celiac disease: One study, two points of view. *Dig Dis Sci* 1998;43:673-678.
15. Bonamico M, Vania A, Monti S, Ballati G, Mariani P, Pitzalis G, *et al.* Iron deficiency in children with celiac disease. *J Pediatr Gastroenterol Nutr* 1987;6:702-706.
16. Mora S, Barera G, Beccio S, Menni L, Proverbio MC, Bianchi C, *et al.* A prospective, longitudinal study of the long-term effect of treatment on bone density in children with celiac disease. *J Pediatr* 2001;139:516-521.
17. Kalayci A, Kansu A, Girgin N, Kucuk O, Aras G. Bone mineral density and importance of a gluten-free diet in patients with celiac disease in childhood. *Pediatrics* 2001;108:E89.
18. Carroccio A, Iacono G, Lerro P, Cavataio F, Malorgio E, Soresi M, *et al.* Role of pancreatic impairment in growth recovery during gluten-free diet in childhood celiac disease *Gastroenterology* 1997;112:1839-1844.
19. Carroccio A, Iacono G, Montalto G, Cavataio F, Lorello D, Greco L, *et al.* Pancreatic enzyme therapy in childhood celiac disease. A double-blind prospective randomized study. *Dig Dis Sci* 1995;40:2555-2560.
20. Wu TT, Hamilton SR. Lymphocytic gastritis: Association with etiology and topology. *Am J Surg Pathol* 1999;23:153-158.
21. Mitchison HC, al Mardini H, Gillespie S, Laker M, Zaitoun A, Record CO. A pilot study of fluticasone propionate in untreated coeliac disease. *Gut* 1991;32:260-265.
22. Vaidya A, Bolanos J, Berkelhammer C. Azathioprine in refractory sprue. *Am J Gastroenterol* 1999;94:1967-1969.
23. Wahab PJ, Crusius JB, Meijer JW, Uil JJ, Mulder CJ. Cyclosporin in the treatment of adults with refractory coeliac disease—An open pilot study. *Aliment Pharmacol Ther* 2000;14:767-774.

KE Elizabeth

41 Nutritional Support in Cystic Fibrosis

INTRODUCTION

Cystic fibrosis (CF) is one of the most common autosomal recessive diseases, especially among the whites. It is characterized by maldigestion, malabsorption, intestinal obstruction, chronic airway disease, superadded infections and sometimes, endocrine pancreatic dysfunction like diabetes. Over 800 mutations are known. The defective gene is such a common gene among the whites that it occurs even among offsprings of nonconsanguineous parents. The high frequency of this defect is ascribed to its resistance to morbidity and mortality due to cholera. The CF gene located in chromosome 7 codes for a protein with 1480 amino acids, called the CF transmembrane regulator (CFTR). The defect leads to failure to clear mucus secretions, a paucity of water in mucus secretions, an elevated salt content of sweat and other secretions and increased susceptibility to infections like pseudomonas.

BACKGROUND

Nutritional support plays a key role in the management of CF.[1] In 1930s 'fibrotic disease of the pancreas' was described and was attributed to vitamin A deficiency. In 1940s, it was recognized as a genetic disorder. In 1940s to 1960s, the diet advised was high protein, low fat and moderate starch. Vegetables, fruit and sugar also were encouraged and vitamin E supplementation was introduced. In 1970s, liberalized diets with 30-40 g fat were introduced depending upon tolerance. The Allan Diet is an example. Beef serum hydrolysate, glucose polymer and medium chain triglycerides (MCT) were advocated. Low fat diets were abandoned as per the observations of the Toronto CF clinic.[2] In 1980s increasing involvement of dieticians and the introduction of enteric-coated enzymes revolutionized the nutritional support in CF. Availability of CF Milk formula, glucose polymers and lifting of fat restrictions brought a new trend in this context.

Various workers have demonstrated positive association of nutritional support with survival and improvement in both weight and height.[1, 2] Growth failure was identified as a highly significant independent prognostic indicator of survival in a large sample of 2773 cases included in the UK National CF Registry.[1] Wasting also is an independent predictor of mortality in patients with cystic fibrosis . Weight for height, weight for age and height for age have been shown to be significantly associated with pulmonary function at 6 years.[3]

NUTRITIONAL SUPPORT

It is very important in view of the increased energy expenditure on one side and malabsorption on the other side.[4] Energy, protein and fluid should be given liberally as per the RDA. Fat should be given as per tolerance and with enzyme replacement. Factors that are considered in planning nutritional support are the following:

- Age at diagnosis.
- Nutritional status at diagnosis.
- Degree of pancreatic involvement.
- Respiratory involvement.
- Hypoalbuminemia.
- Anemia.
- Fat soluble vitamin deficiency and EFA deficiency.
- Electrolyte depletion.
- Degree of stool energy losses.
- Degree of anorexia.

1. Type of Feed

Breast milk or whey-based formula are suitable for young infants. In those with growth failure, energy supplementation with protein hydrolysate or nasogastric feeding may be needed. In those with short bowel disease following surgery for meconium ileus, pre-digested protein hydrolysate preparations like Pregestimil, Peptijunior are beneficial.

Breastfeeding

Breast milk is optimum for most babies.[1] The advantages of breast milk include:

1. The lipase and amylase present in it partially compensating for the pancreatic insufficiency.
2. Optimal fatty acid profile.
3. Optimal amino acid profile including taurine, which is needed for bile salt synthesis and fat absorption.
4. Immunological properties including immunoglobulins, lysozymes, lactoferrin, epidermal growth factors, secretory IgA etc., that offer protection against infection and development of cow's milk allergy.
5. Bioavailability of micronutrients like iron, calcium, phosphorus etc.
6. Hormonal factors.
7. Psychological benefit.

In spite of all these well-known benefits of human milk, only a small proportion of CF babies are breastfed upto 4-6 months of age. The discrepancy between those who are capable and those who succeed may pinpoint weakness amongst those who support them rather than the women themselves.[5] Breastfeeding is a hormonally controlled supply and demand process. The more the infant suckles, the more milk will be produced. Slow weight gain among the breastfed can be corrected by increasing the feeding frequency.

Artificial Feeding

Many babies need artificial feeding due to various reasons. A whey-based formula is recommended. Those who have persistent symptoms even after enzyme therapy may be having cow's milk allergy. In such cases, protein hydrloysate formula is better in view of additional soya intolerance.[6]

Age of Weaning

Weaning can be introduced at 4-6 months of age. There is no advantage of early weaning. Weaning on to low energy pureed rice, fruits and vegetables may slow weight gain. Milk based feeds should be given throughout to promote weight gain. Introduction of solids and cow's milk based formula require an increase in pancreatin therapy.

Sodium Supplementation

This is especially important in hot countries. The normal requirements is 2-4 mmol/kg. Na content of breast milk low and standard infant formulae, 200 ml/kg supply 1.6 mmol/kg. Protein hydrolysate, and 200 ml/kg supply 2.8 mmol/kg. Supplementation is required in growth failure and negative sodium balance on monitoring.[6] 600 mg sodium chloride = 10 mmol Na.

Medium Chain Triglycerides (MCT)[6]

MCT supplementation in formula and addition of MCT oil like coconut oil and cottonseed oil may be useful. MCT will be directly absorbed into portal vein even during fat malabsorption and promote weight gain. Upto 10% of the energy intake can be given as visible MCT oil.

2. Oral Supplements[6]

Some may need oral supplements in addition to usual diet. The examples are energy/calorie only (Duocal, Maxijul, Polycal), protein-calorie, (Scandishake), fruit-based (Enlive, Fortijuice), milk-based nutritionally complete (Ensure Plus, Entera, Fortisip), etc.

3. Micronutrients

Vitamin A

Vitamin A deficiency is anticipated in CF. It may be multifactorial and not simply due to malabsorption. There may be faecal loss of vitamin A unrelated to the degree of fat loss.[7] Vitamin A status correlates with plasma retinal binding protein (RBP) rather than plasma retinal level. The latter is dependent on the former and the retinal level may be depressed in acute infections. Five to ten times the requirement i.e. about 5000-10,000 IU/ day, may be given. Loading doses of vitamin A may cause hypervitaminosis.

Vitamin D

Even though clinical evidence of vitamin D deficiency is uncommon, but reduced plasma levels of 25-Dihydroxy cholecalciferol have been documented in CF. Reduced bone mineral density (BMD) and increased fragility of bones may occur in CF.[8] Almost 10 times the requirement, 400-800 IU of vitamin D is required to maintain normal blood level of 25 Dihydroxy vitamin D in most cases. Hypervitaminosis D has not been reported in CF.

Vitamin E

Symptomatic vitamin E deficiency has been noted in CF.[9] Vitamin E is very important in slowing the lung disease and in offering protection against free radical disease, erythrocyte survival and nerve conduction. Vitamin E level correlates better with erythrocyte vitamin E level rather than plasma level. Large doses, 10-200 mg/day may be needed. Adverse effects are not usually seen, except the possibility of necrotizing enterocolitis especially in very young infants.

Vitamin K

Vitamin K deficiency as evidenced by Protein induced in vitamin K absence (PIVKA) is the rule in CF. Deficiency is due to fat malabsorption, bile salt deficiency, liver disease and antibiotic therapy. Overt bleeding is rare, but osteopenia and osteoporosis due to decreased formation of osteocalcin may occur.[10] Various workers recommend daily or at least weekly supplementation. Hypervitaminosis K has not been reported in CF. The suggested dose is 1 mg/ year to a maximum of 10 mg/dose. The natural kenadione preparation may be better than synthetic menadione preparation.

Water Soluble Vitamins

Routine supplementation is needed if the intake is poor. Vitamin B_{12} injections are needed in children with short bowel disease following intestinal surgery for obstruction.

4. Pancreatic Enzyme Replacement Therapy (PERT)[1]

PERT is needed when there is fat malabsorption. Obvious symptoms include fatty stools and weight loss between birth and diagnosis or poor weight gain. Steatorrhoea should be confirmed by direct microscopy for fat globules. Indirect pancreatic function tests like faecal Pancreatic elastase –1 (PE-1) measurement and chymotrypsin is also useful. A concentration PE-1 less than 100 mcg/g is indicative of severe pancreatic insufficiency.[11] Most babies develop significant insufficiency by one year of age. As approximately 50% of the energy in infants is through fat, PERT is absolutely beneficial in them.

Principles of PERT

1. Use microsphere or mini-microsphere enzyme preparations that are acid resistant especially in infants.
2. The dose should be adjusted up to Lipase 10,000 IU/kg/day.
3. Pancreatin should be mixed with only small quantity of food or drink immediately before feeding.
4. As PERT enhances vitamin absorption, vitamins may be given along with meals and pancreatin.

The various enzyme preparations are given in Table 41.1.

The microsphere and microtablets contain porcine pancreatin coated with a thin layer of acid resisting phthalate. The initial dose can be 1/4-1/3 Creon 10000 (2500-3333 IU lipase) for infants, 1/2 scoop Creon for children (2500 IU lipase) or 1/3-1/2 Pancreas (1666-2500 IU lipase) per fed. These doses equate to approximately 400-800 IU lipase/g fat.[1] Mix enzymes with formula/expressed breast milk or fruit puree and give from a spoon directly at the beginning of the feed. The dose can be gradually increased according to objective assessment of absorption, growth and clinical symptoms. Enzyme dose should be varied according to the fat content of the weaning food. Because of the multiple factors affecting enzyme efficacy dose requirements can vary between 500-4000 IU/g fat.

Powdered enzyme preparations e.g. Pancrex V Forte. This can be mixed with a small amount of feed or water and given by mouth or syringe down tube. >90% activity may be destroyed by gastric acid and if this is used, give acid suppression preferably a proton pump inhibitor.

Advantages

1. Highly water soluble.
2. Rapid release of lipases.
3. Absorption through gastric mucosa in neonates.
4. Bile salts not required for absorption.

Table 41.1: The various pancreatic enzyme preparations

Product	*Manufacturer*	*Lipase*	*Protease*	*Amylase*
Enteric-coated Microsphere				
Nutrizym GR	Merck	10,000	650	10,000
Pancrease	Jassen Cilag	5,000	330	2,900
Enteric-coated Minimicrosphere				
Creon	Solvay	10,000	600	8,000
Enteric-coated Microtablets				
Nutrizym 10	Merck	10,000	500	9000
Pancrease HL	Jassen Cilag	25,000	1250	22,500
Cotazym S	Organon	8,000	30,000	30,000
Others				
Enteric-coated tablets				
Pancrex V	Paine & Byrne	1900	110	1700
Enzox Plus	Tidal	4800	305	4600
Festal N	Aventis	6000	300	4500
Farizym Forte	Organon	6000	350	4000
Pankreoflat	Duphar	6500	400	5500
Capsules	Paine & Byrne	8000	430	9000
Pancrex V				
Buff powder	Paine & Byrne	25,000	1400	30,000
Pancrex V				
Coated granule	Paine & Byrne	5000	300	4000
Pancrex V				

5. Carnitine Independent Passage

The disadvantages include incomplete oxidation, thermogenic effect, ketogenic effect and poor deposition in adipose tissue. Gastro-oesophageal reflux disease (GERD) and failure to thrive (FTT) are common associated problems. GERD has increased incidence in CF. It compounds poor weight gain, aggravates respiratory symptoms. Treatment includes antacids, PPIs, motility stimulants and feed thickeners. Failure to thrive can be tackled by energy supplementation via High-energy formula and enteral or parenteral nutrition. Is dense formula that supply 1Kcal/1ml is well tolerated.

Enteral Tube feeding

Intermittent or overnight continuous infusions should be tried in those less than 2 years with—FTT despite oral supplements. In 2-18 years enteral feeding is needed in those with either % weight/height <85 or weight falling below 2 major centile positions or no weight gain for 6 months. In those >18 years, this may be useful in those with BMI <18.5 Kg/m^2 or >5% weight loss over <2 months.

Upto 150% of the RDA of energy requirement may be given and also upto 200 ml/kg of fluid can be given under supervision. The choices are normal milk based feed with 1.5-2.0 Kcal/ml and enzymes given at the beginning and at the end of feeding. Overnight continuous infusions are the most beneficial and convenient.

Short-term benefits are increase in weight, body fat, and lean body mass and muscle mass. Long-term benefits are increase in weight and height, improved well-being and slower progression in respiratory function. Younger patients have a more successful outcome. Those with a positive outlook to feeding have a better outcome.

Routes of Feeding

The preferred routes are via nasogastric (NG) tubes or gastrostomies that are sited operatively or percutaneously by endoscopic placement (PEG). These are well suitable for long-term nutritional support. Poly vinyl chloride (PVC) NG tubes are used in short-term cases and they need to be changed every week. Polyurethane or silicone tubes are used for long-term cases and may remain for a month. Intermittent bolus gravity assisted feeding mimics physiological conditions, but may induce vomiting by reverse peristalsis, whereas continuous feeds do not evoke vomiting. No. 6 French gauge pediatric incubator tubes or 8 French gauge fine bore feeding tubes are suitable for feeding. Blocked tubes can be flushed with 20 ml water with or without ¼ tsp sodabicarb or pancreatic enzyme powder.

Percutaneous endoscopic gastrostomies (PEGs) may be retained for 2 years without replacement. Newer style balloon buttons called the Mickey's gastrostomy buttons can be inserted into a ready formed track and changed by pulling the existing PEG and simply inserting the button.[12] The complications of gastrostomies are pain following insertion and rarely peritonitis.

Type of Feeds

Elemental/semi-elemental feeds include MCT and Pepdite ranges. Polymeric feeds include Fortini, Nutrini, Pediasure, Novasource Junor and so on. The requirement of enzymes with elemental dirt is not fully settled. Some may need special feeds such as Pulmocare (Abbott) in those with severe pulmonary disease and Generaid in those with hepatic disease. Timing of feeding can be adjusted as per the lifestyle of the patient.

Parenteral Nutrition[13]

It is an option for short-term nutritional support especially following abdominal surgery. Proper fluid electrolyte balance and monitoring supervised by the TPN team is essential for success of such interventions.

6. CF-Related Diabetes Mellitus (CFRD)[14]

As the survival in CF has improved, CFRD is becoming increasingly common. It may also be precipitated by steroid therapy and may need short term insulin therapy. Conflicts between CF and DM diet should be resolved in favour of the CF diet. High-energy diet based on complex starch with modifications like avoidance of refined sugars and drinks that cause rapid rise in blood sugar is advisable.

7. Nutritional Complications[15,16]

Distal intestinal obstruction syndrome (DIOS), an equivalent of meconium ileus, fibrosing colonopathy with proximal colon strictures, pancreatitis, growth faltering and multiple deficiencies are some of the complications of nutritional support in CF.

8. Celiac Disease[18-19]

Occasionally, celiac disease may complicate CF. High index of suspicion and rapid diagnosis and timely treatment with withdrawal of gluten-containing foodstuffs is important in such children.

9. Behavioral Problems

More than 70% of parents of children with CF identified mealtimes as problematic. Mealtimes were the most frequently cited management problem for parents of pre-school children with CF.[1]

Solutions

1. Set rules and expectations at mealtimes as with healthy children.
2. Limit mealtimes to 30 minutes.
3. Make food attractive and fun.
4. Encourage positive and discourage negative statements about eating.
5. Decide on a goal and split it into manageable tasks.
6. Implement reward systems for "good" eating behaviour. These should be consistent and immediate. Bad behaviour should be ignored.
7. Avoid empty threats, unless threatened punishment is carried out discipline is meaningless.
8. Give parents information about child's developmental abilities so that they can focus on the child to increase their responsibility.
9. Dietary supplements should be taken in addition to diet to improve total energy intake and improve weight gain rather than blame the child.

10. Growth Monitoring

Growth monitoring with appropriate weight, height, weight for height and BMI charts form the corner stone in the follow-up of children with CF. The minimum goals of therapy are weight and height above 5th centile or weight for age >80%, height for age >90% and weight for height >85%.[17-19]

CONCLUSIONS

Our understanding of the treatment of the nutritional needs of patients with CF continues to evolve. Early nutritional intervention to prevent or resolve malnutrition is most effective. Meticulous attention to both the quantitative and qualitative aspects of the diet is essential for improving survival and quality of survival in cystic fibrosis.

REFERENCES

1. UK Cystic Fibrosis Trust Nutrition Working Group. *Nutritional Management of Cystic Fibrosis.* London: CF Trust 2002.
2. Corey M, Mc Laughlan FJ, Williams M, Levison H. A comparison of survival, growth and pulmonary function in patients with cystic fibrosis in Boston and Toronto. *J Clin Epidemiol* 1998; 41:583-591.
3. Steinkamp G, Von der Hardt H. Improvement of nutritional status and lung function after long-term nocturnal gastrostomy feedings in cystic fibrosis. *J Pediatr* 1994;124: 244-249.
4. Shepherd RW, Holt TL, Vasques-Velasquez L *et al.* Increased energy expenditure in young children with cystic fibrosis. *Lancet* 1988;1:1300-1303.
5. Raj VK, Plichta SB. The role of social support in breastfeeding promotion: A literature review. *J Human Lactation* 1998; 14: 41-45.
6. Mc Donald A. Nutritional management of cystic fibrosis. *Arch Dis Child* 1996; 74: 81-87.
7. Ahmed F, Ellis J, Murphy J, *et al.* Excessive fecal losses of vitamin A in cystic fibrosis. *Arch Dis Child* 1990; 65: 589-593.
8. Henderson RC, Madsen CD. Bone density in children and adults with cystic fibrosis. *J Pediatr* 1996; 128:28-34.
9. Bye AME, Muller DPR< Wilson J *et al.* Symptomatic vitamin E deficiency in cystic fibrosis. *Arch Dis Child* 1985; 60: 162-164.
10. Budhikanok GS, Lim J, Marcus R, *et al.* Correlates of osteopenia in patients with cystic fibrosis. *Pediatrics* 1996; 97: 103-111.
11. Cade A, Walters MP, Mc Ginley N *et al.* Evaluation of fecal pancreatic elastase-1 as a measure of pancreatic exocrine function in children with cystic fibrosis. *Pediatr Pulmomol* 2000; 29: 172-176.
12. Griffiths M. Single stage percutaneous gastrostomy button insertion—A leap forward. *J Parenter Enter Nutr* 1996; 20: 237-239.
13. Lester LA, Rothberg RM, Dawson G *et al.* Supplemental parenteral nutrition in cystic fibrosis. *J Parenter Enter Nutr* 1986;10:280-295.
14. Wilson DC, Kalnins D, Stewart C, *et al.* Challenges in the dietary treatment of cystic fibrosis related diabetes. *Clin Nutr* 2000; 19: 87-93.
15. Hodson ME, Mearns MB, Batten JC. Meconium ileus equivalent in adults with cystic fibrosis. *BMJ* 1976; ii: 790-791.
16. Rubinstein S, Moss R, Lewiston N. Constipation and meconium ileus equivalent in patients with cystic fibrosis. *Pediatrics*1986; 78: 473-479.
17. Lai HC, Kosorok MR, Sondel SA, *et al.* Growth status in children with cystic fibrosis based on the National CF patient registry data: Evaluation of certain criteria used to identify malnutrition. *J Pediatr* 1998; 132: 478-485.
18. Gupte S, Anderson RA. Pediatric gastroenterology. In: Gupte S (ed): *The Short Textbook of Pediatrics*, 11th edn. New Delhi: Jaypee 2004: 443-478.
19. Sharma M, Singh M. Nutritional management of children with cystic fibrosis. *Indian Pediatr* 2003;40:1055-1063.

Lalit Bharedia • Priyanka Rohtagi

42 Nutrition in Liver Disease

INTRODUCTION

'Life depends upon the liver' is a time-honored saying. The liver is a complex and the largest gland associated with the digestive system in our body. It has several functions in our nutritional wellbeing.

The large size of the liver is matched by its functional complexity and involvement in a diverse array of regulatory mechanisms. An understanding of the basic principles of clinical nutrition is important for the management of patients with diseases of the liver. Patients who have liver disease diseases are prone to develop nutritional abnormalities because the major function of the gastrointestinal tract, to process and absorb nutrients, is impaired. In addition, anorexia, dietary restrictions, medications, increased losses and altered nutrient requirements can compromise nutritional status.

LIVER AND METABOLISM

The liver is a "workhorse" for metabolic activity, as illustrated in the Figure 42.1. The liver consumes approximately 20% of resting energy requirements while constituting only 2% of body weight. It receives dual blood supply: approximately 20% of the blood flow is oxygen-rich blood from the hepatic artery, and 80% is nutrient-rich blood from the portal vein arising from the stomach, intestines, pancreas, and spleen. Patients who have significant liver disease demonstrate impaired hepatic metabolic function as well as extrahepatic alterations in glucose (insulin resistance and impaired glucose tolerance), lipid (increased lipolytic rates), and protein (decreased protein synthesis and increased amino acid oxidation rates) metabolism.[1]

LIVER AND NUTRITION

Dietary and nutrient adequacy can be evaluated by dietary history, examination of growth data, physical examination, and laboratory testing. Nutritional assessment and therapy are particularly important for the recognition, treatment, and prevention of nutritional complications of gastrointestinal (GI) disease in infants and children.

Malnutrition is a relevant feature of advanced liver disease. A large proportion of patients with cirrhosis show signs of protein-energy malnutrition, which is associated with a higher prevalence of complications and poor prognosis. The prevalence of malnutrition depends on patients' selection and on the etiology of the disease and is higher in cirrhosis of alcoholic origin. A large Italian population survey reported a significant reduction of fat stores and/or muscle mass in 30% of cases, whereas 29% of females and 18% of males appeared to be over nourished.[2]

Malnutrition contributes to poor prognosis and complications.[3] It was selected as a component of the score predicting severity of liver disease and death risk after portacaval anastomosis by Child *et al.*[4] Hence, the relevance of a correct diagnosis, a thorough analysis of pathogenic causes and prompt treatment is essential. There can be various potential causes of malnutrition in liver diseases as shown in Figure 42.2.

Anthropometric Assessment of Nutritional Status in Children with Liver Disease

In children with chronic liver disease, both acute and chronic malnutrition are nearly universal.[5] There are, however, few studies that have characterized, in a prospective, chronological fashion, anthropometri information defining the nutritional status in children with differing types of liver disease. Several excellent studies do provide general information about nutritional risks in various types of pediatric liver disease and improve the accuracy of interpreting anthropometric assessment result.

Sokol and Stall[6] studied a group of children with chronic liver disease, where onset was clinically apparent before the age of 6 months. Children were compared with an age-matched, normal control population. Cirrhosis was present in the majority of patients, although all were clinically stable and none was considered to be an active candidate for liver transplantation at the time of evaluation. Normalized z scores were used to analyze the data sets. The data demonstrated that both acute (wasting) and chronic (stunting) malnutrition are nearly universal consequences of early childhood liver

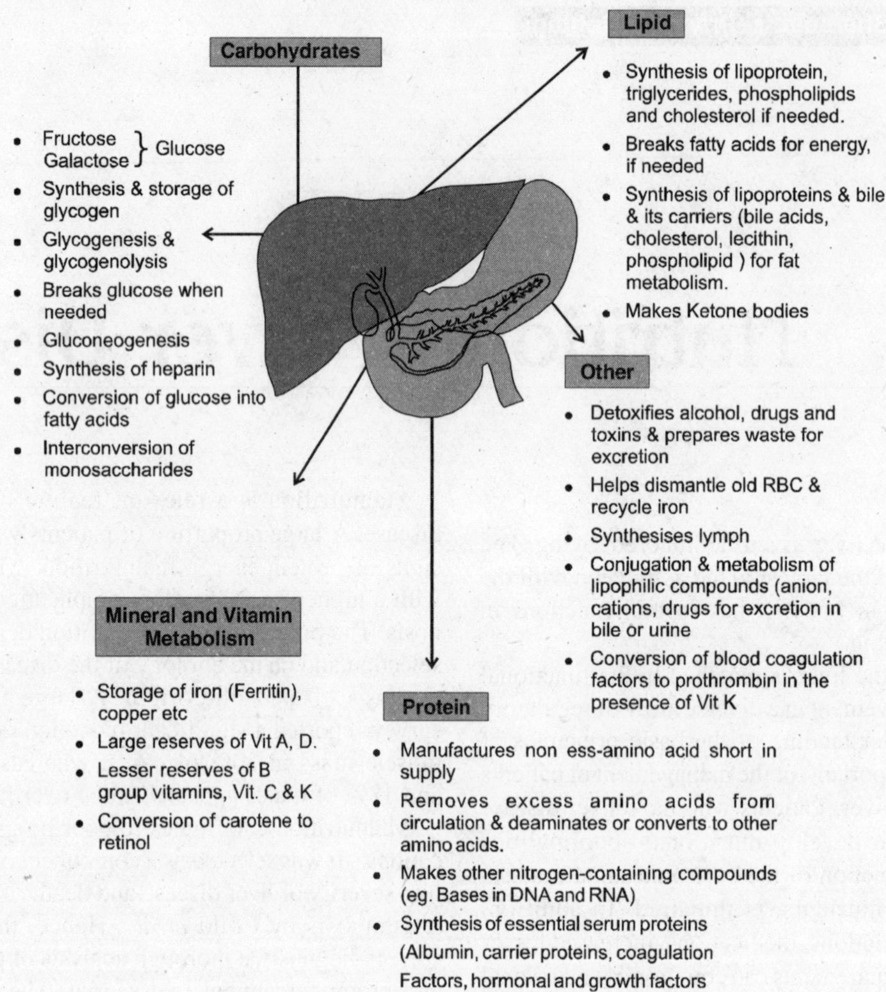

Fig. 42.1: Liver, the "work-horse" for metabolism

disease. A comparison of z scores for weight and height erroneously suggested that although children with chronic liver disease are stunted linear growth, they are well-nourished. This misinterpretation probably results from the increased body weight due to the organomegaly and/or ascites, which may exist even when not detected clinically. Reconfirmation of the imprecision of using a weight/height index versus a triceps skin-fold (TSF) measurement for nutritional assessments comes from a study, done within a month of transplantation, of adult patients with end-stage liver disease.[7]

Acute malnutrition, therefore, is best estimated by a triceps skin-fold determination. Although weight-for-height is generally used to ascertain acute malnutrition, in children with chronic liver disease the increase in body weight resulting from the enlargement of the liver and the spleen may mask the extent of weight loss. Chronic malnutrition (stunting), which occurs over time, is best determined by a height/age index.[8-10]

Nearly all nutritional studies have been cross-sectional or prevalence rather than longitudinal. Future studies are needed to confirm the possible immediate benefit of nutritional intervention in children with chronic liver disease.

There are various factors affecting the interpretation of nutrition assessment tests in patients with end-stage liver disease which have been illustrated in the Table 42.1.

The tool used for the assessment shall comprise the following parameters as illustrated in the Table 42.2.

There are many nutritional risk factors associated with chronic liver diseases as illustrated in the Table 42.3.

To understand the nutritional role or liver, effects of the hepatobiliary damage, and its management it is essential to understand the normal nutrient metabolism, the alternations in the nutrient metabolism due to the liver damage and the possible remedial measures to be taken as shown below in Table 42.4.

Nutritional factors causing liver disease:

An adequate balanced nutrition is essential to maintain body mass, support organ function and allow growth and development of the infant of child. Any devotion from normal nutrition is likely to affect hepatobiliary function.

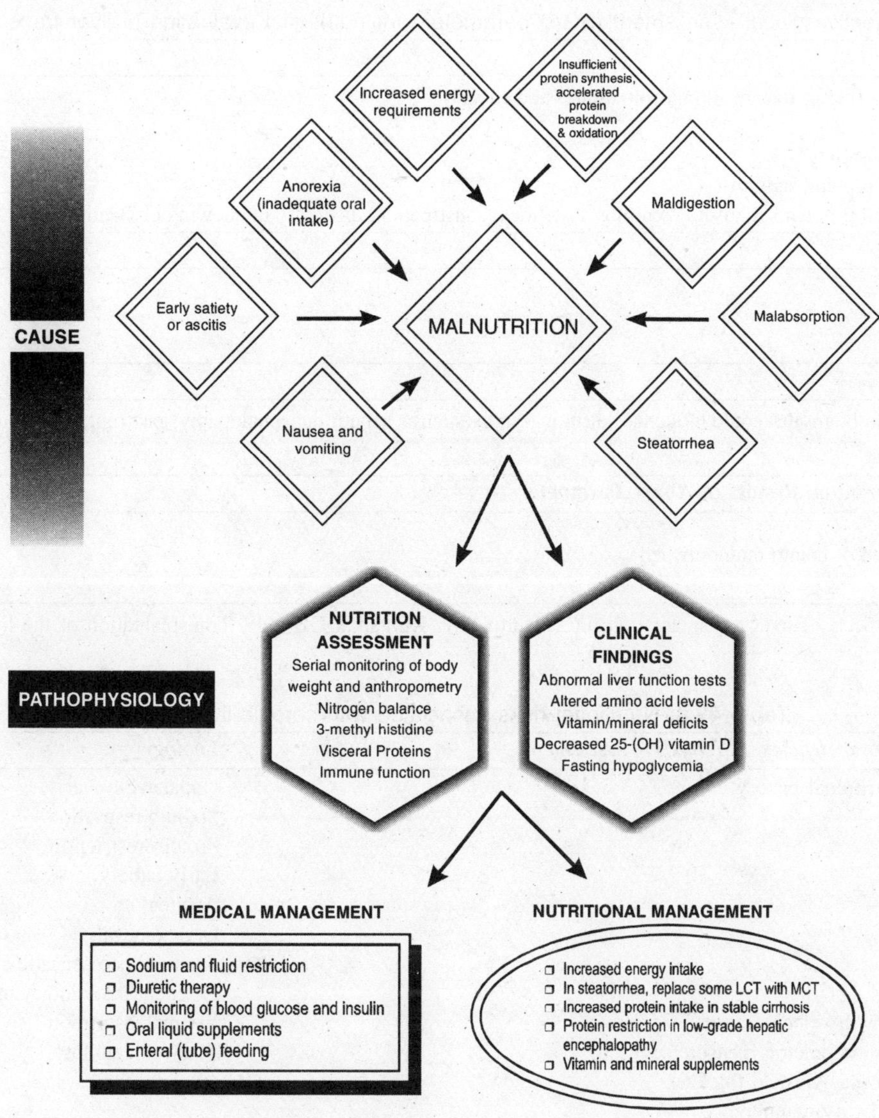

Fig. 42.2: Malnutrition in liver disease

Table 42.1: Factors that affect interpretation of nutrition assessment tests in patients with end-stage liver disease

Parameter	*Factors affecting interpretation*
Body weight	• Affected by edema, ascites, and diuretic use.
Anthropometric measurement	• Questionable sensitivity, specificity, and reliability. • Multiple sources of error. • Question if skinfold measurements reflect total body fat.
Creatinine-height index	• Affected by malnutrition, aging, decreased body mass, and protein intake. • Affected by renal function. • Creatinine is a metabolic end product of creatine, which is synthesized in the liver, therefore severe liver disease alters creatinine synthesis rates.
Nitrogen balance studies	• Nitrogen is retained in the body in the form of ammonia. • Hepatorenal syndrome can affect the excretion of nitrogen.
3-Methyl histidine excretion	• Affected by dietary intake, trauma, infection, and kidney function.
Visceral protein levels	• Synthesis of visceral proteins is decreased. • Affected by hydration status, malabsorption, and kidney insufficiency.
Immune function tests	• Affected by liver failure, electrolyte imbalances, infection, and kidney insufficiency.

(Hasse J. Nutritional aspects of liver transplantation. In: Busuttil RW, Klintamal GB (eds) Transplantation of the liver, Philadelphia: WB Saunders, 1996;359)

Table 42.2: Subjective global assessment (SGA) parameters for nutritional evaluation of liver transplant candidates

History
Weight change (consider fluctuations resulting from ascites and edema) Appetite Taste changes and early satiety Dietary recall (calories, protein, sodium) Persistent gastrointestinal problems (nausea, vomiting, diarrhoea, constipation, difficulty in chewing or swallowing)
Physical
Muscle wasting Fat stores Ascites or edema
Existing Conditions
Disease state and other problems that could influence nutritional status such as hepatic encephalopathy, gastrointestinal bleed, renal insufficiency, infection
Nutritional Rating (Based on Results of Above Parameters)
Well nourished Moderately (or suspected of being) malnourished Severely malnourished

(Hasse J. Nutritional aspects of liver transplantation. In: Busuttil RW, Klintamal GB (eds) Transplantation of the liver. Philadelphia: WB Saunders, 1996, P367)

Table 42.3: Nutritional risks associated with chronic liver disease

Nutritional risks	*Signs of deficiency/Methods of assessment*	*Etiology*
Anorexia	Nutritional history	Unpalatable diet Sodium restriction Protein restriction Early satiety Ascites Organomegaly Altered taste sensation Frequent infections/ antibiotics
Growth failure	Growth velocity curve Anthropometric measurement Triceps skin-fold thickness Midarm circumference Midarm muscle mass area (MAMA) History of drugs that bind bile acids or interfere with Mucosal function	Fat malabsorption 72-hour fecal fat
Hypoproteinemia	Assess nutritional intake and Distributions of calories, carbohydrates, protein, and fat Clinical examination to edema ascites, muscle wasting Anthropometry	Therapeutic maneuvers to control ascites (e.g. fluid withdrawal) GI protein loss Fecal a1-antitrypsin excretion And/or clearance Increased catabolism, decreased Synthesis due to infection, Hepatic dysfunction
Fat-soluble vitamin deficiency	Dermatitis, night blindness, osteomalacia, serum vitamin A and retinol ester Determination (HPLC)	Fat malabsorption, neomycine, cholestyramine, alcoholism, glucorticoids
Vitamin A	Retinol-binding protein, transthyretin (prealbumin) concentrations Functional assessment, dark field adaptation studies (difficult to perform in children)	
Vitamin E	Edema, peripheral neuropathy, serum vitamin E level (HPLC) Vitamin E/total lipid ratio Vitamin E absorption test Biochemical evidence for vitamin E deficiency	Fat malabsorption, cholestyramine

Contd.

Contd.

	Clinical evidence for vitamin E deficiency Neurological dysfunction DTRs diminished Wide-based gait Occular palsy Spinocerebellar degeneration Anemia/hemolysis	
Vitamin D	Assessment of dietary intake of vitamin D and calcium Determine serum 25-OH vitamin D level, absorption study Radiographic studies of bone/bone densitometry Serum alkaline phosphatase Determination/bone fraction Determine 25-OH vitamin D level	Fat malabsorption Increased requirements due to interaction with pharmacologic agents (e.g.phenobarbital, neomycin, cholestyramine)
Vitamin K	Bleeding, Prothrombin time/vitamin K challenge clotting factor levels	Fat malabsorption, cholestyramine Use of antibiotics (neomycin, bile sequestering acids)
Mineral deficiency (Iron, magnesium and zinc)	Neuromuscular irritability, hypokalemia, hypocalcemia, Stomatitis, anemia, malaise, impaired taste acuity, Poor wound healing Document adequate supplementation Determination of serum Magnesium level/urinary excretion Serum iron, total iron-binding capacity, ferritin levels Plasma zinc determination Serum alkaline phosphatase level Urinary excretion	Chronic bleeding Use of bile acid sequestering agents

Deitz WH. Nutritional requirements and feeding of the handicapped child. In grand RJ, Sutphen JL, Deitz WH eds. Pediatric nutrition: Theory and practice.
Boston: Butterworth, 1987;387-392
Merritt RJ. Nutritional requirements. In: Walker WA, *et al.* eds, Pediatric gastrointestinal disease, pathophysiology, diagnosis management, vol 2 Philadelphia, Toronto: BC Decher 1981; 1579-1596.

Table 42.4: Liver damage and the possible remedial measures

Role of liver in nutrient metabolism	*Effect of damage of liver on nutrient metabolism*	*Remedial measures*
Energy		
Liver plays a central role in energy balance and fuel homeostasis, so that changes in the presence of acute and chronic liver disease, Liver effectively stores energy in the form of glycogen preventing the depletion of fat and protein reserves	In chronic liver disease, 15-20% may be hypermetabolic, while 15-20% may be hypometabolic patients. Hypo/hypermetabolic patients represent high risk population with greater hemodynamic changes and to have a poorer outcome following transplantation. Capacity to store hepatic glycogen decreases in cirrhotic patients.	Provision of small frequent meals throughout the waking hours, together with a late night snack improves the fuel utilization and nitrogen economy in these patients. Hence, a small frequent meal pattern (4-7 small meals) should the encouraged with a late night snack of complex carbohydrates.
Carbohydrates		
Liver is responsible for the maintenance of euglycemia, gluconeogenesis, glycogen synthesis and breakdown. Synthesis of heparin.	In fulminant hepatic failure hypoglycemia is common, impaired gluconeogenesis, glucogen synthesis and breakdown.	Infusion of 10% glucose intravenously at the rate of 1.5 to 2.0 litres daily of 20% glucose delivered centrally if fluid restriction is necessary, blood sugar levels should be monitored constantly as hypoglycemia may be asymptomatic. 15-37% of cirrhotics have frank diabetes from complex carbohydrates and low GI and high soluble fibre.
Fat		
Liver synthesis bile salts, lipoproteins, phospholipids and cholesterol, ketone bodies.	In parenchymal liver disease or chronic cholestasis flow of bile salts reduces and interferes with fat emulsification and triglyceride hydrolysis by pancreatic lipase.	Dietary supplementation with poly unsaturated fatty acids could be justified in the decompensated cirrhotic patients who are malnourished.

Contd.

Contd.

Conversion of fatty acids, carbohydrate and protein intermediate to fats.	This steatorrhoea is usually modest. The micelle formation is disrupted which impairs absorption of fat soluble vitamins. Total plasma fatty acid concentration may be increased in patients with CLD but concentration of polyunsaturated fatty acids are usually reduced, which may result in impaired prostaglandin synthesis Xanthelasma may develop in patients with primary biliary cirrhosis.	
Proteins		
Synthesis of plasma proteins, carrier proteins (transferrin) and coagulation factors. Deamination and transamination of amino acid. Urea formation.	In severe viral hepatitis and fulminant hepatic failure, requirements are increased depending upon degree of hepatic decompensation. Blood urea concentrations may be low in chronic liver disease reflecting a reduction in urea in urea. Synthesis rate. But, blood ammonia concentrations may be elevated secondary to ammonia concentrations may be elevated secondary to impaired hepatic function and portal systemic shunting of blood. Increase in circulating ammonia concentrations implicates the genesis of hepatic encephalopathy. Significant changes in plasma amino acid concentrations. Branched chain amino acids are predominantly metabolised by muscle. Hence, plasma concentration of branched chain amino acids are decreased, while concentrations of one or both of the aromatic amino acids (Phenylalanine and tyrosine) are increased together with methionine.	It's important to provide protein of high biological value to ensure their maximum utilisation preferably supplemented with proteins with vegetable origin which are rich in branched chain amino acids. Whey proteins should be the proteins of choice.

Malnutrition: Nutrition affects the course and the prognosis of liver disease hence nutritional status is included in child's score for cirrhosis.

Hepatic necrosis and fibrosis can be produced in experimental animals by appropriate diets, particularly those low in protein and essential amino acids (Table 42.5).[11]

The most clearly defined syndrome is kwashiorkor, but this represents only one end of the malnutrition spectrum the liver is often grossly enlarged in children with kwashiorkor, containing 30-50% fat by weight, predominantly in the form of neutral fat or triglyceride. If the malnutrition is severe and off long-standing hepatic fibrosis may be observed. The hepatic changes in the alcoholic may be, at least in part, nutritional.[12]

In starvation and hunger oedema, the liver shrinks, increased lipochrome pigment is seen in the liver cells, but there is no fatty change.[13] Liver biopsies from malnourished children show a reduction in liver protein.[14] Previous malnutrition may 'condition' the liver to toxic and infective agents, but this has not been proved. Increased mortality from virus hepatitis, particularly in pregnancy, may occur in protein-deficient communities.

Fatty Liver

This is defined as fat, largely triglyceride, exceeding 5% of the liver weight. It is caused by failure of normal hepatic fat metabolism either due to a defect within the hepatocyte or to delivery of excess fat, fatty acid or carbohydrate beyond the secretory capacity for lipid of the liver cell. Liver biopsy and imaging procedures, such as ultrasound and CT, are resulting in increasing numbers of patients being identified with excess fat in the liver.

Theoretically fatty liver could accumulate through at least four mechanisms:

Table 42.5: Amino acids commonly altered in liver disease

Aromatic amino acids-Serum levels increased	*Branched-chained amino Acids-serum levels decreased*	*Other amino acids-serum levels increase*
Tyrosine	Valine*	Methionine*
Phenylalanine*	Leucine*	Glutamine
Free tryptophan*	Isoleucine*	Asparagine
		Histidine*

* Essential amino acid.

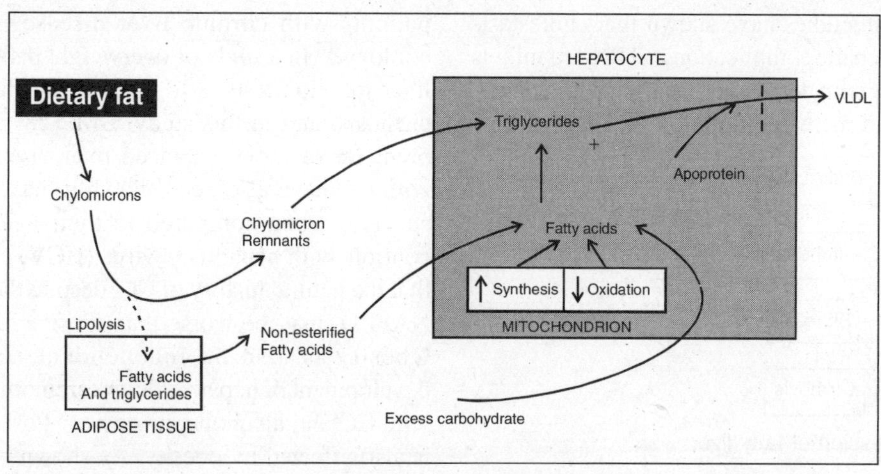

Textbook of liver and biliary disease, Sheila Sherlok 9th edition, Fig. No. 427

Fig. 42.3: Factors in fatty liver

1. Increased delivery of dietary fat or fatty acids to the liver. Dietary fat is transported in the circulation mainly as chylomicrons Figure 42.3. Lipolysis in adipose tissue liberates the fatty acids. These are incorporated into triglyceride within the adipocyte but some fatty acids may be released into the circulation and taken up by the liver. The chylomicron remnants also enter the liver.
2. Increased mitochondrial synthesis of fatty acids or reduced oxidation. Both augment triglyceride production.
3. Impaired export of triglyceride out of the liver cell. Export of triglycerides from the hepatocyte depends upon packaging with apo-protein, phospholipid and cholesterol to form very low density lipoprotein (VLDL). This process may be inhibited. Excess carbohydrate delivered to the liver may be converted to fatty acids.

Nonalcoholic fatty liver disease (NAFLD), Hepatic steatosis (Fatty Liver), and nonalcoholic steatohepatitis (NASH).

Fatty liver can be separated into two categories based on whether the fat droplets in the hepatocytes are macrovesicular or microvesicular (Table 42.6). In addition, fatty infiltration may be accompanied by necroinflammatory activity, a condition designated nonalcoholic steatohepatitis, a form of NAFLD. Although prospective data on natural history are limited, there is increasing evidence that patients may progress through several histologically distinct stages beginning with fatty liver and culminating in cirrhosis with intervening states of steatohepatitis and steatohepatitis with fibrosis.

Table 42.6: Causes of hepatic steatosis

Macrovesicular (large fat droplets in hepatocytes)	*Microvesicular (small fat droplets in hepatocytes)*
Nutritional	
Malnutrition (Kwashiorkor)	Reye's syndrome
Obesity*	
Prolonged parenteral nutrition*	Acute fatty liver of pregnancy
Metabolic diseases	Drugs, e.g. valproic acid, tetracycline, nucleoside analogues
Drug-related	Environmental hepatotoxins (e.g. phosphorus, petrochemicals)
Inflammatory bowel disease	

Textbook of liver and biliary disease, Sheila Sherlok 9th edition, Page No. 429.

Parenteral Nutrition and Liver

The use of the vascular system to supply nutrient requirements can be an important and even life-saving therapy. The complications associated with the use of parenteral nutrition can be divided into mechanical, vascular, infectious, metabolic, and gastrointestinal.

Hepatobiliary Complications of TPN

Hepatic abnormalities are the most common gastrointestinal complications associated with TPN. However, it is difficult to establish a true causal relationship between the use of TPN and many of the reported liver abnormalities because of the paucity of prospective randomized trials. Many of the hepatic abnormalities in patients receiving TPN might have been caused by clinical factors unrelated to the use of TPN itself. Patients who require TPN often have serious illnesses that are associated with liver disease or have received hepatotoxic therapy, which can cause liver disease.

Hepatic abnormalities are more frequent and more severe in infants receiving TPN than in adults. The first report of TPN-associated liver disease, published in 1971, was of a premature infant who developed cholestatic jaundice, bile duct proliferation, and cirrhosis after 71 days of TPN therapy.[20] Subsequent studies have shown that cholestasis is the most frequent hepatic complication in TPN-fed infants and correlates directly with decreased gestational age, decreased birth weight, and increased duration of TPN therapy.

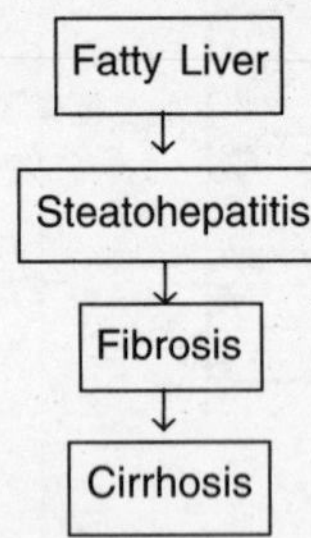

Progression of fatty liver

Obesity and its Impact on Liver Disease and Transplantation

Obesity is twice as common in patients with cryptogenic cirrhosis compared to those with other chronic liver disease.[15] Obesity is also a negative prognostic predictor in patients with chronic liver disease irrespective of the etiology.[16] In a study of overweight patients with abnormal liver function tests, 30% had septal fibrosis and 11% had cirrhosis, and in this study, BMI>28 was an independent predictor of more advanced liver disease. Obese patients with CC have also been shown to have a relatively lower survival when compared to their age and sex matched controls with hepatitis C virus (HCV) cirrhosis suggesting that the natural history of CC, despite the indolent nature of NAFLD, may be worse than those with HCV cirrhosis.[17] Obesity is also an independent risk factor for the development of hepatocellular carcinoma (HCC) in patients with CC and alcoholic cirrhosis.[18] Post-transplant survival is also affected by obesity. As shown by our group where patients with BMI>35 had a significantly lower 5-year survival compared to less obese transplant recipients.[19]

Hypervitaminosis A and Liver

Vitamin A is a dose-dependent hepatotoxin, and severe liver disease may result from hypervitaminosis A.[25]

Food borne liver illness

Disease and organism	*Source*	*Prevention methods*
1. Hepatitis (Hepatitis A & E virus)	Raw vegetable Contaminated water	Sanitary handling of foods Use of pure drinking water Adequate sewage disposal Adequate cooking
2. Hydatid cyst (Echinococcus granulosus)	Salad, vegetable contaminated dog feces containing embryonated egg	Sanitary handling of foods Adequate sewage disposal Adequate cooking
3. Amebic liver abscess (E. histolytica)	Fecally contaminated water, food or hands	Sanitary handling of foods Use of pure drinking water
4. Hepatobiliary ascariasis (Ascaris lumbricoides)	Contaminated vegetables, salads, pickle	Sanitary handling of foods Adequate sewage disposal Adequate cooking
5. Cholangiocarcinoma (Clonorchis sinensis)	Raw or inadequately cooked fresh water fish	Adequate cooking

Toxins causing liver illness

Agent	*Type of exposure*	*Nature of liver injury*
1. Pyrrolizidine alkaloids	Herbal and bush teas; contaminated crop	Veno-occlusive disease, cirrhosis
2. Vitamin A	Health tonic; skin disorder (no longer appropriate: massive ingestion of liver	Noncirrhotic portal hypertension, hepatic fibrosis, liver failure with or without cirrhosis, peliosis hepatitis
3. Amanita phalloides, other toxic mushrooms	Accidental ingestion, as little as one mushroom	Fulminant hepatic failure
4. Aflatoxin	Contaminated crops, foodstuffs, groundnuts	Hepatocellular carcinoma (p53 deletions)
5. Arsenic	Nonproprietary medications; contaminated water supply; industrial exposure (pesticides, herbicides)	Hepatic fibrosis, cirrhosis, noncirrhotic portal hypertension, angiosarcoma

The clinicopathologic spectrum of hypervitaminosis A-related liver disease includes minor changes with abnormal liver tests and stellate cell hyperplasia, noncirrhotic portal hypertension with perisinusoidal fibrosis, cirrhosis, or fatal chronic liver disease with hepatocellular failure in the absence of cirrhosis.[26]

Gradual improvement occurs after discontinuation of vitamin A ingestion, but deterioration may continue in cases of severe intoxication, particularly when cirrhosis is present. Features of liver failure and established cirrhosis is present. Features of liver failure and established cirrhosis at diagnosis indicate a poor prognosis; most patients die or require hepatic transplantation.[27] There is a need for better public education to prevent hypervitaminosis A.

Hepatobiliary complications of total parenteral nutrition	
Cholestasis	Biliary sludge
Cholelithiasis	Fibrosis
Cirrhosis	Hepatocellular carcinoma

The mechanisms involved in the pathogenesis of hepatic complications are not well understood. Many potential contributing factors have been proposed as being responsible for TPN-associated liver disease: those associated with the patients' clinical condition or therapy, the TPN solution itself (excessive glucose calories, excessive lipid infusion, amino acid degradation products, aluminum toxicity), nutritional deficiencies (essential fatty acid deficiency, choline deficiency, carnitine deficiency), and gut factors (intestinal bacteria or endotoxin translocation, bacterial overgrowth, bacterial metabolism of bile acids). Three types of biliary complications have been associated with the use of TPN acalculous cholecystitis, gallbladder sludge, and cholelithiasis. Biliary complications usually occur in patients receiving more prolonged (more than 4 weeks) courses of TPN. Acalculous cholecystitis has been reported to occur in about 5%,[21] cholelithiasis in about 30% (Pitt HA, King W, Mann L, *et al*. Increased risk of cholelithiasis with prolonged total parenteral nutrition. Am J Surg 145:106, 1983) and gallbladder sludge in up to 100% of patients receiving prolonged TPN. The pathogenesis of acalculous cholecystitis is unclear, but it occurs in the setting of bile stasis and increased bile lithogenicity and is associated with major trauma, severe systemic illness, and major operative procedures. The pathogenesis of gallbladder sludge and stones is related to gallbladder stasis caused by the absence of enteral feeding in TPN-fed patients. Most TPN-related gallstones are pigment stones containing large amounts of calcium bilirubinate.[22]

The development of gallbladder sludge appears to be a prerequisite for the development of gallstones. Stimulating gallbladder contraction and emptying with either enteral feedings[23] or cholecystokinin injections[24] has been shown to reduce or completely prevent gallbladder sludge and gallstone formation.

GOALS FOR NUTRITIONAL INTERVENTION

The ultimate goals of nutritional intervention in children with chronic liver disease are nutritional homeostasis, deposition of lean body mass, and enhanced growth. This is accomplished by (a) nutritional supplementation, which corrects existing deficits and meets ongoing losses; and (b) establishing nitrogen deposition while decreasing hepatic encephalopathy. Special attention must be directed toward infants and young children, the largest group of young patients requiring liver transplantation.[28]

Nutritional formulas adequate to promote catch-up growth must contain approximately 150% of the recommended dietary allowances (RDA) for height and age. Infant formulas, which contain a balanced lipid composition to maximize absorption in the face of cholestasis and deficient lipolysis (e.g. 40% of lipid calories as medium chain triglycerides) and yet have sufficient linoleic acid to prevent essential fatty acid deficiency, have been recommended.[29] Protein intake adequate to promote growth and to maintain positive nitrogen balance is essential.

Studies that have examined nitrogen balance while reducing hepatic encephalopathy through the use of branch-chain amino acids have conflicting results.[30] The use of branch-chain amino acids in children with liver failure has been recommended, the potential benefits being an increased utilization rate of branch chain amino acids by skeletal muscle, which would promote net energy uptake and possibly reduce the potential for hepatic encephalopathy. To date, the high cost of these formulations and limited information demonstrating efficacy preclude their routine use in children with cholestasis and/or liver disease. Chronic malabsorption and deficiency of fat-soluble vitamins are nearly universal in children with chronic liver disease.[31] Careful assessment of current status and monitoring of vitamin intake to avoid toxicity are essential.

METHOD OF FEEDING IN LIVER DISEASE

Many patients with chronic liver disease are anorexic or suffer from nausea or abdominal distension. Maintenance of an adequate oral intake may prove difficult under these circumstances. Patients should be encouraged to eat, and also to modify, their eating pattern in order to take four to seven small meals throughout the day, including a late night snack, as this reg is better tolerated and improves nitrogen balance and substrate utilization.

It is often difficult, however, to sustain oral intake in patients with persistent anorexia and nausea, or to increase oral intake beyond a certain limit in malnourished patients.

If oral intake remains inadequate despite supplementation, then enteral feeding via a fine-bore nasogastric tube should be instituted at the earliest opportunity. Depending on the degree of malnutrition, nighttime infusions alone may be sufficient to maintain growth.[32] if abdominal distension and vomiting continue then the nasogastric tube can be endoscopically repositioned in the jejunum. Standard, proprietary feeds, providing 1 kcal/ml, are suitable for use in the majority of patients but the volume of feed required to supply daily requirements may be excessive in those who are fluid overloaded. Under these circumstances, more concentrated feeds providing 1.5 or 2.0 kcal/ml can be used, the choice being determined by the amount of protein required. The rate of feed administration and osmolarity can be manipulated to optimize tolerance.

Every attempt should be made to feed these patients either orally or enterally; the use of parenteral feeding should be avoided if at all possible for a number of reasons: these patients may be fluid intolerant so that the volume infused may need to be restricted to one liter or less. It may also be necessary to modify the amino acid solutions used. In addition many of the formulations used in patients with liver disease are nutritionally incomplete or else contain quantities of amino acids, such as glycine, proline, lysine, threonine, and arginine, which may not be adequately cleared when the liver's ureagenic capacity is limited.

Lipid solutions can be used safely in these patients; long-chain and medium-chain triglycerides are equally well tolerated. Thus, if patients with liver disease require parenteral nutrition there is no contraindication to providing energy as glucose and fat, the latter constituting 35-50% of the non-protein calories, and nitrogen as conventional amino acids.

Essential dietary principles in liver diseases[33]

Calories/day	: 1.2-1.4 times resting energy expenditure (REE)
Proteins/day	: 1.2-1.5 g/kg of ideal body weight (IBW)
Fats/day	: 20-40% of non-protein calories
Carbohydrates/day	: Rest of the calories.

NUTRITIONAL MANAGEMENT OF INDIVIDUAL LIVER DISEASE

Fatty Liver

Fatty liver is known as the disease of the decade, it may or may not be associated with obesity.

Nutritional therapy: Weight management with low-fat diet rich in polyunsaturated and monounsaturated fatty acids is recommended.

Non-alcoholic steatohepatitis (NASH)/Non Alcoholic fatty liver disease (NAFLD): Non-alcoholic steatohepatitis (NASH) is thought to be an intermediate stage of the disease which is characterized by the presence of hepatic inflammation, injury and cell death in conjunction with steatosis in the absence of any other attributable causes including alcohol, drugs, or any other identifiable causes. The spectrum of non-alcoholic fatty liver disease (NAFLD) extends from steatosis (fatty liver) without inflammation or fibrosis at the most benign end to cirrhosis at the opposite end.

It represents a spectrum of conditions. Is generally associated with obesity, diabetes and hypertension.

Nutritional therapy: Dietary treatment is based on the associated illness. Management involves regular physical exercise, weight maintenance with low fat diabetic diet and salt restriction for hypertension. Saturated fats are to be replaced with polyunsaturated or monounsaturated fats in limited quantity.

Acute Hepatitis

Acute hepatitis is usually a self-limiting inflammatory condition. It is most commonly caused by viruses, and can also be caused by various other agents such as alcohol, drugs, or toxins. Alcoholic hepatitis is frequently accompanied by protein-calorie malnutrition, which increase the risk for clinical severity and poor prognosis.

Nutritional Therapy

The principles of diet therapy relate to the liver's function in metabolizing each of the nutrients:

1. *Adequate protein:* Protein is essential for liver cell regeneration. It also provides lipotropic agents such as methionine and choline for the conversion of fats to lipoproteins and removal from the liver, thus preventing fatty infiltration. The diet should supply from 1.2 to 1.5 gms/kg.b.wt./day of high-quality protein.
2. *High carbohydrate:* Sufficient available glucose must be provided to restore protective glycogen reserves and meet the energy demands of the disease process. Also, adequate glucose for energy ensure the use of protein for vital tissue regeneration. The diet should supply from 50 to 55 % calories from carbohydrate.
3. *Moderate fat:* A moderate amount of fat makes the food more palatable and therefore encourages the anorexic patient to eat. Some easily used fat, such as whole milk, cream, butter, margarine, mayonnaise, and vegetable oil, is beneficial. The diet should supply about 20 to 25 % of the total calories/day.
4. *High energy:* From 1.5 times of the total caloric requirement per day are needed to furnish energy demands of the tissue regeneration process, to compensate for losses from fever and debilitation, and to renew strength and recuperative powers.
5. *Meals and feedings:* The problem of supplying a diet adequate to meet the increased nutritive demands for a patient whose illness makes food almost repellent calls for creativity and supportive encouragement. The food may need to be in liquid form at first, using concentrated commercial or blended formulas for frequent feedings.

As the patient improves, appetizing and attractive food is needed. Since nutritional therapy is the key to recovery, a major nutrition and nursing responsibility requires devising ways to encourage the increased amounts of food intake needed. The clinical nutritionist and the nurse will work together closely to achieve this goal.

In the recovery stage after the subacute stage when the enzymes begin to fall, a normal diet is recommended the diet should have normal proteins and normal fat content as tolerated.

Cirrhosis

Studies have shown that there is a direct relationship between calorie intake and mortality in patients with cirrhosis.

Mendenhall's analysis:[33]

Calorie intake	*Mortality at 6 months*
< 1000 kcal/day	90%
1000 - 2000 kcal/day	50%
> 2000 kcal/day	20%

It shows that mortality decrease with high calorie diet. Malnutrition is common in cirrhosis and severity of liver diseases is correlated with severity of malnutrition, therefore, it is very essential to feed these patients.

Sample diet plan for a child with Hepatitis

Weight = 10 kg

Sex = Male

Food Habit—Non vegetarian

Food groups	*Amt*	*Household measure*
Cereals	200 gm	8 chapatis
Pulses	50 g	2 katon cooked dal
Milk	750 ml	3 glass
Meat	1 piece	
Vegetables	200 g	½ k cooked
Fruits	250 gm	2 fruits
Fats	40 g	8 tsp
Sugar	30 g	6 tsp
Nutritive value	Normal	Modified
Total calories	1240 kcals	Increased upto 1½ times 1800 kcals
Proteins	22 gms	Increased upto 1½ times 33 gms
Fat	25 gms	38 gms

Sample Menu	
Early morning	1 cup milk
	2 biscuits
Breakfast	1 katori porridge with milk with sugar
	1 fruit (Pear)
Mid morning	Sprout chat
	Sprouted dal + cucumber and potatoes
Lunch	1½ katori vegetable khichdi with veg. raita
Mid afternoon	2 rasgulla
Evening	Fruit juice
Dinner	1 katori Rice pulao + Dal + 1 katori
	1 paneer chapati + 1 katori vegetable
Bedtime	Rice Kheer

Chronic liver disease may advance to the chronic stage of cirrhosis.

Nutritional Therapy: Therapy is usually aimed at correcting fluid and electrolyte problems and providing nutritional support for hepatic repair as much as possible. Nutritional therapy for cirrhosis should include the following principles:

Optimal general nutrition: The remaining overall diet principles outlined for hepatitis are continued for cirrhosis for the same reasons. Kilocalories, carbohydrates, and vitamins are supplied according to individual need and deficiency. Moderate fat is used. Alcohol is strictly forbidden.

1. *Protein according to tolerance:* In the absence of impending hepatic coma, about 1.2 to 1.5 gms/kg.b.wt./day of protein is needed to correct severe undernutrition, regenerate functional liver tissue, and replenish plasma protein. However, if signs of hepatic coma appear, protein must be adjusted to individual tolerance.
2. Fats should be about 30 to 35% of the total calories preferably derived from fats rich in unsaturated fatty acids with adequate essential fatty acids.
3. 55-60% of energy as complex carbohydrates with low glycemic index (GI), foods rich in soluble fibers, as according to WHO criteria 60-80% of patients with cirrhosis have impaired glucose tolerance.
4. *Low sodium:* Sodium 2-2.5 g/day is permitted, which would be supplied from 5 gms i.e. 1 tsp of the common table salt. Sodium is restricted to help reduce fluid retention. If low sodium affects the palatability of food then low sodium salt preparation can also be used.
5. *Texture:* If esophageal varices develop, it may be necessary to give soft foods that are smooth in texture to prevent danger of rupture and hemorrhage, but the presence of esophageal varices is not a contraindication to the use of nasogastric tubes although they should be used with caution in the presence of post-injection sclerotherapy esophageal ulceration
6. Liberal amounts of vitamins and minerals with an exception in copper, sodium, iron in cases of Wilson's disease, ascites and hemochromatosis respectively.
7. Fluid as per the ascites status has to be restricted.

NUTRITIONAL MANAGEMENT OF COMPLICATION OF LIVER DISEASE

(I) Fluid Retention:

Nature of disease: Fluid loss and weight change are directly related to sodium balance in patients with portal hypertension related ascites.

Nutrition: In the presence of avid renal retention of sodium, dietary sodium restriction is essential. The patient and the food preparer should be educated about a sodium-restricted diet by a dietitian. Severe sodium-restricted diets

Suggested nutritional management of persistent cholestasis

Clinical impairment	*Management*
Malnutrition resulting from malabsorption of dietary long-chain triglyceride	Replace with dietary formula or supplements containing medium chain triglycerides
Fat soluble vitamin malabsorption	
Vitamin A deficiency Night blindness, thick skin)	Replace with 10,000-15,000 IU/day as Aquasol A (water soluble)
Vitamin E deficiency (Neuromuscular degeneration)	Replace with 50-400 IU/day as oral α-tocopherol
Vitamin D deficiency (Metabolic bone disease)	Replace with 5,000-8,000 IU/day of D2, or 3-5 ug/kg/day of 25-hydrocholecalciferol
Vitamin K deficiency (Hypoprothrombinemia)	Replace with 2.5 to 5.0 mg every other day as water-soluble derivative or menadione
Micronutrient deficiency	Calcium, phosphate, or zinc supplementation
Deficiency of water-soluble vitamins	Supplement with twice and recommended daily allowance
Retention of biliary constituents such as bile acids and cholesterol (itch or xanthomata)	Administer choleretics
Progressive liver disease	Interim management (control bleeding; salt restriction; spironolactone)
Portal hypertension (variceal bleeding, ascites, hypersplenism)	Transplantation
End-stage liver disease (liver failure)	

Nelson Textbook of Pediatrics 15th Edition. Pg. # 1137

(e.g. 500 mg or 22 mmol/day of sodium) are feasible (but not palatable) in an inpatient setting but are unrealistic for outpatients. The dietary sodium restriction that the author recommends for inpatients and outpatients is 2 g/day (88 mmol/day).[34]

Fluid restriction: An indiscriminate fluid restriction in treating the patient with cirrhotic ascites is inappropriate; hypernatremia may result. It is the sodium restriction, not the fluid restriction, that results in weight loss; fluid follows sodium passively. The chronic hyponatremia usually seen in patients with cirrhotic ascites is seldom morbid. Attempts to rapidly correct hyponatremia in this setting can lead to more complications than occur with hypontremia itself. Indiscriminate fluid restriction serves only to alienate patients, nurses, and dietitians.

Bed rest: Although it is traditional to order bed rest, there are no controlled trials to support this practice.

(II) Hepatic Encephalopathy:

Nature of the disease: As cirrhotic changes continue in the liver, the portal blood circulation diminishes and liver functions begin to fail. The normal liver has a major function of removing ammonia from the blood by converting it to urea for excretion. The failing liver can no longer inactivate or detoxify substances or metabolize others. A key factor involved in the progressive disease process is an elevated blood level of ammonia. The resulting hepatic encephalopathy, sometimes called hepatic coma, brings changes in consciousness, behavior, and neurologic status.

Clinical symptoms: Typical response involves disorders of consciousness and alterations in motor function. There is apathy, confusion, inappropriate behavior, and drowsiness, progressing to coma. The speech may be slurred or monotonous. A coarse, flapping tremor is observed in the outstretched hands. The breath may have a fecal odor.

Basic treatment objectives: The fundamental objective of treatment is two-fold :

1. Removal of the sources of excess ammonia, and
2. Provision of nutritional support.

Medical and nutritional therapy are involved. Parenteral fluid and electrolytes are used to restore normal balance. Two drugs may be used to control ammonia-lactulose and neomysin. Lactulose is a nonabsorbable synthetic disaccharide that reduces the absorption of intestinal ammonia. Neomysin is an antibiotic that reduces the population of urea-splitting organism within the bowel that produce ammonia. To stop bleeding into the intestine as another source of intestinal ammonia, a Sengstaken Blakemore tube may be used.

Nutritional therapy: Special parenteral and enteral nutritional support may include use of branched-chain amino acids. These three essential amino acids leucine, isoleucine, and valine are not catabolized by the liver but are taken up by other tissues. Thus they can be metabolized without depending on healthy liver tissue, as is the case with other amino acids. Solutions of these branched—chain amino acids, for example, hepatamine, have therefore been used successfully to maintain adequate nitrogen balance and reduce the encephalopathy.

General nutritional support for hepatic encephalopathy is based on the following principles of dietary management:

1. *Low protein:* Protein intake is reduced as individually necessary to restrict the dietary sources of nitrogen

in amino acids. The amount of restriction will vary with the circumstances. The unconscious patient will receive no protein, but the usual amounts given range from 15 to 50 g/day, depending on whether symptoms of ammonia intoxication are severe or mild. A simple method for controlling dietary protein uses a base meal pattern containing approximately 15 g protein, adding small items of protein foods according to the level of protein desired.

2. *Kilocalories and vitamins:* Adequate energy intake is crucial to the patient's recovery, especially through the impact of caloric intake on liver glycogen reserves and their protective role in the healing process. The amounts of kilocalories and vitamins are prescribed according to need. About 2000 kcal/day is needed to prevent tissue catabolism, which would be as source of more amino acids and available nitrogen and urea. Sufficient carbohydrate is essential as the primary energy source, with some fat as tolerated. Vitamin K is usually given parenterally, along with other vitamins and minerals that may be deficient.
3. *Fluid intake:* Fluid intake—output balance is carefully controlled.

Gallbladder Disease

The basic function of the gallbladder is to concentrate bile 5 to 10 fold and store.

Nutritional preventive measure: There is no specific dietary treatment to prevent cholelithiasis in susceptible individuals. Nutritionally related factors include obesity and severe fasting and these should be corrected where possible. In cholecystitis, dietary treatment includes a low fat diet to prevent gallbladder contractions. Two additional modifications usually found in traditional diets for gallbladder disease concern restriction of foods containing cholesterol and foods labelled "gas formers". Neither modification has a valid rationale. The body synthesizes daily several times more cholesterol than is present in an average diet. Thus restriction of dietary cholesterol has little effect in reducing gallstone formation. Total dietary fat reduction is more to the point. As for the use of so- called "gas formers", such as legumes or cabbage or fiber, blanket restriction seems unwarranted, since food tolerances in any circumstances are highly individual.

Acute Cholecystitis

In an acute attack, oral feedings are discontinued. Parenteral nutrition may be indicated if the patient is malnourished and it is anticipated that he or she will be NPO for a prolonged period of time. When feedings are resumed, a low fat diet is recommended to decrease gallbladder stimulation. A hydrolyzed low fat formula or an oral diet consisting of 30 to 45 g fat per day can be given. Studies have failed to show a relationship between dietary cholesterol and gallstone formation.

Chronic Cholecystitis

Patients with chronic conditions may require a long-term low fat diet that contains 25% to 30% of total kilocalories as fat. Stricter limitation is undersirable because fat in the intestine is important for some stimulation and drainage of the biliary tract.

The degree of food intolerance varies widely among individuals with gallbladder disorders, but bloating. It is best to determine with the patient any foods that should be eliminated for this reason.

Administration of water-soluble forms of fat soluble vitamins may be of benefit in individuals with chronic gallbladder conditions or in those in whom fat malabsorption is suspected.

Perioperative Nutrition: There is a paucity of data evaluating the usefulness of perioperative nutritional support in patients with liver disease. The results of one PRCT suggested that early postoperative enteral feeding may be beneficial in patients undergoing liver transplantaion.[35] Nasojejunal tube feeding started 12 hours after transplant surgery was well tolerated and allowed increased protein and energy intake during the first 4 postoperative days. Early tube feeding was associated with a significant reduction in postoperative viral infections and a trend toward a decrease in bacterial infections. However, these results may be biased, because one third of the patients who entered the study failed to complete their assigned protocol and were not included in the final analysis. Another PRCT found that pretransplant enteral supplementation improved grip strength and other nutritional parameters but did not affect clinical outcome.[36]

One PRCT evaluated the clinical efficacy of perioperative CPN, given as a BCAA-enriched solution for 7 days before and 7 days after hepatectomy for hepatocellular carcinoma.[37] Patients randomized to receive CPN head better postoperative hepatic function and significantly fewer postoperative complications (mostly pulmonary infection and ascites).

NUTRITIONAL ASPECT OF LIVER TRANSPLANTATION

Liver Transplantation (Table 42.7)

Better outcome is seen in patients with a good pre-transplant nutritional status, especially so in the survival rate. So all transplant patients should be well-fed in terms of calories and proteins.

Free Radicals and Antioxidants in Liver Diseases

Although the liver is well endowed with endogenous enzymatic antioxidants, it is also the organ with active

Table 42.7: Nutrition care guidelines for liver transplantation

	Pretransplantation	*Immediate post-transplantation First 2 post-transplantation mo*	*Long-term post-transplantation*
Calories	High calorie (basal + 20% or more)	Moderate calorie (basal + 15-30%)	Weight maintenance (basal + 10-20%)
Protein	Moderate protein (1-1.5 g/kg/day-minimize needed for restriction)	High protein (1.2-1.75 g/kg/day)	Moderate protein (1g/kg/day)
Fat	As needed	20-30% of non-protein calories	Low fat (< 30% of calories)
Carbohydrate	High carbohydrate (complex and simple)	70% of non-protein calorie	Reduced simple carbohydrate
Sodium	2-4 g/day (as indicated)	2-4 g/day (as indicated)	2-4 g/day (as indicated)
Fluid	Restrict to 1000-1500 mL/day (as indicated)		As needed 1200-1500 mg/day
Calcium	800-1200 mg/day	800-1200 mg/day	Daily multivitamin/mineral supplement to RDA levels for first post-transplant year
Vitamins	Daily multivitamin/mineral supplement to RDA levels; additional water and fat soluble vitamins as indicated	Daily multivitamin/ mineral supplement to RDA levels; additional water and fat-soluble vitamins as indicated	

microsomal and mitochondrial systems that generate oxygen free radicals during normal metabolic processes. When this balance is upset, however, tissue damage may occur. Free radical injury has been implicated in a variety of hepatic disorders.[38]

Taking these data into account a new antioxident solution has been developed (the Carolina rinse solution) for liver allograft preservation that contains antioxidants (e.g., Allopurinol, deferosamine, and glutathione), compounds to prevent activation of Kupffer cells, and precursors of ATP generation (adenosine, glucose, and fructose). Improved outcome of allografts after liver transplantation with use of this solution has been reported.[39]

Oxidative stress has been demonstrated in alcohol-induced liver injury because of altered NADH/NAD^+ ratios in hepatocytes that favor generation of free radicals from mitochondria and microsomal P_{450} systems and alter ferritin chelation of iron.

The possible use of antioxidant therapy in alcoholic liver disease now is being studied; however, Lieber's group has provided data in nonhuman primates, cautioning against the use of beta carotene in this condition.[40]

Copper and iron storage diseases are strongly linked to oxidant damage of hepatocytes and mitochondria. In Wilson's disease livers removed at liver transplantation, in vivo evidence of oxidant injury and reduced concentrations of vitamin E and glutathione have been demonstrated. The possible use of antioxidants as adjunct therapy, in addition to reducing the iron or copper burden in these disorders, needs investigation. In addition, the possible targeting of antioxidants to the mitochondria should be explored. Recently, an antioxidant "cocktail" (including vitamin E, selenium, deferoxamine, prostaglandin E, and N-acetyl cysteine) apparently has reversed the previously fatal liver failure of neonatal iron storage disease in at least eight infants.[41] Whether such an approach will prove useful in acute iron ingestions in young children awaits trials. Also use of n-acetyl cysteine as an anti-oxidant in non-paracetamol induced acute liver failure is being studied.

Finally, in cholestatic liver disorders, possible pro-oxidant compounds are retained in the hepatocyte, such as copper and hydrophobic bile acids. These bile acids seem to be mitochondrial toxins, causing morphologic swelling of mitochondria, inhibition of normal respiration and electron flow through the respiratory chain, and increased H_2O_2 generation by mitochondria. The final consequences of bile acid toxicity consist of ATP depletion, increased intracellular cytosolic calcium levels, protease activation, and cell necrosis. Sokol and co-workers showed that *in vitro* anti oxidants (e.g. SOD catalase, deferoxamine, and alpha tocopherol) protect the isolated hepatocyte from hydrophobic bile acid toxicity. In addition vitamin E treatment to the intact rat prevents hepatic injury and oxidant damage to hepatic mitochondria after the intravenous infusion of taurochenodeoxycholic acid).

The possible role of anti-oxidant therapy in cholestasis is under investigation. It should be pointed out that the fat malabsorption cosequent to cholestasis leads to malabsorption and deficiency of vitamin E, betacartene and selenium. This perhaps sensitizes the hepatocyte to oxidative injury.

Table 42.8 lists the immunosuppressant medications that are commonly employed after the liver transplantation along with possible side-effects and proposed nutrition therapy.

Galactosemia

Metabolic defect: This genetic disease, also caused by a missing cell enzyme, galactose-1 phosphate uridyl transferase or galactokinase which affects carbohydrate

Table 42.8: Medications commonly used after liver transplantation

Immunosuppressant Drug	*Possible side-effects*	*Proposed nutrition therapy*
Azathioprine	Macrocytic anemia	Folate supplements
	Mouth sores	Soft foods if needed
	Nausea, vomiting, diarrhoea, anorexia, sore throat, stomach pain, decreased taste acuity	Adjust food/meals as needed, monitor intake
Antithymocyte globulin	Nausea, vomiting	Adjust food/meals as needed,monitor intake
Cyclosporine	Sodium retention	Decrease sodium intake
	Hyperkalemia	Decrease potassium intake
	Hyperlipidemia	Limit fat and simple carbohydrate intake
	Hyperglycemia	Decrease simple carbohydrate intake
	Decreased serum magnesium level	Increase magnesium intake; give magnesium supplement
	Nausea, vomiting	Adjust food/meals as needed; monitor intake
Glucocorticoids	Sodium retention	Decrease sodium intake
	Hyperglycemia	Decrease simple carbohydrate intake
	Hyperlipidemia	Limit fat and simple carbohydrate intake
	False hunger	Avoid overheating
	Protein wasting with high doses	Increase protein intake
	Decreased absorption of calcium and phosphorus	Increase calcium and phosphorus intake; give supplement as needed
Muromonab-CD3	Nausea, vomiting, anorexia	Adjust food/meals as needed; monitor intake
Mycophenolate mofetil	GL symptoms, nausea, vomiting diarrhoea	Adjust food/meals as needed; monitor intake
Sirolimus	Possible hyperglycemia	Decrease simple carbohydrate intake
	Possible GL symptoms	Adjust food/meals as needed; monitor intake
	Hyperlipidemia	Limit fat and simple carbohydrate intake
Tacrolimus	Hypertension	Adjust food/meals as needed; monitor intake
	Hyperglycemia	Decrease simple carbohydrate intake
	Hyperkalemia	Decrease potassium intake
	Nausea, vomiting	Adjust food/meals as needed; monitor intake
	GL symptoms (diarrhoea)	Adjust food/meals as needed; monitor intake
15-Deoxysperagualin	GL symptoms	Adjust food/meals as needed; monitor intake

Ref.: Hasse J. Role of the dietitian in the nutrition management of adults after liver transplantation J. Am Diet Assoc. 91:199.

metabolism. The missing enzyme controls the conversion of galactose, which is derived from lactose, to glucose. Milk, the infant's first food, contains a large amount of the precursor lactose (milk sugar). After galactose is initially combined with phosphate to begin the metabolic conversion to glucose, it cannot proceed further in the galactosemic infant. Galactose rapidly accumulates in the blood and in various body tissues.

Nutritional therapy—Galactose free diet

The main indirect source of dietary galactose is the lactose in milk. Therefore all forms of milk and lactose must be removed from the diet. In this instance a galactose free diet is used. Any needed amount of galactose for certain body structures can be synthesized by the body. A soy-base formula, is used. Breast-feeding, of course, cannot be used. Later, as solid foods are added to the infant's diet at about 6 months of age, careful attention must be given to avoiding lactose from other food sources. Parents quickly learn to check labels carefully on all commercial products to detect any lactose or lactose-containing substances.

Liver function improves following exclusion of galactose from the diet unless liver failure or cirrhosis has developed. Galactose elimination is lifelong. The long-term outcome is disappointing. Learning difficulties and growth disturbance are described, and 75% of girls develop ovarian failure. Detection of galactosemia in a neonatal screening program will lead to early detection except for infants who present with fulminant hepatitis. Antenatal diagnosis is possible by chorionic villus sampling.

(Williams, essentials of nutrition and diet therapy, 5th edition, times mirror/Mosby College Publishing, Pg. No. 454).

Hereditary Tyrosinaemia

This autosomal recessive disorder is due to lack of the enzyme fumaryl acetoacetate hydrolase, an enzyme that catalyses the last step of tyrosine degradation. Abnormal metabolites of tyrosine accumulate, which are toxic to both liver and kidney. The main clinical features are progressive live disease and renal tubular abnormalities.

The acute type, usually seen in early infancy, results in death from hepatic failure within the first year of life. The chronic form leads to growth retardation, cirrhosis, severe hypophosphatemic rickets, renal tubular defects and a derangement of tyrosine metabolism with hyperamino-acidaemia. Hepato-cellular carcinoma is a complication occurring in over 40% of patients.

The chronic type will respond to dietary avoidance of aromatic amino acids and methionine but this does not prevent the liver disease or the appearance of hepato-cellular carcinoma. Without liver transplantation death occurs within the first decade of life.

Diagnosis is confirmed by the presence of elevated plasma and urinary tyrosine, phenylalanine and methionine levels and increased levels of succinyl acetone in the urine.

Liver transplantation for both acute and chronic disease can be successful and virtually corrects the metabolic disease. A mild metabolic abnormality persists probably due to continued abnormal renal metabolism but this is not a clinical problem. Because of the high risk of hepato-cellular carcinoma with increasing age, liver transplantation should be seriously considered for children aged more than 2 years.[42]

Dietary treatment recommended for tyrosinemia is low phenylalanine and tyrosine diet.

Phenylalanine and tyrosine content in food items

Eat in moderation		*Avoid*		*Foods allowed freely*	
Beans	Orange	Meat	Chicken	Sugar	Spices
Beetroot	Pineapple	Lamb	Fish	Jam	Fruit juice
Cabbage	Apple	Eggs	Cheese	Squash	Soda
Cauliflower	Melon	Wheat	Wheat products	Cornflour	Custard
Carrot	Grapes	Spinach	Soya	Sago	Oils
Mushroom	Peach	Pulses	Dry fruits	Vinegar	
Cucumber	Pear	Jelly	Ice Cream		
Onion	Plum				
Radish	Banana				
Tomato	Turnip				
Milk	Potato				
Corn/wheat	Oats				
Rice	Peas				
Chocolate (milk)					

Hereditary Fructose Intolerance

This autosomal recessive condition is caused by mutations in the gene for aldolase B on chromosome 9[1]. Deficiency of this enzyme impairs the cleavage of fructose 1-phosphate in liver, renal cortex and intestinal epithelium. Exposure to fructose induces cytoplasmic accumulation of fructose 1-phosphate and hence fructose intoxication.[2]

The acute syndrome is marked by abdominal pain, vomiting and hypoglycemia. The chronic syndrome is one of severe metabolic derangement with failure to thrive, vomiting, hepatomegaly and liver and renal tubular dysfunction. Fructosemia, fructosuria and hypophosphatemia are features. Diagnosis is confirmed by the intravenous fructose tolerance test or by direct assay of fructaldolase activities in tissue biopsy samples. Hepatic histology shows similar findings to galactosemia with the ultimate development of cirrhosis.

Treatment is by a diet without sucrose and fructose. Sometimes the symptoms persist in older children and are marked by growth retardation when even more strict fructose restriction may be necessary.[43]

Older children learn to avoid fructose and sucrose and isolated hepatomegaly may be the only abnormality.

Familial Hypercholesterolaemia

This is an autosomal dominant disease due to absence of a gene which codes for the LDL receptor on cell membranes. The liver contains 60% of such receptors. Sufferers have increased plasma total cholesterol and LDL from birth, cutaneous xanthomas develop and most homozygotes die from coronary artery disease before the age of 30.

Hypercholesterolaemia is controlled by reduction in dietary saturated fats and administration of bile acid sequestrants such as cholestyramine. One child has been successfully treated by simultaneous heart transplant for the coronary disease and liver transplant to provide low-density lipoprotein receptors.[44] Follow-up showed decrease in LDL and plasma cholesterol.

Hepatic Porphyrias

Porphyrias are caused by defects in the biosynthesis of heam. Broadly they are classified as hepatic or erythropoietic depending on the major site in which there is excess production of porphyrin or its precursors. Lack of heam results in increased ALA and PBG production because of greater ALA-synthetase activity. The major symptoms and signs are from involvement of the skin and/or neurological system.

The acute hepatic porphyrias include acute intermittent porphyria, hereditary copropophyria and variegate porphyria, which have autosomal dominant inheritance. All are marked by neuropsychiatric attacks with vomiting, abdominal colic, constipation and peripheral neuropathy. All are exacerbated by countless enzyme-inducing drugs including barbiturates, sulphonamides, oestrogens, oral contraceptives, griseofulvin, chloroquine and possibly alcohol.

Hormones are impotrant inducers and women develop attacks in pregnancy and pre-mensturually.

During the attacks, large amounts of the colourless porphyrin precursors, porphobilinogen and delta amino-laevulinic acid (ALA), are excreted in the urine. In all three, an acute attack is treated by glucose loading. Infusions of haematin which repress or inhibit hepatic ALA synthetase may also be valuable.

Haem arginate which suppresses overproduction of haem precursors and improves hepatic oxidative metabolism may be useful.

The fourth type of hepatic porphyria, porphyric cutanea tarda, is probably hereditary and may be associated with hepato-cellular disease. It is not exacerbated by barbiturates and acute neurological attacks are not seen.

Hepato-cellular carcinoma occurs in 8% during long-term follow-up.

Glycogen Storage Disease

Salient Features

Stored sugar or glycogen cannot be accessed.
Infants cannot go for longer than 3-4 hours without feeding.
After 3-4 hours, hypoglycemia occurs.

Glycogen cannot be broken down but just accumulates in the liver, causing liver enlargement.

Some GSD types cannot be treated, while others are relatively easy to control through symptom management. In more severe cases, receiving an organ transplant is the only option. In the most severe cases, there are no available treatments and the victim dies within the first few years of life.

Of the treatable types of GSD, many are treated by manipulating the diet. The key to managing GSD I is to maintain consistent levels of blood glucose through a combination of nocturnal intragastric feeding (usually for infants and children), frequent high-carbohydrate meals during the day, and regular oral doses of cornstarch (people over age 2). Juvenile and adult forms of GSD II can be managed somewhat by a high protein diet, which also helps in cases of GSD III, GSD VI and GSD IX. GSD V and GSD VII can also be managed with a high protein diet and by avoiding strenuous exercise. Overnight continuous gastric high-carbohydrate feedings; frequent daytime feedings with energy distributed as 65% carbohydrate, 10% to 15% protein, and 25% fat; and supplements of uncooked cornstarch. In GSD III, though glycogenolysis is impeded, gluconeogenesis is enhanced to help maintain endogenous glucose production. In contrast to treatment for GSD I, advocated treatment for GSD III comprises frequent high-protein feedings during the day and a high-protein snack at night; energy is distributed as 45% carbohydrate, 25% protein, and 30% fat. Patients with GSD IV, VI and IX have benefited from high-protein diets similar to that recommended for patients with GSD III.

The recommended distribution of calories in GSD

	GSD-I	*GSD-II*
Protein	10-15	25%
Carbohydrate	65	45%
Fat	25	30%

Uncooked cornstarch is a complex carbohydrate that provides a slow and continuous glucose source and may delay gastric emptying. Uncooked cornstarch controlled the glucose shifts, resolved most of the symptoms, allowed bolus feedings, and enhanced weight gain in these children.

For GSD cases in which dietary therapy is ineffective, organ transplantation may be the only viable alternative. Liver transplants have been effective in reversing the symptoms of GSD IV.

Prognosis

People with well-managed, treatable types of GSD can lead long, relatively normal lives. This goal is accomplished with the milder types of GSD, such as Types VI, IX and X. As

Name		*Affected organs system*
Type O	Liver, muscle	Enlarged liver with accumulation of fat inside the liver cells (fatty liver); episodes of low blood sugar levels (hypoglycemia) when fasting
von Gierke's disease (Type IA)	Liver, kidney	Enlarged liver and kidney; slowed growth; very low blood sugar levles abnormally high levels of acid, fats, and uric acid in blood
Type IB	Liver, white blood cells	Same as in von Gierke's disease but may be less severe; low white blood cell count; recurring mouth and intestinal infections or Crohn's disease
Pompe's disease (Type II)	All organs	Enlarged liver and heart, muscle weakness
Forbes' disease (Type III)	Liver, muscle, heart, white blood cells	Enlarged liver or cirrhosis; low blood sugar levels, muscle damage and heart damage in some people
Andersen's disease (Type IV)	Liver, muscle, most tissues	Cirrhosis in juvenile type; muscle damage and heart failure in adult (late-onset) type
McArdle disease (Type V)	Muscle	Muscle cramps or weakness during physical activity
Hers' disease (Type VI)	Liver	Enlarged liver; episodes of low blood sugar when fasting; often no symptoms
Tarui' disease (Type VII)	Skeletal muscle, red blood cells	Muscle cramps during physical activity; red blood cell destruction (hemolysis)

the GSD type becomes more severe, a greater level of vigilance against infections and other complications is required.

Wilson disease: Normal daily dietary intake of copper is 4 mg of which 2 mg is absorbed and excreted in bile, so that body maintains balance. In Wilson disease only 0.2 to 0.4 mg can be excreted in bile with 1 mg in the urine so that a positive copper balance develops. Diet in Wilson disease should be of low copper.

Indian childhood cirrhosis (ICC): ICC though rare these days is strongly associated with habit of storage and or boiling of milk in copper or brass utensils. Stoppage of use of copper and brass utensils and low copper diet are recommended apart from standard therapy.

Copper content of diet

> 0.1 mg/portion	*0.1 portion*
High to moderate copper rich food	Commonly use low copper food
Avoid	Eat
All organ meal	Beef, Cheese, Paners, eggs, all dairy products
Soya milks, cocoa soyabeans, lentils and pulses, wheat germ, bran, mushroom	Bread, pastas, wheat flour, all other vegetables except mushrooms all other dried fruits
Dried fruits–raisins, dates, prunes	Lemonade
Mango, pineapple, papaye	Jams, gellies, candies, made from allowed fruits
Mineral water, alcohol chocolates	

Medium-chain triglycerides (MCTs)

Medium-chain triglycerides (MCTs) contain only fatty acids with 6-12 carbon atoms. They are rare in nature. They have been fractionated from coconut oil. They are composed of :

75% caprylic acid (8 C)
22-23% caprylic acid (10 C)
1% caprylic acid (6 C)
1% caprylic acid (12 C)

Traces of other fatty acids such as linoleic, stearic, and palmitic acids are also present.

Importance of MCTs

Since MCTs are liquid at room temperature, they are more soluble in water than natural triglycerides. MCTs are easily digested by pancreatic lipase and do not require bile salts for absorption. Once absorbed, they enter the portal vein and into the liver as fatty acids and do not go through the lacteal system.

Synthetic MCTs are also popular in the treatment of intestinal diseases, especially malabsorption such as steatorrhea, sprue and pancreatic insufficiency. They are a ready source of energy and prevent starvation from lack of absorbed calories.

Uses of MCTs

1. When pancreatic enzymes and/or bile salts are either absent or present in very small amounts.
2. When the lymphatic system has an obstruction especially in the branches leaving the intestinal walls.
3. When the intestinal mucosa is infective.

Problems of MCT Therapy

Because MCTs are easily absorbed, any excessive consumption forces their increased degradation. As a result, formation of acetone, acetoacetic acid and hydroxbutyric acid may increase and acidosis may occur. Patients susceptible to hepatic encephalopathy may react adversely to MCTs that reach the liver directly from the gut.

All vitamins especially the B-complex vitamins should be given in plenty. Sodium may be restricted if swelling is seen. There are restrictions on spices, chillies and oily preparations.

Nutrients and Nutriceuticals

The importance of the liver in the metabolism of ingested nutrients and drugs suggests that hepatic function can be influenced by dietary manipulations. Less obvious is the potential role of specific nutrients in ameliorating the natural history of various chronic liver diseases or toxic exposures. Preliminary evidence supports the use of several nutriceutical agents in the treatment of liver diseases for which conventional therapies are limited.

Silymarin

Silymarin is derived from the seeds of Sily-bum marianum (milk thistle). The extract contains a group of chemical compounds in the flavonoid family. There is a long history of its use in traditional medical systems for treatment of liver disease and manifestations of portal hypertension .[45]

The hepatoprotective effects of silymarin have been demonstrated in animal studies and in cell culture, the principal mechanism of which appears to be the prevention of lipid peroxidation. A randomized trial in patients with alcoholic cirrhosis reported no benefit with regard to either clinical course of the disease of survival of patients over 3 years.[46] The authors of this trial noted the possibility of benefit in patients with hepatitis C, as well as the possibility that the trial was underpowered to detect a clinically meaningful survival benefit.

Cell culture study suggests that silymarin acts independently of the cytochrome P-450 enzyme system, with free radical scavenging the dominant action accounting for hepatoprotection. The possibility of toxic effects on the hepatocyte membrane and cytoskeleton is suggested and requires further investigation.

Antifibrotic effects of silymarin have been shown in a rat model suggesting a role in cirrhosis.[47]

Evidence supporting a role for silymarin in viral hepatitis, drug-induced and toxin-induced hepatitis, and alcoholic liver disease has been summarized.[48] To date, there is no evidence of toxicity in humans. Well controlled studies of silymarin are small and the populations studied heterogeneous, the historical experience and promising results from studies to date indicate a need for additional well-controlled trials.

Branched-chain Amino Acids

Impairment in amino acid metabolism in cirrhosis results in accumulation of aromatic ring amino acids and depletion of branched chain amino acids. An imbalance in the amino acid distribution has been implicated in the development of hepatic encephalopathy.[49]

Impairment in amino acid metabolism in cirrhosis results in accumulation of aromatic ring amino acids and depletion of branched-chain amino acids. An imbalance in the amino acid distribution has been implicated in the development of hepatic encephalopathy. There is preliminary evidence that supplementation with branched-chain amino acids benefits patients with chronic hepatic encephalopathy.

Branched-chain Ketoacids

The ketoacid analogues of branched-chain amino acids offer the putative advantage of providing a substrate for protein synthesis devoid of the amine group. Metabolic advantages of such preparations have been well described, but the evidence of clinical benefit in advanced liver disease is limited. Use of branched-chain ketoacids in patients intolerant of standard protein is reasonable in light of available evidence, although additional study of this intervention is needed.

Vegetable Protein

Benefits from a diet deriving protein from plant sources have been reported to reduce the incidence of hepatic encephalopathy in patients with cirrhosis. Such diets often are poorly tolerated, however, because of their high fiber and high total food volume. To the extent that protein derived from plant sources is tolerated by individual patients, its use is reasonable.[50]

Glutamine

Glutamine is a nonessential amino acid. Because of abnormal intestinal permeability, endotoxemia in cirrhosis accelerates turnover of skeletal muscle. Glutamine is the predominant amino acid in muscle, and its consumption in cirrhosis may result in the need for dietary replacement. Although plausible, the benefits of glutamine supplementation are unproved.

Amino Acids

Cysteine and tyrosine are no essential amino acids the synthesis of which hepatocytes is impaired in chronic liver disease. Inclusion of these amino acids in the diet may become essential when liver disease is advanced.

Vitamins and Trace Elements

Reduction in the serum levels of zinc and selenium attributable to chronic liver disease has been reported in patients with chronic hepatitis C, with or without cirrhosis. Zinc supplementation has been shown to improve hepatic encephalopathy in alcoholic patients. Zinc is also recommended in few subsets of Wilson disease. Thiamine supplementation is indicated in all alcoholic patients.

Use of a multivitamin supplement is advocated for all patients with chronic liver disease.[51]

SUMMARY

Malnutrition is a nearly universal component of chronic liver disease in children. Causal factors are multi-factorial so that careful nutritional assessment, identification of important risk factors, and specific deficiency states and/or excessive losses are essential to good management and for achievement of nutritional rehabilitation. Attention to the limited ability of the child with chronic liver disease to withstand a prolonged fast, plus alleviation and treatment of ascites or infection, which may increase energy expenditure or precipitate nutritional deficiencies, are essential. The increased success of programs for pediatric liver transplantation has demonstrated the importance of good nutritional rehabilitation prior to transplantation: the pretransplant nutritional status appears to impact on postoperative morbidity, expense, time in hospital and most importantly, survival.

REFERENCES

1. Romijn JA, Klein S: Extrahepatic metabolic consequences of cirrhosis. *Gastroenterology* 1992;102:2175.
2. Italian Multicentre Cooperative Project on Nutrition in Liver Cirrhosis. Nutritional status in cirrhosis. *J Hepatol* 1994;21: 317-25.
3. Merli M, Riggio O, Dally L, Nutrizione PI. Cirrhosis. Does malnutrition affect survival in cirrhosis ? *Hepatology* 1996;23: 1041-1046.
4. Child CG, Turcotte JG. Surgery and portal hypertension. In: Child CG (ed): *The Liver and Portal Hypertension*, 3rd edn. Philadelphia: Saunders 1964: 50-51.
5. Hellerstein MK, Munro HN. Interaction of liver and muscle in the regulation of metabolism in response to nutritional and other factors. In: Arias IM, Jacoby WB Popper H, Schacter D, Schafritz DA (eds): *The Liver Biology and Pathobiology*, 2nd edn. New York: Raven Press 1988.
6. Sokol RJ, Stall C. Anthropometric evaluation of children with chronic liver disease. *Am J Clin Nutr* 1990; 52:203-208.
7. Hehir DJ, Jenkins RL, Bistrian BR. Blackbrun GL. Nutrition in patients undergoing orthotopic liver transplant. *J Parenter Enteral Nutr* 1985;9:695-700.
8. Hasse J. Nutritional aspects of liver transplantation. In: Busuttil RW, Klintamal GB (eds): *Transplantation of the Liver*. Philadelphia: WB Saunders: 1996:359.

9. Deitz WH. Nutritional requirements and feeding of the handicapped child. In:Grand RJ, Sutphen JL, Dietz WH (eds): *Pediatric Nutrition: Theory and Practice*. Boston: Butterworth 1987; 387-392.
10. Merritt RJ. Nutritional requirements. In: Walker WA, *et al.* (eds): Pediatric gastrointestinal disease, pathophysiology, diagnosis management, vol 2. Philadelphia: BC Decher 1991; 1579-1596.
11. Himsworth HP, Glynn LE. Massive hepatic necrosis and diffuse hepatic fibrosis acute yellow atrophy and portal cirrhosis: Their production by means of diet. *Clin. Sci* 1944; 5: 93.
12. Sherlock S. Nutrition and the Alcoholic. *Lancet* 1984;1: 436.
13. Sherlock S, Walshe VM. *Studies of Undernutrition*, Wuppertal. London: Medical Research Council 1951:111-113.
14. Waterlow JC, Cravioto J, Stephen JML. Protein malnutrition in man. *Adv Protein Chem* 1960; 15 : 130-133.
15. Poonawala A, Nair SP, Thuluvath PJ. Prevalence of obesity and diabetes in patients with cryptogenic cirrhosis: A case-control study. *Hepatology* 2000;32:689-692.
16. Ratziu V, Giral P, Charlotte F, *et al.* Liver fibrosis in overweight patients. *Gastroenterology* 2000;118:1117-23.
17. Ratziu V, Bonyhay L, Di Martino V, *et al.* Survival, liver failure, and hepatocellular carcinoma in obesity related cryptogenic cirrhosis. *Hepatology* 2002;36:150-155.
18. Nair S, Mason A, Eason J, Loss G, Perrillo RP. Is obesity an independent risk factor for hepatocellular carcinoma in cirrhosis. *Hepatology* 2002;36:150-155.
19. Nair S, Verma S, Thuluvath PJ. Obesity and its effect on survival in patients undergoing orthotopic liver transplantation in the United States. *Hepatology* 2002;35:105-109.
20. Peden VH, Witzleben CL, Skelton MA.Total parenteral nutrition. *J Pediatr* 1971; 78:180-185.
21. Roslyn JJ, Pitt HA, Mann LL, *et al.* Gallbladder disease in patients on long-term parenteral nutrition. *Gastroenterology* 1983; 84:148.
22. Pitt HA, Lewinski MA, Muller EL, *et al.* Ileal resection-induced gallstones: Altered bilirubin or cholesterol metabolism? Surgery 1984; 96:154.
23. Roslyn JJ, Den Besten L, Thompson JE Jr. Effects of periodic emptying of gallbladder on gallbladder function and formation of cholesterol gallstones. *Surg Forum* 1979; 30:403-406.
24. Sitzmann JV, Pitt HA, Steinborn PA, *et al.* Cholecystokinin prevents parenteral nutrition induced biliary sludge in humans. *Surg Gynecol Obstet* 1990;170:25.
25. Friis, H., and Andreasen, P. B. Drug-induced hepatic injury: An analysis of 1100 case reports to The Danish Committee on Adverse Drug Reactions between 1978 and 1987. *J. Int. Med* 1992; 232:133.
26. Farrell, G.C., Bhathal, P.S., and Powell, L.W. Abnormal liver function in chronic hypervitaminosis A. *Am. J Dig. Dis 1977;* 22:724.
27. Geubel AP, De Galoesy, C., Alves, N, *et al.* Liver damage caused by therapeutic vitamin A administration: Estimation of dose—related toxicity in 41 cases. *Gastroenterology* 1991; 100:1701-1702.
28. Sokol RJ, Stall C. Anthropometric evaluation of children with chronic liver disease. Am J Clin Nutr 1990;52:203-208.
29. Kaufman SS, Murray ND, Wood P, Shaw BW, Vanderhoof JA. Nutritional support for the infant with extrahepatic biliary atresia. *J Pediatr* 1987; 110:697-686.
30. Weber FL, Bagby BS, Licate L, Kelsen SG. Effects of branched-chain amino acids on nitrogen metabolism in patients with cirrhosis. *Hepatology* 1990:11:1942-950.
31. Linscheer WG, Vergroesen AJ. Lipids. In: Shils ME, Young VR (eds): *Modern Nutrition in Health and Disease*. Philadelphia: Lea nad Febiger 1988: 72-107.
32. Kaufman SS, Murray ND, Wood P, Shaw BW, Vanderhoof JA. Nutritional support for the infant with extrahepatic biliary atresia. *J Pediatr* 1987; 110:697-686.
33. Sharma R. *Diet Management*, 3rd edn. New Delhi: Elsevier 1995: 21-23.
34. Gupte S, Anderson RA. Pediatric hepatology. In: Gupte S (ed): *The Short Textbook of Pediatrics*, 11th edn. New Delhi: Jaypee 2004:481-504.
35. Hasse JM, Blue LS, Liepa GU, *et al.* Early enteral nutrition support in patients undergoing liver transplantation. *J Parenter Enteral Nutr* 1995; 19: 437-438.
36. Le Cornu KA, McKiernan FJ, Kapadia SA, Neuberger JM. A prospective randomized study of preoperative nutritional supplementation in patients awaiting elective orthotopic liver transplantation. *Transplantation* 2000; 69:1364-1371.
37. Fan ST, Lo CM, Lai ECS, *et al.* J. Perioperative nutritional support in patients undergoing hepatectomy for hepatocellular carcinoma. *N Eng J Med* 1994; 331:1547-1548.
38. Rosser BG, Gores GJ . Liver cell necrosis: Cellular mechanisms and clinical implications. *Gastroenterology* 1995;108:252-275.
39. Sanchez-Urdazpal L, Gores GJ, Lemasters JJ, *et al.* The Carolina rinse solution decrease liver injury during clinical liver transplantation. *Transplant Proc* 1993; 25:1574-1575.
40. Lieber CS . Alcohol and the liver: 1994 update. *Gastroenterology* 1994;106: 1085-1105.
41. Shamieh I, Kibort PK, Suchy FJ, *et al.* Antioxidant therapy for neonatal iron storage disease (NISD). (Abstract) *Pediatr Res* 1993; 33:109A.
42. Editorial Hereditary Tyrosinemia, *Lancet* 1990; 335: 1500.
43. Mock Dm, Perman JA Thaler Mmetal Chronic fructose intoxication after infancy in children with hereditary fructose intolerance: A cause of growth retardation. *N Engl J Med* 1983;309:764.
44. Starzl TE, Bilheimer DW, Bahnson HT *et al.* Heart-liver transplantation in a patient with familial hypercholesterolaemia. Lancet 1984; i : 1382-1384.
45. Utrilla MP. Natural products with hepatoprotecting action. *Meth Find Exp Clin Pharmacol* 1996. 18 [suppl]:11-20.
46. Pares A, Planas R, Torres M *et al.* Effects of silimarin in alcoholic patients with cirrhosis of the liver results of a controlled, double-blind, randomised and multicenter trial. *J Hepatol* 1998:28:615-616.
47. Boigk G, Stroedter L, herbst H, *et al.* Silymarin biliary fibrosis secondary to complete bile duct obliteration in rats. *Hepatology* 1997;26:643-645.
48. Flora *K, Hahn M, Rosen H, et al. Milk thistle (Silybum marianum) for the therapy of liver disease. Am J Gastroenterol* 1998;93: 139-140.
49. Siriboonkoom W, Gramlich L, Nutrition and chronic liver disease. *Can J Gastroenterol* 1998, 12:201-209.
50. Munoz SJ. Nutritional therapies in liver disease *Semin Liver Dis* 1991;11:278-281-289.
51. Levinson MJ. A practical approach to nutritional support in liver disease. *Gastroenterologist* 1995;3:234-236.

Kara Feigenbaum

43 Nutritional Management of Diabetes in Children

INTRODUCTION

Diabetes mellitus is a chronic disease in which the body does not make or properly use insulin, a hormone needed to convert glucose to energy. Worldwide, the prevalence of diabetes was estimated to be 2.8% in 2000 with projections of 4.4% in 2030.[1] The increasing number of diabetes cases can be attributed to an aging population, urbanization, obesity, and physical inactivity.

Type 1 diabetes, which affects approximately 10% of the diabetic population, is usually caused by an autoimmune destruction of the beta cell resulting in insulin deficiency. Decreased tissue sensitivity to insulin and inadequate beta cell function characterize type 2 diabetes, which accounts for 90% of diabetes cases. Type 1 is primarily diagnosed in childhood and adolescence. It is one of the most common and increasingly prevalent chronic diseases in the pediatric population.[2,3] Progressively more problematic, however, is the rapidly growing number of children developing type 2 diabetes worldwide.[4]

Consistent diet and lifestyle modification is key for both type 1 and type 2 diabetes in prevention of such long-term complications as neuropathy, retinopathy, nephropathy, peripheral vascular disease, hyperlipidemia, hypertension, atherosclerosis, and coronary artery disease. A multidisciplinary team approach to diabetes education and treatment is recommended. Ideally, this would include a physician, diabetes educator, social worker, psychologist and dietitian trained in the care of children with diabetes.[5] With support and involvement from family and diabetes team, children and adolescents can improve and maintain metabolic control through self-management.[6,7] Consideration of the patient's age, eating patterns and food preferences, physical activity, past medical history, school or work schedule, home environment, personality, and cultural factors should all be integrated into education process.[5]

NUTRITIONAL GOALS

Box 43.1 summarizes the goals of diet in diabetes mellitus.

Box 43.1: Nutrition goals for diabetes management

- Achieve normal growth and development.
- Maintain healthy weight.
- Maintain optimal blood pressure, blood glucose and lipid levels to help prevent/delay both short- and long-term medical problems and complications.

Energy

The diet for diabetes focuses on providing adequate energy to achieve or maintain a healthy and realistic body weight and support growth. Caloric requirements are personalized, based on weight, height, ideal body weight, activity level, and average energy allowance. Several predictive equations are available to calculate calorie needs in children. Indirect calorimetry may also be helpful in the obese population.

Carbohydrates

Carbohydrates are the primary energy fuel source for the body. They make up approximately 50-60% of caloric intake and supply 4 calories per gram. Types of carbohydrates include sugar, starch and fiber. Carbohydrates have the greatest influence on blood glucose levels. Glycemic response most closely reflects the total amount of carbohydrates consumed. Although dietary carbohydrate increases postprandial blood glucose levels, eliminating carbohydrates from the diet in diabetes will not maintain blood glucose levels in the normal range, since glucose will be produced by the body from protein and fat if dietary carbohydrate intake is restricted. The brain and central nervous system and several other body organs depend on a steady supply of glucose for fuel. Carbohydrate-containing foods are also the most important dietary source of fiber and water-soluble vitamins and minerals. Restricting total carbohydrate intake to <130 grams is not recommended.

Protein

Protein provides about 10-20% of total calories in the diabetic diet. One gram of protein supplies 4 calories. Adequate intake is needed for growth, development, maintenance of lean body mass, and cell function and metabolism. Although protein is not the primary stimulus for insulin release, it does augment insulin release when ingested with a carbohydrate, increasing glucose clearance from blood in type 2 diabetics.[8]

Fat and Cholesterol

Fat makes up approximately 30% of total calories and provides 9 calories per gram. Of the 30%, no more than 10% should come from saturated and trans fats, upto 10% should come from polyunsaturated sources, and 10-15% from monounsaturated fat.[9] Dietary fat is needed to supply energy and essential fatty acids, and for absorption of fat-soluble vitamins. In diabetes management, fat affects blood glucose response by delaying the glucose peak when ingesting a mixed fat and carbohydrate meal.[10] Because of the increased risk of cardiovascular disease in diabetes, it is recommended that cholesterol and triglyceride levels be maintained as near to normal range as possible. Dietary fat goals should focus on decreasing intake of saturated and trans fats by limiting fast foods and convenience foods and choosing lean protein sources. Use of monounsaturated fats such as peanut, olive, and canola oils are encouraged to replace saturated and trans fats in the diet. Overall fat restriction may be necessary to decrease total caloric intake when weight loss is needed. National Cholesterol Education Program (NCEP) guidelines recommend restriction of saturated fat to <7% of total calories and cholesterol intake <200 mg/dl for treatment of elevated LDL cholesterol levels (Box 43.2).[9]

Box 43.2: Consensus guidelines for diagnosis of dyslipidemia in children[9]

Total Cholesterol	Borderline ≥170 mg/dL Abnormal ≥200 mg/dL
LDL Cholesterol	Borderline ≥100 mg/dL Abnormal ≥130 mg/dL
HDL Cholesterol	Abnormal <40 mg/dL
Triglycerides	Abnormal ≥200 mg/dL

Fiber

Fiber is an important dietary component in blood glucose and cholesterol control. Fiber is a category of carbohydrates that are not fully digested or absorbed. There are two types of fiber, soluble and insoluble. Gum, mucilage, and pectin comprise soluble fiber, which bind to fatty substances in the gut and are excreted through the stool. Consuming soluble fiber has been proven to lower cholesterol and LDL levels.[11] Insoluble fiber, including cellulose, hemicellulose, and lignan, add bulk to foods, which may help with satiety for weight management. Insoluble fiber also plays a key role in bowel regularity. Recommended fiber intake for children over age 2 is (age in years + 5 grams) however individualized recommendations are warranted for children who are at high risk of or already have diseases or conditions that may require adjustments in dietary fiber intake.[12]

Non-nutritive Sweeteners

Also referred to as "sugar substitutes" or "artificial sweeteners", the non-nutritive sweeteners provide a sweet taste to foods with little or no effect on blood sugar levels. Common non-nutritive sweeteners include saccharin, aspartame, acesulfame potassium (or acesulfame K), sucralose, and neotame. In a position statement by the American Dietetic Association, it was concluded that both children and adults can safely enjoy a range of nutritive and nonnutritive sweeteners when consumed in a diet that is guided by current federal nutrition recommendations as well as individual health goals.[13] In a recent study of children with type 1 diabetes, intake of nonnutritive sweeteners was common, but risk of excessive intake was low.[14]

In addition to its minimal effect on blood glucose levels, non-nutritive sweeteners also provide little to no calories. As part of a healthy, low fat diet, replacement of concentrated sugar beverages with those containing non-nutritive sweeteners are recommended for diabetic and obese children.

Sugar alcohols, or polyols, are another form of low calorie sweetener. Sugar alcohols include sorbitol, mannitol, xylitol, erythritol, lactitol, maltitol, isomalt, maltitol syrup, and hydrogenated starch hydrolysates. Most sugar alcohols provide approximately 2 calories per gram and should be counted as providing half the calories by weight of other carbohydrates when carbohydrate counting. Sugar alcohols are absorbed slowly and incompletely from the intestine by passive diffusion. Therefore, amounts greater than 50 grams of sorbitol and or 20 grams of mannitol should be avoided in children due to its laxative effect.

ASSESSMENT OF FOOD NEEDS

Glycemic Index

The glycemic index (GI) is a concept that assesses foods based on postprandial blood glucose response. It is defined as the area under the glucose response curve after consumption of a 50 gram carbohydrate containing test food divided by the area under the curve after consumption of 50 grams of carbohydrate from a control food (white bread or glucose).[15] Factors determining the glycemic index of a food include carbohydrate type and variety,[16] fiber,[17] protein,[18] fat[19] and method of preparation and storage.[20,21] The usefulness of glycemic index in the treatment of diabetes has been controversial. In a recent meta-analysis, a low GI diet was shown to improve blood glucose control and decrease total cholesterol and triglycerides in subjects with type 2 diabetes.[22]

Carbohydrate Counting

Carbohydrate counting is a flexible and effective way to allow a variety of foods to fit into the meal plan of children with diabetes.[23] When counting carbohydrates, it is important to look at the portion size and total grams of carbohydrate in the product. Use of measuring cups and spoons are recommended to ensure accurate portion size. Reference books and food labels are used to obtain number of grams in a specific food or beverage.

TREATMENT STRATEGIES FOR TYPE 1 DIABETES

Meal planning for children with type 1 diabetes is highly individualized, based on lifestyle and insulin regimen. Use of rapid acting insulin with meals and long acting background insulin is a popular and effective treatment option in the pediatric population.[24] Also referred to as a multiple daily injection (MDI) regimen, children are allowed more flexibility in the number of carbohydrates consumed and the timing of consumption than with traditional diabetes management plans. A dose of rapid acting insulin is given with each meal, calculated using a personalized insulin to carbohydrate ratio, along with a correction formula, or sliding scale, to cover premeal hyperglycemia. Children on this regimen are required to check blood sugar before each meal and at bedtime. Use of a correction formula and insulin to carbohydrate ratio (Table 43.1) are also used for continuous subcutaneous insulin infusion (CSII) regimens.

For those children who wish to initiate MDI and CSII therapy they or their caregiver must be able to accurately count carbohydrates and measure and weigh portions, demonstrate adequate math skills for calculating insulin dose, and be willing to keep a blood sugar log to assess trends.[25]

Plasma blood glucose and A1C goals for type 1 diabetes by age group are given in Table 43.2.

For children whose diabetes is being managed according to a more traditional regimen, such as twice-daily injections of a combination of intermediate- and rapid-acting insulins, consistent carbohydrate intake is stressed to maintain normoglycemia. These children work with a dietitian to develop daily carbohydrate goals based on calorie requirements. The total number of carbohydrates suggested is then distributed throughout the day for meals and snacks.

TREATMENT STRATEGIES FOR TYPE 2 DIABETES

There is a direct correlation between the increasing incidence of obesity and type 2 diabetes in children and adolescents.[26,27] Impaired glucose tolerance associated with insulin resistance is common.[28] Children who are obese are more likely to become obese adults and parental obesity more than doubles the risk of adult obesity among both obese and nonobese children under 10 years of age.[29] Strategies for prevention and treatment of obesity and type 2 diabetes focus on lifelong healthy food choices,[30] portion control,[31,32] and physical activity.[33] Education should be aimed at both child and family, rather than child alone.[34,35]

Table 43.1: Determining insulin dose using insulin: Carbohydrate ratio and correction formula

Sample Meal	*Grams (g) of carbohydrate*	
8 oz juice	27 g	Premeal blood sugar: 320
Bagel	60 g	Sample insulin to carb ratio: 1:15
1 tbsp butter	0 g	Sample correction formula:
4 oz milk	6 g	Blood sugar–120/50
8 oz coffee	0 g	
Total carbs consumed:	93 g	

Units of insulin to cover blood sugar: 320 – 120/50 = 4 units
Units of insulin to cover meal: 93/15 = 6.2 units
Total insulin dose: 4 + 5.2 = 10.2 or 10 units

Table 43.2: Plasma blood glucose and A1C goals for type 1 diabetes by age group[5]

	Plasma blood glucose goal range (mg/dl)		
Values by Age	*Before meals*	*After meals*	*A1C(%)*
Toddlers and preschoolers (<6 years)	100-180	110-200	<8.5(but >7.5)
School age (6-12 years)	90-180	100-180	<8
Adolescents and young adults (13-19 years)	90-130	90-150	<7.5 (or <7.0 if achieved without excessive hypoglycemia)

When evaluating patients with type 2 diabetes, a thorough diet history should be obtained. It is important to assess the child's usual food intake, eating behaviors, and family eating habits.

Treatment strategies are personalized, based on diet and pharmacological therapies. Children are often instructed on how to count carbohydrates and maintain a consistent carbohydrate intake throughout the day. Portion control should be stressed, focusing on appropriate portion sizes for age. Calorie restriction may be needed to attain and maintain a healthy weight. Recent studies by Gannon *et al.* have shown an improved glycemic response and decreased glycosylated hemoglobin levels when a lower carbohydrate, higher protein diet is consumed by type 2 diabetics. No significant change in renal function was noted.[36, 37] A carbohydrate to protein to fat ratio of 40:30:30 may be favorable. However, caution must be exercised in generalizing the findings of adult studies with type 2 diabetes to children. Long-term studies are also warranted.

Physical activity, in conjunction with diet modification, is essential for type 2 diabetes management to achieve a healthful weight and increase insulin sensitivity. A recently published study showed that obese pediatric subjects who participated in an interdisciplinary nutrition, exercise, and behavioral program demonstrated a prolonged decrease in weight, body mass index, body fat, total cholesterol and LDL levels at three months and one year. Subjects also showed continued physical activity participation in the 12 months following the study.

During the 3-month intervention, subjects and parents attended four lectures on childhood obesity, general nutrition, a therapeutic nutritional approach for childhood obesity, and exercise. Participants met with the dietitian six times and received a balanced hypocaloric diet. Participants also took part in a twice-weekly training program and were instructed to add an extra 30 to 45 minutes of walking or other weight-bearing sport activity at least once per week.[33-38]

SUMMARY AND CONCLUSIONS

The diet for diabetes parallels a healthy diet for all people in amounts and types of nutrients consumed. Intake of fruits, vegetables, whole grains, low fat and nonfat dairy products, beans, fish, and lean meat is recommended.[38] Saturated and trans fats should be replaced with monounsaturated sources whenever possible. Non-nutritive sweeteners are most beneficial when used to replace calorie-dense and nutrient-diluted products such as soda and fruit flavored beverages. Convenience foods should be limited and portion control is stressed to avoid excessive weight gain and achieve normal linear growth. Teaching strategies for nutrition are individualized based on each patient's treatment goals and desired outcomes. The education process should include both child and caregiver.

Section 10

REFERENCES

1. Wild S, Roglic G, Green A, Sicree R, King H. Global Prevalence of Diabetes. *Diabetes Care* 2004;27:1047-1053.
2. LaPorte R, Matsushima M, Chang Y. Prevalence and incidence of insulin dependent diabetes. In: *Diabetes in America*, 2nd edn. Washington, DC: National Institutes of Health, NIDDK 1995:37-46.
3. Onkanmo P, Vaananen S, Karnoven M, Tuomilehto J. Worldwide increase in incidence of type 1 diabetes: The analysis of the data on published incident trends. *Diabetologia* 1999;42: 1395-1403.
4. Fagot-Campagna A. Emergence of type 2 diabetes mellitus in children. *J Pediatr Endocrinol Metab* 2000;13(Suppl 6):1395-1402.
5. American Diabetes Association: Standards of Medical Care in Diabetes. *Diabetes Care* 2005; 28(Suppl 1): S4-S36.
6. Anderson B, Ho J, Brackett J, Finkelstein D, Laffel L. Parental involvement in diabetes management tasks: Relationships to blood glucose monitoring adherence and metabolic control in young adolescents with insulin dependent diabetes mellitus. *J Pediatr* 2005;130: 257-265.
7. Wolfsdorf J. Improving Diabetes control in adolescents. *Diabetes Care* 2005;22: 1767-1768.
8. Floyd J, Fajans S, Pek S, Thiffault C, Knopf R, Conn J. Synergistic effect of essential amino acids and glucose upon insulin secretion in man. *Diabetes* 1970;19: 109-115.
9. *National Cholesterol Education Program*. Place: The National Heart, Lung and Blood Institute (NHLBI).
10. Collier G, McLean A, O'Dea K. Effect of coingestion of fat on the metabolic responses to slowly and rapidly absorbed carbohydrates. *Diabetologia* 1984;26: 50-54.
11. Brown L, Rosner B, Willett W, Sacks F. Cholesterol-lowering effects of dietary fiber: A meta-analysis. *Am J Clin Nutr* 1999;69: 30-42.
12. Williams C, Bollella M, Wynder E. A New Recommendation for Dietary Fiber in Childhood. *Pediatrics* 1995;96: 985-988.
13. American Dietetic Association Position Statement. Use of nutritive and nonnutritive sweeteners. *Journal of the American Dietetic Association* 2004;104: 255-275.
14. Garnier-Sagne I, Leblanc J, Verger P. Calculation of the intake of three intense sweeteners in young insulin-dependent diabetics. *Food Chem Toxicol* 2001;39:745-749.
15. Jenkins D, Thomas D, Wolever T, *et al*. Glycemic index of foods: A physiological basis for carbohydrate exchange. *Am J Clin Nutr* 1981;34: 362-366.
16. Wolever T, Bolognesi C. Prediction of glucose and insulin responses of normal subject after consuming mixed meals varying in energy, protein, fat, carbohydrate and glycemic index. *J Nutr* 1996;126: 2807-2812.
17. Bjorck I, Granfeldt Y, Liljeberg H, Tovar J, Asp N. Food properties affecting the digestion and absorption of carbohydrates. *A J Clin Nutr* 1994; 59: 699S-705S.
18. Krezowski PA, Nuttall FQ, Gannon MC, Bartosh NH. The effect of protein ingestion on the metabolic response to oral glucose in normal individuals. *Am J Clin Nutr* 1986;44: 847-856.
19. Welch I, Bruce C, Hill S, Read N. Duodenal and ileal lipid suppresses postprandial blood glucose and insulin response in man: Possible implications for the dietary management of diabetes mellitus. *Clin Sci* 1987;74: 209-219.

20. Thorne MJ, Thompson LU, Jenkins D. Factors affecting starch digestibility and the glycemic response with special reference to legumes. *A J Clin Nutr* 1983;38: 481-488.
21. Foster-Powell K, Miller J. International tables of glycemic index. *Am J Clin Nutrition* 1995;62: 871S-890S.
22. Opperman A, Venter C, Oosthuizen W, Thompson R, Vorster H. Meta-analysis of the health effects of using the glycemic index in meal planning. *Br J Nutr* 2004;92: 367-381.
23. The DCCT Research Group. Nutrition interventions for intensive therapy in the diabetes control and complications trial. *J Am Dietet Assoc* 1993;93: 768-772.
24. Alemzadeh R, Ellis J, Holzum M, Parton E, Wyatt D. Beneficial effects of continuous subcutaneous insulin infusion and flexible multiple daily insulin regimen using insulin glargine in type 1 diabetes. *Pediatrics* 2004;114: e91-e95.
25. Gillespie S, Kulkarni K, Daily A. Using carbohydrate counting in diabetes clinical practice. *Journal of the American Dietetic Association* 1998;98: 897-905.
26. Pinhas-Hamiel O, Dolan L, Daniels S, Standiford D, Khoury P, Zeitler P. Increased incidence of non-insulin dependent diabetes mellitus among adolescents. *J Pediatr* 1996;128 (5 Pt 1):608-615.
27. Rosenbloom A, Roe J, Young R, Winter W. Emerging epidemic of type 2 diabetes in youth. *Diabetes Care* 1999;22: 345-354.
28. Sinha R, Fisch G, Teague B, Tamborlan W, *et al*. Prevalence of impaired glucose tolerance among children and adolescents with marked obesity. *N* Engl J Med 2004;346: 802-810.
29. Whitaker R, Wright J, Pepe M, Seidel K, Dietz W. Predicting obesity in young adulthood from childhood and parental obesity. *N Engl J Med* 1997;337: 869-873.
30. Gidding S, Dennison B, Birch L, *et al*. Dietary recommendations for children and adolescents. *Circulation* 2005;112: 2061-2075.
31. Nielsen S, Popkin B. Patterns and Trends in Food Portion Sizes, 1977-1998. *JAMA* 2003;289: 450.
32. Fisher J, Rolls B, Birch L. Children's bite size and intake of an entrée are greater with large portions than with age-appropriate or self-selected portions. *Am J of Clin Nutr* 2003;77: 1164.
33. Nemet D, Barkan S, Epstein Y, Friedland O, Kowen G, Eliakim A. Short and long term beneficial effects of a combined dietary-behavioral-physical activity intervention for the treatment of childhood obesity. *Pediatrics* 2005;115: e443-e449.
34. Epstein L, Valoski A, Wing R, McCurley J. Ten-year follow-up of behavioral, family-based treatment for obese children. *JAMA* 1990;264: 2519-2523.
35. Epstein L. Family-based behavioral intervention for obese children. *Int J Obes Relat Metab Disord* 1996;20 (suppl 1): S14-21.
36. Gannon M, Nuttall F, Saeed A, Jordan K, Hoover H. An increase in dietary protein improves the blood glucose response in persons with type 2 diabetes. *Am J Clin Nutr* 2003;78: 734-741.
37. Gannon M, Nuttall F. Effect of a high protein, low carbohydrate diet on blood glucose control in people with type 2 diabetes. *Diabetes* 2004;53: 2375-2382.
38. Kavey R, Daniels S, Lauer R, Atkins D, Hayman L, Taubert K. American Heart Association. American heart association guidelines for primary prevention of atherosclerotic cardiovascular disease beginning in childhood. *Circulation* 2003; 107: 1562-1566.

Sabeena Farhath • Millie Boettcher • Karoly Horvath

44 Nutrition in Inflammatory Bowel Disease

INTRODUCTION

Inflammatory bowel disease (IBD) is a nonspecific, chronic inflammation that includes two diseases, Crohn's disease (CD) and ulcerative colitis (UC). It is accepted that IBD is the result of an inappropriate response by the gut-associated immune system to bacterial and nutritional factors; however, the trigger of this reaction is unknown.

This chapter focuses on the nutrition in IBD, summarizing the nutritional problems and providing practical guidelines for the nutritional therapy in this disease.

ETIOLOGIC ASPECTS

While CD can occur in any part of the digestive tract from the mouth to the anus and characterized by patchy, *transmural* inflammation with skip areas interspersed between actively diseased segments, UC involves only the superficial layers of the *mucosa* with continuous lesions starting in the rectum and it is limited to the colon (Fig. 44.1A and 1B).

Four factors play a role in the pathogenesis of IBD, namely

- Mucosal immune system
- Bacterial flora
- Diet
- Genetic background

Immune System

The immune dysregulation in IBD involves both the innate and adaptive immunity. The defect in innate immunity is the result of the damage in the epithelial barrier, which is the first line defense against pathogenic organisms. The exaggerated host response to luminal antigens leads to chronic inflammation and increased secretion of pro-inflammatory cytokines.[1] Antigen presenting cells *and* macrophages play an important role in *this process.*

Bacterial Flora

The distal ileum and colon contain high concentrations of bacteria (>10^{12} organisms/g). These may include pathogens and bacterial factors that could be directly responsible for initiating IBD. The role of bacterial flora in the pathogenesis is supported by indirect data, such as beneficial response to antibiotics (Cipro, metronidazole) and the positive effect

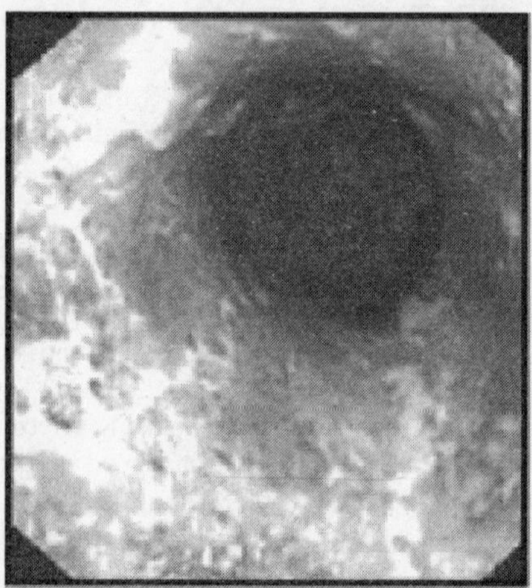

A. Ulcerative colitis

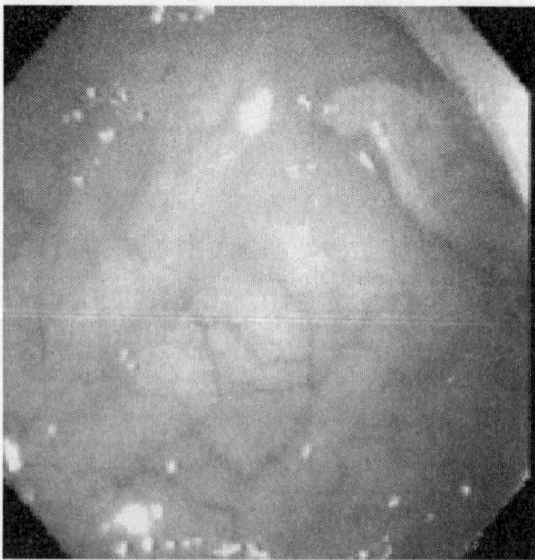

B. Crohn's disease

Fig. 44.1: Endoscopic pictures of children with IBD (A) Ulcerative colitis showing diffuse involvement of the colon; (B) Crohn's disease with typical ulceration and skip area (See for colour figure Plate 4)

of probiotics in cases with CD. There are no specific bacteria identified as the trigger of abnormal immune response.

Diet

Dietary antigens represent a daily challenge to the gut-associated immune system; therefore diet is logically implicated in the pathogenesis of IBD. However, there are no specific dietary antigens identified as etiologic factors in either UC or CD.[2] Differences in diet might explain the significant geographical differences in the prevalence of IBD. A study conducted in Sweden found that the incidence of UC and CD were higher in urban than in rural areas.[3] Another study examining the association between diet and IBD found that the relative risk associated with consumption of fast foods at least two times a week was estimated at 3.4 (95% confidence interval=1.3-9.3) for CD and 3.9 (95% confidence interval=1.4-10.6) for UC.[4] A Japanese study reported that the combined consumption of Western foods (bread for breakfast, butter, margarine, cheese, meats, and ham and sausage) was associated with an increased risk of UC (p=0.04). Among individual foods, consumption of margarine was positively associated with UC (p=0.005).[5,6] A recent study reported from England identified meat, especially red meat consumption as a factor in the increased relapse in UC patients.[7] However, the results of these epidemiological studies have to be confirmed by further investigations.

Genetic Background

Most of the evidence for genetic background in inflammatory bowel disease is derived from family and twin studies. The concordance rate for monozygotic twins for CD and UC are approximately 58.3% and 18.2% respectively, while the rates for dizygotic twins are 0% and 4.5% respectively.[8] On genetic analysis of families with high incidence of CD specific chromosomal regions with significant degrees of genetic linkage have been identified. One of them is the CARD15/NOD2 gene.[9]

The typical management of children with IBD includes the use of steroids, anti-inflammatory medications (5-ASA preparations), immunosuppressants (mercaptopurine, azathioprine, methotrexate), biological agents (anti-TNF) and nutritional therapy.

GROWTH OF CHILDREN WITH IBD

Generally, children with CD have growth failure, vitamin and mineral deficiencies, delayed bone age and decreased bone density then those with UC. This is due to the differences between these two diseases (Table 44.1).

Growth Failure

It had been described decades ago that growth failure is one of the main initial manifestations of IBD. It is much more prevalent in children with CD. The prevalence varies from 10 to 50% in the reported studies partially due to the different criteria used. Short stature may develop years before the manifestations of digestive symptoms. Kanof *et al.*[10] reported decreased height velocities in 42 per cent of children with CD before the digestive symptoms manifested and in 88 percent at the time of diagnosis. Markowitz *et al.*[11] followed the growth patterns of 48 children with

Table 44.1: Comparison of Crohn's disease and ulcerative colitis

		Crohn's Disease	*Ulcerative Colitis*
Extent of the disease	Localization	From mouth to anus	Colon
	Transmural involvement	Common	Unusual
	Ileum involvement	Frequent	Absent (only blackwash ileitis)
	Rectal involvement	Occasional	Universal
Extraintestinal involvement	Fistula/stricture	Common	Absent
	Intraabdominal/ perianal abscess	Common	Absent
	Mouth ulcers	Common	Rare
	Erythema nodosum	Common	Less common
	Pyoderma gangrenosum	Less frequent	More frequent
	Iritis, iridocyclitis	More frequent	Less common
	Clubbing	Common	Less frequent
	Sclerosing cholangitis	Less frequent	More frequent
Endoscopic finding	Skip lesions	Common	Absent
	Diffuse inflammation	Less common	More common
Histology	Granuloma	30-50%	Unusual
	Crypt abscess	Less common	Common
Bleeding/ diarrhea	Rectal bleeding	Less common	Common
	Diarrhea	Less common	Always present
Growth/ nutrition	Growth failure	Common	Less frequent
	Delayed puberty	Common	Less common
	Nutritional deficiencies	Common	Less frequent
	Osteopenia	Common	Less frequent

inflammatory bowel disease from adolescence to adulthood and found that 31 percent had permanent growth failure. Growth failure is less prevalent and present only in 6-10% of children with Ulcerative colitis.

As one of the peak ages when IBD manifests is the teenage period a delay in sexual maturation (delayed puberty) is an important feature of the CD in children.

Failure to gain weight is also an initial symptom while weight loss becomes a significant feature at the time of diagnosis. Gryboski and Spiro reported weight losses of 2 to 11kg at the time of diagnosis in 86 patients with CD.[12]

Bone age can be delayed by more than 2 years of the actual chronological age at presentation of CD.

The etiology of growth failure associated with IBD is multifactorial. It includes inadequate intake, increased loss, malabsorption and increased energy requirement.

Malnutrition and inflammation can change the Insulin–like growth factor-1 (IGF-1) blood level. GF-1 is produced by the liver in response to growth hormone (GH) stimulation and it mediates the effects of growth hormone on the growth plate of bones. The association between impaired growth in CD and low IGF-1 levels has been reported two decades ago.[13] The factors influencing IGF-1 levels are malnutrition,[13] direct cytokine effects[14] and chronic corticosteroid therapy[15] (Fig. 44.2).

Nutrient deficiency may result in altered cellular immunity with increased risk of infection and delayed wound healing.

Box 44.1: Factors affecting the nutritional status in IBD

- **Decreased nutrient intake**
  - Anorexia
  - Fear of eating due to nausea, vomiting or crampy pain
  - Feeling of early fullness (early satiety)
  - Difficulty in swallowing
  - Side-effects of medications
  - Oral aphthous ulcerations
  - Diminished taste acuity (zinc deficiency)
- **Increased nutrient loss**
  - Vomiting
  - Diarrhea
  - Protein losses from the inflamed, ulcerated mucosa
  - Bleeding
- **Malabsorption/Maldigestion**
  - Extensive small bowel disease
  - Small bowel bacterial overgrowth
  - Bile salt-losing enteropathy
  - Surgical resection/short gut syndrome
  - Fat and fat soluble vitamin malabsorption
- **Increased calorie/nutrient requirements**
  - Increased calorie need for catch-up growth
  - Increased vitamin and mineral needs
  - Fever, stress
  - Abscess, fistula
  - Repletion of losses.

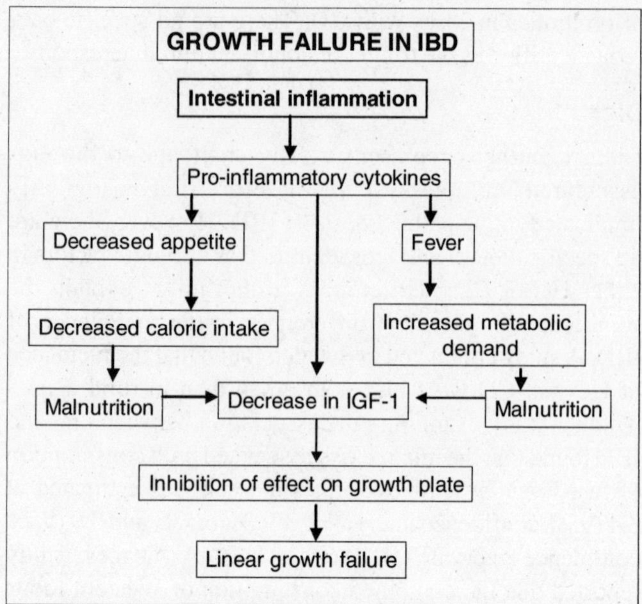

Fig. 44.2: Pathogenesis of linear growth failure in children with CD

Assessment of Nutritional Status

A good history and physical examination are the best clinical tools to assess the nutritional status of a patient. Although malabsorption is less prevalent in UC due to the absence of small intestinal involvement the nutritional status is affected in this disease as well. Assessment of nutritional status includes:

- History.
- Physical examination.
- Laboratory testing.
- Imaging studies.

History

It is very important to obtain growth charts showing the weight, height, and growth velocity in the previous years, especially in children suspected of having CD. The history should include questions related to appetite, diet and eating habits. Early fullness, eating small meals, pain during or after eating, and taste sensation changes are all associated with CD. A 24-hour dietary history, which is analyzed by a clinical nutritionist or a registered dietitian, can provide useful and more objective information. CD can start as a silent disease with gradual growth failure and may take years to develop gastrointestinal symptoms. Patients with UC typically have a shorter history, although frequently they have episodes of diarrhea with or without blood in stool months before the full-blown symptoms develop.

It is also important to document the list of medications, nutritional supplements, including vitamins and minerals and also to ask questions about the use of alternative and complementary medicines. Clinical symptoms of vitamin and nutritional deficiencies associated with IBD should be asked.

Physical Examination

The next part of nutritional evaluation is the physical examination. The general appearance of children (malnutrition, weight loss) should be documented. The actual weight, height, weight/height ratio and body mass index (BMI) should be plotted in standard national growth charts. As part of the systematic organ system examinations the stage of sexual maturation (Tanner stage, onset of menses) should be recorded. In addition to the detailed gastrointestinal examination a special attention should be paid for the extraintestinal manifestations of IBD (Box 44.2).

Box 44.2: Extraintestinal manifestations of IBD

- **Eyes:** Uveitis, episcleritis
- **Mouth:** Aphthous ulcers
- **Skin:** Anemia, erythema nodosum, pyoderma gangrenosum, perianal skin tag
- **Joints:** Reactive arthritis, ankylosing spondylitis, sacroilitis
- **Extremities:** Clubbing
- **Liver:** Cholelithiasis (RUQ tenderness), primary sclerosing cholangitis (jaundice)
- **Renal:** Nephrolithiasis

Many nutritional deficiencies are characterized clinically in changes involving the skin, eyes, oral cavity, skeletal system and neuromuscular system. Nutritional deficiencies of vitamins and minerals have specific clinical symptoms and signs (Box 44.3).

Box 44.3: Manifestations of vitamin and mineral deficiencies

• Vitamin A	: Keratomalacia, night blindness, xerophthalmia
• Vitamin D	: Rickets, osteomalacia, bone pain, muscle weakness, tetany
• Thiamine (B_1)	: Anorexia, confusion, edema, cardiac failure
• Riboflavin	: Cheilosis, glossitis, photophobia, angular stomatitis
• Folic acid	: Sore mouth, glossitis, forgetfulness
• Vitamin B_{12}	: Megaloblastic anemia, paresthesias, ataxia
• Iron	: Microcytic anemia, fatigue
• Calcium	: Osteopenia, osteoporosis, tetany
• Magnesium	: Tremor, muscle weakness, arrhythmias, confusion, seizures
• Zinc	: Growth failure, acrodermatitis, diarrhea, hair loss, hypogeusia

Simple measures such as triceps skinfold thickness and mid-arm circumference can be used to estimate body fat and muscle mass.

Laboratory Tests

Laboratory tests can provide an objective measure of nutritional deficiencies suspected by the history and physical findings. They can also be used to monitor the nutritional therapy. However, the results can be influenced by the underlying illness and not necessarily reflect the nutritional reserve of the patient (Box 44.4).

Box 44.4: Laboratory test in IBD

Commonly Used Tests
- CBC with differential
- Albumin
- Prealbumin
- Serum iron/ferritin
- Transferrin

Tests for Specific Micronutrient Deficiencies
- Retinol binding protein
- Serum 25-hydroxy vitamin D
- Serum vitamin E
- Prothrombin time (for vitamin K)
- Red blood cell folate
- Serum vitamin B_{12}
- Plasma zinc
- Serum calcium
- Serum magnesium
- Serum phosphorus
- Serum copper
- Plasma selenium

Imaging Studies

Studies of bone age and bone density are useful in the evaluation of children with IBD.

Bone Age: An X-ray of the left hand and wrist to evaluate bone age may be obtained to assess skeletal maturation, and may be repeated over time if needed. It provides information about the relationship between chronologic age and skeletal maturation.

Bone Mineral Density: IBD patients, especially those with CD require Dual Energy X-ray Absorptiometry (DEXA) to assess bone mineral density. Bone demineralization, accelerated bone loss and osteopenia are a significant problem in patients with CD.

Factors contributing to the bone abnormalities are inadequate nutrition (vitamin D and calcium deficiency), poor absorption, reduced physical activity and the use of corticosteroids. Recent studies suggested that circulating pro-inflammatory cytokines produced in the inflamed bowel can effect the bone metabolism, particularly bone resorption.[14]

The reasons for hypovitaminosis include inadequate intake, small intestinal involvement, chronic steroid therapy and limited exposure to sunlight. Corticosteroids affect bone mineralization by inhibiting osteoblasts, impairing intestinal calcium absorption and antagonizing the biological activity of growth hormone.[15]

NUTRITIONAL MANAGEMENTS IN IBD

Nutritional support should be an integral part of the management of all children with IBD. The nutritional management starts with a nutritional assessment as described above. Nutritional therapy should be individualized to each patient depending on the nutritional status at the time of diagnosis. Management goals should include:

- Achieve a catch-up growth.
- Correction of nutritional deficits.
- Continuous monitoring of growth and nutritional parameters.

The nutritional management is more challenging in the newly diagnosed then in the established patients. Evidently malnutrition, characterized by weight loss, growth failure and micronutrient depletion are the main problems in the newly diagnosed children. Good control of intestinal inflammation and appropriate nutritional support are important for the enhancement of linear growth and achieve a catch-up weight gain. Children with CD generally have greater nutrient needs, based on age, gender, and weight, than do children with UC.

Nutritional intervention not only improves the body mass but it potentially improves the inflammation through the modulation of pro- and anti-inflammatory cytokine profiles.[16] Bannerje *et al.*[17] reported significant improvements in inflammatory parameters (ESR, IL-6) by day 3 and in Pediatric Crohn's disease activity index, CRP, and IGF-1 by day 7 in 12 children on enteral nutrition. These changes preceded any significant changes in nutritional parameters.

Nutrition in patients with IBD has been used as primary therapy and as supplemental therapy.

Nutrition as Primary Therapy

Patients stop eating regular foods and receive all calories either as elemental or polymeric formula by mouth, through nasogastric or gastric tube or in the form of total parenteral nutrition. Enteral nutrition costs less than parenteral nutrition, maintains gut integrity, stimulates immunocompetence, and helps to control symptoms and overall disease activity.

Enteral Nutrition (EN)

EN has been used successfully as primary therapy in children. It has been hypothesized that enteral formulas decrease the stimulation of the gut-associated immune system. Over the past two decades, a number of studies supported that EN as primary therapy able to induce remission and control disease activity in patients with CD. Various forms of EN have been evaluated, including elemental, hypoallergenic and polymeric formulas based on their protein content. The elemental diets contain amino acids, semi elemental diet has oligopeptides and polymeric diet consists of whole proteins. Studies in children supports that elementary formulas do not have advantage over polymeric ones, in fact a multicenter randomized controlled trial reported that children with CD ingesting polymeric formula gained more weight.[18] It seems that the type of formula used did not make difference in response as both elemental and polymeric diets were associated with improved disease activity scores, histologic healing, and down-regulation of pro-inflammatory cytokines.[16] Clinical indications of enteral nutrition are given in Box 44.5.

Box 44.5: Indications of EN in IBD

Proven indications
- Reversing growth failure by avoiding steroid use
- Steroid resistant
- Steroid dependent

Potential indications
- Postoperatively developed fistula
- Perianal disease
- Intestinal stricture
- Maintenance of remission

Meta-analysis published in the mid-1990s concluded that enteral nutrition as primary therapy for CD is less effective than corticosteroids to induce clinical remission.[6,19] A recent meta-analysis of four trials that included 130 patients treated with enteral nutrition and 123 treated with steroids yielded a pooled OR (odds ratio) of 0.30 favoring steroid therapy (95% CI: 0.17, 0.52).[20]

However, pediatric studies support the concept that EN is equal to steroid therapy.[21] The choice between EN and steroid therapy for a child with newly diagnosed CD is straightforward from medical point of view. Because both therapies have a similar efficacy, but EN has no side-effect, has beneficial effects on growth, leads to a rapid nutritional restitution; therefore most pediatricians have no difficulty to recommend it. Due to the poor palatability of elemental solutions they have to be given via feeding tube as continuous night time feeding. It requires either the passage of the feeding tube every evening or long-term placement of feeding tube. However, the permanent presence of tube makes it socially unacceptable especially for teenagers. Although polymeric diet is easier to digest still many families and children do not consider it.

Feeding through gastrostomy tube is an option. There is no risk of fistula formation based on a retrospective study on 25 patients with CD who underwent surgical or endoscopic gastrostomy tube placement.[22] A study conducted in children confirmed the safety of PEG tubes and indicated that they were more tolerable than nasogastric tubes.[23] Gastric tube placement can be considered in children with severe malnutrition whose compliance with an EN is poor.

There are special formulas developed for patients with IBD. Transforming growth factor beta (TGF-α) is a polypeptide that modulates intestinal epithelial cell growth and development and has anti-inflammatory effects. In a trial with polymeric diet with added TGF-α2 (Modulen, Nestle) 79% of patients achieved remission within 8 weeks.[16]

Total Parenteral Nutrition (TPN)

Enteral route should be the preferred method of nutrition whenever possible. It has significantly less complications and costs much less than TPN. TPN is justified in severely malnourished CD patients who are unable to tolerate enteral feeding or in whom enteral feeding is contraindicated (Box 44.6).

Box 44.6: TPN as primary therapy in IBD

- Enteral route cannot be used
- Enteral route is ineffective in maintaining nutritional support
- Extensive small bowel disease
- In children before and after surgery
- Severely undernourished children with short bowel syndrome
- Toxic megacolon
- Intestinal obstruction
- Perforation
- Severe perianal disease
- Fistulizing disease.

Both bowel rest and TPN reduce intestinal inflammation and decrease disease activity in selected patients with CD. However, in UC it does not have any advantage over EN with polymeric formula.[24]

TPN has some effect on the closure of intestinal fistula(s) in patients with CD. The initial closure rate was 44% and of these only 37% remains closed for an extended period of time.[25]

Nutrition as Supplemental Therapy

Calorie Intake

Children with CD have greater nutrient needs, based on age, gender, and weight, than children with UC. The excess caloric needs depend on the disease activity. Resting energy expenditure (REE) in well-nourished children with CD is not different from values obtained in healthy children. The apparent increase in REE in children with CD is a result of their lower fat-free mass.[26] These changes in REE are reversible and sustainable with aggressive enteral feeding. An expert panel of NASPGHAN recommends that the energy needs may be increased above recommended dietary intakes by 5% to 35% in children with CD depending on their nutritional status and the degree of inflammatory disease activity.[27]

In some children with active CD, who are unable to increase their enteral intake night time continuous feeding is needed to provide adequate amount of calories for a catch-up growth. Foods and formulas can be enriched with medium-chain-triglyceride (MCT) oils that have a better absorption. However, a care should be taken not to exceed the threshold dose. MCT oil upto 50 g/day mixed with foods or formula can be introduced gradually into the diet.

Protein Intake

There is an increase in the protein turnover especially with systemic inflammation and infections[28] due to losses from inflammation of the intestinal tract, and increased catabolism. It requires additional protein supplementation above the normal daily requirement. There is no clear recommendations for protein intake,[27] so it should be individualized. A glutamine-enriched enteral nutrition formula diet did not offer advantage over a low-glutamine diet in children with CD in a double-blind randomized controlled trial.[29]

Nutritional Supplements

A recent placebo controlled randomized study in adults reported decreased steroid use ($p<0.01$) in patients with UC who received 18 oz of the oral supplement enriched with fish oil, fructooligosaccharides, gum arabic, vitamin E, vitamin C, and selenium compared with those who received a carbohydrate-based placebo formula each day for 6 months.[30] The following paragraph describes various nutritional supplements and they effect on the disease activity in IBD.

***Folic acid/B_{12}*:** Medications used to treat IBD, such as methotrexate, a folate antagonist, and sulphasalazine, which interferes with folic acid absorption, may result in deficiency. Typically 1mg/day of folic acid supplementation is given to children with IBD. The best indicator of folic acid status is red blood cell folate content. Some past studies showed decreased relapse rate in patients receiving folate supplementation. Hyperhomocysteinemia is significantly more common in patients with IBD compared to healthy controls and is associated with lower levels of vitamin B_{12} and folate.[31] Increased levels are inversely proportionate to folate levels (and to a lesser degree with B_{12} levels). While the clinical significance is uncertain, elevated homocysteine levels have been associated with a hypercoagulable state, thus possibly contributing to the hypercoagulability that has been observed in patients with IBD. There is an association between hyperhomocysteinemia and osteoporosis, which also support the practice of folic acid supplementation.

Vitamin B_{12} deficiency can be due to decreased factor production, inflammation or resection of the terminal ileum, which is the site of absorption. It occurs upto one third of the patients. Serum methylmalonic acid is a more sensitive indicator of cobalamin deficiency than serum vitamin B_{12}. A nasal gel form of B_{12} is now available but it is much more expensive compared with monthly IM administration.

Multivitamins with Minerals: Vitamin and mineral deficiencies have been well documented in IBD.[32] The list of the reported deficiencies are: vitamin A, D, E, thiaminc, riboflavin, folate, vitamin B_{12}; iron; calcium; magnesium;

potassium; and zinc.[33] Fat soluble vitamin deficiency (vitamins A, D, E and K) can occur secondary to decreased bile acid pool and fat malabsorption in patients with CD. Patients with IBD are advised to take multivitamin supplements, although there are no controlled trials to support this practice. The multivitamin/mineral preparations have all water and fat-soluble vitamins and minerals such as iron, zinc, magnesium, calcium, selenium etc.

Calcium: Risk factors for low body calcium include corticosteroids, vitamin D deficiency, malabsorption, and systemic inflammation.[34] Assessment of adequate calcium and vitamin D intake is important in all patients with IBD and supplementation is needed if the diet is found deficient. Osteoporosis is present in approximately 30% of children with CD. DEXA scan is recommended to evaluate bone density. In adolescent 1200-1500 mg of calcium and a multivitamin containing 400 IU of Vitamin D is recommended per day. Given, the lack of data on biphosphonates use in children, this therapy is not recommended at the present time. Osteopenic patients should undergo monitoring of vitamin D and calcium status and bone density.

Iron: Iron deficiency results from excessive iron loss due to chronic, occult, or gross bleeding and from proximal intestinal disease leading to malabsorption of iron.

Upto 66 percent of patients with ulcerative colitis and 25 to 40 percent of those with CD are iron-deficient. Concerns about intolerance, lack of efficacy, or worsening of disease state due to supplemental iron therapy among patients with IBD have not been substantiated in clinical studies.

***Zinc*:** Patients with IBD can have excessive stool losses and urine excretion of zinc. Clinical signs of deficiency include acrodermatitis, peeling of palms and soles of feet. Serum measurement is less reliable indicator of zinc status then e.g. measurement from hair samples. A deficient state is often reflected by a decreased serum alkaline phosphatase concentration, as it is a zinc metalloenzyme. Excessive losses of zinc may be observed in patients with ostomies, fistulas, and profuse diarrhea.

Magnesium: Magnesium deficiency in patients with IBD may result from decreased oral intake, malabsorption, and increased intestinal losses, and may contribute to osteopenia. Oral supplementation with magnesium can lead to diarrhea. If magnesium supplementation is needed magnesium gluconate has a higher degree of solubility, making it a better choice for intestinal supplementation.

Selenium: Selenium occurs naturally in meats, cereals and fish. It is an essential part of the antioxidant glutathione peroxidase. Selenium concentration in whole blood and glutathione peroxidase activity can be decreased in patients with IBD. Selenium deficiency may result in a potentially fatal but reversible cardiomyopathy.

***Fish oil*:** Fish oil contains n-3-PUFA (poly-unsaturated fatty acid), which inhibits production of proinflammatory cytokines and has some benefit in the treatment of CD. Fish oils have been used as complementary nutritional therapy in IBD. In addition their known beneficial effect on vascular epithelium they influence the leukotriene balance by shifting LTB4 production to LTB5, which much less pro-inflammatory. Fish oil have anti-inflammatory effects exerted through several potential mechanisms: (1) reduced production of leukotriene B4 and thromboxane-A2, (2) inhibition of inflammatory cytokines such as interleukin-1 and tumor necrosis factor, and (3) scavenging of free radicals.[35] A double-blinded, placebo controlled one-year study in adult patients receiving 2.7 g of n-3 fatty acids per day reported decreased relapse rate compared with the placebo group (28% vs. 69%).[36]

A reduction in disease activity and a corticosteroid sparing effect was noted in patients with UC, but not CD when they received treatment with omega–3 long chain fatty acids.[37] However, in other study there was no difference in relapse rates between the treatment and placebo groups.[39]

Nutritional Modification of Intestinal Bacterial Flora

***Prebiotics*:** Prebiotics are oligosaccharides that cannot be hydrolyzed by human digestive enzymes, therefore they reach the colon and metabolized by bacteria. The two main groups of prebiotics are fructooligosaccharides (FOS), such as inulin, lactulose and galactooligosaccharides (GOS). They are naturally present in our foods including onions, garlic, asparagus, leeks, bananas, artichokes and chicory root. The quantity of prebiotics cannot be high as studies showed that ingestion of prebiotics over 10 grams per day can cause increased diarrhea and cramping.[38] Recently enteral tube feeding formulas are available that containing FOS (Peptamen with FOS, Jevity Plus and Nepro).

In the next few years, important advances are expected in understanding the interactions between prebiotics, intestinal flora and the colonic mucosa in health and diseases, which may lead to improvement of therapy and nutritional management of susceptible individuals.[39]

There are increasing evidences suggesting that some components of the enteric flora play role the pathogenesis of IBD. Probiotics are living organisms that favorably modify the bacterial flora in the colon. They help re-establishing the normal intestinal flora by creating an environment that is unfavorable to potential pathogenic bacteria and maintain the integrity of the gut mucosal barrier. The mechanism of these actions is not fully understood, but may include direct effect on bacteria, changes in the colonic pH and stimulation of the intestinal immune system by enhancing macrophage and natural killer activities and proliferation of lymphocytes. Lactobacillus strains and bifidobacterium are the most frequently used probiotics.

Clinical trials on patients with CD and postoperative pouchitis demonstrated a significantly benefit of probiotic therapy compared to the control groups.[40] The three trials involving patients with UC found no significant difference in relapses.

There are yoghurts with live cultures that have high concentration of probiotics and can be used as alternative to probiotic capsules or tablets. In addition they provide extra calories.

Dietary Restrictions in IBD

Dietary restrictions should be avoided unless intestinal obstruction or specific abnormalities of digestion or absorption exist.

Dietary lactose only restricted if patients have symptoms associated with dietary intake or has a positive breath hydrogen test. Since dairy products are excellent source of calcium the use of lactase enzyme supplement is recommended rather than a full elimination of milk. The prevalence of lactose malabsorption in IBD patients is estimated to be between 10% and 20%.[41] Lactose restrictions should only be employed in patients exhibiting symptoms, such as crampy pain, gas and diarrhea after consuming dairy products.

Levenstein *et al.*[42] reported that *ad libitum diets* were equally as effective as *low residue diets* in maintaining remission in adults with CD. Soluble fiber metabolized to short chain fatty acids like butyrate is the preferred fuel for colonocytes. The diet of IBD should be a balanced diet with appropriate fiber content. The typical daily fiber in a balanced diet is approx. 0.5 g/kg/day. There is often confusion between low fiber and low residue diets. Low fiber diet reduces fiber intake while a low residue diets limit fiber as well as any other food known to leave a residue in the GI tract (such as milk products, prune juice, etc). "Diet as tolerated" is still remains the recommendation to patients with IBD.

In patients with *strictures* it may be prudent to avoid such fiber containing food as broccoli, raw carrot, grapes, nuts, seeds, mushrooms, popcorn, celery and all fruits with skins as they are potentially able to cause obstruction. It is important to warn patients to chew their foods well if strictures are present. Some patients may need to rely on liquids as the sole source of nutrition if strictures or narrowing do not allow passage of normal foods, however, in these cases surgical management should be considered. Figure 44.3 shows the barium study of a child with CD who developed stricture in the ascending colon and required resection and ileostomy.

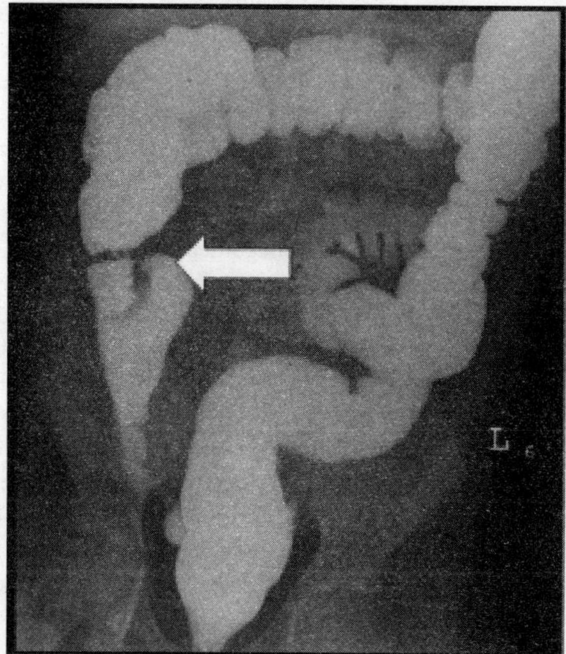

Fig. 44.3: Barium enema study of a child with CD who developed a stricture in the ascending colon and required surgical resection and temporary ileostomy

Patients with new *ileostomies* represent a special category. They are instructed to avoid the high fiber foods listed above for a period of 2-4 weeks to allow post-operative swelling to subside. Fiber-containing foods typically are added back slowly beginning with water-soluble fibers (e.g. oatmeal, banana, rice and apple sauce) followed by insoluble fibers (wheat, bran, corn or nuts) as tolerated. However, this practice is not based on research data.

Patients with ileostomies may require additional fluid and electrolytes due to losses.

Low oxalate diet is required in patients with terminal ileum resection or with significant fat malabsorption, because these patients have the propensity for oxalate kidney stones.

IBD AND PREGNANCY

Since an increasing proportion of teenagers are getting pregnant, a word on IBD and pregnancy should be in order.

Fertility is reduced in patients with CD compared to UC. Women are naturally concerned about the effects of IBD on fertility, pregnancy and fetus and how pregnancy may affect their disease activity. UC and CD behave in a similar manner with a relapse rate of approximately 30-35% during gestation. Most pregnant women are concerned about the risks of drugs to the fetus. There are controversies regarding medical therapy in pregnant IBD patients. Nutritional support is an important adjunct during the pregnancy in IBD patients. Drug therapies and the disease by itself may lead to vitamin deficiency states. It is very important that folate supplementation be reinforced as it has a protective effect on neural tube defects.

SUMMARY AND CONCLUSIONS

Multiple factors contribute to the pathogenesis of growth failure and malnutrition in IBD including reduced nutrient intake, malabsorption, increased energy expenditure, and enteral losses. Nutritional management is essential for the care of children with IBD, as it can help prevent growth failure and improves mucosal healing. It should include the assessment of dietary intake, body composition, determination of bone age, and routine laboratory studies, including specific testing for micronutrient deficiencies.

Nutritional support should be an integral part of the management of children with IBD. Growth failure is frequent in newly diagnosed children and it requires additional enteral supplementation for a catch-up growth. Adequate nutrition results in an improvement in the well-being, nutritional status, and growth and also leads to a reduction in the biochemical and histologic markers of disease activity and potentially reduces corticosteroid use, particularly in CD.

Enteral diets alone are effective to induce remission in children with active CD. There is no advantage to use the more expensive elemental formulas because polymeric ones are also effective. Fish oils that are rich in omega-3 long-chain fatty acids are able to reduce disease activity and corticosteroid use.

Periodic nutritional assessment of children with IBD and appropriate nutritional therapy provides an effective complementary therapy in inflammatory bowel diseases.

REFERENCES

1. Strober W, Fuss IJ, Ehrhardt RO, Neurath M, Boirivant M, Ludviksson BR. Mucosal immunoregulation and inflammatory bowel disease: New insights from murine models of inflammation. *Scand J Immunol* 1998;48:453-458.
2. Griffiths AM. Inflammatory bowel disease. *Nutrition* 1998;14:788-791.
3. Ekbom A, Montgomery SM. Environmental risk factors (excluding tobacco and microorganisms): Critical analysis of old and new hypotheses. *Best Pract Res Clin Gastroenterol* 2004;18:497-508.
4. Persson PG, Ahlbom A, Hellers G. Diet and inflammatory bowel disease: A case-control study. *Epidemiology* 1992;3:47-52.
5. Beattie RM, Schiffrin EJ, Donnet-Hughes A, Huggett AC, Domizio P, MacDonald TT, *et al.* Polymeric nutrition as the primary therapy in children with small bowel Crohn's disease. *Aliment Pharmacol Ther* 1994;8:609-615.
6. Fernandez-Banares F, Cabre E, Esteve-Comas M, Gassull MA. How effective is enteral nutrition in inducing clinical remission in active Crohn's disease? A meta-analysis of the randomized clinical trials. *JPEN J Parenter Enteral Nutr* 1995;19:356-364.
7. Jowett SL, Seal CJ, Pearce MS, Phillips E, Gregory W, Barton JR, *et al.* Influence of dietary factors on the clinical course of ulcerative colitis: A prospective cohort study. *Gut* 2004;53:1479-1484.
8. Orholm M, Binder V, Sorensen TI, Rasmussen LP, Kyvik KO. Concordance of inflammatory bowel disease among Danish twins. Results of a nationwide study. *Scand J Gastroenterol* 2000;35:1075-1081.
9. Duerr RH. Update on the genetics of inflammatory bowel disease. *J Clin Gastroenterol* 2003;37:358-367.
10. Kanof ME, Lake AM, Bayless TM. Decreased height velocity in children and adolescents before the diagnosis of Crohn's disease. *Gastroenterology* 1988;95:1523-1527.
11. Markowitz J, Grancher K, Rosa J, Aiges H, Daum F. Growth failure in pediatric inflammatory bowel disease. *J Pediatr Gastroenterol Nutr* 1993;16:373-380.
12. Gryboski JD, Spiro HM. Prognosis in children with Crohn's disease. *Gastroenterology* 1978;74(5 Pt 1):807-817.
13. Kirschner BS, Sutton MM. Somatomedin-C levels in growth-impaired children and adolescents with chronic inflammatory bowel disease. *Gastroenterology* 1986;91:830-836.
14. Hyams JS, Wyzga N, Kreutzer DL, Justinich CJ, Gronowicz GA. Alterations in bone metabolism in children with inflammatory bowel disease: An in vitro study. *J Pediatr Gastroenterol Nutr* 1997;24:289-295.
15. Hyams JS, Moore RE, Leichtner AM, Carey DE, Goldberg BD. Relationship of type I procollagen to corticosteroid therapy in children with inflammatory bowel disease. *J Pediatr* 1988;112:893-898.
16. Fell JM, Paintin M, Arnaud-Battandier F, Beattie RM, Hollis A, Kitching P, *et al.* Mucosal healing and a fall in mucosal pro-inflammatory cytokine mRNA induced by a specific oral polymeric diet in paediatric Crohn's disease. *Aliment Pharmacol Ther* 2000;14:281-289.
17. Bannerjee K, Camacho-Hubner C, Babinska K, Dryhurst KM, Edwards R, Savage MO, *et al.* Anti-inflammatory and growth-stimulating effects precede nutritional restitution during enteral feeding in Crohn disease. *J Pediatr Gastroenterol Nutr* 2004;38:270-275.
18. Ludvigsson JF, Krantz M, Bodin L, Stenhammar L, Lindquist B. Elemental versus polymeric enteral nutrition in paediatric Crohn's disease: A multicentre randomized controlled trial. *Acta Paediatr* 2004;93:327-335.
19. Griffiths AM, Ohlsson A, Sherman PM, Sutherland LR. Meta-analysis of enteral nutrition as a primary treatment of active Crohn's disease. *Gastroenterology* 1995;108:1056-1067.
20. Zachos M, Tondeur M, Griffiths AM. Enteral nutritional therapy for inducing remission of Crohn's disease. *Cochrane Database Syst Rev* 2001:CD000542.
21. Heuschkel RB, Menache CC, Megerian JT, Baird AE. Enteral nutrition and corticosteroids in the treatment of acute Crohn's disease in children. *J Pediatr Gastroenterol Nutr* 2000;31:8-15.
22. Mahajan L, Oliva L, Wyllie R, Fazio V, Steffen R, Kay M. The safety of gastrostomy in patients with Crohn's disease. *Am J Gastroenterol* 1997;92:985-988.
23. Cosgrove M, Jenkins HR. Experience of percutaneous endoscopic gastrostomy in children with Crohn's disease. *Arch Dis Child* 1997;76:141-143.
24. Gonzalez-Huix F, Fernandez-Banares F, Esteve-Comas M, Abad-Lacruz A, Cabre E, Acero D, *et al.* Enteral versus parenteral nutrition as adjunct therapy in acute ulcerative colitis. *Am J Gastroenterol* 1993;88:227-232.

25. Han PD, Burke A, Baldassano RN, Rombeau JL, Lichtenstein GR. Nutrition and inflammatory bowel disease. *Gastroenterol Clin North Am* 1999;28:423-443.
26. Zoli G, Katelaris PH, Garrow J, Gasbarrini G, Farthing MJ. Increased energy expenditure in growing adolescents with Crohn's disease. *Dig Dis Sci* 1996;41:1754-1759.
27. Kleinman RE, Baldassano RN, Caplan A, Griffiths AM, Heyman MB, Issenman RM, *et al.* Nutrition support for pediatric patients with inflammatory bowel disease: A clinical report of the North American Society for Pediatric Gastroenterology, Hepatology And Nutrition. *J Pediatr Gastroenterol Nutr* 2004;39:15-27.
28. Thomas AG, Miller V, Taylor F, Maycock P, Scrimgeour CM, Rennie MJ. Whole body protein turnover in childhood Crohn's disease. *Gut* 1992;33:675-677.
29. Akobeng AK, Miller V, Stanton J, Elbadri AM, Thomas AG. Double-blind randomized controlled trial of glutamine-enriched polymeric diet in the treatment of active Crohn's disease. *J Pediatr Gastroenterol Nutr* 2000;30:78-84.
30. Seidner DL, Lashner BA, Brzezinski A, Banks PL, Goldblum J, Fiocchi C, *et al.* An oral supplement enriched with fish oil, soluble fiber, and antioxidants for corticosteroid sparing in ulcerative colitis: A randomized, controlled trial. *Clin Gastroenterol Hepatol* 2005;3:358-369.
31. Romagnuolo J, Fedorak RN, Dias VC, Bamforth F, Teltscher M. Hyperhomocysteinemia and inflammatory bowel disease: Prevalence and predictors in a cross-sectional study. *Am J Gastroenterol* 2001;96:2143-2149.
32. Graham TO, Kandil HM. Nutritional factors in inflammatory bowel disease. *Gastroenterol Clin North Am* 2002;31:203-218.
33. Kelly DG, Fleming CR. Nutritional considerations in inflammatory bowel diseases. *Gastroenterol Clin North Am* 1995;24:597-611.
34. Arden NK, Cooper C. Osteoporosis in patients with inflammatory bowel disease. *Gut* 2002;50:9-10.
35. Belluzzi A, Brignola C, Campieri M, Camporesi EP, Gionchetti P, Rizzello F, *et al.* Effects of new fish oil derivative on fatty acid phospholipid-membrane pattern in a group of Crohn's disease patients. *Dig Dis Sci* 1994;39:2589-2594.
36. Belluzzi A, Brignola C, Campieri M, Pera A, Boschi S, Miglioli M. Effect of an enteric-coated fish-oil preparation on relapses in Crohn's disease. *N Engl J Med* 1996;334:1557-1560.
37. Aslan A, Triadafilopoulos G. Fish oil fatty acid supplementation in active ulcerative colitis: A double-blind, placebo-controlled, crossover study. *Am J Gastroenterol* 1992;87:432-437.
38. Bouhnik Y, Vahedi K, Achour L, Attar A, Salfati J, Pochart P, *et al.* Short-chain fructo-oligosaccharide administration dose-dependently increases fecal bifidobacteria in healthy humans. *J Nutr* 1999;129:113-116.
39. Delzenne N, Cherbut C, Neyrinck A. Prebiotics: Actual and potential effects in inflammatory and malignant colonic diseases. *Curr Opin Clin Nutr Metab Care* 2003;6:581-586.
40. Fedorak RN, Madsen KL. Probiotics and prebiotics in gastrointestinal disorders. *Curr Opin Gastroenterol* 2004;20:146-155.
41. Mishkin B, Yalovsky M, Mishkin S. Increased prevalence of lactose malabsorption in Crohn's disease patients at low risk for lactose malabsorption based on ethnic origin. *Am J Gastroenterol* 1997;92:1148-1153.
42. Levenstein S, Prantera C, Luzi C, D'Ubaldi A. Low residue or normal diet in Crohn's disease: A prospective controlled study in Italian patients. *Gut* 1985;26:989-993.

Swati Gadewar • Karoly Horvath

45 Nutritional Management in HIV

INTRODUCTION

During the last two decades, there has been a significant improvement in our scientific knowledge in virology, antiretroviral therapies, management of chronic psychosocial problems and multisystem disorders related to human immunodeficiency virus (HIV) infection in the last two decades. Parallel with these changes, the nutritional management of human immunodeficiency virus (HIV) infection has also demonstrated a steadily progress. It was recognized at the beginning of the HIV epidemic that malnutrition is common and it is one of the earliest complications of AIDS. It was further appreciated that malnutrition plays a significant and independent role in the morbidity and mortality of HIV infection.

PATHOGENESIS OF MALNUTRITION IN HIV

World Health Organization (WHO) defines malnutrition as *"the cellular imbalance between supply of nutrients and energy and the body's demand for them to ensure growth, maintenance, and specific functions"*.

Malnutrition is associated with adverse consequences, irrespective of the level of immune status. The pathogenic mechanisms of malnutrition in HIV are multifactorial:

- Decreased calorie and nutrient intake.
- Poor appetite.
- Malabsorption.
- Diarrhea.
- Opportunistic infection with increased requirement.
- Metabolic disturbances.
- Psychosocial factors.

The nutritional implications of HIV infection for children are more devastating because children have additional nutritional demands for growth and development. Periods of rapid growth increase the demands of muscle and other organs. If the supply of any essential nutrient does not meet the demand, growth retardation and other functional deficits may occur. Poor weight gain, failure to thrive and short stature are common in children with untreated HIV infection and AIDS.

It has been reported that nutrition by either enteral nutrition (tube feeding) or parenteral nutrition improves the immunity (CD4 count) and intestinal function in HIV-infected children.[1] This underlines the importance of proper nutrition in immune function. The clinical and biochemical association between malnutrition and altered immune function is well established.

Recent advances in antiretroviral therapy have decreased the prevalence of opportunistic infections and malnutrition. However, the introduction of highly active antiretroviral therapy (HAART) results in body fat redistribution problems in a substantial proportion of HIV-infected children.

Figure 45.1 focuses on the GIT-cum-nutritional manifestations of HIV.

GROWTH FAILURE IN HIV-INFECTED CHILDREN

The CDC defined wasting in HIV-infected children based on their age:[2]

- <13 years of age a weight loss of more than 10% of baseline.
- A decline of at least 2 percentile lines on the weight-for-age chart in a child aged 1 year or older; or
- Less than the 5th percentile on the weight-for-height chart on two consecutive measurements at least 30 days apart.
- Plus chronic diarrhea or documented fever for at least 30 days, whether intermittent or constant.

A change in body composition, particularly a decline in body cell mass (loss of cells) should raise the suspicion of HIV-related wasting in the absence of other explanations for weight loss. HIV-infected children experience wasting of lean body mass over time without significant change in fat mass.[3] The identification and treatment of wasting is critical to ensure long-term survival and quality of life in children with HIV infection. The consequences of malnutrition are the following:

- **Shortened survival:** Death from wasting in AIDS is related to the degree of tissue depletion. Progressive depletion of body cell mass occurs in patients near death.[4]

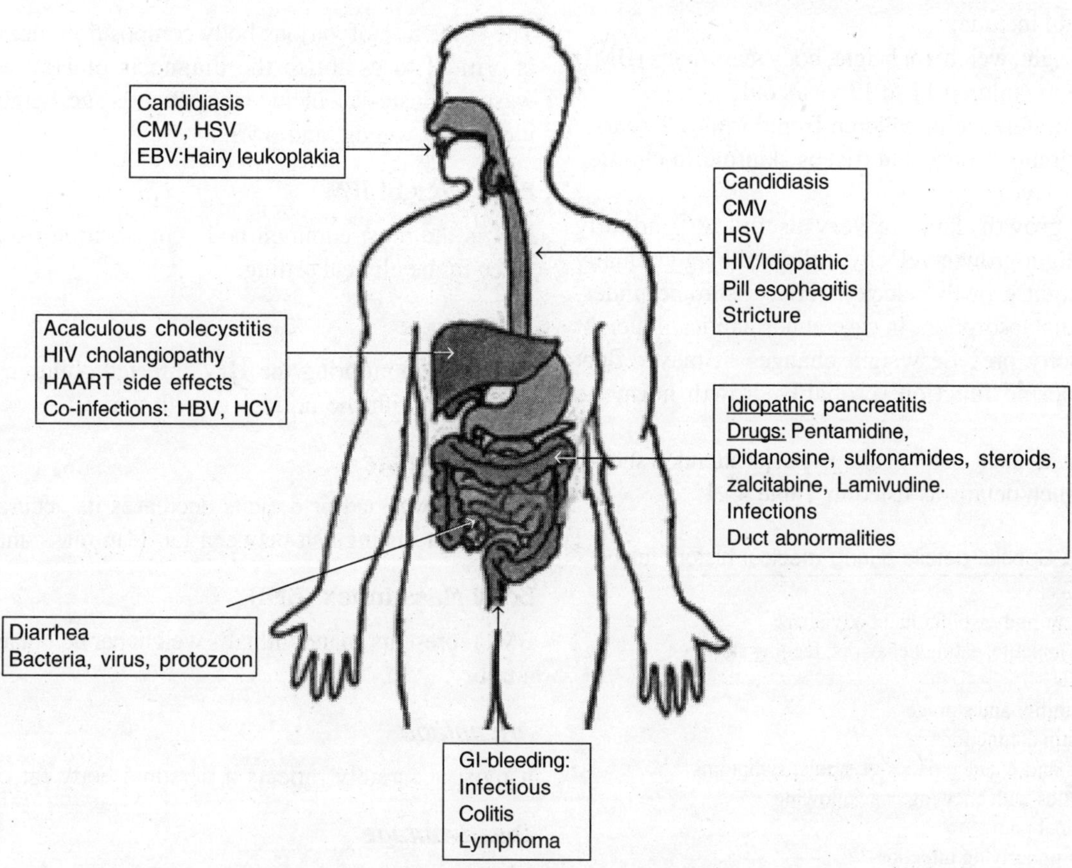

Fig. 45.1: GIT and nutritional manifestations of HIV infection

- **Decreased quality of life**: Weight loss is significantly associated with a decline in functioning and quality of life.[5]
- **Immune dysfunction**: Malnutrition is associated with a rapid decrease in CD4 cell numbers. Nutritional intervention may be able to improve intestinal absorption and result in increase in the CD4 cell numbers.[1]
- **Increase in opportunistic infections**: Weight loss can increase the risk of opportunistic infections by as much as 61% to 176%.[6]

With the introduction of HAART, there have been dramatic declines in AIDS-related morbidity and mortality in populations that have access to these new treatments.[7]

NUTRITIONAL ASSESSMENT OF A PATIENT WITH HIV

Every child who is infected with HIV should receive a complete baseline nutritional assessment within 3 months of diagnosis in order to assess the need for early nutritional intervention. Follow-up assessment should be conducted every 1 to 6 months, depending on the child's age and nutritional status.[8]

History and Physical Examination

All children with HIV should first have a comprehensive history and physical examination (Fig. 45.2). Clothing often masks subtle signs of wasting, such as abdominal, gluteal, and limb atrophy. Therefore, the patient should be comple-

History (travel, medications, antibiotics, lactose intolerance.

↓

Physical examination
Height, weight, oral, skin, abdominal and rectal (occult blood)

↓

LAB Tests
CBC and CD4 count; if CD4 < 75. Stool: culture for bacteria and C. difficile toxin; AFB stain, O/P or EIA for Giardia and cryptosporidium

↓ If all negative

Colonoscopy, upper endoscopy or both with biopsies and aspiration

Fig. 45.2: History and physical examination and investigations for nutritional management of the HIV infection

tely undressed for the examination The triage of these patients should include:

- Weight, height, weight for height, body mass index (BMI) percentile in children 11 to 17 years old.
- Head circumference in children from birth to 3 years.
- Midarm circumference and triceps skinfold in children older than 1 year.

Previous growth data are very useful. A gradually declining weight growth velocity, followed by a gradually declining height growth velocity, reflects chronic undernutrition or malabsorption. In case abnormalities in height growth velocity precede weight changes, it may reflect altered endocrine function (probably growth hormone deficiency).[9]

During the medical history taking, special attention should be given to such details as listed in Table 45.1.

Table 45.1: Special details during medical history taking

- Caloric intake
- Alterations in body weight and body shape
- Changes in appetite, eating behaviors, feeding skills
- Eating habits
- Food availability and storage
- Gastrointestinal function
  - Number and characteristics of stools, symptoms
  - Difficulties with chewing or swallowing
  - Abdominal pain
- Presence of underlying infection
- Other medical problems
- Functional status (including physical activity)
- Perceived levels of weakness, fatigue
- Medications
- Use of nutritional supplements: vitamin and mineral supplements, and herbs
- Use of complementary treatments
- Social history

Table 45.2: Laboratory and clinical tests

- Plasma HIV RNA
- CD4:CD8 ratio
- CBC with differential
- Serum iron, total iron-binding capacity
- Serum glucose
- Fasting cholesterol, and triglycerides (especially on HAART)
- Liver function tests
- Serum vitamin A and E
- Serum zinc
- Thyroid function tests if clinically warranted
- Stool examination for opportunistic pathogens in patients with diarrhea.
- Blood cultures if case of fever
- Chest radiography
- Pulse oximetry if there is breathing problem
- Barium radiography
- Upper gastrointestinal endoscopy and colonoscopy with biopsy
- A 24-hour recall or diet record should be obtained and compared with estimated needs to assess adequacy of intake

Estimation of Body Fat Content

The collection of various body composition measurements is critical to establish the diagnosis of HIV-associated wasting. Basic data include the patient's age, height, weight, ideal body weight, and BMI.

Body Weight (BW)

BW is the most common body composition measurement taken in the clinical setting.

Advantage

Useful in monitoring the HIV infected children's growth compared with the normal growth curves.

Disadvantage

- Fluid overload or deficits decreases its accuracy.
- Cannot distinguish between fat, lean mass and water.

Body Mass Index (BMI)

BMI represents an individual's weight per height as an index number.

Advantage

It most accurately reflects a person's body fat content.

Disadvantage

BMI cannot differentiate between lean tissue and either fat or extracellular water. Clinicians therefore, should not rely solely on BMI as their only measurement technique.

Skinfold Measurements

It provides estimates of fat and fat-free mass only. Measuring skinfold thickness is the most widely used technique for estimating fat mass.

Advantage

- Useful in identifying individuals with HIV associated fat redistribution.
- Readily available and inexpensive

Disadvantages

- Observer error is possible.
- There may also be errors because of inter individual variability in fat redistribution.
- Hard to standardize.
- Not efficient for small changes.

Cross-sectional Imaging

Advantage

Magnetic resonance imaging (MRI) and computed tomography are the most precise of the available measures that allow differentiation of subcutaneous adipose tissue and visceral adipose tissue and can measure changes in these compartments.[10]

Disadvantage

It needs expensive equipments and experienced technicians.

Dual-energy X-ray Absorptiometry (DEXA)

Reflects regional body composition, especially in the limbs.[11]

Advantage

- Very accurate
- Brief scanning time
- Safe radiation level.

Disadvantage

- High equipment cost
- Not portable
- Hydration status affects results.

Bioelectrical Impedance Analysis (BIA)

BIA uses the electrical impedance of body tissues to estimate body composition. It provides an estimate of the total body water by measuring changes in a low electrical current passed between electrodes placed on the upper and lower extremities. The sizes of other body compartments (including body cell mass) are then calculated using equations based on assumptions about the relationships between different body compartments and total body water. The validity and reliability of the results depend on the correct placement of the electrodes, room temperature, patient exercising, hydration status and the equations used to estimate body cell mass.

Loss of body cell mass, as measured by BIA, occurs early in the course of HIV infection, even in patients who are otherwise asymptomatic and is an independent adverse prognostic marker of clinical progression and survival.[12]

Advantages

- Rapid and easy to perform
- Portable and therefore can be used in clinical settings and hospitals.

COMPLEX NUTRITIONAL MANAGEMENT OF CHILDREN WITH HIV INFECTION

Because HIV can be transmitted through breast milk, the CDC recommends that HIV antibody-positive women in the United States avoid breast-feeding and use commercially available formulas for their child.

Children with HIV infection may be at increased nutritional risk because of the energy and micronutrient demands necessary to compensate for infection as well as support growth and development. Although the management should focus on the compliance to medications and nutrition but it should address additional measures. It is evident that patients who are compliant with HAART are less likely develop opportunistic infection and wasting.

The nutritional management of HIV infected children includes

- Implementation of nutritional support
- Drug therapy
- Oral care
- Nutritional aspects of highly active antiretroviral therapy (HAART)
- Follow up assessments

Implementation of Nutritional Support

Nutrition plays an essential role in supporting the health and quality of life of children with HIV disease. Nutrition intervention should begin soon after diagnosis. For optimal care, a nutritionist should perform an initial nutrition evaluation and periodic follow-ups.

For many children, nutritional status is often directly related to their socioeconomic status and it is an important determinant of overall nutritional status and growth.

Oropharyngeal and esophageal abnormalities associated with AIDS should be addressed before any nutritional intervention. If children have any signs of oral candidiasis, aphthous ulcers, gingivitis, poor dentition, leukoplakia, herpetic lesions they need to be treated. In such cases, high-calorie, smooth, nonirritating foods should be offered frequently throughout the day to maintain adequate total caloric intake.

Up to 75% of HIV-infected children have mild to severe developmental delay. HIV-associated encephalopathy not only results in delayed acquisition or loss of developmental milestones but also may affect oral motor skills. If poor feeding skills are suspected, the oral motor and self-feeding skills should be observed at the clinic and referral to an occupational therapist for evaluation should be made. If the possibility of aspiration is raised videofluoroscopic swallowing study should be ordered.

Several medications commonly used in the treatment of HIV disease, especially antiretroviral agents, macrolide antibiotics and chemotherapy, may cause anorexia, nausea or vomiting. In addition, drug interactions can increase serum levels of offending medications, exacerbating the problem.

Antiretroviral medications, especially the protease inhibitors, are unpalatable and difficult to administer to younger children. It is recommended adding the medication to a small amount of cold food (ice cream, shakes, fruit ices) or thick, sweet foods (honey, jellies, frozen juice concentrate) or small amounts of peanut butter, pudding, applesauce, or yogurt can make it palatable. These medications should be added to small quantities of food in order to be completely swallowed and the full dose be taken. In infants the placement of medication into a full bottle of formula should be avoided because the infant may not ingest the whole formula.

There is a great variation of nutritional requirements and feeding modes in HIV infection. There is a high prevalence of malabsorptive disorders in untreated HIV-infected children.[13] In case of suspected or proven malabsorptive disorders, protein hydrolysate and elemental formulas are better tolerated. All children with HIV and AIDS require high-energy, high-protein, nutrient-dense diets. The protein intake should be between 100% and 150% of the recommended daily allowance (RDA) in order to support the immune system and avoid muscle wasting. Caloric and protein needs should be adjusted for fever, infections, viral load, catch-up growth, and activity level.

The first step should be a trial with dietary manipulation. The caregivers should be counseled on food choices, frequency of meals and snacks, and methods of increasing caloric density. Commercially available nutritional supplements, high calorie drinks are cheaper than special high calorie formulas and still provide high-nutrient addition to the diet.

If the oral route fails to provide enough calorie and nutrients, supplemental enteral nutrition (EN) should be the next step. Enteral supplementation can improve weight and fat mass in HIV-infected children when other oral supplements fail.[14] EN improves not only weight, but also triceps skinfold thickness and decreases the number of hospital admission days.

A trial of nasogastric (NG) feeding is easily available and it may prove that a child is able to gain weight. The disadvantages of NG-tube feeding are complications such as sinusitis, worsening esophageal candidiasis. Additional limitations include the inability of the caregiver to maintain the NG feeding or a non-cooperative child.

The next step can be the endoscopic or surgical placement of a gastrostomy feeding tube. Miller *et al.*[14] reported that a low weight for height at the initiation of gastrostomy tube feedings predicts a good response to enteral supplementation. An additional benefit of a gastrostomy tube in HIV infected young children is that it eases administration of unpalatable antiviral liquid medications. The advantages, disadvantages and complications of enteral feeding and the indications of various feeding formulas are discussed in details in the previous volume of this book.[15]

Nutritional deficiencies should be addressed. Commonly deficient nutrients include thiamine mononitrate (vitamin B_1), riboflavin (vitamin B_2), pyridoxine hydrochloride (vitamin B_6), cyanocobalamin (vitamin B_{12}), folate, ascorbic acid (vitamin C), tocopherol (vitamin E), vitamin A, selenium, and zinc.

Adolescents and young adults often have lifestyle and eating habits that lead to poor-quality diets. Obesity is a common nutrition problem for both HIV-infected and uninfected teenagers. In addition, HIV-infected teenagers are at increased risk of developing metabolic abnormalities[16] and micronutrient deficiencies, and at highest risk of being deficient in vitamins A and E and zinc.[17] It was reported that supplemental vitamin A[18] and zinc[19] can decrease the frequency of respiratory and diarrheal illnesses. Experimental studies have suggested that high serum levels of vitamin E may be associated with slower disease progression.[20]

Micronutrients play important roles in maintaining immune function and neutralizing the reactive oxygen intermediates produced by activated macrophages and neutrophils in their response to microorganisms. Micronutrient status reflects the efficiency of the body's cellular functions. Insufficient dietary intake, malabsorption, diarrhea, and impaired storage and altered metabolism of micronutrients can contribute to the development of micronutrient deficiencies. In addition, infection and its evolution likely lead to an increased requirement for nutritional micronutrients, especially antioxidants.

Although the mechanisms are not known, micronutrient deficiencies may exacerbate the oxidative stress induced by HIV. Because young children have difficulty taking pills or capsules, a single complete multivitamin and mineral supplement in liquid or powdered form is ideal for them.

Drug Therapy

Appetite Stimulants

If diet with supplements does not lead to the desired weight gain, appetite stimulants can be considered as a short-term approach to reversing malnutrition. *Megestrol acetate,* an agent used for the treatment of metastatic breast cancer, is associated with appetite stimulation and weight gain. It has been shown in anorectic patients to improve appetite, quality of life and total body weight.[21] Megestrol acetate-induced weight gain is primarily the result of an increase in body mass.[22] It is a relatively non-toxic drug with a low incidence of side effects. A dose of 20 to 40 mg of megestrol acetate daily may improve weight gain in children. The adult dose is up to 800 mg/day.

Disadvantages

- No survival benefit or decrease in morbidity has been seen.
- Therapy is costly.
- May cause loss of lean body mass in some patients.
- Decreases serum testosterone levels.[23]

Anabolic Agents

Androgen deficiency is a common endocrine abnormality among adult men and women with HIV infection. Low testosterone concentrations are associated with lower CD4 cell count, advanced stage of illness, medication use, and weight loss. Androgens—particularly oxandrolone (Oxandrin), nandrolone (DecaDurabolin), oxymetholone (Anadrol-50) and testosterone have been used to increase body cell mass in patients with wasting syndrome. However, there are no accepted standards for indications, dosages and duration of therapy. In addition to its effects on body composition, testosterone treatment results in improved mood and libido in HIV-infected women and increased bone mineral density in HIV-infected men.[24] Anabolic agents have not been studied in children infected with HIV but has been studied in children with severe burns, which showed that long-term administration of oxandrolone safely improves Lean body mass, bone mineral content, and bone mineral density.[25]

Recombinant Human Growth Hormone (rhGH)

Body shape abnormalities are the side effect of highly active antiretroviral therapy (HAART), therefore has been great interest in potential interventions. Recombinant human growth hormone therapy is approved by the US Food and Drug Administration (FDA) and it is highly effective therapy for increasing lean body mass. rhGH treatment may enable patients with wasting to perform activities of daily living that would be exhausting.[26] However, the safety and efficacy of long-term rhGH therapy and its impact on survival are unknown. At this stage the use of rhGH is reserved for patients who are undergoing unexplained significant weight loss, have not responded to other therapies or require short-term treatment to maintain body cell mass during acute infection.

Oral Care

Studies have estimated that majority of persons with HIV infection will have at least one oral manifestation at some time during the course of their disease. Over 30 different oral manifestations of HIV disease have been reported since the beginning of the AIDS epidemic, which include infections, tumors, conditions caused by direct HIV activity, as well as adverse side-affects of antiretroviral and other antimicrobial drugs.

Patients with HIV infection may not have dental care. Patients should be examined for oral diseases and be treated. The medical staff plays an important role in educating the patient about good oral hygiene and the prevention and treatment of these conditions.

Nutritional Aspects of Highly Active Antiretroviral Therapy (HAART)

The presentation of the nutritional problems of HIV-infected children has changed since the implementation of the HAART. While the early reports on HIV infection mainly discussed the problems of malnutrition and wasting, the introduction HAART therapy in developed countries has added two additional nutritional problems, which are truncal obesity and insulin resistance, to the management of HIV-infected children. Miller *et al.*[27] reported that protease inhibitor therapy improves weight, weight for height, and muscle mass of HIV-infected children, independent of the concurrent decrease in HIV-1 viral load and improved CD4 T-lymphocyte counts.

Body Morphology Changes and Lipid Abnormalities

Lipodystrophy (LD) is a general term used to describe varying degrees of fat redistribution, including fat loss or lipoatrophy and fat accumulation or lipohypertrophy, Fat accumulation includes dorsocervical fat accumulation ("buffalo hump"), visceral adiposity, and breast enlargement. Fat loss includes facial-fat and limb-fat loss. Though LD was observed in persons with HIV infection before highly active treatment regimens were developed, the prevalence of LD has increased drastically with the widespread use of more active therapies. It has been reported mostly in adult but there is report in children.[28]

Clinical fat redistribution is significantly associated with older age, duration of antiretroviral treatment and highly active antiretroviral therapy and hypertriglyceridaemia.[29] The clinical importance of these is demonstrated by the increased prevalence of cardiovascular disease and diabetes in adult HIV infected persons. Many studies have suggested a link between the use of protease inhibitors (PI)[30,31] and nucleoside analogues[32] and LD.

There is ongoing research to diminish the clinical and biochemical features of fat redistribution syndrome. Therapeutically, oral hypoglycemic agents, such as metformin[33] and troglitazone,[34] and exercise training have been tried.[35]

Follow up Assessments

Reassessment of nutritional status is part of the management of HIV infected children. The extent of nutritional evaluation during follow up visits in addition to the routine developmental measures depends on the progress of a child.

Development and Body Mass Assessments

Weight and height growth velocities should be monitored every 3 to 6 months. Head circumference reflects brain growth and it should be monitored monthly for the first 3 years of life. A deviation from that normal growth warrants further investigation. Chronic malnutrition will eventually compromise brain growth and cognitive development.

Body composition measurements provide a more accurate assessment of nutritional status than weight and weight changes alone. In HIV-positive adults, bioelectric impedance analysis (BIA) is the method often used to assess lean body mass, adipose tissue, and fluid changes, however, there are no generally accepted BIA standards for children. It is more difficult due to changes in fluid status and lean body mass distribution in growing children.

Routine subscapular skinfolds compared with triceps skinfolds or routine abdominal girth may help identify children with changes in body shape or emerging lipodystrophy. Serial measurement of mid-arm circumference and skinfold can be an indicators of nutritional status if serially measured in the same children by the same person. Mid-arm circumference, triceps and subscapular skinfolds, and a calculated arm muscle area should be measured at a child's initial assessment and at least every 6 months.

Laboratory Tests

In addition to the routine blood and immunological tests, markers of nutritional status should be periodically measured during follow up visits. Serum prealbumin or transferrin are sensitive markers of nutritional change and it is recommended to monitor them serially.

Because deficiency of numerous micronutrients have been identified in patients with HIV infection, folate, zinc selenium, iron, and vitamins A, C, B_6, and B_{12} may need to be monitored in selected patients, especially in children who refuse or avoid one or more food groups.

Children on antiretroviral and nucleoside analogue therapies need fasting serum glucose and lipids monitoring routinely in order to detect possible antiretroviral-induced changes.

SUMMARY

Optimal nutritional status is very important in HIV infected children as it supports immune function and improves the quality of life. Initial nutritional assessment followed by regular clinical nutritional reassessment should be an integral part of the management of these children. The dietary treatment is often challenging due to HIV related diseases, medication side effects, psychosocial factors and age related nutritional problems in children. The goal of nutritional management is to optimize the child's growth, prolong and improve the quality of life.

REFERENCES

1. Guarino A, Spagnuolo MI, Giacomet V, Canani RB, Bruzzese E, Giaquinto C, *et al.* Effects of nutritional rehabilitation on intestinal function and on CD4 cell number in children with HIV. *J Pediatr Gastroenterol Nutr* 2002;34:366-371.
2. Prevention CfDCa. Revised classification system for human immunodeficiency virus infection in children less than 13 years of age. *MMWR* 1994;34(RR-12):1-19.
3. Miller TL, Evans SJ, Orav EJ, Morris V, McIntosh K, Winter HS. Growth and body composition in children infected with the human immunodeficiency virus-1. *Am J Clin Nutr* 1993;57:588-592.
4. Palenicek JP, Graham NM, He YD, Hoover DA, Oishi JS, Kingsley L, *et al.* Weight loss prior to clinical AIDS as a predictor of survival. Multicenter AIDS Cohort Study Investigators. *J Acquir Immune Defic Syndr Hum Retrovirol* 1995;10:366-373.
5. Wilson IB, Cleary PD. Clinical predictors of declines in physical functioning in persons with AIDS: results of a longitudinal study. *J Acquir Immune Defic Syndr Hum Retrovirol* 1997;16:343-349.
6. Wheeler DA. Weight loss and disease progression in HIV infection. *AIDS Read* 1999;9:347-353.
7. Palella FJ, Jr., Delaney KM, Moorman AC, Loveless MO, Fuhrer J, Satten GA, *et al.* Declining morbidity and mortality among patients with advanced human immunodeficiency virus infection. HIV Outpatient Study Investigators. *N Engl J Med* 1998;338:853-860.
8. Heller LS. Nutritional Support for Children With HIV/AIDS. *AIDS Read* 2000;10:109-114.
9. Matarazzo P, Palomba E, Lala R, Ciuti E, Altare F, de Sanctis L, *et al.* Growth impairment, IGF I hyposecretion and thyroid dysfunction in children with perinatal HIV-1 infection. *Acta Paediatr* 1994;83:1029-1034.
10. Ross R, Leger L, Morris D, de Guise J, Guardo R. Quantification of adipose tissue by MRI: Relationship with anthropometric variables. *J Appl Physiol* 1992;72:787-795.
11. Mazess RB, Barden HS, Bisek JP, Hanson J. Dual-energy x-ray absorptiometry for total-body and regional bone-mineral and soft-tissue composition. *Am J Clin Nutr* 1990;51:1106-1112.
12. Schwenk A, Beisenherz A, Romer K, Kremer G, Salzberger B, Elia M. Phase angle from bioelectrical impedance analysis remains an independent predictive marker in HIV-infected patients in the era of highly active antiretroviral treatment. *Am J Clin Nutr* 2000;72:496-501.
13. Miller TL, Orav EJ, Martin SR, Cooper ER, McIntosh K, Winter HS. Malnutrition and carbohydrate malabsorption in children with vertically transmitted human immunodeficiency virus 1 infection. *Gastroenterology* 1991;100(5 Pt 1):1296-1302.
14. Miller TL, Awnetwant EL, Evans S, Morris VM, Vazquez IM, McIntosh K. Gastrostomy tube supplementation for HIV-infected children. *Pediatrics* 1995;96(4 Pt 1):696-702.
15. Gadewar S, Horvath K. Enteral nutrition. *In: Gupte S (ed) Recent Advances in Pediatrics* 2005;14:1-26.
16. Kruzich L, Marquis G, Wilson C, Stephensen C. HIV-infected US youth are at high risk of obesity and poor diet quality: A challenge for improving short- and long-term health outcomes. *J Am Diet Assoc* 2004;104(10):1554-1560.
17. Kruzich L, Marquis G, Carriquiry A, Wilson C, Stephensen C. US youths in the early stages of HIV disease have low intakes of some micronutrients important for optimal immune function. *J Am Diet Assoc* 2004;104:1095-1101.
18. Julien MR, Gomes A, Varandas L, Rodrigues P, Malveiro F, Aguiar P, *et al.* A randomized, double-blind, placebo-controlled clinical trial of vitamin A in Mozambican children hospitalized with nonmeasles acute lower respiratory tract infections. *Trop Med Int Health* 1999;4:794-800.
19. Bhutta ZA, Bang P, Karlsson E, Hagenas L, Nizami SQ, Soder O. Insulin-like growth factor I response during nutritional rehabilitation of persistent diarrhoea. *Arch Dis Child* 1999;80:438-442.

20. Wang Y, Huang DS, Liang B, Watson RR. Nutritional status and immune responses in mice with murine AIDS are normalized by vitamin E supplementation. *Jf Nutrition* 1994;124:2024-2032.
21. Von Roenn JH. Randomized trials of megestrol acetate for AIDS-associated anorexia and cachexia. *Oncology* 1994;51(Suppl 1):19-24.
22. Loprinzi CL, Schaid DJ, Dose AM, Burnham NL, Jensen MD. Body-composition changes in patients who gain weight while receiving megestrol acetate. *J Clin Oncol* 1993;11:152-154.
23. Geller J, Albert J, Yen SS, Geller S, Loza D. Medical castration of males with megestrol acetate and small doses of diethylstilbestrol. *J Clin Endocrinol Metab* 1981;52:576-580.
24. Dobs A. Role of testosterone in maintaining lean body mass and bone density in HIV-infected patients. *Int J Impot Res* 2003;15(Suppl 4):S21-25.
25. Murphy KD, Thomas S, Mlcak RP, Chinkes DL, Klein GL, Herndon DN. Effects of long-term oxandrolone administration in severely burned children. *Surgery* 2004;136:219-224.
26. Evans WJ, Kotler DP, Staszewski S, Griffin GE, Isgaard J, Gertner JM, *et al.* Effect of recombinant human growth hormone on exercise capacity in patients with HIV-associated wasting on HAART. *AIDS Read* 2005;15:301-314.
27. Miller T, Mawn B, Orav E, Wilk D, Weinberg G, Nicchitta J, *et al.* The effect of protease inhibitor therapy on growth and body composition in human immunodeficiency virus type 1-infected children. *Pediatrics* 2001;107:E77.
28. Arpadi SM, Cuff PA, Horlick M, Wang J, Kotler DP. Lipodystrophy in HIV-infected children is associated with high viral load and low CD4+ -lymphocyte count and CD4+ -lymphocyte percentage at baseline and use of protease inhibitors and stavudine. *J Acquir Immune Defic Syndr* 2001;27:30-34.
29. Sanchez Torres AM, Munoz Muniz R, Madero R, Borque C, Garcia-Miguel MJ, De Jose Gomez MI. Prevalence of fat redistribution and metabolic disorders in human immunodeficiency virus-infected children. *Eur J Pediatr* 2005;164:271-276.
30. Negredo E, Paredes R, Bonjoch A, Tuldra A, Fumaz CR, Gel S, *et al.* Benefit of switching from a protease inhibitor (PI) to nevirapine in PI-experienced patients suffering acquired HIV-related lipodystrophy syndrome (AHL): interim analysis at 3 months of follow-up. *Antivir Ther* 1999;4(Suppl 3):23-28.
31. Francis S, Taylor M, Strickland A. Needs and preference assessment for an in-home nutrition education program using social marketing theory. *J Nutr Elder* 2004;24:73-92.
32. Saint-Marc T, Partisani M, Poizot-Martin I, Bruno F, Rouviere O, Lang JM, *et al.* A syndrome of peripheral fat wasting (lipodystrophy) in patients receiving long-term nucleoside analogue therapy. *AIDS* 1999;13:1659-1667.
33. Hadigan C, Corcoran C, Basgoz N, Davis B, Sax P, Grinspoon S. Metformin in the treatment of HIV lipodystrophy syndrome: A randomized controlled trial. *JAMA* 2000;284:472-477.
34. Inoue OJ, Freeman DE, Wallig M. Effects of hypochlorous acid and ascorbic acid on conductance, permeability, and structure of equine colonic mucosa in vitro. *Am J Vet Res* 1998;59:82-87.
35. Roubenoff R, Weiss L, McDermott A, Heflin T, Cloutier GJ, Wood M, *et al.* A pilot study of exercise training to reduce trunk fat in adults with HIV-associated fat redistribution. *AIDS* 1999;13:1373-1375.

Swati Gadewar • Anjali Malkani • Karoly Horvath

46 Enteral Nutrition

INTRODUCTION

Children have low energy reserves and higher energy and nutrient needs making them more susceptible than adults to malnutrition. Nutritional support should be considered if the recommended daily requirements will not be met for one to three days in infants, three to five days in children and more than seven days in older children and adults.

Patients who have swallowing dysfunction, food refusal, gastrointestinal diseases or are unable to maintain their nutritional needs due to underlying chronic disease or increased energy needs are prone to have poor growth or develop nutritional deficiencies. Enteral nutrition is useful not only to maintain the calorie and nutrient needs but also to provide additional calories for normal or catch-up growth. In certain clinical situation, feeding tubes are used primarily for the administration of fluids, e.g. patients who aspirate thin liquids or for the administration of medications, e.g. in children with HIV.

It is widely recognized that maintenance or improvement of nutritional status has a positive effect on the treatment outcomes in children. In the last few decades, there has been a significant advance in enteral feeding, which has led to the development of new formulas, feeding tubes, and endoscopic tube placement techniques allowing home enteral nutrition (HEN) after a short hospital stay. HEN has resulted in reduction of health care costs. Parental interest in HEN has increased as a result of the ongoing advances in technology for safe nutrient delivery, as well as the growth of support structures in the community. HEN has significant impact on the management of certain diseases, e.g. patients with short-gut syndrome or intestinal transplantation.

Enteral feeding is possible in all patients who have a functioning gastrointestinal tract. Typically, enteral nutritional support is initiated in the hospital setting and transitioned to the patient's home. If enteral tube feeding is not possible, parenteral nutrition (PN) should be initiated. Parenteral nutrition is efficient in providing nutritional support but is associated with significant complications, such as line sepsis, cholestasis, steatohepatitis, pneumothorax and venous thrombosis. It is expensive due to the high cost of preparation of sterile parenteral solutions and the longer hospital stay required initiating it. Hence, parenteral nutrition is limited to those patients who cannot be fed enterally. The basic rule is that if the intestine works it should be used.

This chapter discusses enteral nutrition (EN) via tube feeding and includes the indications of tube feeding, tube placement techniques, formula selection criteria and associated complications.

ADVANTAGES OF ENTERAL NUTRITION

Box 46.1 gives the precise advantages of enteral nutrition.

Box 46.1: Advantages of enteral nutrition

- Safer than parenteral nutrition.
- Physiologic way of feeding.
- Less expensive than parenteral nutrition.
- Easier to administer by caregiver.
- Supplies gut-preferred fuels like glutamine, glutamate, and short chain fatty acids.
- Can provide other beneficial compounds, such as fibers, fructo-oligosaccharides and probiotics that are not present in parenteral formulations.
- Maintains the mucosal integrity of the small and large intestine and prevents atrophy not only of the intestinal mucosa but also the pancreas.
- Preserves the normal function of the gut-associated immune system.
- Prevents cholelithiasis by stimulating gallbladder motility.

INDICATIONS OF TUBE FEEDING

Enteral nutrition *via* tube feeding is indicated in various clinical settings. Tube feeding is necessary to meet the nutritional needs of premature babies until they are able to meet their nutritional requirement orally. Children with gastrointestinal diseases, such as short-bowel syndrome, feeding disorders, inflammatory bowel disease, malabsorption, severe intestinal dysmotility, chronic liver disease, eosinophilic gastroenteritis, hepatic failure also require enteral feeding. Children with non-gastrointestinal diseases, such as congenital heart disease, pulmonary disease (cystic fibrosis, bronchopulmonary dysplasia, respiratory failure), chronic renal insufficiency, neurological disability (cerebral palsy), malnutrition/failure-to-thrive, cancer, post bone marrow transplantation, trauma and burns also may need tube feeding.

Table 46.1 summarizes the indications of tube feedings and lists clinical conditions and diseases when the appropriate enteral tube feeding is a reasonable approach.

The only absolute contraindications to enteral feeding are intestinal obstruction and a non-functioning gastro-intestinal tract. Relative contraindications include severe vomiting, enteric fistula, severe intrac diarrhea, upper gastrointestinal bleeding and significant intestinal dysmotility.

In certain clinical situations particular enteral feeding methods are not indicated, e.g. nasogastric tube placement contraindicated in children with critical illness, facial fractures, severe coagulopathy or esophageal strictures.

Nasogastric tubes should not be used if there is significant gastro-esophageal reflux, delay in gastric emptying, or altered gag reflex with the risk of aspiration. Although naso-gastric feeding is inexpensive and easy, there are potential drawbacks. They are often pulled out and have to be replaced, may worsen oral aversion, and have body image issues associated with it for both caregivers and older children.

Table 46.1: Typical indications for tube feeding

Tube feeding	*Indication*	*Disease/Disorder*
	Short-term feeding	
Nasogastric and Orogastric	Short-term feeding in patient with no reflux and normal gastric motility	Postoperative patients Premature infants Food refusal Miscellaneous causes of inadequate caloric intake After bone marrow transplant
Nasojejunal and Orojejunal	Short-term feeding in patients with significant reflux, risk of aspiration, abnormal gastric	Acute respiratory distress in critically ill patients Acute pancreatitis Severe gastroesophageal reflux disease Superior mesentery artery syndrome
	Long-term feeding	
Gastrostomy	Long-term feeding in patients who have normal gastric motility and do not have significant reflux	Oro-motor dysfunction Pharyngo-esophageal dysfunction Swallowing abnormalities (e.g. aspiration with clear liquids) Chronic lung disease without aspiration Proximal GI tract obstruction (head and neck injury, malignancy) Miscellaneous causes of inadequate caloric intake requiring long-term feeding Crohn's disease Chronic liver disease (e.g. Biliary atresia) Short bowel syndrome Severe food allergy and eosinophilic gastroenteropathy Metabolic diseases (e.g. glycogen storage disease) Trauma Burns Cancer patients Acquired immune deficiency disease Neurological impairment Chronic renal disease Severe congenital heart disease Bronchopulmonary dysplasia Cystic fibrosis
Transpyloric	Long-term feeding in patients with significant reflux and risk of aspiration	Severe gastric dysmotility Chronic lung disease with aspiration Superior mesentery artery syndrome Critical care patients with long-term feeding needs

ENTERAL FEEDING SELECTION

The appropriate tube feeding method depends on the clinical situation. For short-term use, usually orogastric and nasogastric tubes are used, however, if long-term feeding is necessary, more permanent tubes are placed endoscopically, radiologically or surgically.

Box 46.2 provides information helpful in the selection of the tube feeding method:

Box 46.2: Selection criteria for tube feeding

- Age of the patient (e.g., orogastric feeding is preferred in neonatal age group as they are obligate nasal breathers).
- Patient's diagnosis (e.g., severe reflux, failure to thrive, chronic illness, neurological impairment).
- Physical examination (severe scoliosis, surgical scar in epigastrium etc.).
- Past medical history.
- Surgical history, e.g. previous abdominal surgery; ventriculoperitoneal shunt, pacemakers, splenectomy etc.
- Prior imaging studies (upper gastrointestinal studies to rule out esophageal stricture, malrotation or other anatomical problems).
- The results of pH probe study if clinically indicated.
- Risk of aspiration (jejunal feeding or transpyloric feeding preferred over gastric feeding in this situation).
- Previous endoscopy histology results.
- History of allergy (e.g. in case of latex allergy silicon tubes should be used; allergy to milk or soy protein etc.).
- Feeding history: Previous nutritional interventions, volume of oral intake, tolerance to the previous feeding regimen.
- Patency, motility and function of the gut (e.g. jejunal feeding preferred over gastric feeding if there is history of gastroparesis).

Based on the above listed information it is possible to make decisions regarding the:

- Expected duration of tube feeding (short or long term).
- Gastric versus transpyloric tube feeding.
- Method of formula administration (bolus feeding, gravity or continuous feeding).

Expected Duration of Tube Feeding

In patients requiring short-term feeding, which is usually less than 30 days, nasally placed tubes (nasogastric or nasojejunal tubes, depending on the indication) are recommended because of their low cost, ease of placement, and lower complication rate. Long-term gastric tube feeding is the most common method for enteral nutrition support in patients with chronic diseases. In certain situations a G-J tube or a jejunostomy tube is indicated, which is discussed later.

Gastric or Transpyloric Tube Feeding

If there is no contraindication, gastric feeding is preferred over jejunal feeding because it is more physiological. In addition, gastric acid has bactericidal activity. All transpyloric feeds require the use of a feeding pump, which increases the cost of enteral feeding. Transpyloric tubes are more difficult to maintain and use than nasogastric tube (NGT) due to their ability to get dislodged and move back into the stomach. Transpyloric feeding is administered continuously via a pump with an iso-osmolar formula in order to avoid hyperosmolar diarrhea. Bolus feeds must not be given since it results in vomiting, distention, and diarrhea.

Fig. 46.1 shows an algorithm for tube feeding method selection.

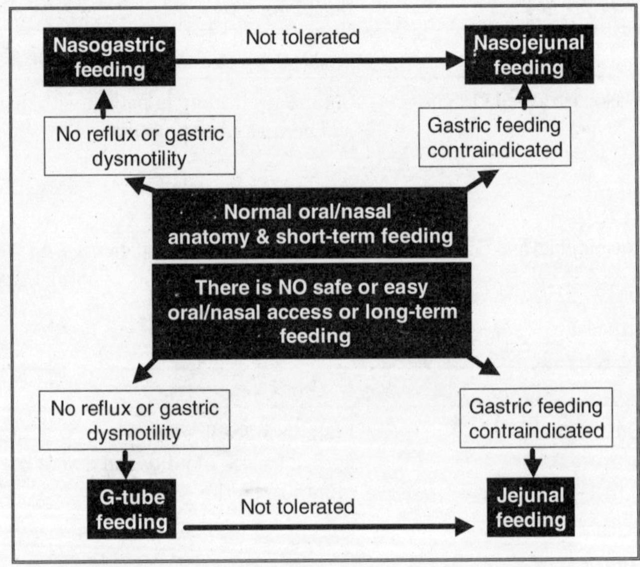

Fig. 46.1: A guide for tube feeding method selection

Nasogastric Tube Feeding (NGT): NGT is the simplest method of enteral feeding. It can be placed at the bedside and at home by the caregiver. Larger caliber tubes are used when decompression of the stomach, monitoring gastric pH or administration of thicker medications are needed in addition to feeding. In infants and young children, NG tubes may be changed once a month; in older school-going children they may be placed every night and removed in the morning.

Gastrostomy Tube (GT) Feeding: When a patient requires prolonged tube feeding (usually more than 30 days) gastrostomy tube placement should be considered. However, before the placement of a gastric tube, it is recommended to prove that the patient tolerates the feeding regimen with a temporary NGT. GT can be placed endoscopically, radiologically or surgically.

Transpyloric Tube Feeding: Transpyloric feeding delivers formula continuously into the small intestine. *Naso-duodenal or nasojejunal* tube feeding is indicated whenever there is a risk of aspiration, history of significant reflux, evidence of gastric dysmotility, acute pancreatitis or superior mesenteric artery syndrome. Tubes placed into the third portion of the duodenum or beyond the ligament of Treitz are associated with a decreased risk of aspiration, preventing gastric distension and allowing improved respiratory function. Hence transpyloric feeding is an invaluable and well-tolerated method of feeding in the critically ill child.

Jejunostomy Tube (JT) Feeding: If long-term transpyloric feeding is required jejunostomy tube placement should be considered. Jejunostomy tube feeding is indicated in children with aspiration, gastroparesis, inadequate stomach size due to previous resection and superior mesentery artery syndrome. Alternatives are endoscopic, radiological or surgical jejunostomy tube placement. In patients who already have a gastrostomy tube (GT) this can easily be converted to a gastrojejunostomy (GJ) tube.

Method of Formula Administration

Enteral feedings can be delivered intermittently as bolus or gravity feeding or as continuous feeding using feeding pump. Bolus and gravity feeding are used in gastric feeding only. Continuous feeding is mandatory when transpyloric tubes are used and is optional with gastric feeds.

Bolus feeding or intermittent feeding is the administration of formula, usually by syringe over a 5-15 minutes period every few hours. Caregivers can learn to administer bolus feeds and this does not require the use of a feeding bag or pump. It also allows the patient to continue with their regular activity. Bolus feeding is more physiologic than continuous feeds and is the method of choice, when tolerated. The advantages and disadvantages are listed in Table 46.2.

Table 46.2: Advantages and disadvantages of intermittent feeding

Advantages of intermittent feedings	*Disadvantages of intermittent feedings*
• Do not require infusion pumps	• Diarrhea
• More convenient for the parents	• Vomiting
• Permits patient mobility	• Aspiration pneumonia
• More physiologic	• Reflux

Gravity feedings can be delivered via intermittent or continuous drip. The rate of delivery is more accurate than with bolus feeding. It usually requires the use of a feeding bag. The risk of reflux and aspiration is the same as with bolus feeding.

Continuous feedings: Infants who cannot tolerate bolus feeds are switched to continuous gastric or duodenal/jejunal feeds. It requires a feeding pump with a source of power. The pump allows the delivery of formula either via an intermittent or continuous schedule. The delivery rate is accurately controlled.

Continuous intragastric feeding is safer, with fewer episodes of diarrhea and decreased risk of aspiration compared to intermittent feeding. If the clinical situation permits, continuous feeding can be converted to intermittent feeding. There is no defined protocol for this change. The gastric feeding rate can be gradually compressed depending on the patient's age and condition.

Continuous feeding is associated with less thermal energy loss. Caloric goals can also be achieved quickly with continuous feeding. However, continuous duodenal perfusion of liquid formulas has been shown to cause sequestration of bile acids as a result of incomplete emptying of the gallbladder.[1]

Independent of the feeding method, the bag with formula should hang no longer than 8 hours and the bag should be changed every 24 hours.

SELECTION OF THE FEEDING TUBE

A variety of tubes are available for each method of enteral feeding. Feeding tubes are usually made of ***polyethylene, polyurethane or silicone***. Polyethylene tubes stiffen and hence increase the risk of mucosal erosions or perforation; therefore, should be used only for a few days. The small and softer silicone or polyurethane nasogastric tubes are generally preferred as they provide more patient comfort, less local nasal complications, gastroesophageal reflux and aspiration pneumonia. They are more sui for long-term use.

Because latex allergy has become more prevalent in the last decade, patients with suspected or proven latex allergy should not get latex containing tubes.

The main determinant in the tube size selection is the viscosity of formula. The smallest necessary size should be selected to increase patient comfort. Typically an 8 Fr tube is used for commercial formulas. However, larger diameter is needed when using blenderized formulas (12-14 Fr).

Figures 46.2 and 46.3 show different gastric and transpyloric feeding tubes.

TECHNIQUES OF TUBE PLACEMENTS

Orogastric or Nasogastric Tube Placement

Estimating the length of the tube: The first step in nasogastric intubation is estimating the length of the tube to be inserted. A simple method to calculate this is to extend the distal end of the tube from the tip of the patient's nose to the earlobe and then from there to the xiphoid process and then add 10-15 cm (6 inches). A more accurate measurement for the distance between the nares and

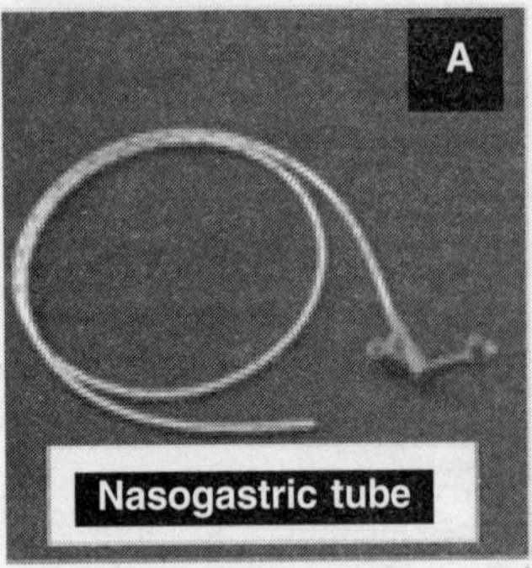

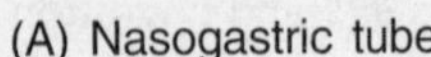
(A) Nasogastric tube

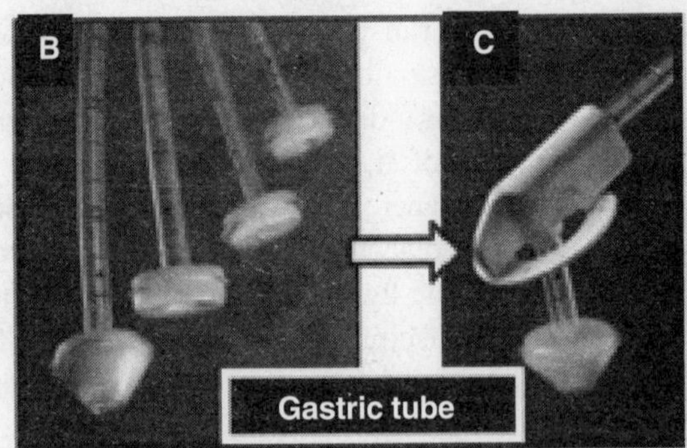

(B) Bumpers of the G-tube (C) Skin level lock

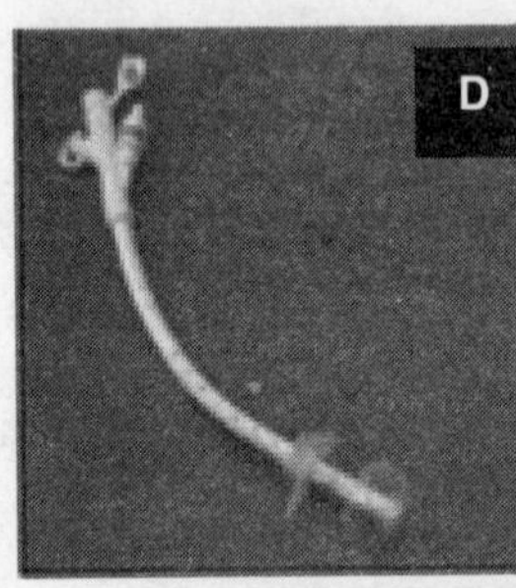

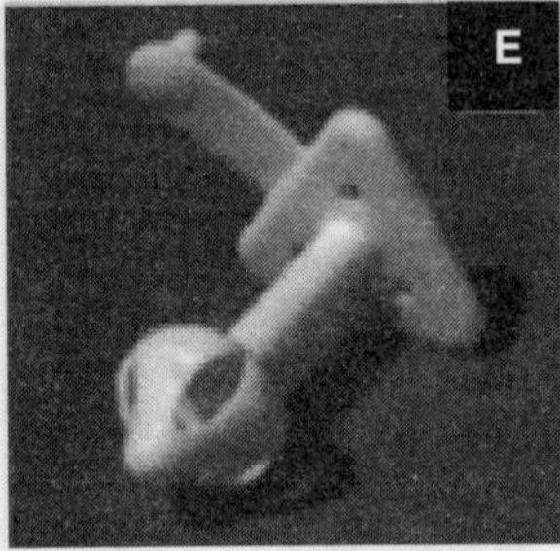

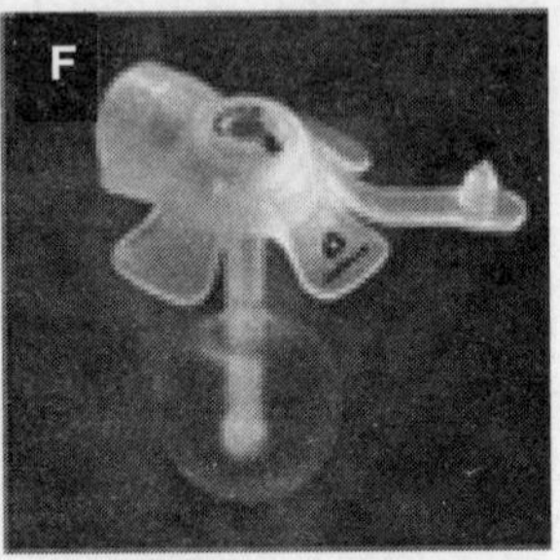

Low profile tubes for the replacement of the G-tube

Figs 46.2A to F: Feeding tubes for the transfer of formula to the stomach. (A) Nasogastric tube; (B) Internal bumpers of the gastrostomy tubes; (C) Gastrostomy tube with the external lock; (D) Long low profile balloon tube; (E) Short low profile tube needs stretching device to remove; (F) Short balloon type replacement tube

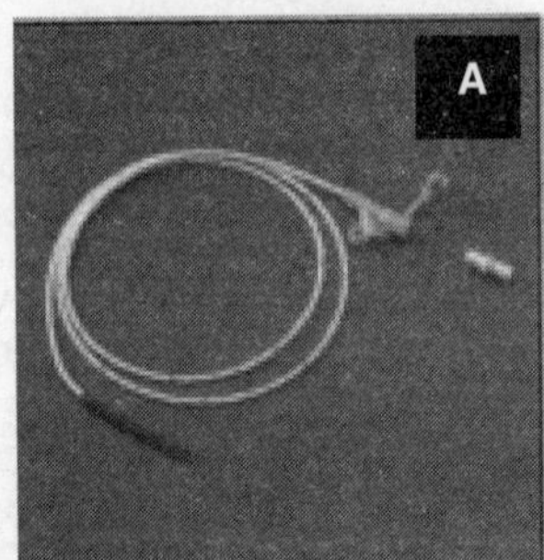

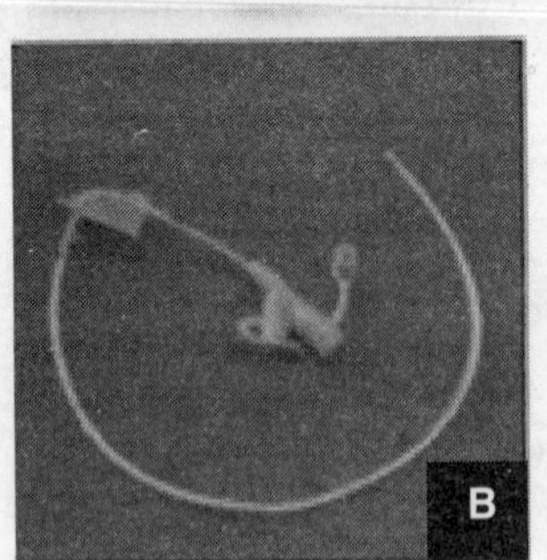

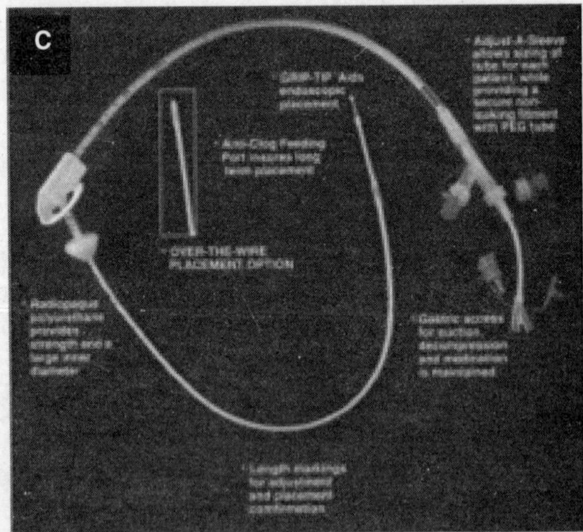

Fig. 46.3: Feeding tubes for the transfer of formula to the duodenum/jejunum. (A) Nasojejunal tube; (B) Surgical jejunal tube; (C) Gastro-jejunal tube with the conversion of the tube seen in Figure 46.2C

Section 11

gastroesophageal junction is the following formula used for pH probe: 0.25 × height [cm] + 5 cm.

Local anesthesia: The nares should be checked for obstruction and the tube passed down the more patent side. When necessary topical vasoconstrictors, such as phenylephrine (Neo-Synephrine 0.5%), or oxymetazoline (Afrin 0.05%) should be sprayed into the nasal passages, at least 3 to 5 minutes before the procedure. In order to avoid gagging, the nares, nasopharynx and oropharynx, should be anesthetized at least 5 minutes before the procedure. However, in infants the local anesthetic may trigger cough and laryngeal spasm. The tube is then lubricated with viscous lidocaine or lidocaine jelly prior to insertion.

Insertion: The tube is inserted along the floor of the nose. Mild resistance may occur in the posterior nasopharynx, but only gentle pressure should be required to overcome this resistance. Bleeding or dissection into retropharyngeal tissue may occur if force is used. Flexing the neck also tends to direct the tube into the esophagus. Excessive choking, gagging, coughing, change in voice, or the appearance of condensation in the lumen of the tube are signs of misplacement into the trachea and prompt withdrawal into the oropharynx is necessary. In patients who cannot cooperate or cannot cough (e.g. infants with chronic aspiration) extra precautions should be taken to avoid misplacement. The pharynx should be inspected after placement to exclude coiling of the tube. Tube position lateral to the midline suggests correct position in the esophagus. Once the tube is in the esophagus, it should be advanced rapidly to the previously determined depth.

Confirmation of tube position: Before securing the NG tube, its position should be confirmed (Box 46.3).

Box 46.3: Confirmation of tube position

- Injecting approximately 20cc of air through the tube and auscultating in the epigastric region for a gurgling sound is a simple way of confirming tube placement in the stomach. If the patient burps immediately after air instillation, the tube is probably in the esophagus and needs to be advanced further.
- Aspirating gastric contents is also a good way of checking the tube placement.
- If the patient is able to talk, the tube most likely is not coiled in the pharynx or in the trachea.
- If there is any doubt an X-ray is the most definitive way to confirm the position of an NG tube.

Nasojejunal Tube Placement

Successful placement of a nasojejunal tube depends on individual's skill and experience. The tube placement can be attempted at the bedside, under fluoroscopic view or endoscopically. Simple bedside placement is the preferred method. The initial phase of tube placement is the same as the nasogastric tube placement. Endoscopically or fluoroscopically guided tube placement should be reserved for those patients for whom bedside techniques have not been successful.

Nasojejunal tubes are available from 8F to 16F in diameters and in 90 to 240 cm in lengths. There are various tubes; some have a removable stylet and others have a weighted radio-opaque tip.

Nasojejunal tubes are available from 8F to 16F in diameters and in 90 to 240 cm in lengths. There are various tubes; some have a removable stylet and others have a weighted radio-opaque tip. Tubes with multiple side holes are less likely to become clogged. There are special tubes with a double lumen and double port allowing access to both the stomach and small intestine.

Transpyloric placement (duodenum, jejunum) of the feeding tube can be difficult and time consuming. There is no significant difference in the passage rate between tubes with or without weighted tips.[2,3] In one of the study, patients were placed in right lateral decubitus position and the passage of the tube into the small intestine was followed by auscultation.[4] This technique resulted in a successful transpyloric placement in 83% of the 103 patients, but only 44 of 103 of the tubes (43%) were in the preferred position, which is the third portion of the duodenum or beyond.

Prokinetic medications that increase antral motility are helpful for bedside and fluoroscopic insertions. Erythromycin stimulates gastric migrating motor complexes via the release of motilin, which then increases gastric motility.[5] Another useful prokinetic agent is metoclopramide, which is a cholinergic agonist and dopamine antagonist. It increases the amplitude of gastric contractions and promotes synchronization of peristalsis. In a study comparing weighted vs. unweighted 8F tubes, metoclopramide was given as an intravenous bolus 10 minutes before tube placement. The combination of preinsertion metoclopramide treatment and unweighted tube placement was significantly better, as after 4 hours, 84% of unweighted tubes passed into the duodenum compared to 36% of the weighted tubes.[2] When other methods fail I.V. erythromycin (3 mg/kg as infusion, an hour before tube placement) can help the passage of the tube into the duodenum.[6]

Although intravenous prokinetic administration may help, experience of the physician correlates better with successful tube placement than the administration of medications.[6] Ozdemir *et al.*[7] reported 88% success with the use an external magnet to direct a tube with a magnetic end through the pylorus.

If blind bedside insertion is not successful, fluoroscopic guidance may be used to advance the feeding tube into the jejunum, with a success rate of 86% to 90%. If this fails, nasojejunal tube can be placed with endoscopic guidance, which has a success rate as high as 98%.[8]

Maintenance of chronic transpyloric jejunal feeding catheters is more difficult than NG tubes. Upto one-third of patients require reinsertion because of jejunostomy tube malfunction or misplacement.[9]

Gastrostomy Feeding Tube Placement

Gastrostomy placement is the most frequently used method for long-term enteral feeding. It can be placed endoscopically, radiologically and surgically. Endoscopic placement is the preferred method over surgical placement as it is faster, cheaper and the feeding can start few hours after the procedure. Contraindications to endoscopic GT placement are listed in Box 46.4.

Box 46.4: Contraindications to endoscopic GT placement

1. Pharyngeal or esophageal obstruction.
2. Gastrointestinal fistulas.
3. Microsgastria or previous gastric surgery.
4. Gastric varices.
5. Hepatomegaly.
6. Morbid obesity.
7. Coagulopathy.
8. Neutropenia.
9. Portal hypertension.
10. Large ascites

Due to a high suspicion of intervening bowel loop endoscopic placement must not proceed when:

1. It is not possible to approximate gastric wall and abdominal wall.
2. Insertion site cannot be localized with finger palpation and transillumination.

Percutaneous Endoscopic Gastric (PEG) Tube Placement

In contrary to surgically placed G-tubes, percutaneous endoscopic placement of gastrostomy tubes do not require general anesthesia and has a shorter recovery period. PEG tube can be changed to a low-profile device when the track matures in approximately 8-12 weeks. One-step low profile PEG is an alternative, but it requires measuring the thickness of abdominal and stomach walls before selecting the length of the device. Either a water-filled balloon or a collapsible "dome" that can be stretched for insertion and removal anchors the low profile device internally. The low profile tube is almost at skin level and has cosmetic advantages since it can be concealed under the child's clothing.

Antibiotic prophylaxis: Since PEG tube placement requires the passage of the tube through the mouth, it is not a sterile procedure, and therefore the risk for tube-site infection is greater compared to an open gastrostomy. Administration of prophylactic antibiotic therapy reduces the incidence of infection[10] and is cost-effective.[11]

Procedure: Figure 46.4 shows the steps of the procedure. The pull technique is usually performed. A standard upper gastrointestinal endoscope is introduced into the stomach. The stomach is slightly distended by insufflation of air. A site for PEG placement is identified with the combination of *transillumination and finger indentation* on the abdominal wall. In most cases the insertion site is along an imaginary line drawn from the umbilicus to the left anterior axillary line in the subcostal region and, is at the junction of the upper and the middle third of this line. After an aseptic field is created, *local anesthetic* (1% Lidocaine) is injected into the selected area. The anesthetic syringe is advanced into the stomach lumen and can be seen by the endoscope. While withdrawing the needle aspiration is recommended. The appearance of *air bubbles* while the needle tip is in the wall may indicate the presence of an intervening hollow organ between the stomach and abdominal wall. If the illumination and the indentation are adequate and there is no suspicion of an intervening bowel loop, a *skin incision* is made to accommodate the PEG tube. The length of incision depends on the size of feeding tube. The next step is the *insertion of a trochar* through the incision into the stomach. It should be done with a brief, forceful thrust. This way the trochar does not push the anterior gastric wall away from the anterior abdominal wall. A *guide wire* is then advanced through the trochar into the stomach and it is *grasped with a snare* or forceps and withdrawn along with the endoscope through the mouth. The PEG tube (12-20 Fr) is hooked to the guide wire, lubricated with sterile jelly and is pulled through the mouth and esophagus into the stomach, and finally through the abdominal wall. The endoscope is passed into the esophagus and stomach again to inspect for mucosal trauma and to evaluate the PEG tube's position against the anterior abdominal wall of the stomach.

A modification of the pull technique is the push technique. In push technique a percutaneously inserted wire is used as a guide and the feeding catheter is threaded over the wire, pushed into the stomach and finally pushed out through the abdominal wall.

An external plastic positioner (crossbar) secures the PEG on the outside and prevents its inward migration into the stomach. It also keeps the tube in close approximation to the skin and inner part closer to the stomach wall. Once the PEG is fixed in place, the tube, which is originally approximately 3 feet long, is shortened and an adapter is attached to its end.

A "one-step button" tube is also available (Surgitek, One-Step button). If it is used, the thickness of the abdominal wall should be assessed before insertion. It is a compressed button tube, which opens after "peeling off" the plastic line.

The adapters of all tubes have ports for feeding pumps

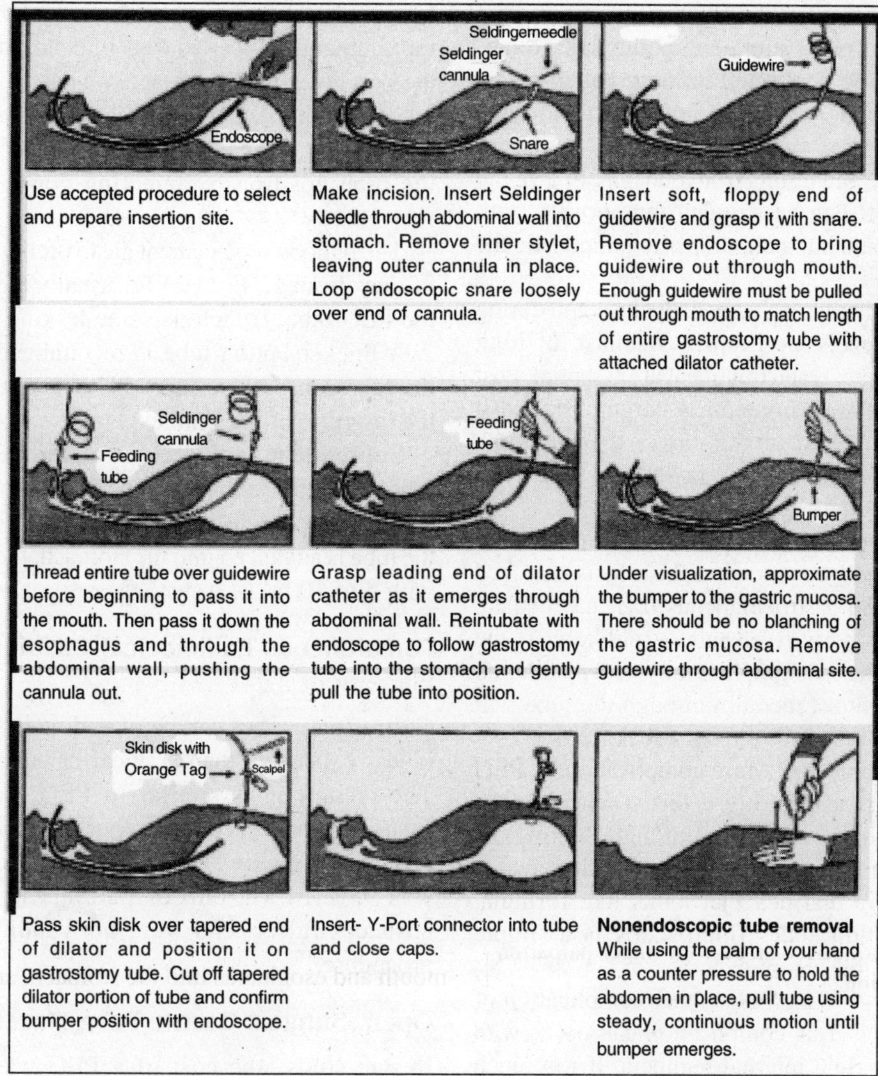

From the catalogue of the Ross Product Division of Abbott Laboratories

Fig. 46.4: Steps of the pull-through endoscopic gastric tube placement

and extension tubing for the administration of formula and medications.

Pain Management: The discomfort and pain after PEG placement can be relieved usually with acetaminophen (through G-tube or rectal suppository) or with intravenous non-steroid anti-inflammatory drugs (NSAIDs). Intravenous narcotics should be avoided for pain as they may induce a pharmacological ileus.

Feeding after Placement: There is no uniformly accepted recommendation for the time when tube feeding can be started after PEG placement. In our practice, we start infusing small volume of formula 6-8 hours after the procedure if the intestinal motility is normal and there is no significant gastric residuum. Our protocol includes the ventilation of the tube for 6 hours and a repeat dose of antibiotic 6 hours post procedure.

The volume is increased every 2-3 hours as continuous feeding and usually the patients reach the full volume of feeding within 24 hours after the procedure. Most patients are discharged 24 hours after the procedure.

If the patient does not tolerate feeds, they should be stopped and restarted at the initial volume 3 hours later. There is edema at the PEG site post procedure, which usually resolves in 24 hours. Once the edema resolves, the plastic crossbar is repositioned to provide a good fit against the abdomen. The gastrostomy site can be cleaned with soap and water or alcohol pad. Full strength hydrogen peroxide should be avoided because it contributes to the formation of granulation tissue.

Complications of Gastrostomy Placement: Peristomal wound infection is the most common complication of PEG placement. Treatment usually includes local care, and rarely oral antibiotic therapy. Necrotizing fasciitis often requires surgical debridement in addition to IV antibiotic therapy.

Other possible complications of PEG tube placement are hemorrhage, intestinal perforation, and peritonitis. Radiographic study should be performed in those patients who develop abdominal pain, vomiting, fever, or abdominal distention.

Hemorrhage is rare and results from puncture of a vessel in the gastric wall. It can be stopped temporarily with increased traction on the internal bumper to tamponade the tract.

Perforation of another viscus, especially the colon during the procedure may cause peritonitis. Because of high mortality, prompt diagnosis and treatment are essential. Post PEG procedure pneumoperitoneum is common[12] and it occurs in more than 1/3rd of the cases, therefore the presence of free air on abdominal X-ray cannot be used to diagnose perforation.

Peritonitis soon after PEG placement occurs in less than 1% of patients. It usually occurs when the tube is removed prematurely before the gastrocutaneous tract has healed. Leakage around a properly fixed tube is unlikely. If the PEG tube is still present, radiographic study with instillation of a water-soluble contrast medium through the tube will localize the tip of the tube and rule out a leak.

A colo-cutaneous fistula is a rare complication of PEG tube placement.[13] It is usually not detected until months after the initial placement, and often not until the original tube is replaced with a low-profile device. In these cases feeding causes severe diarrhea that looks like formula. Contrast administration under fluoroscopy is a simple method to recognize this complication.

"Buried bumper syndrome" is another complication of PEG tube placement.[14] This complication can occur with PEG tubes that have rigid internal bumpers. If too much pressure is maintained between the inner and outer bumper, it results in pressure necrosis and ulceration leading to tube migration slowly from the stomach into the gastrocutaneous tract.

Replacement of Gastrostomy Tube: Several methods are used to remove PEG tubes, depending on the configuration of the inner bumper. Some tubes are designed such that they can be directly pulled through the stoma, whereas stiff or rigid bumpers are best managed by endoscopic removal. Among the many available tubes we prefer using the Cor-Pak tube system, which has a collapsible intragastric disk (bumper), which is easy to remove by traction without endoscopy. Additional advantage of the Cor-Pak system is that it can be converted to gastro-jejunal feeding if needed at the time of PEG placement or later. Simply cutting the tube externally at skin level and allowing the tube to pass through the gastrointestinal tract is not recommended, as it can cause intestinal obstruction requiring surgical intervention.

The initial PEG tube is changed after 2-3 months, when the tract has matured. Skin level gastrostomy tubes (e.g., low profile button-type) are commonly used as PEG replacement devices placed into the mature tract. When the skin level tube is in place, we pass a small (5Fr) feeding tube through it and aspirate gastric juice to confirm proper positioning. If there is any doubt we recommend checking the tube position by injecting contrast material under fluoroscopy.

The balloon replacement gastrostomy tubes are available in sizes from 12 Fr to 24 Fr, usually the same diameter as the PEG tube. If there is some leaking around the PEG a 2 Fr thicker button tube is recommended. The length of the tube can be assessed with a measuring device before the insertion of the skin level tube.

Subsequent replacement of the balloon gastrostomy tubes is simple and may be performed by trained nurses or caregivers through the established gastrostomy tract. Once the tube is advanced into the stomach, the balloon is inflated with 5 to 10 ml of water.

Percutaneous Radiological Gastric (PRG) Tube Placement

Gastrostomy tubes can be placed under fluoroscopy. PRG is less expensive than surgical or endoscopic placement. The technique is similar to PEG placement, and the gastrostomy tube is pulled or pushed over a fluoroscopically placed guide wire. The success rate for PRG placement was 98% in a group of patients in whom PEG was unsuccessful or who were not candidates for the PEG procedure.[15]

Open, Surgical Gastric Tube Placement

In one study, the cost of a PEG was $ 700 less than operative gastrostomy. However, this advantage narrowed to approximately $100 if the tube required repeat endoscopy for a tube change and skin level device insertion.[16] There are fewer side-effects with PEG placement than with surgical GT. Patients can be fed sooner with a PEG, and general recovery is quicker as there is no laparotomy involved.

Surgical placement of GT may be combined with a Nissen fundoplication in children with severe reflux. Surgical placement of a gastrostomy tube may be required when PEG or PRG is contraindicated or not available. It can be accomplished with either open or laparoscopic technique. Surgical gastrostomy also should be used when PEG cannot be performed safely, e.g. in patients with extensive intra-abdominal adhesions or if an intestinal loop is positioned in between the stomach and abdominal wall.

Jejunostomy Feeding Tube Placement

Endoscopic Jejunal Feeding Tube Placement

Percutaneous endoscopic jejunostomy and gastrojejunostomy were originally reported in 1984. It is more difficult and time-consuming than G-tube placement. Contraindications are the same as PEG tube placement. Jejunostomy is most commonly used to reduce the risk of aspiration. It is frequently used in critically ill patients to avoid total parenteral nutrition. Aspiration cannot be fully prevented with jejunal feeding. However, its incidence is substantially reduced when it is combined with gastric decompression.

The indirect endoscopic method is used when the patient has an existing PEG tube. The jejunal tube is inserted through the gastrostomy (PEG/J). The jejunal tube is then advanced into the jejunum either over a guide wire or pushed into the jejunum with the endoscope. A simple technique is to attach a suture at the end of the J-tube. The tube is then inserted into the stomach through the gastrostomy and the suture is grasped by forceps. The endoscope is advanced into the small bowel with the tube along its side. Once in position, the suture is released and the endoscope is slowly removed to avoid withdrawal of the jejunal tube.

The advantage of the combined tube is that the gastric port can be used for gastric decompression, and the jejunal port used for feeding. Use of 10 to 12 F jejunal tubes substantially decreases the possibility of tube clogging.

Direct endoscopic jejunostomy is an alternative method. It is indicated in patients who had their stomach removed or altered. Usually an enteroscope or pediatric colonoscope is used for this procedure. The endoscope should be advanced into the jejunum near the ligament of Treitz. The abdominal wall in illuminated and a percutaneous endoscopic jejunostomy tube is inserted with a technique similar to that for PEG tube placement. Success rates with this approach have been in the range of 72% to 100%, with few complications.

Percutaneous Radiologic Jejunostomy (PRJ) Tube

The percutaneous jejunostomy (PRJ) feeding tube is placed under fluoroscopic guidance. The tube can be inserted through an existing gastrostomy tube and advanced into the jejunum over a guide wire (indirect method). It can also be inserted into the jejunum by direct percutaneous puncture near the ligament of Treitz.

Surgical Jejunostomy

Open surgical and laparoscopic techniques have been used with success to obtain jejunostomy access.

Jejunal feeding tubes are easily dislodged requiring frequent X-ray to confirm its position, bolus feedings cannot be given through jejunal tube, and higher rates of infusion can cause diarrhea. There is a high incidence of formula intolerance manifesting as diarrhea, nausea and cramps.

COMPLICATIONS OF TUBE FEEDING

Tube feeding patients should be monitored closely, especially in the initial stages for gastric residuals, reflux, vomiting, pulmonary symptoms, abdominal distention, urinary output, and stool frequency and consistency.

Clogged Tube: Precipitation of formulas is an important factor in the occlusion of gastrostomy and NG feeding tubes. Tubes are easily clogged if the:

1. Caliber of the tube is small.
2. Length of the tube is long.
3. Tube is in the stomach.
4. Feeding is continuous as opposed to bolus feedings.
5. Gastric residual volume is measured frequently.
6. Medication is administered through the tube.
7. Bulking agents such as psyllium fiber or resins, such as cholestyramine are given through the tube. In order to prevent tube clogging it is recommended to administer medications orally whenever possible. Flushing the tube every 6 to 8 hours prevents tube occlusion during continuous feedings and it is also recommended after every feed and medication administration (Box 46.5).

Box 46.5: Management of a clogged tube

- Instill warm water and clamp the tube for a few minutes, then instill air.
- In a prospective study the best declogging agent was a pancreatic enzyme concentrate mixed with bicarbonate to optimize the pH.[17]
- If applying the declogging solution with a syringe fails, a catheter can be passed through the tube to directly apply the solution at the clogged site.
- Most clogged tubes should be replaced.
- Tubes that have been unclogged by using force should be radiographed after water-soluble contrast injection to check for internal leaks.

Complications at the Insertion Site

Local irritation: Transnasally placed tubes can cause nasopharyngeal erosions, soreness of the nose, sinusitis and otitis media. Changing the side of tube insertion may resolve these problems.

Granulation tissue: Leaking of gastric juice around the G-tube site indicates that the internal part is not covering the tract completely. This leads to maceration and irritation of the skin predisposing to local infection and also promotes the development of granulation tissue. The management of this problem is listed in Box 46.6.

Box 46.6: Management of granulation tissue

- Inflate the balloon so that it sits firmly on the surface covering the tract. If needed change to a bigger size tube.
- An antacid can be applied on the surface to prevent maceration, or an acid suppressing medication may be administered.
- Granulation tissue can be treated with silver nitrate at the time of dressing changes.

Bleeding: It is rare complication of G-tube feeding. Management involves tightening the external bumper against the abdominal wall so it compresses the G-tube tract. The compression should be released within 48 hours to avoid tract wound breakdown. Surgical intervention is rarely necessary.

Deterioration of the tube: This can be recognized if there is pitting, ballooning, and a characteristic smell. It does not present a real risk to the patient; however, the tube can break, develop leaks or come out while the patient is sleeping. If the latter occurs, the tube site shrinks within hour and often tract dilatation is necessary to replace the same size. In our practice we replace the low profile tubes every 3-4 months. Microscopic examinations have demonstrated that fungal colonization is an important cause of G-tube failure.[18]

Complication at the End of the Tube

Ulceration: Ulcer may develop below the internal PEG tube bolster or on the opposite gastric wall. Loosening of the external bolster releases the bolster from the gastric mucosa and helps healing. Ulcers occur more frequently with rigid bolsters. Plastic and larger diameter tubes may cause esophageal and gastric erosions especially if they are used to check gastric residuum due to the force of negative pressure.

Dislodgement of tubes: The tip of the nasogastric, nasojejunal and gastrojejunal feeding tubes may move back during procedures, patient care, coughing etc. When dislodgement of the feeding tube is suspected, feeding should be stopped immediately and a radiograph obtained to verify the position of the tube prior to restarting the feeding. In case of G-tube if it comes out the gastrocutaneous tracts may close in as little as 24 hours; thus these tubes should be replaced promptly. A Foley catheter can be used temporarily to maintain a patent fistulous tract if low profile tube is unavailable.

Gastric obstruction: A longer balloon non button-type G-tube may migrate distally into the stomach and obstruct the gastric outlet if the external crossbar is not properly positioned. Patient may then present with vomiting, high residual volume or regurgitation.

Jejunal tube: Jejunal tubes are more prone for dislodgement as it is difficult to anchor them. Small intestinal ischemia and necrosis may develop. This more likely occurs in patients who are hemodynamically uns.

Nutritional Complications

Refeeding syndrome: This occurs in approximately 25% of patients who have limited oral intake or in whom feeding is introduced rapidly. Signs of refeeding syndrome are glucose intolerance, fluid retention, and electrolyte imbalance (hypophosphatemia, hypomagnesaemia, and hypokalemia). These signs are usually observed during the first few days after initiation of feeding. In these patients daily monitoring of electrolytes may be necessary until nutritional goals are achieved and the electrolytes and glucose are s. If the condition is left untreated or unrecognized, paralysis, respiratory failure, and even death can occur.

Aspiration: Aspiration is a risk in children with severe gastroesophageal reflux disease who are on nasogastric or gastrostomy feeding. Confirming the position of the tube radiographically before initiating the feeding and also when displacement is suspected can reduce the incidence of aspiration. Reflux precautions, including elevation of the head of the bed by 20-30 degrees during feeding and using continuous feeding reduce the risk of this complication. In high-risk patients nasojejunal, gastrojejunal or jejunostomy feeding should be used temporarily. In patients with severe gastroesophageal reflux, funduplication with gastrostomy tube provides a long-term resolution to avoid aspiration.

Table 46.2 summarizes feeding tube related problems and gives recommendations for the resolution.

ENERGY REQUIREMENTS IN CHILDREN

Estimating the caloric and nutritional requirement is one of the criteria to decide on the preferred route of EN. The following two *tables* (Tables 46.3A and 46.3B) show the energy requirement in children, which consists of the resting energy expenditure multiplied with various stress and activity factors.

TUBE FEEDING FORMULA SELECTION

Feeding should not be started until the proper placement of the feeding tube is verified. The most important goal of tube feeding is to meet nutritional needs of the patient. When selecting the appropriate formula, the factors to consider are included in Table 46.4.

The formula selection depends on the age, clinical diagnosis and gastrointestinal function of the child. In general, "intact" formulas containing unaltered components (proteins, carbohydrates, fat) are suitable for most patients and "elemental" or "predigested" formulas are used for patients with malabsorption, critical illness, allergic enteropathy, or other gastrointestinal impairments.

Age-specific formulas exist for premature infants, term infants, toddlers, and children upto 10 years of age. As a general rule adult formulas for enteral nutrition can be used in children >10 years of age. Below 10 years of age pediatric formulas are recommended. Infants under 12 months should be given breast milk, a standard infant formula or a special infant formula. For most children 1-10 years of age, pediatric enteral formulas (Pediasure, Resource, Kindercal) are designed specifically to meet their nutrient requirements.

In premature infants, who are unable to coordinate sucking, swallowing, and breathing, orogastric (or

Table 46.2: A short guide to manage symptoms associated with tube feeding

Problem	Possible cause	Possible solution
Constipation	Inadequate fluid intake	Use more water to flush
	Low fiber diet	Use fiber containing formula; add soluble fiber supplement to the formula
	Lack of activity	Physiotherapy; exercise
Cramping	Cold formula	Room temperature formula
	Tube in wrong place	Reposition
	Too fast feeding	Reduce the feeding rate
Diarrhea	Rapid transpyloric feeding	Reduce the feeding rate
	Formula intolerance	Change formula
	Lactose intolerance	
	Concentrated formula	Start with lower caloric density formula (20Kal/oz) and gradually increase the concentration in 3-5 days
	Medication	Use alternate medication with less osmolality
		In case of antibiotic administration check stool for C. difficile toxins
Gas, bloating	Air in the tube, plus same causes as diarrhea	Clamped the tube between intermittent feedings.
		Remove all air from the delivery system before feeding
		Ventilate stomach before G-tube feeding starts
Nausea	Delayed gastric emptying	Try prokinetic medications
	Stomach distention	Ventilate stomach via GT before feeding
	Too cold formula	Use room temperature formula
Reflux and Vomiting	Physiological reflux	Elevate the head side of the bed Thicken feeds (add cereal to the formula)
		Pharmacotherapy for reflux
	Too rapid feedings	Slow feeding rate
	Tube is too large	Use smaller sized tube
	Improper tube placement	Reposition
	Large residual in stomach	Change to continuous drip infusion
		Consider adding a prokinetic agent
		Use isotonic formula
		Change to transpyloric feeding
	Medications given with feeding	Give medication before or >1 hour after feeding

nasogastric) feeding should be initiated. Breast milk or a special formula can be administered by continuous infusion or bolus delivery every two to three hours. Healthy premature infants tolerate bolus feeding, while infants with pulmonary problems or gastrointestinal abnormalities may tolerate continuous feeding better.

Table 46.3A: Estimated Resting Energy Expenditure (REE; Kcal/day) for children

Age (years)	1–3	3–10	10–18
Female	61*W – 51	22.5*W + 499	12.2*W + 746
Male	60.9*W – 54	22.7*W + 495	17.5*W + 651

W = weight in kg

Adapted from WHO: Energy and protein requirements, Technical Report Series 724:71, 1985.

Table 46.3B: Stress/activity factors affecting energy needs

REE X 1.3	• Well-nourished child at bed rest • Mild-to-moderate stress minor surgery
REE X 1.5	• Normally active child with mild-to-moderate stress • Inactive child with severe stress • Sepsis, cancer, extensive surgery • Minimally active child with malnutrition and need for catch-up growth
REE X 1.7	• Active child needing catch-up growth • Active child with severe stress

* Multiply REE adjustment factor for estimated daily energy requirements.

REE= Resting energy expenditure.

Adapted from Department of Pharmacy Services: Pharmacy Handbook and Formulary, Hudson, OH, 1997, Lexi-comp, Inc., 375.

Table 46.4: Factors affecting the formula selection

Patient Related	Age Underlying diagnosis Digestive and absorptive capacity of the GI tract Fluid, nutrient and caloric needs Activity level History of food intolerance or allergy
Formula Related	Caloric density Osmolality, viscosity and nutrient content of the formula Ease of preparation
Expense	Cost Insurance coverage

Protein and calorie requirements are age-dependent. In certain clinical situations higher protein intake is necessary (e.g. intestinal loss) or higher caloric intake is required for a catch-up growth.

Infants with intolerance to milk and/or soy protein should get hydrolyzed, hypoallergenic formula. If hypoallergenic formula is not tolerated, an amino acid based formula should be considered (e.g. Neocate).

The presence of gastrointestinal disease may require special formulas, e.g. medium chain triglyceride (MCT) containing formulas are used in patients with pancreatic, biliary, or intestinal diseases when the digestion and absorption of long-chain fat is impaired or when there is problem with lymphatic flow.

There are new components added to formulas in the last few years. These include nucleotides, soluble fiber, glutamine, arginine, and fructo-oligosaccharides.

The availability and price of special formulas can be a limiting factor in the selection. Generally it is better to use original formulas without modifications in order to avoid errors. If after estimating energy needs additional nutrients are required, formulas can easily be supplemented with modular components.

Sometimes parents modify formulas without physician approval, which may result in altered caloric or protein intake (e.g. mixing formula with juice reduces protein content etc). It is important to reassure parents that the appropriately selected formulas meet their child's nutritional needs.

Types of Formulas

Complete or Standard Formulas

Standard formulas are nutritionally complete and made of complex proteins, fats, carbohydrates, and contain adequate vitamins and minerals. They are appropriate for patients who have normal digestion and absorption but unable to ingest adequate calories and nutrients. The advantages of complete formulas are that they have low osmolality, are palatable, easy to use, and are sterile. Some of the complete formulas have "fiber containing" versions which helps in regulating bowel movements and preventing constipation, which is a frequent problem in neurologically impaired or postoperative patients.

Elemental Formulas

One form of elemental formulas contains hydrolyzed (predigested) protein and is called hypoallergenic formulas. Other, real elemental formulas have only amino acids as the protein component. In addition, they usually have different ratios of medium-chain triglycerides to long chain triglycerides, along with essential fatty acids, vitamins and minerals.

The elemental formulas require less digestion, result in lower stool volume and cause less stimulation of bile and pancreatic secretions. The disadvantage of elemental formulas is that they have higher osmolality. Higher infusion rate may cause cramping and osmotic diarrhea. The most frequent clinical indications for the use of elemental formulas include short gut syndrome, malabsorption syndromes, severe food allergies, inflammatory bowel disease and gastrointestinal fistulas. They are much more expensive than standard formulas, therefore should not be given to children with normal digestive function and no food allergies.

Home-Prepared Formulas

Home-prepared, blenderized formulas can be administered through low profile gastrostomy tubes. They cost less than standard commercial formulas and require more time to prepare. Homemade preparations are more viscous and may contain chunks, which could easily block the tube. They are not sterile and run the risk of bacterial contamination during preparation and storage. In addition there is a risk that they are nutritionally incomplete unless a pediatric dietitian closely supervises them. This is an economic option in developing countries where pre-made formulas are expensive.

Modular Formulas

Modular formulas contain only specific nutrients. They are added to commercial or home-prepared formulas to meet specific nutrient needs. Examples of modular formulas are the following:

- Medium-chain triglycerides (e.g., MCT oil) provide fat calories in an easily digestible and absorbable form.
- Readily-digested carbohydrates (e.g., Moducal or Polycose) used for additional calories.
- Protein and specific amino acid preparations (e.g., Casec or ProMod) to increase the protein content.

Special Formulas

Various specialized formulas are available for children with special needs, such as premature infants, children with renal failure or inborn errors of metabolism. The treating physician and dietitian who are familiar with the products and their indication select these formulas.

MONITORING PATIENTS ON LONG-TERM TUBE FEEDING

The measures are listed in Box 46.7.

Box 46.7: Measures for monitoring children on long-term tube feeding

- Weigh every other day until stable, then weekly for acute care and monthly for long-term care. Daily weights may be required in intensive care settings. Monitor weight for height. Evaluate the need for reducing caloric intake in case of low energy needs due to low activity and adjust the calories accordingly.
- Basic electrolytes plus calcium, magnesium, and phosphorous, complete blood count initially then every 10 days. These should be monitored more frequently in intensive care situations. Do monthly or at least quarterly in long-term home care.
- Albumin initially then every month.
- Monitor glucose readings until feeding is at final rate and blood sugars are stable.
- Evaluate if formula is meeting the requirements for fluids, calories, protein, vitamins, minerals and electrolytes.
- Replace the tube as needed.

SUMMARY

Enteral tube feeding is widely used both in the inpatient and outpatient setting to meet the nutritional requirements in patients who otherwise cannot maintain these needs for various reasons. It is a valuable modality of treatment in acute and chronic illnesses. Complications can usually be avoided if appropriate care is taken. Patients should be monitored for tolerance, complications and assessed for a possible return to oral feeding.

REFERENCES

1. Rutgeerts P, Ghoos Y, Vantrappen G. The enterohepatic circulation of bile acids during continuous liquid formula perfusion of the duodenum. *J Lipid Res* 1983;24:614-619.
2. Lord L, Weiser-Maimone A, Pulhamus M, Sax H. Comparison of weighted vs unweighted enteral feeding tubes for efficacy of transpyloric intubation. *JPEN J Parenter Enteral Nutr* 1993;17:271-273.
3. Levenson R, Turner W, Dyson A, Zike L, Reisch J. Do weighted nasoenteric feeding tubes facilitate duodenal intubations? *JPEN J Parenter Enteral Nutr* 1988;12:135-137.
4. Ugo P, Mohler P, Wilson G. Bedside postpyloric placement of weighted feeding tubes. *Nutr Clin Pract* 1992;7:284-287.
5. Komenaka I, Giffard K, Miller J, Schein M. Erythromycin and position facilitated placement of postpyloric feeding tubes in burned patients. *Dig Surg* 2000;17:578-580.
6. Heiselman D, Hofer T, Vidovich R. Enteral feeding tube placement success with intravenous metoclopramide administration in ICU patients. *Chest* 1995;107:1686-1688.
7. Ozdemir B, Frost M, Hayes J, Sullivan D. Placement of nasoenteral feeding tubes using magnetic guidance: Retesting a new technique. *J Am Coll Nutr* 2000;19:446-451.
8. Ott D, Mattox H, Gelfand D, Chen M, Wu W. Enteral feeding tubes: Placement by using fluoroscopy and endoscopy. *AJR Am J Roentgenol* 1991;157:769-771.
9. Albanese C, Towbin R, Ulman I, Lewis J, Smith S. Percutaneous gastrojejunostomy versus Nissen fundoplication for enteral feeding of the neurologically impaired child with gastroesophageal reflux. *J Pediatr* 1993;123:371-375.
10. Lockett M, Templeton M, Byrne T, Norcross E. Percutaneous endoscopic gastrostomy complications in a tertiary-care center. *Am Surg* 2002;68:117-120.
11. Kulling D, Sonnenberg A, Fried M, Bauerfeind P. Cost analysis of antibiotic prophylaxis for PEG. *Gastrointest Endosc* 2000;51:152-156.
12. Gottfried E, Plumser A, Clair M. Pneumoperitoneum following percutaneous endoscopic gastrostomy. A prospective study. *Gastrointest Endosc* 1986;32:397-399.
13. Berger S, Zarling E. Colocutaneous fistula following migration of PEG tube. *Gastrointest Endosc* 1991;37:86-88.
14. Klein S, Heare B, Soloway R. The "buried bumper syndrome": A complication of percutaneous endoscopic gastrostomy. *Am J Gastroenterol* 1990;85:448-451.
15. Ho S, Marchinkow L, Legiehn G, Munk P, Lee M. Radiological percutaneous gastrostomy. *Clin Radiol* 2001;56:902-910.
16. Stiegmann G, Goff J, Silas D, Pearlman N, Sun J, Norton L. Endoscopic versus operative gastrostomy: Final results of a prospective randomized trial. *Gastrointest Endosc* 1990;36:1-5.
17. Marcuard S, Stegall K. Unclogging feeding tubes with pancreatic enzyme. *JPEN J Parenter Enteral Nutr* 1990;14:198-200.
18. Iber F, Livak A, Patel M. Importance of fungus colonization in failure of silicone rubber percutaneous gastrostomy tubes (PEGs). *Dig Dis Sci* 1996;41:226-231.

Deonath Mahto • B Vishnu Bhat

47 Parenteral Nutrition

INTRODUCTION

Parenteral nutrition (PN) is a method of providing nutritional support to an individual whose gastrointestinal tract is either not functioning or is inaccessible. It may be total or supplementary, central or peripheral.

In the year 1968 Dudrick *et al.*[1] reported that growth and development could be sustained with long term PN in an infant who could not be fed via gastrointestinal tract. Subsequently, numerous reports were published documenting the feasibility of supporting normal growth with this technique.[2,3] However, this new technology was not without problems. Several nutritional deficiency syndromes were reported, including trace element deficiency[4-6] and essential fatty acid deficiency.[7,8] Even biotin deficiency was documented in an infant receiving inadequate amount of biotin which is rarely seen in individuals having normal diet.[9]

Hence, PN should be provided only when clearly indicated. When PN is essential to administer, every effort should be made to provide at least a minimum amount of nutrients enterally to preserve the integrity and function of gastrointestinal tract, unless there is an absolute contraindication.

INDICATIONS OF PARENTERAL NUTRITION[10,11]

The primary goal of PN is to maintain or improve the nutritional and metabolic status of patients who, for a critical period of time, cannot be adequately nourished by oral or enteral route. Following clinical conditions may benefited from PN:

1. Very low birthweight premature infants when enteral feeding is inadequate.
2. Necrotizing enterocolitis.
3. Short bowel syndrome.
4. Gastroschisis.
5. Persistent ileus.
6. Severe intestinal obstruction.
7. Critically ill patients with hypercatabolic state, where enteral nutrition has failed.
8. During intensive care / ventilatory support.
9. Severe persistent vomiting induced by drugs, intracranial tumors or other diseases.

VASCULAR ACCESS FOR PN

PN can be administered through central vein or peripheral vein. In children who are relatively well nourished requiring PN not more than 7-10 days, peripheral veins can be used successfully.[12] For long-term administration of PN, central route is preferred. For administration of PN, following routes were used by various workers Table 47.1.

Table 47.1: Route of venous access

Sl. No.	*Route of Administration*	*Authors*	*Year*
1.	Peripheral vein (Percutaneous approach)	Stokes MA *et al.*[13]	1993
		Kearns PJ *et al.*[14]	1996
2.	Jugular vein (Internal or external) (Percutaneous approach)	Dudrick SJ *et al.*[15]	1969
3.	Jugular vein (Internal or external) surgical approach	Jeejeebhoy KN *et al.*[16]	1973
4.	Subclavian vein or tributary (Surgical approach)	Broviac JW *et al.*[17]	1973
5.	Subclavian vein or tributary (Percutaneous approach)	Dudrick SJ *et al.*[15]	1969
6.	Portal vein	Joyeux J *et al.*[18]	1974
7.	Anteriovenous fistulas		
	Internal	Zincke H *et al.*[19]	1974
	External	Heizer WD *et al.*[20]	1977
		Shils ME *et al.*[21]	1977
8.	Common facial vein	Jeejeebhoy KN *et al.*[16]	1973
9.	Inferior epigastric vein	Krog M *et al.*[22]	1983
10.	Saphenous vein	Fonkalsrud EW *et al.*[23]	1982
11.	Right atrium	Oram-Smith JC *et al.*[24]	1979

Among these routes, jugular vein (internal or external) percutaneous approach is the preferred one for central PN. Other vascular approaches may be used when the usual vessels are not patent or unavailable.[11]

COMPONENTS AND REQUIREMENTS

PN solutions supply basic nutrients including fluid, carbohydrates, protein, fat, minerals, tarce elements and vitamins. These components can be given together as an admixture termed "total nutrient admixture" (TNA) or the lipid component may be given separately. Typically, PN solution for infants contain 2.5% amino acids, 10-25% and dextrose electrolytes, vitamins and minerals in amount sufficient to meet patients estimated daily requirements. The proportion of calories from each of the major nutrients should approach the percentage in the average enteral diet e.g. 50-60% carbohydrate, 30-40% fat and 10-15% protein.[12]

FLUID REQUIREMENTS

Fluid needs are based on water losses from skin, respiration, urine and stool, water accumulation in newly formed tissues and water produced from carbohydrate oxidation.[25,26] Because the body surface area per unit weight is greater in children than in adults, evaporative losses are increased, which results in greater fluid requirements per unit weight in children. Maintenance fluid requirements in children, except preterm neonates, can be calculated from equations described by Holliday and Segar as per Table 47.2.[27]

Table 47.2: Maintenance fluid needs

Weight	*Fluid requirement*
Upto 10 kg	100 ml/kg
11 to 20 kg	1000 ml + (weight – 10) x 50 ml
> 20 kg	1500 ml + (weight – 20) x 20 ml

Patients with excessive fluid losses (e.g. gastric drainage, diarrhoea, vomiting, chest tube drainage, burn or wound exudates, fistula drainage, or patients under radiant warmer, UV light or with fever) require additional fluids to compensate for these losses. These outputs should be replaced with fluids that are similar in volume and electrolyte composition.

ENERGY REQUIREMENTS

When patients are on PN, no energy is used in nutrient absorption. These factors account for at least 7% of energy in the diet of the enterally fed subject. Hence, average energy requirement is at least 7% less in children on PN.[28] Parenteral calorie requirement in infants and children is given in Table 47.3.

CARBOHYDRATE SOURCES OF ENERGY

Dextrose is used almost exclusively as the carbohydrate calorie source. With increasing age, maximum exogenous glucose oxidation rates decrease approximately from 12.5 mg/kg/min in infants to about 5 mg/kg/min in older children.[12]

Table 47.3: Parenteral calorie requirement in children[12]

Age of the child	*Calorie requirement (Kcal / kg / day)*
Preterm neonate	85 – 130
Infant	90 – 120
1-6 yr	75 – 90
7-12 yr	50 – 75
13-18 yr	30 – 50

Neonates, particularly premature neonates, are less glucose tolerant and are at risk for developing hyperglycemic induced hyperosmolar coma and intra ventricular hemorrhage.[29] With very high glucose intakes (>40 Kcal/Kg/day) which saturate glucose oxidation, the excess is converted to fat.[30] High carbohydrate intake may also increase Co_2 production, aggravating impaired respiratory function causing difficulties in 'weaning', ventilated patients.

Excessive hepatic lipogenesis can produce 'fatty liver' or TPN liver: This usually occurs when glucose is given as the sole energy source.[31]

Septic and traumatized patients can develop peripheral insulin resistance due to the altered hormonal profile that is associated with stress.[32,53]

LIPID SOURCES OF ENERGY

Lipids as energy source in PN are given as emulsions. Lipid emulsions are available as 10% (1 Kcal / ml) or 20% (2 Kcal / ml) solutions. The 20% concentration is usually used instead of the 10% concentration to diminish the total fluid volume. Commercially available intravenous lipid emulsions (IVLE) products contain two principal families of essential fatty acids derived from vegetable oil long chain fatty acids (LCFA) - W-6 and W-3 fatty acids.[33] Egg yolk phospholipid is used as an emulsifying agent and glycerin is added to achieve isotonicity.[34]

IVLE, is used to provide energy and to avoid essential fatty acid deficiency, which can develop within 2 weeks if patients are given parenteral nutrition without lipids. At least 5% of the total energy infused should be provided as lipid to avoid essential fatty acid deficiency. Parenteral lipid enters the blood stream directly as chylomicron or very low density lipoprotein like particle, which can then be hydrolyzed by the endothelial lipoprotein lipase. Lipid infusion at higher rates exceeding the capacity for clearance by lipoprotein lipase, leads to accumulation of triglyceride rich particles that are likely to interfere with pulmonary diffusion and leukocyte function.[34,35]

Altered pulmonary hemodynamic is believed to arise from metabolic breakdown products of the long-chain polyunsaturated fatty acids, such as prostaglandin, leukotrienes and thromboxanes.[36] When IVLE are administered rapidly (> 0.12 gm/kg/hr), an increased production of vasoconstrictive prostaglandins (PGF_2a, TXA_2) may result, causing hypoxemia in selective lung areas with pre-existing low ventilation perfusion ratio. Indeed, the majority of studies demonstrating changes in oxygenation infused IVLE at rates faster than 0.12 g/kg/hr.[37] A predominance of vasodilating prostaglandins was reported by Hunt *et al.* with a slow infusion of lipid emulsion, whereas an increase in vasoconstrictive prostaglandins was observed with rapid infusion.[38]

Reports of alterations in immune function have been associated with excessive infusion rates or doses of IVLE. Early experimental studies suggested that IVLE containing primarily long chain fatty acids (LCFAs) impaired the bactericidal and migratory functions of polymorphonuclear cells and decreased bacterial clearance by the mononuclear phagocyte system.[39] Large bolus infusions of IVLE administered over 1 to 6 hours were given in these studies. To date controlled clinical trials using recommended infusion rates have failed to demonstrate clinically significant alterations in neutrophil or monocyte/ macrophage function in patients receiving IVLE containing LCFAs. Studies assessing the influence of LCFA based IVLE on cellular immunity have yielded variable results.[40-44] No clinical trials have shown significant alterations in components of humoral immunity, such as serum immunoglobulin or complement factor concentrations as a result of LCFA based IVLE.[40,45,46]

American Academy of Pediatrics (AAP) recommends that IVLE should be initiated at 0.5 g/kg/day in premature neonates. Term infants and infants older than one month can usually be started at 1g/kg/day. If serum triglyceride or free fatty acid concentrations are within acceptable limits, the fat emulsion dosage can be increased by 0.25 to 0.5 g/kg/day upto 3 g/kg/day in preterm neonates and by 0.5 to 1 g/kg/day upto maximum of 4 g/kg/day in term and older infants.[47]

NEWER INTRAVENOUS LIPIDS

Medium chain triglycerides (MCT) derived from coconut oil, mixed long chain triglycerides and MCTs, short chain fatty acids, W-3 fatty acids are all currently under study as lipid fuels in PN.[48]

Protein Requirements

Parenteral protein requirements in children is greater on a per kilogram basis than adults because of increased tissue anabolism. Guidelines for parenteral protein requirements in children are given in Table 47.4.

Preterm and term neonates also require qualitatively different amino acids for optimal growth and development.[49-51] Enzyme immaturity in the transsulfuration pathway prevents conversion of methionine to cysteine and cysteine to taurine. Similarly, phenylalanine hydroxylase insufficiency may limit the conversion of phenylalanine to tyrosine. Thus, cysteine, taurine, tyrosine, and histidine are conditionally essential aminoacids for preterm infants and neonates.[12]

Table 47.4: Protein requirement in children[12]

Age Group	*Protein Requirement (g/kg/day)*
Preterm	2.5–3.0
Term neonates	2.0–2.5
Older infants	1.5–2.0
Preschool/school age	1.0–1.5
Adolescent	0.8–1.5

Modified amino acid solutions have been developed for specific diseases and conditions.[52] Trophamine[R] and Aminosin PF[R] are modified amino acid solutions that contain adequate concentration of amino acids such as taurine. They are designed to produce serum amino acid concentration similar to those achieved with breast-feeding in healthy infants.[51]

ELECTROLYTE AND MINERAL REQUIREMENTS

Electrolytes in maintenance or therapeutic dosages must be added to the PN each day to maintain electrolyte homeostasis. The daily maintenance electrolyte requirements for neonates, infants and children are given in Table 47.5.

Table 47.5: Daily electrolyte dosages (mEq/ kg/day)[25, 27, 54-58]

Electrolyte	*Preterm Infants*	*Term infants and Children*
Sodium	2 – 8	2 – 5
Potassium	1.4 – 10*	2 – 3
Chloride	1.1 – 5	2 – 3
Magnesium	0.25 – 0.6	0.25 – 0.5
Calcium	2.5 – 3.5	1 – 2
Phosphate (mmol/kg/day)	1.3 – 2	0.5 – 1

* In patients receiving diuretics.

TRACE ELEMENTS REQUIREMENTS

The trace elements constitute less than 0.01% of human body weight.[12] Despite their low body content, trace elements have essential roles in biochemical processes including growth and development. The requirement of premature infants are generally higher as their growth rates are twice that of a term infant and their nervous system is still immature [59,60]

Current recommendations for parenteral dosages of trace element is given in Table 47.6.

VITAMINS

Vitamins are essential dietary components for normal cell maintenance, function and growth. The suggested daily parenteral intake of vitamin in infants and children is given in Table 47.7.

Table 47.6: Daily intravenous requirement (per kg body weight) of trace elements in infants and children[58]

Elements	*Premature infant*	*Full term infants*	*Children*
Zinc (mg)	0.4	0.25 < 3 months 0.1 > 3 months	0.05 (max. 5 / day)
Copper (mg)	20	20	20 (max. 300 / day)
Selenium (mg)	2.0	2.0	2.0 (max. 30 / day)
Chromium (mg)	0.2	0.2	0.2 (max. 5.0 / day)
Manganese (mg)	1.0	1.0	1.0 (max. 50 / day)
Molybdenum (mg)	0.25	0.25	0.25 (max. 5 / day)
Iodide (mg)	1.0	1.0	1.0 (max. 50 / day)

Table 47.7: Daily parenteral requirement of vitamin in infants and children[58]

Vitamins	*Term infants and children (Dose / day)*
A (mg)	700
D (mg)	10
E (mg)	7
K (mg)	200
Ascorbic acid (mg)	80
Thiamin (mg)	1.2
Riboflavin (mg)	1.4
Pyridoxine (mg)	1.0
Niacin (mg)	17
Pantothenate (mg)	5
Biotin (mg)	20
Folate (mg)	140
Cyanocobalamine (mg)	1.0

DELIVERY SYSTEM

In the past, PN formulations consisted of an admixture of dextrose and protein (two in one), and intravenous lipid was added to those solutions. The intravenous admixture of dextrose, amino acids, and fat emulsion is known as total nutrient admixture (TNA).

Creaming and coalescence of the lipid emulsion result when electrolytes are added directly to it. Adding these electrolytes beyond the recommended amounts neutralizes the negative potential at the surface of the emulsion and causes the admixture to coalesce.[61] Hence, TNA must be prepared carefully to ensure stability.[62] PN solutions are usually delivered from bottles as plastic bags via electronic pumps to ensure even flow, thus minimizing likelihood of clotting at the catheter tip.[11]

Dual-chambered plastic bags have been marketed that allows admixture of macronutrients immediately before infusion of PN admixture.[63] Dual-chambered bags are manufactured either empty or with the macronutrients in them (i.e. dextrose in one chamber and amino acids in the other chamber). When lipid is used, the dextrose, amino acids, and electrolytes are added to the bottom chamber of the empty bag and the desired intravenous lipid dose to the upper chamber. This increases stability, because TNA is not prepared with until just before infusion.[11]

CDC RECOMMENDATIONS FOR ADMINISTRATION OF PARENTERAL FLUIDS AND REPLACEMENT OF ADMINISTRATION SET[64]

1. Infusion of lipid containing solution (TNA) should be completed within 24 hours of hanging the solution.
2. IVLE infused separately from dextrose and amino acid PN formulations should be completed within 12 hours of hanging the emulsion.
3. Replacement of administration set and tubing for lipid containing solution should occur within 24 hours of initiating infusion.
4. Administration set and tubing for dextrose and amino acid PN solution do not need to be replaced more frequently than once every 72 hours.

MONITORING

The aim of monitoring is to detect the complications of PN at an early stage so that corrective measures can be instituted. The frequency with which the patient should be monitored depends upon the clinical condition of the patient, the nature of feeding regimen and the results of previous measurements. Guidelines for monitoring of a patient on PN are given in Table 47.8.

Table 47.8: Guidelines for monitoring of a patient on PN[10]

Parameters should be monitored

Daily	*Weekly*	*Monthly*
Weight	X-ray chest	Length
Serum Electrolyte	Blood culture	Arm circumference
Blood urea nitrogen	Coagulation profile	Skin fold thickness
Serum creatinine	Liver function test	X ray of long bones
Serum calcium	Plasma amino acids	Plasma fatty acids
Serum phosphorus	Serum magnesium	Erythrocyte fatty acids
Blood glucose	Serum ferritin	
Urine volume	Urine microscopy for candida	
Urinary electrolyte		
Urinary osmolality		
Urinary glucose		
Nutrients and filters for culture		

The above investigations may be done less frequently when the parameters becomes established and stable.

COMPLICATIONS

Complications of PN may be technical, metabolic or infective.

Technical

The osmolality of PN solution ranges from 800-950 mOsm/kg/H_2O. Thus, phlebitis can occur.[12] Infants and small children who have limited extravascular tissue space and who may not be able to communicate pain adequately are at risk for developing complications, including localized swelling and edema which may progress to necrosis.[65]

Complication that occurs at the time of catheter placement include pneumothorax, vein or cardiac perforation and chylothorax.[66] Catheter may migrate out of the position or be accidentally removed.[67] Catheters located in the right atrium may cause arrythmias by coming in contact with nodal tissue.

Metabolic

Metabolic complications include electrolyte and mineral abnormalities, metabolic bone disease, micronutrient deficiencies, cholestasis, hypersensitivity reactions, acid base abnormalities and alterations in pulmonary and immunologic function.[68]

Infection

Infection is a serious complication associated with central venous catheters and may be blood borne, exit site, or tunnel tract infection.[12] The incidence of central venous line infections is inversely related to age and in pediatric patients ranged from 42-57%.[69] Organism that commonly result in infection in pediatric patients on long-term parenteral nutrition are—*Staphylococcus epidermidis, Klebsiella, Staphylococcus aureus, E.coli* and fungi.[70]

SUMMARY AND CONCLUSIONS

- Normal growth and development can be achieved with parenteral nutrition.
- Even when PN is indicated, every effort should be made to provide at least a minimum amount of nutrients enterally, unless there is absolute contraindication.
- Parentral calorie requirement should be at least 7% less than enteral nutrition.
- Cysteine, taurine, tyrosine and histidine are conditionally essential amino acids in preterm infants and neonates.
- Pediatric parenteral amino acids formulations are designed to produce serum amino acids concentration similar to those achieved with breast feeding in healthy infants.
- The rate of IVLE infusion should be kept to < 0.12 g/kg/hr.
- In healthy infants requiring parenteral nutrition not more than 7-10 days, peripheral venous access is the preferred route.
- Complications associated with PN can be reduced by appropriate monitoring.

Section 11

REFERENCES

1. Dudrick SJ, Wilmore DW, Vars HM, Rhoads JE. Long-term total parenteral nutrition with growth, development and positive nitrogen balance. *Surgery* 1968;64:134-142.
2. Benda GM, Babson SG. Peripheral Intravenous alimentation of the small premature infant. *J Pediatr* 1971;79:494-498.
3. Filler RM, Eraklis AJ, Rubin VG, *et al.* Long-term parenteral nutrition in infants. *N Engl J Med* 1969;281:589-594.
4. Arakawa T, Tamura T, Igarashi Y, *et al.*: Zinc deficiency in two infants during total parenteral alimentation for diarrhoea. *Am J Clin Nutr* 1976; 29:197-204.
5. Heller RM, Kirchner SG, O'Neill JA Jr, *et al.* Skeletal changes of copper deficiency in infants receiving prolonged total parenteral nutrition. *J Pediatr* 1978; 92: 947-949.
6. Kien CL, Ganther HE; Manifestations of chronic selenium deficiency in a child receiving total parenteral nutrition: *Am J Clin Nutr* 1983; 37: 319-328.
7. Caldwel MD, Jonsson HT, Othersen HB. Essential fatty acid deficiency in an infant receiving prolonged parenteral alimentation. *J Pediatr* 1972;81:894-898.
8. Gohlke BC, Fahnenstich H, Kowalewski S: Serum lipids during parenteral nutrition with a 10% lipid emulsion with reduced phospholipid emulsifier content in premature infants. *J Pediatr Endocrinal Metab* 1997;10:505-509.
9. Mock DM, deLorimer AA, Liebman WM *et al.* Biotin deficiency: An unusual complication of parenteral alimentation. *N Engl J Med* 1981; 304: 820-823.
10. Smart AEW. *Textbook of Parenteral Nutrition*, 2nd edn. London: Smithson 2003.
11. Shils ME, Brown RO. Parenteral Nutrition. In: Maurice E Shils, *et al* (eds): *Modern Nutrition in Health and Disease.* Philadelphia: Lippincott Williams and Wilkins 1999:1657-1688.
12. Hak EB, Helms RA. Pediatric and neonatal nutrition. In : Herfindal ET, Gourley DR (eds): *Textbook of Therapeutics, Drug and Disease Management.* Philadelphia: Lippincott Williams and Wilkins 2000: 1969-1992.
13. Stokes MA, Hill GL. Stokes MA, Hill GL, Peripheral parenteral nutrition a preliminary report on its efficacy and safety. *J Parenter Enteral Nutr* 1993;17:145-147.
14. Kearns PJ, Coleman S, Wehner JH. Complications of long arm-catheters: A randomized trial of central Vs peripheral tip location. *J Parenter Enteral Nutr* 1996;20:20-24.
15. Dudrick SJ, Wilmore DW, Vars HM, *et al.* Can entravenous feeding as the sole means of nutrition support growth in the child and restore weight loss in adult? An affirmative asnwer. *Ann Surg* 1969; 169: 974-984.
16. Jeejeebhoy KN, Zohrab WJ, Langer B, *et al.* Total parenteral nutrition at home for 23 months, without complication, and with good rehabilitation. A study of technical and metabolic features. *Gastroenterology* 1973;65:811-820.
17. Broviac JW, Cole JJ, Scribner BH. A silicone rubber atrial catheters for prolonged parenteral alimentation. *Surg Gynecol Obstet* 1973; 136: 602-606.
18. Joyeux J, Astruc B, Martin G, *et al.* Experimental parenteral nutrition via the portal vein. Techniques and results. *J Chir (Paris)* 1974;107:335-366.
19. Zincke H, Hirsche BL, Amamoo DG, *et al.* The use of bovine carotid grafts for hemodialysis and hyper alimentation. *Surg Gynecol Obstet* 1974;139:350-352.
20. Heizer WD, Orringer EP. Parenteral nutrition at home for 5 yrs via arteriovenous fistulae. Supplemental intravenous feeding for a patient with severe short bowel syndrome. *Gastroenterology* 1977; 72: 527-532.

21. Shils ME, Wright WL, Turnbull A, *et al.* Long-term parenteral nutrition through an external arteriovenous shunt. *N Engl J Med* 1970; 283: 341-344.
22. Malt RA, Kempster M, Direct azygos vein and superior vena cava cannulation for parenteral nutrition. *J Parenter Enteral Nutr* 1983; 7: 580-581.
23. Fonkalsrud EW, Berquist W, Burke M, *et al.* Long-term hyperatimentation in children through saphenous central venous catheterization. *Am J Surg* 1982; 143: 209-211.
24. Oram-Smith JC, Mullen JL, Harken AH, *et al.* Direct right atrial catheterization for total parenteral nutrition. *Surgery* 1978; 83: 274-276.
25. Costarino A, Baumgart S. Modern fluid and electrolyte management of the critically ill premature infant. *Pediatr Clin North Am* 1986;33:153-178.
26. Heely AM, Talbot NB. Insensible water losses per day by hospitalized infants and children. *Am J Dis Child* 1955; 90:251-256.
27. Holliday MA, Segar WE, The maintenance need for water in parenteral fluid therapy. *Pediatrics* 1957;19:823-832.
28. Nancy F, Krabs K, Hambidge M. Normal childhood nutrition and its disorders. In: Hay WW Jr, Hayward AR, Levin MJ, Sondheimer JM (eds): *Current Pediatric Diagnosis and Treatment*. New York: Lange/McGraw Hill 2003:277-307.
29. Thomas DB, Hyperosmolality and intraventricular haemorrhage in premature babies. *Acta Pediatr Scand* 1976; 65:429-432.
30. Grimble GK, Payne-James JJ, Rees RG, Silk DBA. TPN: Novel energy substrates. *Intens Ther Clin Monitor* 1989;10:108-113.
31. Baker AL, Rosenberg IH. Hepatic complications of total parenteral nutrition. *Am J Med* 1986; 82:489-497.
32. Stoner HB, Little RA, Fnayn KN, Elebute AE, Tresaden J, Gross E. The effect of sepsis on the oxidation of carbohydrate and fat: *Br J Surg* 1983; 70:32-35.
33. Sacks GS. Enhancing the response to parenteral nutrition in critical care. *Nutr Clin Pract* 2003;19:226-234.
34. Michail S, Vanderhoof JA. Parenteral nutrition in clinical practice. *Annales Nestle* 1996; 54:53-60.
35. Barr LH, Dunn GD, Brennan MF. Essential fatty acid deficiency during total parenteral nutrition. *Ann Surg* 1981;193:304-311.
36. Mayer K, Grimm H, Grimminger F, Seeger W. Parenteral nutrition with n-3 lipids in sepsis. *Br J Nutr* 2002, 87 (suppl 1): S69-S75.
37. Faucher M, Bregeon F, Gainnier M, Thirion X Auffray J.P. Paperzian L. Cardiopulmonary effects of lipid emulsions in patients with ARDS. *Chest* 2003;124:285-291.
38. Hunt CE, Pachman LM, Hageman JR, Cobb MA, Klemka L. Liposyn infusion increases plasma prostaglandin concentrations. *Pediatr Pulmonal* 1986;2:154-158.
39. Pulmblad J. Intravenous lipid emulsions and host defense: A critical review. *Clin Nutr* 1991;10:303-308.
40. Ota DM, Jessup JM, Babcock GF, *et al.* Immune function during intravenous administration of soyabean oil emulsion. *J Parenter Enteral Nutr* 1985;9:23-27.
41. Helms RA, Herrod HG, Burckart GJ, Christensen ML. E-rosette formation, total T – cells, and lymphocyte transformation in infants receiving intravenous safflower oil emulsion. *J Parenter Enteral Nutr* 1983;7:541-545.
42. Monson JR, Ramsden CW, Macfile J, Brennan TG, Guillou PJ. Immunorestorative effect of lipid emulsions during TPN. *Br J Surg* 1986; 73: 843-846.
43. Gogos CA, Kalfarentzos FE, Zoumbos NC. Effect of different types of TPN on T. Lymphocyte subpopulations and NK cells. *Am J Clin Nutr* 1990;51:119-122.
44. Sedman PC, Somers SS, Remsden CW, Brennan TG, Guillou PJ. Effects of different lipid emulsions on lymphocyte function during TPN. *Br J Surg* 1991;78:1396-1399.
45. Strunk RC, Murrow BW, Thilo E, Kunke KS, Johnson EG. Normal macrophage function in infants receiving intralipid by low dose intermittent administration. *J Pediatr* 1985; 106: 640-645.
46. Dahlstrom KA, Goulet OJ, Roberts RL, Ricour C, Ament ME. Lipid tolerance in children receiving long-term parenteral nutrition: A biochemical and immunologic study. *J Pediatr* 1988; 113: 985-990.
47. American Academy of Pediatrics. Committee on nutrition, AAP: Commentary on parenteral nutrition. *Pediatrics* 1983;71:547-552.
48. Furst P. New parenteral substrates in clinical nutrition Part II. New substrates in lipid nutrition. *Eur J Clin Nutr* 1994;48:681-691.
49. Helms RA, Christensen ML, Mayer EC, *et al.* Comparison of pediatric versus standard amino acid formulation in preterm neonates requiring parenteral nutrition. *J Pediatr* 1987; 110:466-470.
50. Adamkin DH, McClead RE, Desai NS, *et al.* Comparison of two neonatal intravenous amino acid formulations in preterm infants: A multicenter study. *J Perinatol* 1991; 11:375 -382.
51. Heird WC, Dell RB, Helms RA *et al.* Amino acid mixture designed to maintain normal plasma amino acid patterns in infants and children requiring parenteral nutrition. *Pediatrics* 1987; 80: 401-408.
52. Cochran EB, Phelps SJ, Helms RA. Parenteral nutrition in pediatric patients. *Clin Pharm* 1988;7:351-366.
53. Lemoyne M and Jeejeebhoy KN. Total parenteral nutrition in the critically ill patient. *Chest* 1986;89:568-575.
54. Heird WC, Winters RW. Total parenteral nutrition. *J Pediatr* 1975; 86:2-16.
55. Bell EF, Oh W. Fluid and electrolyte balance in very low birth weight infants. *Clin Perinatal* 1979; 6:139-150.
56. Perkin RM, Levin DL. Common fluid and electrolyte problems in the pediatric intensive care unit. *Pediatr Clin North Am* 1980;27:567–586.
57. Arnald WC. Parenteral nutrition and fluid and electrolyte therapy. *Pediatr Clin North Am* 1990;37:449-461.
58. Greene HL, Hambidge KM, Schanler R, *et al.* Guidelines for the use of vitamins, trace elements, calcium, magnesium, and phosphorus in infants and children receiving total parenteral nutrition. *Am J Clin Nutr* 1988;48:1324-1342.
59. Zenk KE, Husetable RF, Dunaway D. Advisable daily vitamin intake for preterm infants. *J Parenter Enteral Nutr* 1981;5:447-448.
60. James BE, Hendry PG, MacMahon RA. Total parenteral nutrition of premature infants. 2 Requirement for micronutrient elements. *Aust Pediatr J* 1979;15:62-71.

61. Rex O. Brown. Parenteral nutrition in adult patients. In: Eric T. Herfinalal, Dick R. Growley (eds): *Textbook of Therapeutics, Drug and Disease Management.* Philadelphia: Lippincotts/ Williams and Wilkins 2000:193-211.
62. National Advisory Group on Standards and Practice. Guidelines for parenteral nutrition: Safe practices for parenteral nutrition formulations. *J Parenter Enteral Nutr* 1998;22:49-66.
63. Tripp MG, Menon SK, Mikrut BA, Stability of total nutrient admixtures in a dual-chamber flexible container. *Am J Hosp Pharm* 1990;47:2496-2503.
64. CDC Guidelines for the prevention of intravascular catheter-related infections *MMWR* 2000; 51 (RR–10):1-28.
65. Brown AS, Hoelzer DJ, Piercy SA. Skin necrosis from extravasation of intravenous fluids in children. *Plastic Reconstruct Surg* 1979; 64: 145-150.
66. Ruggiero RP, Caruso G. Chylothorax–A complication of subclavian vein catheterization. *J Parenter Enteral Nutr* 1985; 9:750-753.
67. Gutcher G, Cutz E. complications of parenteral nutrition. *Semin Perinatal* 1986; 10:196-207.
68. Baker SS, Dwyer E, Queen P. Metabolic derangements in children requiring parenteral nutrition. *J Parenter Enteral Nutr* 1986;10:279-281.
69. Vargas JH, Ament ME, Berquist WE. Long-term home parenteral nutrition in pediatrics. Ten years of experience in 102 patients. *J Pediatr Gastroenteral Nutr* 1987;6:24-37.
70. Buchman AL, Moukarzel A, Goodson B, *et al.* Catheter related infections associated with home parenteral nutrition and predictive factors for the need for catheter removal in their treatment. *J Parenter Enteral Nutr* 1994;18:297-302.

A I Innocent Declaration on Protection, Promotion and Support of Breastfeeding

The famous and historic Innocenti Declaration on the promotion, protection and support of breastfeeding was produced and adapted by participants at the WHO/UNICEF policymakers' meeting on "Breastfeeding in the 1990s: A global initiative" cosponsored by the United States Agency for International Development (AID) and the Swedish International Development Authority (SIDA), held at the Spedale degli Innocenti, Florence; Italy, on July 30-August 1, 1990. As many as 32 countries, including India, are signatories to it.

The goals of the Declaration included a call to the various governments in the world to act and create an environment enabling all women to practise exclusively breastfeeding from birth of the baby till he/she is 4 to 6 months old, and to continue breastfeeding with adequate complementary foods for upto two years.

The Declaration made a commitment that each country would develop a national strategy to implement the recommendations made in it.

OPERATIONAL TARGETS

All Governments by the Year 1995 should have:

- Appointed a national breastfeeding coordinator of appropriate authority, and established a multisectoral national breastfeeding committee composed of representatives from relevant government departments, non-governmental organizations, and health professional associations.
- Ensured that every facility providing maternity services fully practises all ten of the *Ten Steps to Successful Breastfeeding* set out in the joint WHO/UNICEF statement "Protecting, promoting and supporting breastfeeding: the special role of maternity services."
- Taken action to give effect to the principles and aim of all Articles of the International Code of Marketing of Breastmilk Substitutes and subsequent relevant World Health Assembly resolutions in their entirety; and
- Enacted imaginative legislation protecting the breastfeeding rights of working women and established means for its enforcement.

We also Call upon International Organizations to:

- Draw up action strategies for protecting, promoting and supporting breastfeeding, including global monitoring and evaluation of their strategies.
- Support national situation analyses and surveys and the development of national goals and targets for action; and
- Encourage and support national authorities in planning, implementing, monitoring and evaluating their breastfeeding policies.

A II National Task Force Baby Friendly Hospital Initiative

MODEL BREASTFEEDING POLICY FOR NURSING HOMES MATERNITY HOSPITALS

Preamble

For recognition as a Baby Friendly Hospital (BFH), it is mandatory to implement the 'Ten Steps to Successful Breastfeeding' effectively as described in the joint WHO/ UNICEF statement, protecting, promoting and supporting breastfeeding.

To achieve effective implementation of this policy, the hospital should have training for health personnel, employed in the maternity ward.

This policy has been suggested in sequence of Ten Steps for Successful Breastfeeding.

Step 1

Have a written breastfeeding policy that is routinely communicated to all health care staff.

POLICY

Breastfeeding policy document will be displayed. In the OPD, maternity ward, antenatal ward, antenatal clinic and be also available in the office and in the maternity service. The document should be translated in regional languages.

The breastfeeding policy will be communicated to all nurses and resident doctors also in addition to Pediatrician and Gynaecologist.

Step 2

Train all healthcare staff in skills necessary to implement the policy.

POLICY

Training will be implemented to Resident Doctors and Nursing staff and others posted in maternity wards on advantages of breastfeeding, management of lactation problems, on promotion of breastfeeding communication skills and art of counselling.

Senior doctors should emphasize various aspects of breastfeeding management when on rounds and will take extra care that this is discussed with Resident Doctors/ Nursing staff.

Step 3

Inform all pregnant women about the benefits and management of breastfeeding.

POLICY

Antenatal Clinic

Every pregnant mother should receive clear advice with a written leaflet on breastfeeding at least once during her antenatal visits in II/III TRIMESTER from Resident or the nurse.

This advice should include:

1. Nutritional, protective, psychological benefits for the newborn from breastfeeding.
2. Benefits to the mother from breastfeeding.
3. Benefits of exclusive breastfeeding for the first 4 months and homemade weaning foods thereafter.
4. Normal positioning and attachment, importance of demand feeding and rooming in.
5. Maternal diet during pregnancy and lactation.

Obstetricians conducting antenatal clinic will examine breasts of all pregnant women to foresee problems about breastfeeding and also to advice corrective action.

All mothers should bring antenatal cards at the time of delivery.

Step 4

Help mothers initiate breastfeeding.

POLICY

1. In case of normal delivery:
   – The baby should be mopped, dried and after tying the cord placed on mother's chest for skin to skin contact

at birth, an attendant should help the mother to put the baby to breast, within first half hour of birth.
- The newborn baby must not be separated from her mother, at least during the first hour. During this period it is preferable that breastfeeding be initiated and maintained.
- Colostrum should not be discarded, it is first, immunization of the child.

2. In case of baby born of cesarean section:
   - The baby should be given to be held by the mother for skin to skin contact as soon as the mother is conscious and able to respond to the baby.
   - The birth attendant should help mother to put the baby to breast for breastfeeding and ensure correct positioning and proper latchin at the breast for sucking within 4 hours of birth.
3. In cases of unstable premature babies, the baby is sent to special care unit immediately.

Step 5

Show mothers how to breastfeed and how to maintain lactation even if they should be separated from their infants.

POLICY

Mothers are allowed to enter special care unit after usual precautions to see and touch her baby even offer the child non-nutritive suckling at the breast for milk formation and milk ejection.

Nothing except breast milk will be given to premature babies and sick newborns. Vitamin and mineral supplementations will be given only when really indicated.

Premature babies and sick babies will be put to breast as early as possible.

Mothers whose babies cannot be put to breast, will be taught the art of expressing milk manually and using breast pump whenever required. It shall be ensured that every such mother expresses milk at least eight times in a 24-hour period.

Step 6

Give newborn infants no food or drink other than breast milk unless medically indicated.

POLICY

No food or drink other than breast milk be given. No water, glucose water, animal milk, gripe water, honey and indigenous medicine be given. Nursing staff should ensure that nothing except breast milk be given.

No vitamin/mineral drops/syrups need be given routinely. Every effort be made that every baby in special care unit is given breast milk only.

Step 7

Practice bedding in and allow mother and infants to remain together 24 hours a day.

POLICY

All babies in postnatal ward will be kept with mother in the same bed 24 hours a day. They will not be kept in the cradle at the footend of the bed.

Step 8

Encourage breastfeeding on demand.

POLICY

Mothers will be advised to practice demand feeding of their babies throughout day and night. They will be told to breastfeed whenever baby cries. Night feeds should be continued.

Step 9

Give no artificial teats or pacifiers to breastfeeding infants.

POLICY

No bottles are allowed. No pacifiers allowed. Nipple shields for woman with flat nipples are not recommended. Expressed breast milk is to be given strictly with spoon and cup.

No display of bottles/pacifiers formula tins in any form including actual bottles/pacifiers/tins, calenders, posters. Literature projecting bottles, pacifiers, infant food are also not permitted in the hospital premises.

Step 10

Foster establishment of mother support group.

It will be explained to all close relatives accompanying a pregnant woman attending an antenatal clinic as well as visitors coming to see her after delivery that she will require all the help and support from household members towards successful breastfeeding of her child. She should be provided all the emotional support.

During the stay in hospital mothers will be encouraged to communicate among themselves in presence of the doctor or nurse and discuss the various myths and problems of breastfeeding. Similar activity will also be carried out in the well baby clinic.

Hospital should also be able to support assistance to mothers having problems in breastfeeding after discharge. Hospitals should form voluntary mothers support groups to help such patients. Hospitals should allot one day for group meetings of antenatal and postnatal mothers and successfully breastfeeding mothers should discuss and solve the problem in presence of a facilitator (Nurse/Doctor).

For further information contact Secretary National Task Force Baby Friendly Hospital Initiative, IMA, Indraprastha Marg, New Delhi-1.

A III The Infant Milk Substitutes, Feeding Bottles and Infant Food Act, 1992

BACKGROUND

Ever since 1981 when the World Health Assembly adopted the "International Code for the Marketing of Breastmilk Substitutes", India has been associating with the international efforts to protect breastfeeding against the overwhelming onslaught of the infant food industry. In 1983, we adopted the "Indian National Code for Protection and Promotion of Breastfeeding". India has been a party to the Innocenti Declaration, the Convention of Rights of the Child, The World Summit Declaration, and the World Alliance for Breastfeeding Action (WABA).

Notable Provisions

Promotion to Public

- No person shall advertise any kind of infant milk substitutes (IMS) or feeding bottles (FB).
- No person shall take part in the promotion of IMS, FB or infant food (IF).
- No person shall give free samples or gifts of IMS or FB, or gifts of utensils or other articles.
- No person shall offer inducement of any other kind for the purpose of promotion of use or sale of IMS or FB.
- No donation of IMS or FB to any person except to an orphanage shall be made.

Labelling

- Containers of IMS, FB and IF or a label on them should carry certain information prescribed in the Act and rules.
- No picture of an infant or woman or both is allowed on the label or tins of infant milk substitutes.
- No use of words like "humanized" or "maternalized" on the label, container or advertisement of IMS.
- No use of words like "recommended" or "approved" by the medical profession.
- No use of words like "full protein", "complete food", or "energy food" on labels of IF.
  - Not to use educational material or prenatal, postnatal care or infant feeding for the purpose of promoting sale of IMS or FB.

Promotion of Health Care System

- No display of posters or playcards on IMS, FB or IF in the hospitals, etc.
- Information and education material related to IMS and FB can only be distributed by medical practitioners and should have minimum prescribed information as per rules.
- No payment of any kind to a person working in healthcare system by any person producing, supplying, distributing or selling IMS, FB and IF.
- No direct or indirect financial inducement of gifts to health workers.

Company Employees

- No commission to employees on the basis of sales volume by the producer, distributor, supplier or seller of IMS, FB or IF.

Penalty

- Violation of the Act can lead to some fine (upto Rs. 5,000) and or imprisonment upto 3 years.

Monitoring

Health personnel in particular have a particular responsibility to be vigilant that the provisions of the Act are violated in letter and spirit by the infant food industry to promote the use of their products. The violations may be in the form of free samples of infant formulas and other gifts, financial inducements to health personnel, advertisements in the mass media, posters, banners and hoardings in hospitals, etc.

The following non-government organizations (NGOs) are competent to approach the courts of law to seek action for contravention of the provisions of the Act.

- **Indian Council for Child Welfare (ICCW)**
  4, Deendayal Upadhyaya Marg
  New Delhi-110002
- **Central Social Welfare Board (CSWB)**
  B-121, Institutional Area, South of IIT
  Hauz Khas
  New Delhi-110016
- **Association for Consumers Action on Safety and Health (ACASH)**
  Lawyers Chambers, Room No 21
  R.S. Sapre Marg
  Mumbai- 400 002.

A

IV

WHO Child Growth Tables (2006)

Table A-IV.1: Length / Height and weight percentiles for girls and boys aged 0-60 months

Month	*GIRLS*						*BOYS*					
	Length/ height (cm)			*Weight (kg)*			*Length/height (cm)*			*Weight (kg)*		
	3rd	*50th*	*97th*	*3rd*	*50th*	*97th*	*3rd*	*50th*	*97th*	*3rd*	*50th*	*97th*
0	45.6	49.1	52.7	2.4	3.2	4.2	46.3	49.9	53.4	2.5	3.3	4.3
1	50.0	53.7	57.4	3.2	4.2	5.4	51.1	54.7	58.4	3.4	4.5	5.7
2	53.2	57.1	60.9	4.0	5.1	6.5	54.7	58.4	62.2	4.4	5.6	7.0
3	55.8	59.8	63.8	4.6	5.8	7.4	57.6	61.4	65.3	5.1	6.4	7.9
4	58.0	62.1	66.2	5.1	6.4	8.1	60.0	63.9	67.8	5.6	7.0	8.6
5	59.9	64.0	68.2	5.5	6.9	8.7	61.9	65.9	69.9	6.1	7.5	9.2
6	61.5	65.7	70.0	5.8	7.3	9.2	63.6	67.6	71.6	6.4	7.9	9.7
7	62.9	67.3	71.6	6.1	7.6	9.6	65.1	69.2	73.2	6.7	8.3	10.2
8	64.3	68.7	73.2	6.3	7.9	10.0	66.5	70.6	74.7	7.0	8.6	10.5
9	65.6	70.1	74.7	6.6	8.2	10.4	67.7	72.0	76.2	7.2	8.9	10.9
10	66.8	71.5	76.1	6.8	8.5	10.7	69.0	73.3	77.6	7.5	9.2	11.2
11	68.0	72.8	77.5	7.0	8.7	11.0	70.2	74.5	78.9	7.7	9.4	11.5
12	69.2	74.0	78.9	7.1	8.9	11.3	71.3	75.7	80.2	7.8	9.6	11.8
13	70.3	75.2	80.2	7.3	9.2	11.6	72.4	76.9	81.5	8.0	9.9	12.1
14	71.3	76.4	81.4	7.5	9.4	11.9	73.4	78.0	82.7	8.2	10.1	12.4
15	72.4	77.5	82.7	7.7	9.6	12.2	74.4	79.1	83.9	8.4	10.3	12.7
16	73.3	78.6	83.9	7.8	9.8	12.5	75.4	80.2	85.1	8.5	10.5	12.9
17	74.3	79.7	85.0	8.0	10.0	12.7	76.3	81.2	86.2	8.7	10.7	13.2
18	75.2	80.7	86.2	8.2	10.2	13.0	77.2	82.3	87.3	8.9	10.9	13.5
19	76.2	81.7	87.3	8.3	10.4	13.3	78.1	83.2	88.4	9.0	11.1	13.7

Contd.

Contd.

20	77.0	82.7	88.4	8.5	10.6	13.5	78.9	84.2	89.5	9.2	11.3	14.0
21	77.9	83.7	89.4	8.7	10.9	13.8	79.7	85.1	90.5	9.3	11.5	14.3
22	78.7	84.6	90.5	8.8	11.1	14.1	80.5	86.0	91.6	9.5	11.8	14.5
23	79.6	85.5	91.5	9.0	11.3	14.3	81.3	86.9	92.6	9.7	12.0	14.8
24	80.3	86.4	92.5	9.2	11.5	14.6	82.1	87.8	93.6	9.8	12.2	15.1
25	80.4	86.6	92.8	9.3	11.7	14.9	82.1	88.0	93.8	10.0	12.4	15.3
26	81.2	87.4	93.7	9.5	11.9	15.2	82.8	88.8	94.8	10.1	12.5	15.6
27	81.9	88.3	94.6	9.6	12.1	15.4	83.5	89.6	95.7	10.2	12.7	15.9
28	82.6	89.1	95.6	9.8	12.3	15.7	84.2	90.4	96.6	10.4	12.9	16.1
29	83.4	89.9	96.4	10.0	12.5	16.0	84.9	91.2	97.5	10.5	13.1	16.4
30	84.0	90.7	97.3	10.1	12.7	16.2	85.5	91.9	978.3	10.7	13.3	16.6
31	84.7	91.4	98.2	10.3	12.9	16.5	86.2	92.7	99.2	10.8	13.5	16.9
32	85.4	92.2	99.0	10.4	13.1	16.8	86.8	93.4	100.0	10.9	13.7	17.1
33	86.0	92.9	99.8	10.5	13.3	17.0	87.4	94.1	100.8	11.1	13.8	17.3
34	86.7	93.6	100.6	10.7	13.5	17.3	88.0	94.8	101.5	11.2	14.0	17.6
35	87.3	94.4	101.4	10.8	13.7	17.6	88.5	95.4	102.3	11.3	14.2	17.8
36	87.9	95.1	102.2	11.0	13.9	17.8	89.1	96.1	103.1	11.4	14.3	18.0
37	88.5	95.7	103.0	11.1	14.0	18.1	89.7	96.7	103.8	11.6	14.5	18.3
38	89.1	96.4	103.7	11.2	14.2	18.4	90.2	97.4	104.5	11.7	14.7	18.5
39	89.7	97.1	104.5	11.4	14.4	18.6	90.8	98.0	105.2	11.8	14.8	18.7
40	90.3	97.7	105.2	11.5	14.6	18.9	91.3	98.6	105.9	11.9	15.0	19.0
41	90.8	98.4	106.0	11.6	14.8	19.2	91.9	99.2	106.6	12.1	15.2	19.2
42	91.4	99.0	106.7	11.8	15.0	19.5	92.4	99.9	107.3	12.2	15.3	19.4
43	92.0	99.7	107.4	11.9	15.2	19.7	92.9	100.4	108.0	12.3	15.5	19.7
44	92.5	100.3	108.1	12.0	15.3	20.0	93.4	101.0	108.6	12.4	15.7	19.9
45	93.0	100.9	108.8	12.1	15.5	20.3	93.9	101.6	109.3	12.5	15.8	20.1
46	93.6	101.5	109.5	12.3	15.7	20.6	94.4	102.2	109.9	12.7	16.0	20.4
47	94.1	102.1	110.2	12.4	15.9	20.8	94.9	102.8	110.6	12.8	16.2	20.6
48	94.6	102.7	110.8	12.5	16.1	21.1	95.4	103.3	111.2	12.9	16.3	20.9
49	95.1	103.3	111.5	12.6	16.3	21.4	95.9	103.9	111.8	13.0	16.5	21.1
50	95.7	103.9	112.1	12.8	16.4	21.7	96.4	104.4	112.5	13.1	16.7	21.3
51	96.2	104.5	112.8	12.9	16.6	22.0	96.9	105.0	113.1	13.3	16.8	21.6
52	96.7	105.0	113.4	13.0	16.8	22.2	97.4	105.6	113.7	13.4	17.0	21.8

Contd.

Contd.

53	97.2	105.6	114.1	13.1	17.0	22.5	97.9	106.1	114.3	13.5	17.2	22.1
54	97.6	106.2	114.7	13.2	17.2	22.8	98.4	106.7	115.0	13.6	17.3	22.3
55	98.1	106.7	115.3	13.4	17.3	23.1	98.8	107.2	115.6	13.7	17.5	22.5
56	98.6	107.3	116.0	13.5	17.5	23.3	99.3	107.8	116.2	13.8	17.7	22.8
57	99.1	107.8	116.6	13.6	17.7	23.6	99.8	108.3	116.8	13.9	17.8	23.0
58	99.6	108.4	117.2	13.7	17.9	23.9	100.3	108.9	117.4	14.1	18.0	23.3
59	100.0	108.9	117.8	13.8	18.0	24.2	100.8	109.4	118.1	14.2	18.2	23.5
60	100.5	109.4	118.4	14.0	18.2	24.4	101.2	110.0	118.7	14.3	18.3	23.8

Source: WHO (available at http://www.who.int/childgrowth/standards/en/).

Table A-IV.2: Height and weight percentiles for girls and boys aged 5-10 years

Year : Month	*GIRLS*						*BOYS*					
	Height (cm)			*Weight (kg)*			*Height (cm)*			*Weight (kg)*		
	3rd	*50th*	*97th*	*3rd*	*50th*	*97th*	*3rd*	*50th*	*97th*	*3rd*	*50th*	*97th*
5.1	100.6	109.6	118.6	14.2	18.3	24.3	101.6	110.3	118.9	14.6	18.5	23.8
5.2	101.1	110.1	119.2	14.3	18.4	24.6	102.1	110.8	119.5	14.7	18.7	24.0
5.3	101.5	110.6	119.7	14.4	18.6	24.9	102.6	111.3	120.1	14.8	18.9	24.3
5.4	102.0	111.2	120.3	14.5	18.8	25.1	103.1	111.9	120.7	15.0	19.0	24.5
5.5	102.4	111.7	120.9	14.7	19.0	25.4	103.5	112.4	121.3	15.1	19.2	24.8
5.6	102.9	112.2	121.5	14.8	19.1	25.7	104.0	112.9	121.8	15.3	19.4	25.1
5.7	103.3	112.7	122.0	14.9	19.3	25.9	104.4	113.4	122.4	15.4	19.6	25.3
5.8	103.8	113.2	122.6	15.0	19.5	26.2	104.9	113.9	123.0	15.5	19.8	25.6
5.9	104.2	113.7	123.1	15.2	19.6	26.5	105.4	114.5	123.5	15.7	19.9	25.8
5.10	104.6	114.2	123.7	15.3	19.8	26.7	105.8	115.0	124.1	15.8	20.1	26.1
5.11	105.1	114.6	124.2	15.4	20.0	27.0	106.2	115.5	124.7	16.0	20.3	26.4
6.0	105.5	115.1	124.8	15.5	20.2	27.3	106.7	116.0	125.2	16.1	20.5	26.7
6.1	105.9	115.6	125.3	15.6	20.3	27.5	107.1	116.4	125.8	16.3	20.7	26.9
6.2	106.3	116.1	125.8	15.8	20.5	27.8	107.6	116.9	126.3	16.4	20.9	27.2
6.3	106.8	116.6	126.4	15.9	20.7	28.1	108.0	117.4	126.9	16.5	21.1	27.5
6.4	107.2	117.0	126.9	16.0	20.9	28.4	108.4	117.9	127.4	16.7	21.3	27.8
6.5	107.6	117.5	127.4	16.1	21.0	28.7	108.8	118.4	127.9	16.8	21.5	28.1
6.6	108.0	118.0	127.9	16.3	21.2	28.9	109.3	118.9	128.5	17.0	21.7	28.3
6.7	108.4	118.4	128.5	16.4	21.4	29.2	109.7	119.4	129.0	17.2	21.9	28.6
6.8	108.9	118.9	129.0	16.5	21.6	29.5	110.1	119.8	129.5	17.3	22.1	28.9
6.9	109.3	119.4	129.5	16.6	21.8	29.8	110.5	120.3	130.1	17.5	22.3	29.2
6.10	109.7	119.9	130.0	16.8	22.0	30.1	111.0	120.8	130.6	17.6	22.5	29.5
6.11	110.1	120.3	130.6	16.9	22.2	30.4	111.4	121.3	131.1	17.8	22.7	29.8
7.0	110.5	120.8	131.1	17.0	22.4	30.8	111.8	121.7	131.7	17.9	22.9	30.1
7.1	110.9	121.3	131.6	17.2	22.6	31.1	112.2	122.2	132.2	18.1	23.1	30.4
7.2	111.4	121.8	132.1	17.3	22.8	31.4	112.6	122.7	132.7	18.2	23.3	30.7
7.3	111.8	122.2	132.7	17.5	23.0	31.7	113.0	123.1	133.3	18.4	23.5	31.1
7.4	112.2	122.7	133.2	17.6	23.2	32.2	113.4	123.6	133.8	18.5	23.7	31.4
7.5	112.6	123.2	133.7	17.8	23.4	32.4	113.8	124.1	134.3	18.7	23.9	31.7

Contd.

Contd.

7.6	113.1	123.7	134.3	17.9	23.6	32.8	114.3	124.5	134.8	18.8	24.1	32.0
7.7	113.5	124.1	134.8	18.1	23.9	33.1	114.7	125.0	135.3	19.0	24.3	32.3
7.8	113.9	124.6	135.3	18.2	24.1	33.5	115.1	125.5	135.9	19.1	24.6	32.7
7.9	114.4	125.1	135.9	18.4	24.3	33.8	115.5	125.9	136.4	19.3	24.8	33.0
7.10	114.8	125.6	136.4	18.6	24.5	34.2	115.9	126.4	136.9	19.5	25.0	33.3
7.11	115.2	126.1	136.9	18.7	24.8	34.6	116.2	126.8	137.4	19.6	25.2	33.7
8.0	115.7	126.6	137.5	18.9	25.0	34.9	116.6	127.3	137.9	19.8	25.4	34.0
8.1	116.1	127.0	138.0	19.1	25.3	35.3	117.0	127.7	138.4	19.9	25.6	34.4
8.2	116.5	127.5	138.5	19.2	25.5	35.7	117.4	128.2	138.9	20.1	25.9	34.7
8.3	117.0	128.0	139.1	19.4	25.8	36.1	117.8	128.6	139.4	20.2	26.1	35.1
8.4	117.4	128.5	139.6	19.6	26.0	36.5	118.2	129.0	139.9	20.4	26.3	35.5
8.5	117.9	129.0	140.2	19.8	26.3	36.9	118.6	129.5	140.4	20.5	26.5	35.8
8.6	118.3	129.5	140.7	20.0	26.6	37.4	119.0	129.9	140.9	20.7	26.7	36.2
8.7	118.7	130.0	141.2	20.1	26.8	37.8	119.3	130.4	141.4	20.8	27.0	36.6
8.8	119.2	130.5	141.8	20.3	27.1	38.2	119.7	130.8	141.9	21.0	27.2	37.0
8.9	119.6	131.0	142.3	20.5	27.4	38.6	120.1	131.3	142.4	21.1	27.4	37.4
8.10	120.1	131.5	142.9	20.7	27.6	39.1	120.5	131.7	142.9	21.3	27.6	37.8
8.11	120.5	132.0	143.4	20.9	27.9	39.5	120.9	132.1	143.4	21.4	27.9	38.2
9.0	121.0	132.5	144.0	21.1	28.2	40.0	121.3	132.6	143.9	21.6	28.1	38.6
9.1	121.5	133.0	144.5	21.3	28.5	40.4	121.6	133.0	144.4	21.8	28.3	39.0
9.2	121.9	133.5	145.1	21.5	28.8	40.9	122.0	133.4	144.9	21.9	28.6	39.4
9.3	122.4	134.0	145.6	21.7	29.1	41.3	122.4	133.9	145.4	22.1	28.8	39.8
9.4	122.8	134.5	146.2	21.9	29.4	41.8	122.8	134.3	145.8	22.2	29.1	40.3
9.5	123.3	135.0	146.8	22.1	29.7	42.3	123.2	134.7	146.3	22.4	29.3	40.7
9.6	123.8	135.5	147.3	22.3	30.0	42.7	123.5	135.2	146.8	22.6	29.6	41.1
9.7	124.2	136.1	147.9	22.6	30.3	43.2	123.9	135.6	147.3	22.7	29.8	41.6
9.8	124.7	136.6	148.4	22.8	30.6	43.7	124.3	136.1	147.8	22.9	30.1	42.0
9.9	125.2	137.1	149.0	23.0	30.9	44.2	124.7	136.5	148.3	23.1	30.4	42.5
9.10	125.7	137.6	149.5	23.2	31.2	44.7	125.0	136.9	148.8	23.2	30.6	43.0
9.11	126.1	138.1	150.1	23.4	31.5	45.2	125.4	137.3	149.3	23.4	30.9	43.5
10.0	126.6	138.6	150.7	23.7	31.9	45.7	125.8	137.8	149.8	23.6	31.2	43.9

Source: WHO (available at http://www.who.int/childgrowth/standards/en/).

Table A-IV.3: Head circumference percentiles for girls and boys aged 0-60 months

Month	GIRLS			BOYS		
	3rd percentile	*50th centile*	*97th centile*	*3rd percentile*	*50th centile*	*97th centile*
0	31.7	33.9	36.1	32.1	34.5	36.9
1	34.3	36.5	38.8	35.1	37.3	39.5
2	36.0	38.3	40.5	36.9	39.1	41.3
3	37.2	39.5	41.9	38.3	40.5	42.7
4	38.2	40.6	43.0	39.4	41.6	43.9
5	39.0	41.5	43.9	40.3	42.6	44.8
6	39.7	42.2	44.6	41.0	43.3	45.6
7	40.4	42.8	45.3	41.7	44.0	46.3
8	40.9	43.4	45.9	42.2	44.5	46.9
9	41.3	43.8	46.3	42.6	45.0	47.4
10	41.7	44.2	46.8	43.0	45.4	47.8
11	42.0	44.6	47.1	43.4	45.8	48.2
12	42.3	44.9	47.5	43.6	46.1	48.5
13	42.6	45.2	47.7	43.9	46.3	48.8
14	42.9	45.4	48.0	44.1	46.6	49.0
15	43.1	45.7	48.2	44.3	46.8	49.3
16	43.3	45.9	48.5	44.5	47.0	49.5
17	43.5	46.1	48.7	44.7	47.2	49.7
18	43.6	46.2	48.8	44.9	47.4	49.9
19	43.8	46.4	49.0	45.0	47.5	50.0
20	44.0	46.6	49.2	45.2	47.7	50.2
21	44.1	46.7	49.4	45.3	47.8	50.4
22	44.3	46.9	49.5	45.4	48.0	50.5
23	44.4	47.0	49.7	45.6	48.1	50.7
24	44.6	47.2	49.8	45.7	48.3	50.8
25	44.7	47.3	49.9	45.8	48.4	50.9
26	44.8	47.5	50.1	45.9	48.5	51.1
27	44.9	47.6	50.2	46.0	48.6	51.2
28	45.1	47.7	50.3	46.1	48.7	51.3
29	45.2	47.8	50.5	46.2	48.8	51.4
30	45.3	47.9	50.6	46.3	48.9	51.5

Contd.

Contd.

31	45.4	48.0	50.7	46.4	49.0	51.6
32	45.5	48.1	50.8	46.5	49.1	51.7
33	45.6	48.2	50.9	46.6	49.2	51.8
34	45.7	48.3	51.0	46.6	49.3	51.9
35	45.8	48.4	51.1	46.7	49.4	52.0
36	45.9	48.5	51.2	46.8	49.5	52.1
37	45.9	48.6	51.3	46.9	49.5	52.2
38	46.0	48.7	51.3	46.9	49.6	52.3
39	46.1	48.7	51.4	47.0	49.7	52.4
40	46.2	48.8	51.5	47.0	49.7	52.4
41	46.2	48.9	51.6	47.1	49.8	52.5
42	46.3	49.0	51.6	47.2	49.9	52.6
43	46.4	49.0	51.7	47.2	49.9	52.7
44	46.4	49.1	51.8	47.3	50.0	52.7
45	46.5	49.2	51.8	47.3	50.1	52.8
46	46.5	49.2	51.9	47.4	50.1	52.8
47	46.6	49.3	51.9	47.4	50.2	53.0
48	46.7	49.3	52.0	47.5	50.2	53.0
49	46.7	49.4	52.1	47.5	50.3	53.0
50	46.8	49.4	52.1	47.5	50.3	53.1
51	46.8	49.5	52.2	47.6	50.4	53.1
52	46.9	49.5	52.2	47.6	50.4	53.2
53	46.9	49.6	52.3	47.7	50.4	53.2
54	47.0	49.6	52.3	47.7	50.5	53.3
55	47.0	49.7	52.4	47.7	50.5	53.3
56	47.1	49.7	52.4	47.8	50.6	53.4
57	47.1	49.8	52.5	47.8	50.6	53.4
58	47.2	49.8	52.5	47.9	50.7	53.5
59	47.2	49.9	52.6	47.9	50.7	53.5
60	47.2	49.9	52.6	47.9	50.7	53.5

Courtesy: World Health Organization. Available at: http://www.who.int/childgrowth/standards/en/. Accessed on: 29 June 2011.

Index